Nursing Assistant

A NURSING PROCESS APPROACH

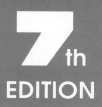

7th
EDITION

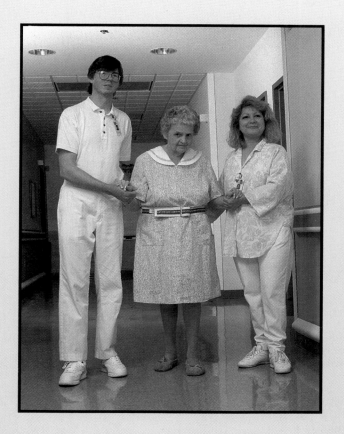

Barbara R. Hegner, MSN, RN
Professor
Nursing and Life Science Department
Long Beach City College (CA)

Esther Caldwell, MA, PhD
Consultant in Vocational Education (CA)

Contributing Author:

Joan F. Needham, MSN, RN
Waubonsee Community College (IL)

Delmar Publishers Inc.™
I(T)P˘ An International Thomson Publishing Company

New York • London • Bonn • Boston • Detroit • Madrid • Melbourne • Mexico City
Paris • Singapore • Tokyo • Albany NY • Belmont CA • Cincinnati OH

NOTICE TO THE READER

Cover design: Timothy J. Conners

Publishing Team

Acquisitions Editor:	Adrianne C. Williams
Editorial Assistant:	Jill Rembetski
Developmental Editor:	Marjorie A. Bruce
Project Editor:	Megan A. Terry
Production Coordinator:	Mary Ellen Black
Art & Design Coordinator:	Timothy J. Conners

COPYRIGHT © 1995
By Delmar Publishers Inc.
an International Thomson Publishing Company
The ITP logo is a trademark under license.

For more information, contact:

Delmar Publishers Inc.
3 Columbia Circle, Box 15015
Albany, New York 12212-5015

International Thomson Publishing
Berkshire House
168–173 High Holborn
London, WC1V7AA
England

Thomas Nelson Australia
102 Dodds Street
South Melbourne 3205
Victoria, Australia

Nelson Canada
1120 Birchmont Road
Scarborough, Ontario
M1K 5G4, Canada

International Thomson Publishing GmbH
Konigswinterer Str. 418
53227 Bonn
Germany

International Thomson Publishing Asia
221 Henderson Bldg. #05-10
Singapore 0315

International Thomson Publishing Japan
Kyowa Building, 3F
2-2-1 Hirakawa-cho
Chiyoda-ku, Tokyo 102
Japan

Printed in the United States of America

2   3   4   5   6   7   8   9   10   XXX   01   00   99   98   97   96   95

Library of Congress Cataloging in Publication Data
Hegner, Barbara R.
    Nursing assistant: a nursing process approach / Barbara R. Hegner, Esther Caldwell. — 7th ed.
      p.   cm.
    Includes index.
    ISBN 0-8273-6223-4
    1. Nurses' aides.   2. Care of the sick.   I. Caldwell, Esther.   II. Title.
    [DNLM: 1. Nurses' Aides.   2. Nursing Care.   WY 193 H4644n 1994]
RT84.H45   1994
610.73'06'98—dc20
DNLM/DLC
for Library of Congress   94-13479
                                  CIP

Study Skills   1

Section 1   INTRODUCTION TO NURSING ASSISTING   7

Unit 1   Community Health Care Facilities   7
Unit 2   Role of the Nursing Assistant   16
Unit 3   Ethical and Legal Issues Affecting the Nursing Assistant   27
Self-Evaluation for Section 1   37

Section 2   SCIENTIFIC PRINCIPLES   39

Unit 4   Basic Anatomy and Physiology   39
Unit 5   Medical Terminology   85
Unit 6   Classification of Disease   95
Self-Evaluation for Section 2   108

Section 3   BASIC HUMAN NEEDS AND COMMUNICATIONS   111

Unit 7   Principles of Observation and Communication   111
Unit 8   Meeting Basic Human Needs   130
Self-Evaluation for Section 3   146

Section 4   INFECTION CONTROL AND SAFETY MEASURES   149

Unit 9   Basic Medical Asepsis   149
Unit 10   Universal Precautions and Isolation Techniques   167
Unit 11   Environmental Control and Safety Measures   179
Self-Evaluation for Section 4   191

Section 5   BODY MECHANICS   193

Unit 12   Principles of Body Mechanics   193
Unit 13   Moving, Lifting, and Transporting Patients   200
Self-Evaluation for Section 5   226

Section 6   MEASURING AND RECORDING VITAL SIGNS, HEIGHT, AND WEIGHT   229

Unit 14   Body Temperature   229
Unit 15   Pulse and Respiration   244
Unit 16   Blood Pressure   250
Unit 17   Measuring Height and Weight   257
Self-Evaluation for Section 6   263

Section 7   PATIENT CARE AND COMFORT MEASURES   265

Unit 18   Admission, Transfer, and Discharge   265
Unit 19   Bedmaking   274
Unit 20   Patient Bathing   287
Unit 21   General Comfort Measures   309
Unit 22   Early Morning and Bedtime Care   325
Self-Evaluation for Section 7   330

Section 8   PRINCIPLES OF NUTRITION AND FLUID BALANCE   335

Unit 23   Nutritional Needs and Diet Modifications   335
Unit 24   Recording Intake and Output and Collecting and Testing Routine Specimens   353
Self-Evaluation for Section 8   368

Section 9   SPECIAL CARE PROCEDURES   371

Unit 25   Heat and Cold Applications   371

Brief Contents

iii

Unit 26   Assisting with the Physical Examination   383

Unit 27   The Surgical Patient   390

Unit 28   Caring for the Emotionally Stressed Patient   409

Unit 29   Long-Term Care of the Elderly and Chronically Ill   421

Unit 30   Death and Dying   461

Unit 31   Nursing Assistant in Home Care   472

Self-Evaluation for Section 9   486

Section 10   BODY SYSTEMS AND RELATED CARE PROCEDURES   489

Unit 32   The Integumentary System and Related Care Procedures   489

Unit 33   The Respiratory System and Common Disorders   502

Unit 34   The Circulatory (Cardiovascular) System and Common Disorders   513

Unit 35   The Musculoskeletal System and Common Disorders   522

Unit 36   The Endocrine System and Common Disorders   538

Unit 37   The Nervous System and Common Disorders   551

Unit 38   The Gastrointestinal System and Common Disorders   570

Unit 39   The Urinary System and Common Disorders   584

Unit 40   The Reproductive System and Common Disorders   596

Self-Evaluation for Section 10   609

Section 11   EXPANDED ROLE OF THE NURSING ASSISTANT   613

Unit 41   The Obstetrical Patient and Neonate   613

Unit 42   The Pediatric Patient   628

Unit 43   Special Advanced Procedures   650

Unit 44   Response to Basic Emergencies   667

Unit 45   Employment Opportunities   678

Self-Evaluation for Section 11   688

Contents

Study Skills   1
    The Learning Process 1; The Textbook 4; Textbook Organization 4

Section 1 — Introduction to Nursing Assisting   7

Unit 1   Community Health Care Facilities   7
    Needs of the Community 8; Community Agencies 8; Health Care
    Facilities 10; Career Opportunities 14; Financing Health Care 14

Unit 2   Role of the Nursing Assistant   16
    The Nursing Team 17; Role of the Nursing Assistant 17; Guidelines for
    the Nursing Assistant 21; Personal Health and Hygiene 21; Personal and
    Vocational Adjustments 22; The Career Ladder 25

Unit 3   Ethical and Legal Issues Affecting the Nursing Assistant   27
    Patient's Rights 27; Ethical/Legal Standards 29; Ethical Questions 29;
    Respect for Life 30; Respect for the Individual 30; Patient Information 30;
    Tipping 31; Legal Issues 32; Safety Devices and Restraints 34

Self-Evaluation for Section 1   37

Section 2 — Scientific Principles   39

Unit 4   Basic Anatomy and Physiology   39
    Basic Anatomy and Related Terminology 41; Body Organization 44;
    The Integumentary System 47; The Respiratory System 49;
    The Circulatory (Cardiovascular) System 52; The Musculoskeletal
    System 56; The Endocrine System 64; The Nervous System 68;
    The Gastrointestinal System 75; The Urinary System 78;
    The Reproductive System 80

Unit 5   Medical Terminology   85
    Word Roots 86; Medical Word Parts 86; Common Abbreviations 91

Unit 6   Classification of Disease   95
    Causes of Disease 96; The Disease Process 99; Diagnosis 101;
    Therapy 103; Body Defenses 104; Medical Specialties 104; Nursing
    Specialties 105

Self-Evaluation for Section 2   108

Section 3 — Basic Human Needs and Communications   111

Unit 7   Principles of Observation and Communication   111
    Communication Skills 112; Observation 116; The Nursing Process 118;
    Factors Influencing Care 123; The Nursing Care Plan 124

Unit 8   Meeting Basic Human Needs   130
    Human Growth and Development 131; Basic Human Needs 136

Self-Evaluation for Section 3   146

Section 4 — Infection Control and Safety Measures   149

Unit 9   Basic Medical Asepsis   149
    Body Flora 151; Characteristics of Microbes 151; Classification of
    Microbes 151; Infectious Disease Process 155; How Pathogens Affect the
    Body 158; Disease Prevention 159

Unit 10   Universal Precautions and Isolation Techniques   167
    Universal Precautions 168; Isolation Systems 170;
    Isolation Technique 172;

Unit 11   Environmental Control and Safety Measures   179
    The Patient Environment 180; Safety Measures 182

Self-Evaluation for Section 4   191

Section 5	**Body Mechanics**	**193**
Unit 12	Principles of Body Mechanics	193
	Body Mechanics for the Nursing Assistant 194;	
	Body Mechanics for the Patient 196	
Unit 13	Moving, Lifting, and Transporting Patients	200
	Introduction to Procedures 200; Moving and Lifting Patients 203;	
	Transporting Patients 220	
	Self-Evaluation for Section 5	226
Section 6	**Measuring and Recording Vital Signs, Height, and Weight**	**229**
Unit 14	Body Temperature	229
	Temperature Values 230; Definition of Body Temperature 230;	
	Temperature Control 231; Measuring Body Temperature 231;	
	Clinical Thermometers 231; Special Situations 241	
Unit 15	Pulse and Respiration	244
	The Pulse 245; Respiration 247	
Unit 16	Blood Pressure	250
	Equipment 251; Measuring the Blood Pressure 252; How to Read the	
	Gauge 253	
Unit 17	Measuring Height and Weight	257
	Self-Evaluation for Section 6	263
Section 7	**Patient Care and Comfort Measures**	**265**
Unit 18	Admission, Transfer, and Discharge	265
	Admission 266; Transfer 269; Discharge 270	
Unit 19	Bedmaking	274
	Operation and Uses of Beds in Health Care Facilities 274; Bedmaking 276	
Unit 20	Patient Bathing	287
	Patient Bathing 288; Century Tub Bathing 297; Dressing a Patient 306	
Unit 21	General Comfort Measures	309
	Oral Hygiene 309; Dentures and Eyeglasses 313; Back Rubs 314;	
	Daily Shaving 316; Daily Hair Care 317; Comfort Devices 318;	
	Elimination Needs 320	
Unit 22	Early Morning and Bedtime Care	325
	Early Morning (AM) Care 325; Bedtime (PM) Care 325	
	Self-Evaluation for Section 7	330
Section 8	**Principles of Nutrition and Fluid Balance**	**335**
Unit 23	Nutritional Needs and Diet Modifications	335
	Normal Nutrition 336; Alternative Nutrition 336; Essential Nutrients 338;	
	The Six Food Groups 339; Basic Facility Diets 342; Special Diets 344;	
	Supplementary Nourishments 346; Changing Water 347;	
	Feeding the Patient 348	
Unit 24	Recording Intake and Output and Collecting and Testing Routine Specimens	353
	Intake and Output 354; Routine Specimens 354	
	Self-Evaluation for Section 8	368
Section 9	**Special Care Procedures**	**371**
Unit 25	Heat and Cold Applications	371
	Therapy with Heat and Cold 371; Types of Heat and Cold 372;	
	Temperature Control Measures 380	
Unit 26	Assisting with the Physical Examination	383

	Positioning the Patient 384; Equipment for Physical Examination 387	
Unit 27	The Surgical Patient	390
	Pain Perception 391; Anesthesia 391; Surgical Care 392; Preoperative Care 392; During the Operative Period 396; Postoperative Care 396	
Unit 28	Caring for the Emotionally Stressed Patient	409
	Mental Health 409; Defense Mechanisms 410; Assisting Patients to Cope 411; The Demanding Patient 411; Alcoholism 412; Maladaptive Behaviors 413	
Unit 29	Long-Term Care of the Elderly and Chronically Ill	421
	Long-term Care of the Elderly and Chronically Ill 422; Types of Long-term Care Facilities 422; Long-term Care Population 422; Legislation Affecting Long-term Care 424; Residents' Rights 424; Role of the Nursing Assistant in Long-term Care 426; Characteristics of the Mature Adult 427; Effects of Aging 427; Sexuality and the Older Adult 430; Nutritional Needs 431; Infection Control in the Long-term Care Facility 432; Safety in the Long-term Care Facility 433; Exercise and Recreational Needs 436; Restorative Care 437; General Hygiene 441; Elimination Needs 447; Communication Needs and Sensory Abilities 449; Psychological Needs 452; Caring for Residents with Dementia 452; Death and Dying in the Long-term Care Facility 458	
Unit 30	Death and Dying	461
	Five Stages of Grief 462; Preparation for Death 464; The Role of the Nursing Assistant 466; Hospice Care 467; Physical Changes as Death Approaches 468; Postmortem Care 468; Organ Donations 469; Postmortem Examination 469	
Unit 31	Nursing Assistant in Home Care	472
	Trends in Health Care 472; Benefits of Working in Home Health Care 473; The Client 473; Home Care Provider 473; Home Health Team 473; The Home Health Assistant and the Nursing Process 474; Characteristics of the Home Care Nursing Assistant and Homemaker Assistant 476; Home Health Care Duties 476; Avoiding Liability 478; Safety in the Home 478; Elder Abuse 478; Infection Control 479; Housekeeping Chores 479; Record Keeping 482	
	Self-Evaluation for Section 9	486

Section 10	**Body Systems and Related Care Procedures**	**489**
Unit 32	The Integumentary System and Related Care Procedures	489
	Common Conditions 490	
Unit 33	The Respiratory System and Common Disorders	502
	Upper Respiratory Infections (URI) 503; Chronic Obstructive Pulmonary Disease 504; Diagnostic Techniques 506; Special Therapies Related to Respiratory Illness 506	
Unit 34	The Circulatory (Cardiovascular) System and Common Disorders	513
	Diagnostic Tests 514; Common Conditions 514; Heart Conditions 518; Blood Abnormalities 519	
Unit 35	The Musculoskeletal System and Common Disorders	522
	Range of Motion 524; Diagnostic Techniques 530; Common Conditions 530	
Unit 36	The Endocrine System and Common Disorders	538
	Diagnostic Techniques 540; Disorders of the Thyroid Gland 540; Disorders of the Parathyroid Gland 541; Disorders of the Adrenal Cortex 541; Diabetes Mellitus 541	
Unit 37	The Nervous System and Common Disorders	551
	Diagnostic Techniques 554; Common Conditions 554	
Unit 38	The Gastrointestinal System and Common Disorders	570

Common Conditions 571; Special Diagnostic Tests 573; Enemas 574;
Rectal Suppositories 582; Care of the Patient With a Colostomy 582

Unit 39   The Urinary System and Common Disorders   584
           Diagnostic Tests 585; Common Conditions 585; Renal Dialysis 587;
           Responsibilities of the Nursing Assistant 587;
           External Drainage Systems (Male) 591

Unit 40   The Reproductive System and Common Disorders   596
           Diagnostic Tests 597; Conditions of the Male Reproductive Organs 597;
           Conditions of the Female Reproductive Organs 599;
           Sexually Transmitted Diseases (STD) 601

Self-Evaluation for Section 10   609

Section 11   Expanded Role of the Nursing Assistant   613

Unit 41   The Obstetrical Patient and Neonate   613
           Prenatal Care 614; Signs of Pregnancy 614; Preparation for Birth 615;
           Prenatal Testing 615; Labor and Delivery 616; Cesarean Birth 619;
           Postpartum Care 620; Toileting and Perineal Care 621; Breast Care 622;
           Neonatal Care 622; Discharge 625

Unit 42   The Pediatric Patient   628
           Pediatric Units 629; Developmental Tasks 630; Caring for Infants
           (Birth–1 Year) 630; Caring for Toddlers (1–3 Years) 640;
           Caring for Preschool Children (3–6 Years) 642; Caring for School-Age
           Children (6–12 Years) 644; Caring for the Adolescent (13–18 Years) 646

Unit 43   Special Advanced Procedures   650
           Sterile Techniques 651; Tracheal Suctioning 656; Urine and Stool
           Tests 656; Collecting a Specimen From a Closed Urinary Drainage
           System 659; Rectal Suppositories 660; Care of the Patient With a
           Colostomy 651; Care of the Patient With an Ileostomy 662

Unit 44   Response to Basic Emergencies   667
           Being Prepared 667; At the Scene 668; Seeking Assistance 668;
           First Aid 668; Emergency Care 669; Choking 670; Bleeding 673;
           Shock 673; Fainting 674; Heart Attack 674; Stroke 675;
           Seizures (Convulsions) 675; Electric Shock 676

Unit 45   Employment Opportunities   678
           Objective 1: Self-Appraisal 678; Objective 2: Search for All Employment
           Opportunities 679; Objective 3: Assemble a Proper Resume 679;
           Objective 4: Validate References 680; Objective 5: Make Specific
           Applications for Work 680; Objective 6: Participate in a Successful
           Interview 685; Objective 7: Keep the Job 685; Objective 8: Continue to
           Grow Throughout Your Career 686; Objective 9: Resign Properly From
           Employment 686

Self-Evaluation for Section 11   688
Comprehensive Final Evaluation   690
Procedure Evaluation   703
Evaluations of Clinical Performance   711
Glossary   712
Index   727

■ Indicates an essential OBRA procedure;   ✔ Indicates a video procedure;
● Indicates a laser disc procedure.

UNIT 9 BASIC MEDICAL ASEPSIS
■ ✔ ● Procedure 1:   Handwashing   159
■ ✔ ● Procedure 2:   Removing Contaminated Disposable Gloves   161
UNIT 10   GUIDELINES FOR UNIVERSAL PRECAUTIONS AND ISOLATION TECHNIQUES
■ ✔ ● Procedure 3:   Putting on a Cover Gown   173
■ ✔ ● Procedure 4:   Removing Contaminated Cover Gown, Gloves, and Mask   174
■ ✔ ● Procedure 5:   Putting on and Taking off a Disposable Paper Face Mask   175
■ ✔   Procedure 6:   Collecting a Specimen in the Isolation Unit   176
■   Procedure 7:   Caring for Linen in the Isolation Unit   176
      Procedure 8:   Transporting the Patient in Isolation   176
UNIT 13   MOVING, LIFTING, AND TRANSPORTING PATIENTS
■ ✔ ● Procedure 9:   Turning the Patient Toward You   203
■   ● Procedure 10:   Turning the Patient Away From You   204
■   Procedure 11:   Assisting the Patient to Sit Up in Bed   205
■   Procedure 12:   Assisting the Patient to Move to the Head of the Bed   206
■ ✔ ● Procedure 13:   Moving a Helpless Patient to the Head of the Bed   207
■   ● Procedure 14:   Using a Transfer (Gait) Belt   208
■ ✔ ● Procedure 15:   Assisting the Patient into a Chair or Wheelchair from Bed   209
■   Procedure 16:   Two Person Transfer With Transfer Belt   210
■ ✔   Procedure 17:   One Person Transfer With Transfer Belt   211
■   Procedure 18:   Independent Transfer, Standby Assist   212
■ ✔ ● Procedure 19:   Assisting the Patient into Bed From a Chair or Wheelchair   212
■ ✔ ● Procedure 20:   One Person Transfer from Wheelchair to Bed   213
■   Procedure 21:   Assisting the Independent Patient From Wheelchair to Bed   214
■ ✔ ● Procedure 22:   Lifting a Patient Using a Mechanical Lift   214
      Procedure 23:   Transferring a Conscious Patient from a Bed to Stretcher   216
      Procedure 24:   Transferring a Conscious Patient from a Stretcher to Bed   217
      Procedure 25:   Transferring an Unconscious Patient or a Patient Unable to Assist
                       from Stretcher to Bed   217
      Procedure 26:   Transferring an Unconscious Patient from a Bed to Stretcher   218
■ ✔ ● Procedure 27:   Log Rolling the Patient   219
■   Procedure 28:   Assisting Patient to Get Out of Bed and Ambulate   220
■   Procedure 29:   Assisting Patient Who is Out of Bed to Ambulate   221
■ ✔ ● Procedure 30:   Care of the Falling Patient   222
■   Procedure 31:   Transporting a Patient by Wheelchair   223
      Procedure 32:   Transporting a Patient by Stretcher   224
UNIT 14   BODY TEMPERATURE
■ ✔ ● Procedure 33:   Measuring an Oral Temperature (Glass Thermometer)   234
■   Procedure 34:   Measuring Temperature Using a Sheath-Covered Thermometer   236
      Procedure 35:   Measuring an Oral Temperature (Plastic Thermometer)   237
■ ✔ ● Procedure 36:   Measuring an Oral Temperature (Electronic Thermometer)   237
■ ✔ ● Procedure 37:   Measuring a Rectal Temperature (Glass Thermometer)   237
■ ✔ ● Procedure 38:   Measuring a Rectal Temperature (Electronic Thermometer)   238
■   Procedure 39:   Measuring an Axillary or Groin Temperature
                       (Glass Thermometer)   239
■   Procedure 40:   Measuring an Axillary Temperature (Electronic Thermometer)   239
    ● Procedure 41:   Cleaning Glass Thermometers   240
UNIT 15   PULSE AND RESPIRATION
■ ✔ ● Procedure 42:   Counting the Radial Pulse Rate   245
      Procedure 43:   Counting the Apical Pulse   247
■ ✔ ● Procedure 44:   Counting Respirations   248
UNIT 16   BLOOD PRESSURE
■ ✔ ● Procedure 45:   Taking Blood Pressure   253
UNIT 17   BLOOD PRESSURE
■ ✔ ● Procedure 46:   Weighing and Measuring the Patient Using an Upright Scale   259
■ ✔ ● Procedure 47:   Measuring and Weighing the Patient in Bed   260
■ ✔   Procedure 48:   Weighing a Patient on the Wheelchair Scale   261
UNIT 18   ADMISSION, TRANSFER, AND DISCHARGE
      Procedure 49:   Admitting the Patient   267
■   Procedure 50:   Transferring the Patient   270
      Procedure 51:   Discharging the Patient   271

Procedures

■ Indicates an essential OBRA procedure;   ✔ Indicates a video procedure;
● Indicates a laser disc procedure.

UNIT 19			BEDMAKING	
■		●	Procedure 52: Making a Closed Bed	276
■			Procedure 53: Opening the Closed Bed	281
■	✔	●	Procedure 54: Making an Occupied Bed	282
			Procedure 55: Making the Surgical Bed	284
UNIT 20			PATIENT BATHING	
■	✔	●	Procedure 56: Assisting With the Tub Bath or Shower	289
■	✔	●	Procedure 57: Giving a Bed Bath	290
■			Procedure 58: Giving a Partial Bath	296
	✔		Procedure 59: Bathing a Patient in a Century Tub	298
■	✔	●	Procedure 60: Giving Female Perineal Care	299
■		●	Procedure 61: Giving Male Perineal Care	300
■		●	Procedure 62: Giving Hand and Fingernail Care	301
■			Procedure 63: Giving Foot and Toenail Care	302
■		●	Procedure 64: Giving a Bed Shampoo	304
■	✔	●	Procedure 65: Dressing and Undressing the Patient	306
UNIT 21			GENERAL COMFORT MEASURES	
■	✔	●	Procedure 66: Assisting With Routine Oral Hygiene	310
■	✔	●	Procedure 67: Assisting With Special Oral Hygiene	312
■			Procedure 68: Assisting Patient to Brush Teeth	312
■	✔	●	Procedure 69: Caring for Dentures	313
■	✔	●	Procedure 70: Giving a Back Rub	314
■	✔	●	Procedure 71: Shaving a Patient	316
■			Procedure 72: Giving Daily Care of the Hair	317
■	✔	●	Procedure 73: Giving and Receiving the Bedpan	320
■	✔	●	Procedure 74: Giving and Receiving the Urinal	322
■		●	Procedure 75: Assisting With the Use of the Bedside Commode	323
UNIT 22			EARLY MORNING AND BEDTIME CARE	
■			Procedure 76: Providing Early Morning (AM) Care	326
■			Procedure 77: Providing Bedtime (PM) Care	328
UNIT 23			NUTRITIONAL NEEDS AND DIET MODIFICATIONS	
■	✔	●	Procedure 78: Assisting the Patient Who Can Feed Self	348
■	✔	●	Procedure 79: Feeding the Helpless Patient	350
UNIT 24			RECORDING INTAKE AND OUTPUT AND COLLECTING AND TESTING ROUTINE SPECIMENS	
■	✔	●	Procedure 80: Measuring and Recording Fluid Intake	355
■	✔	●	Procedure 81: Measuring and Recording Fluid Output	356
			Procedure 82: Collecting a Routine Urine Specimen	357
			Procedure 83: Collecting a Routine Urine Specimen from an Infant	359
	✔	●	Procedure 84: Collecting a Clean-Catch Urine Specimen	360
			Procedure 85: Collecting a Fresh Fractional Urine Specimen	361
	✔	●	Procedure 86: Collecting a 24-Hour Urine Specimen	362
	✔	●	Procedure 87: Collecting a Stool Specimen	364
	✔	●	Procedure 88: Collecting a Sputum Specimen	365
UNIT 25			HEAT AND COLD APPLICATIONS	
	✔	●	Procedure 89: Applying an Ice Bag	373
	✔	●	Procedure 90: Applying a Disposable Cold Pack	374
			Procedure 91: Applying a Warm Water Bag	375
	✔	●	Procedure 92: Applying an Aquamatic-K® Pad	377
	✔	●	Procedure 93: Performing the Warm Foot Soak	378
			Procedure 94: Performing the Warm Arm Soak	378
			Procedure 95: Applying a Moist Compress	379
UNIT 27			THE SURGICAL PATIENT	
			Procedure 96: Shaving the Operative Area	394
			Procedure 97: Assisting Patient to Deep Breathe and Cough	401
			Procedure 98: Performing Postoperative Leg Exercises	403
■	✔	●	Procedure 99: Applying Elasticized Stockings	405
■		●	Procedure 100: Assisting the Patient to Dangle	406
■			Procedure 101: Assisting the Patient in Initial Ambulation	407
UNIT 29			LONG-TERM CARE OF THE ELDERLY AND CHRONICALLY ILL	
■			Procedure 102: Transferring a Resident From Bed to Chair or Chair to Bed (For the Frail Elderly)	442

Indicates an essential OBRA procedure; ✔ Indicates a video procedure;
● Indicates a laser disc procedure.

■ ✔ ● Procedure 103: Assisting the Resident Who Ambulates With a Cane or
                        Walker   443
■   ● Procedure 104: Care of Eyeglasses   452
         Procedure 105: Care of Resident With an Artificial Eye   453
UNIT 30 DEATH AND DYING
■   ● Procedure 106: Giving Postmortem Care   470
UNIT 32 THE INTEGUMENTARY SYSTEM AND RELATED CARE PROCEDURES
         Procedure 107: Giving an Emollient Bath   492
UNIT 35 THE MUSCULOSKELETAL SYSTEM AND COMMON DISORDERS
■ ✔ ● Procedure 108: Performing Range of Motion Exercises (Passive)   525
UNIT 36 THE ENDOCRINE SYSTEM AND COMMON DISORDERS
         Procedure 109: Using a Glucometer 3®   545
         Procedure 110: Using Accu-Chek III®   545
         Procedure 111: Testing Urine for Acetone: Ketostix® Strip Test   548
UNIT 37 THE NERVOUS SYSTEM AND COMMON DISORDERS
■   ● Procedure 112: Applying a Behind-the-Ear Hearing Aid   566
■   Procedure 113: Removing a Behind-the-Ear Hearing Aid   567
UNIT 38 THE GASTROINTESTINAL SYSTEM AND COMMON DISORDERS
   ✔ ● Procedure 114: Giving an Oil-Retention Enema   575
   ✔ ● Procedure 115: Giving a Soapsuds Enema   577
   ✔ ● Procedure 116: Giving a Commercially Prepared Enema   579
         Procedure 117: Giving a Rotating Enema   580
         Procedure 118: Giving a Harris Flush (Return-Flow Enema)   581
         Procedure 119: Inserting a Rectal Tube and Flatus Bag   581
UNIT 39 THE URINARY SYSTEM AND COMMON DISORDERS
■ ✔ ● Procedure 120: Giving Indwelling Catheter Care   589
■ ✔ ● Procedure 121: Disconnecting the Catheter   591
      ● Procedure 122: Replacing a Urinary Condom   592
■   ● Procedure 123: Collecting Urinary Drainage in a Leg Bag   593
■ ✔ ● Procedure 124: Emptying a Urinary Drainage Unit   594
UNIT 40 THE REPRODUCTIVE SYSTEM AND COMMON DISORDERS
      ● Procedure 125: Breast Self-Examination   602
         Procedure 126: Giving a Nonsterile Vaginal Douche   606
UNIT 42 THE PEDIATRIC PATIENT
         Procedure 127: Admitting a Pediatric Patient   630
         Procedure 128: Weighing the Pediatric Patient   633
         Procedure 129: Changing Crib Linens   634
         Procedure 130: Changing Crib Linens (Infant in Crib)   635
         Procedure 131: Measuring Temperature   635
         Procedure 132: Determining Heart Rate (Pulse)   636
         Procedure 133: Counting Respiratory Rate   637
         Procedure 134: Measuring Blood Pressure   637
         Procedure 135: Bottlefeeding the Infant   638
         Procedure 136: Burping (Method A)   639
         Procedure 137: Burping (Method B)   639
UNIT 43 SPECIAL ADVANCED PROCEDURES
         Procedure 138: Opening a Sterile Package   652
         Procedure 139: Putting on Sterile Gloves   654
         Procedure 140: Tracheal Suctioning   656
         Procedure 141: Testing Urine With the HemaCombistix®   657
         Procedure 142: Testing for Occult Blood Using Hemoccult® and Developer   657
         Procedure 143: Testing for Occult Blood Using Hematest® Reagent Tablets   658
         Procedure 144: Collecting a Urine Specimen Through a Drainage Port   659
   ✔ ● Procedure 145: Inserting a Rectal Suppository   660
         Procedure 146: Giving Routine Stoma Care (Colostomy)   662
         Procedure 147: Routine Care of an Ileostomy (With Patient in Bed)   663
         Procedure 148: Routine Care of an Ileostomy (in Bathroom)   664
UNIT 44 RESPONSE TO BASIC EMERGENCIES
■   ● Procedure 149: Heimlich Maneuver—Abdominal Thrusts   670
■   ● Procedure 150: Assisting the Adult Who Has an Obstructed Airway and Becomes
                        Unconscious   671

INTRODUCTION

The passage of the Omnibus Budget Reconciliation Act (OBRA) of 1987, which included the Nursing Home Reform Act, was the first federal legislation to address standards for certification of nursing assistants as health care providers in long-term care. This legislation has influenced both the education and practice of all nursing assistants.

Since the enactment of OBRA, states throughout the nation have made great efforts to develop quality programs to train nursing assistants and prepare them for certification in accordance with the established standards. The National Council of State Boards of Nursing Inc. developed the Nurse Aide Competency Evaluation Program as minimal guidelines in order to meet the specific needs of health care recipients. Many states have exceeded the minimum recommendations of this group.

Previous editions of this best-selling text emphasized the importance of treating those entrusted to care as total individuals who possess dignity, have value, and deserve respect. The continuing goal of this text and supplemental package is to provide the tools that teachers can use to help nursing assistants learn how to offer the correct and compassionate care that will assist clients in reaching an optimum level of comfort, restoration, and wellness.

Nursing assistants are important members of the nursing team. They contribute greatly to the nursing process that the professional nurse follows in assessing the client's needs, planning interventions, implementing care, and evaluating outcomes. Nursing assistants must be helped to see the vital role their accurate observations, reporting skills, and careful following of instructions plays in the overall success of the nursing care plan. Only then can they recognize the full value of their role as part of the nursing team.

The 7th edition of *Nursing Assistant, A Nursing Process Approach*, is designed to help teachers guide students as they achieve the standards that are now legal norms. Materials are also presented to assist those teachers who require more in-depth information and procedural skills to meet their specific community needs.

THE FUTURE

The federal administration is making plans for a comprehensive reform of the health care system in the United States. Under this revised system, it seems that emphasis will be placed on:
- Maintaining wellness
- Limiting length of care in acute care facilities
- Providing basic health care through Health Maintenance Organizations (HMOs)
- Providing short- and long-term rehabilitation and restorative care in more cost-effective settings
- Increasing home care aide services

Regardless of the details of the final health care plan, one fact is very clear. With the increasing population, particularly those of advanced years, restorative care and home care aide services will be major parts of any health program and nursing assistants will provide much of this service. It is essential that nursing assistants be adequately prepared to assume these vital responsibilities.

NEW CONTENT FOR THE SEVENTH EDITION

The following updated and enhanced content addresses the changing character of nursing assistant responsibilities.
- More than 100 new full-color photos highlight skills and emphasize universal precautions
- Most procedures contain one or more symbols to identify the following: *OBRA* indicates a procedure required for certification; *gloves* indicate the required use of universal precautions when performing the procedure; *video symbol* indicates that the proce-

dure appears in *Delmar's Nursing Assistant Procedures Video Series, bar code* for scanning to access the appropriate procedure on Delmar's *Nursing Assistant Laser Discs* which directly correspond to procedures in the text

- New "How To Use This Book" section highlights text elements and relates the text to the supplements to achieve maximum teaching/learning efficiency
- Clarification of nursing assistant responsibilities and scope of practice appear throughout the text
- New procedures

14	Using Transfer (Gait) Belt
16	Two Person Transfer with Transfer Belt
17	One Person Transfer with Transfer Belt
18	Independent Transfer, Standby Assist
20	One Person Transfer from Wheelchair to Bed
21	Assisting the Independent Patient from Wheelchair to Bed
48	Weighing a Patient on the Wheelchair Scale
63	Dressing and Undressing the Patient
123	Collecting Urinary Drainage in a Leg Bag

- New guidelines for the use of postural supports and restraints have been added to clarify correct usage
- New content on Centers for Disease Control (CDC) recommendations and OSHA requirements for preventing transmission of blood-borne diseases in all health care facilities
- Expanded content/procedure on dressing and undressing a client
- New content on the Food Guide Pyramid with guide to daily food choices
- Expanded coverage of cultural diversity and appropriate cultural behavior when providing care
- New content on the use of a body belt by care providers to minimize job-related injuries
- New guidelines for safe client transfers
- Procedures have been revised to correlate more closely with *Delmar's Nursing Assistant Procedures Video Series.*

EXTENSIVE TEACHING/LEARNING PACKAGE

The complete supplement package was developed to achieve two goals:
1. To assist students in learning essential information to permit them to become certified and function as skilled nursing assistants
2. To assist instructors in planning and implementing their instructional program for the most efficient use of time and other resources

Student Workbook

The comprehensive workbook reinforces the text content. It is recommended that the student complete each workbook unit to confirm understanding of essential content.

The workbook content includes:

- Tips on how to study more effectively
- Organization by units with student activities to increase comprehension. Each unit consists of objectives to focus the content for the student, a unit summary to point out key topics, nursing assistant alerts that provide key actions with an explanation of the benefit resulting from the action, and various exercises (review questions, vocabulary exercises and games, and clinical situations). New content in each unit consists of the following sections:

  "Developing Greater Insight" — suggestions for activities and projects to enrich students' understanding of the health care system and their roles as nursing assistants

  "Relating to the Nursing Process" — common nursing assistant actions for which the student is to list the proper nursing process step related to the action

- Student Performance Record — alphabetical listing of 150 text procedures to monitor student completion of return demonstrations
- Competency Checklists for all text procedures to be completed as the student successfully demonstrates each procedure; essential OBRA procedures are indicated. Selected procedures are marked

with a video symbol and/or a bar code for reference to *Delmar's Nursing Assistant Procedures Video Series* or the *Delmar Nursing Assistant Laser Discs*. The perforated checklist pages can be removed from the workbook and placed in student files as a record of competency.

■ Flash cards provide a review of basic medical terms, including combining forms, prefixes, and suffixes. Students can remove the flash card pages and cut them apart to form a deck of individual cards to be used to review medical terminology.

Instructor's Guide

The Instructor's Guide provides the following support:

■ An extensive list of resource materials
■ A list of health care and aging-related organizations providing free or low-cost educational materials
■ Curriculum syllabus for a typical 75–90 hour nursing assistant program
■ Organization by corresponding text unit: instructor objectives, suggested activities, and answers to unit review questions
■ Answers to student workbook exercises
■ Comprehensive final examination (also provided in text) with answers
■ Extra bank of test questions (with answers) to simplify preparation of tests or to provide additional testing material for advanced students
■ Procedures Evaluation Form (A–Z listing for all text procedures) that can be duplicated for each student as a checklist of progress in successfully demonstrating procedures; essential OBRA procedure skills are identified as an aid in monitoring student progress
■ Transparency masters

Computerized Test Bank

An all new computerized testbank (IBM compatible) with more than 1,900 new questions that will give the instructor an expanded capability to create tests. The testbank is available as a separate item or as part of the Instructor's Resource Kit.

Instructor's Resource Kit

This revised supplement provides the instructor with valuable resources to simplify the planning and implementation of the instructional program. It integrates the use of the text, Student Workbook, Instructor's Guide, video series, and laser discs to help the instructor develop an efficient instructional plan.

The complete Instructor's Resource Kit includes the following list of sections, plus the complete Instructor's Guide and the computerized testbank.

Section content:

■ Section A — Teaching Methods and Strategies provides tips on teaching adult learners, including English as a second language (ESL) students
■ Section B — Teaching Resources includes a listing of *Delmar's Nursing Assistant Procedures Video Series*, *Delmar's Nursing Assistant Laser Discs*, other audiovisual aids, software resources, reference texts, models and charts, media sources, and a listing of professional health organizations.
■ Section C — course syllabi for 70 to 90 hour, 120-hour, 300-hour, and 600-hour programs. Each syllabus outlines the number of hours for didactic work and clinical experience and relates these to the use of *Nursing Assistant, A Nursing Process Approach, 7E.*
■ Section D — Lesson Plans in which the supplemental materials and the text are related into a cohesive plan for presenting each topic
■ Section E — Unit Outlines highlight the essential topics for each unit. Suggested activities provide a means of generating student interest and interaction in class to reinforce learning
■ Section F — Competency Checklists and evaluation forms for all text procedures
■ Section G — English-Spanish Flash Cards show common terms and simple phrases in English and Spanish to facilitate communication in the workplace. ESL students can use the flash cards to improve English skills. English speaking students will find them useful in communicating with Spanish-speaking colleagues, patients, and residents

Delmar's Nursing Procedures Video Series

The 12 videos cover 72 essential procedures for nursing assistants. Many of the procedures are core procedures used in acute care, long-term care, and home care situations. Other procedures are designed to meet the unique needs of the elderly in long-term care. The videos average 30 minutes in length and are cross-referenced with symbols in the text and various supplements to help instructors integrate them into the teaching plan.

Delmar's Nursing Assistant Laser Discs

Delmar's Nursing Assistant Laser Discs offer instant accessibility to interactive video segments directly corresponding to essential nursing assistant procedures and bring the text to life. The 5 double-sided laser discs contain approximately 75 essential nursing assistant procedures. Bar codes are included in the text procedures and in the competency checklists within the student workbook. Designed for use on any laser disc player with a bar code reader, a simple swipe of bar codes printed in the text instantaneously plays the specified video procedure.

Delmar's Anatomy and Physiology Transparencies and Slides

Sets of transparencies and slides based on the anatomy drawings from the text and other selected figures provide the instructor with yet another means of promoting student understanding of basic anatomy.

ACKNOWLEDGMENTS

Each new edition bring with it the pleasant task of acknowledging the contributions of a number of individuals. Their enthusiasm, knowledge, and experience all contribute to the continued improvement and success of *Nursing Assistant, A Nursing Process Approach.*

The authors and staff of Delmar Publishers particularly want to thank Joan Fritsch Needham, RN, MSN, who, as contributing author, played a crucial role in the revisions for the seventh edition of the text. Ms. Needham draws from her extensive experience as Director of Education (responsible also for the training of nursing assistants) in a long-term facility and as adjunct faculty at Waubonsee Community College in Sugar Grove, Illinois. In addition to her work on the text, Ms. Needham also revised the Instructor's Guide to accompany the text. The seventh edition reflects Ms. Needham's knowledge, experience, and good humor.

Thanks also to Harry L. McNamara, Administrator, staff, and residents at Bay Harbor Rehabilitation Center, Torrance, CA for their enthusiastic cooperation and assistance during the photo session at the facility.

To Scott Nelson of Van Dyke Photography in Camarillo, CA who worked so well with the Delmar team and the staff and residents at Bay Harbor Rehabilitation Center through the long and intense days of the photo shoot.

To Barbara Acello, Director of Education for the HEA Management Group, Inc., Denton, TX for her invaluable contributions as the author of the completely new computerized testbank and as the revisor of the Instructor's Resource Kit.

To Roberta C. Weiss, LVN, EdD, who contributed content for the Instructor's Resource Kit.

To Joel Ito, Oregon Regional Primate Center, Beaverton, OR, for his anatomy drawings in full color.

The following contributors provided new or extensively revised units, beginning in the fifth edition. Their work was updated and refined for the seventh edition. Appreciation is expressed to:

Judith A. DiNardo, MS, RN (unit 42): Pediatric Staff Education Instructor, New England Medical Center Hospitals, Boston, MA.

Linda M. Donovan, RN, BSN (unit 24): Nurse Manager, Pediatrics Surgical Unit, Boston Floating Hospital for Infants and Children, New England Medical Center Hospitals, Boston, MA.

Mary Jo Conaway, RN, MS (unit 9): Nurse Epidemiologist, Mission Regional Medical Center, Mission Viejo, CA.

The following nursing assistant instructors, consultants, and facility educational supervisors dedicated many hours to reviews of the text manuscript in various stages and the supplements. To each of these individuals, the authors and Delmar Publishers extend a sincere thank you for a job well done.

- Barbara Acello, RN, HEA Management Group, Inc., Denton TX 76201
- Paula E. Baker, RN, Angelina College, Lufkin, TX 75902-1768
- Suzann Balduzzi, MEd, BSN, RN, Western Wisconsin Technical College, LaCrosse, WI
- Jude Franko, St. Paul Technical College, St. Paul, MN 55102
- Patricia Hampton, Escondido Union School District, Escondido, CA 92060-2099
- Laurie Hund-Schieber, Elkhart Area Career Center, Elkhart, IN
- Barbara Kast, Northeast Metro Technical College, White Bear, MN 55110
- Clara E. McElroy, RN, MA, First Call Medical, Inc. and Health Staff, Inc., Bonita Springs, FL
- Carolyn L. Moffett, Superior Career Institute, New York, NY 10011
- Joan F. Needham, MSN, RN, DeKalb County Nursing Home, DeKalb, IL and Waubonsee Community College, Sugar Grove, IL
- Lona Jean Spicer Oates, RN, Manatee Area Vocational and Technical Center, Bradenton, FL 34210
- Pamela S. Porfeli, PRT Vocational-Technical Center, St. Mary's, WV 26170
- Helen Lee Rios, RN, Chula Vista Adult/Del Rey Center, Sweetwater Union High School District, Chula Vista, CA
- Nancy M. Samson, RN, BSN, Licking County Joint Vocational School, Newark, OH 43055
- Davis S. Smith, PhD, Consultant, St. Charles, MO 63304

he seventh edition of *Nursing Assistant, a Nursing Process Approach* has been carefully designed and updated to make the study of nursing assistant tasks and responsibilities easier and more productive. For best results, you may want to become familiar with the features incorporated into this text and accompanying learning tools.

FRONT PAGES

The table of contents lists the major headings for each unit to identify the critical topic areas. A separate listing of procedures includes the unit in which each procedure appears and the procedure number and title. Each procedure is identified as appropriate for

■ 1. essential OBRA procedures that students must master for certification

✔ 2. procedures for which there is a corresponding segment on Delmar's *Nursing Assistant Procedures Video Series*

● 3. procedures included in Delmar's new *Nursing Assistant Laser Discs*

UNITS

A color sidebar on the first page of each unit makes them easy to locate.

LEARNING OBJECTIVES

Each unit begins with specific objectives that direct student learning. They alert students as to what is expected of them. Student success in achieving the objective is measured by the unit end reviews and the section reviews.

VOCABULARY LISTS

Following the objectives, a list of new terms alerts the student to look for each term, note the definition, and be aware of the context in which the term is used. Within the unit, each of these new terms is highlighted in bold type and color. Each new term is defined when it is first used. A *glossary* at the end of the text also defines each of these highlighted terms.

PHONETIC PRONUNCIATION SYSTEM

The glossary also provides a simple phonetic pronunciation for each term. In this easy-to-use "sounds like" system, the word is respelled using standard English letters to create sounds that are familiar. The part of the word that receives the primary emphasis in the pronunciation is in boldface CAPITAL LETTERS. The part or parts of the words that received secondary emphasis is in boldface lower case letters.

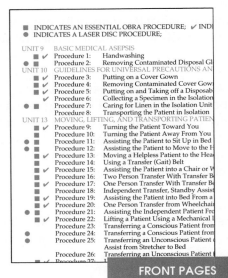

■ INDICATES AN ESSENTIAL OBRA PROCEDURE; ✔ IND
● INDICATES A LASER DISC PROCEDURE;

UNIT 9 BASIC MEDICAL ASEPSIS
■ ✔ Procedure 1: Handwashing
● ■ Procedure 2: Removing Contaminated Disposal Gl
UNIT 10 GUIDELINES FOR UNIVERSAL PRECAUTIONS AN
■ ✔ Procedure 3: Putting on a Cover Gown
■ ✔ Procedure 4: Removing Contaminated Cover Gow
■ ✔ Procedure 5: Putting on and Taking off a Disposab
✔ Procedure 6: Collecting a Specimen in the Isolation
● ■ Procedure 7: Caring for Linen in the Isolation Unit
■ Procedure 8: Transporting the Patient in Isolation
UNIT 13 MOVING, LIFTING, AND TRANSPORTING PATIEN
■ ✔ Procedure 9: Turning the Patient Toward You
■ Procedure 10: Turning the Patient Away From You
● ■ Procedure 11: Assisting the Patient to Sit Up in Bed
● ■ Procedure 12: Assisting the Patient to Move to the H
■ ✔ Procedure 13: Moving a Helpless Patient to the Head
■ Procedure 14: Using a Transfer (Gait) Belt
■ ✔ Procedure 15: Assisting the Patient into a Chair or W
■ Procedure 16: Two Person Transfer With Transfer B
■ ✔ Procedure 17: One Person Transfer With Transfer Be
■ Procedure 18: Independent Transfer, Standby Assist
■ ✔ Procedure 19: Assisting the Patient into Bed From a
■ ✔ Procedure 20: One Person Transfer from Wheelchair
● ■ Procedure 21: Assisting the Independent Patient Fro
■ ✔ Procedure 22: Lifting a Patient Using a Mechanical I
Procedure 23: Transferring a Conscious Patient from
● Procedure 24: Transferring a Conscious Patient from
● Procedure 25: Transferring an Unconscious Patient
Assist from Stretcher to Bed
Procedure 26: Transferring an Unconscious Patient
■ ✔ Procedure 27:

FRONT PAGES

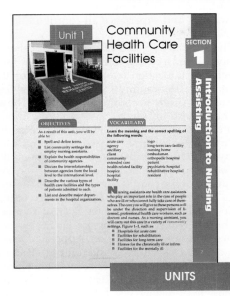

Unit 1

Community Health Care Facilities

SECTION 1

Introduction to Nursing Assisting

OBJECTIVES

As a result of this unit, you will be able to:
■ Spell and define terms.
■ List community settings that employ nursing assistants.
■ Explain the health responsibilities of community agencies.
■ Discuss the interrelationships between agencies from the local level to the international level.
■ Describe the various types of health care facilities and the types of patients admitted to each.
■ List and describe major departments in the hospital organization.

VOCABULARY

Learn the meaning and the correct spelling of the following words:
acute care
agency
ancillary
client
community
extended care
health-related facility
hospice
hospital
facility
logo
long-term care facility
nursing home
ombudsman
orthopedic hospital
patient
psychiatric hospital
rehabilitative hospital
resident

Nursing assistants are health care assistants who play an important role in the care of people who are ill or who cannot fully take care of themselves. The care you will give to these persons will be under the direction and supervision of licensed, professional health care workers, such as doctors and nurses. As a nursing assistant, you will carry out this care in a variety of *community* settings, Figure 1-1, such as
■ Hospitals for acute care
■ Facilities for rehabilitation
■ Facilities for long-term care
■ Homes for the chronically ill or infirm
■ Facilities for the mentally ill

UNITS

B acilli (bah-**SILL**-eye)—rod-shaped bacteria

Bacteria (back-**TEE**-ree-ah)—a form of simple microbes

Bacteriocide (back-**TEE**-ree-oh-side)—agent that destroys bacteria

Balanced suspension skeletal traction (**BAL**-anst sus-**PEN**-shun **SKEL**-eh-tal **TRACK**-shun)—type of traction used to reduce serious fractures in which there is one primary line of traction and extra weight and ropes provide suspension and countertraction

Bargaining (**BAR**-gan-ing)—stage of the grieving process in which the individual seeks to form a pact that will delay death

Barrier (**BAIR**-ee-er)—gown, mask, or gloves or combination of these articles worn by health care providers to prevent contact with pathogens spread by blood and other body fluids

Baseline assessment (**BAYS**-line ah-**SESS**-ment)—initial observ

GLOSSARY

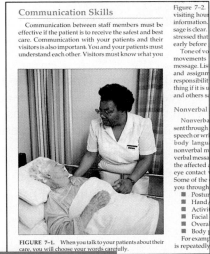

Communication Skills

Communication between staff members must be effective if the patient is to receive the safest and best care. Communication with your patients and their visitors is also important. You and your patients must understand each other. Visitors must know what you

Figure 7–2. visiting hour information. sage is clear. stressed that early before

Tone of vo movements message. Lis and assignm responsibilit thing if it is u and others sa

Nonverbal

Nonverba sent through speech or wr body langu nonverbal m verbal messa the affected eye contact Some of the you through
■ Postu
■ Hand,
■ Activi
■ Facial
■ Overa
■ Body
For examp is repeatedly

FIGURE 7–1. When you talk to your patients about their care, you will choose your words carefully.

COLOR PHOTOS

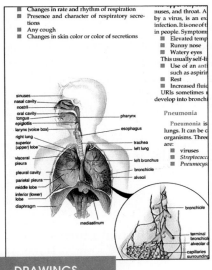

■ Changes in rate and rhythm of respiration
■ Presence and character of respiratory secretions
■ Any cough
■ Changes in skin color or color of secretions

nuses, and throat. A by a virus, is an ex infection. It is one of t in people. Symptom
■ Elevated temp
■ Runny nose
■ Watery eyes
This usually self-li
■ Use of an anti such as aspirin
■ Rest
■ Increased fluid
URIs sometimes develop into bronchi

Pneumonia

Pneumonia is lungs. It can be c organisms. Three are:
■ viruses
■ Streptococc
■ Pneumocys

sinuses
nasal cavity
nostril
oral cavity
tongue
epiglottis
larynx (voice box)
right lung
superior (upper) lobe
visceral pleura
pleural cavity
parietal pleura
middle lobe
inferior (lower) lobe
diaphragm
pharynx
esophagus
trachea
left lung
left bronchus
bronchiole
alveoli
mediastinum
bronchiole
terminal bronchiol
alveolar d
capillaries surroundi

DRAWINGS

position on bed protector.
13. Assist patient to gradually place arm in basin.
14. Check temperature every 5 minutes. Use pitcher to get additional water and add to arm-soak basin to maintain temperature.

20.

PROCEDURE 91   SIDE 3

APPLYING A MOIST COMPRESS

1. Carry out each beginning procedure action.
2. Remember to wash your hands, identify the patient, and provide privacy.
3. Assemble equipment needed:
   ■ Disposable gloves
   ■ Asepto syringe
   ■ Bed protector
   ■ Compresses
   ■ Bath thermometer
   ■ Binder or towel
   ■ Pins or bandage
   ■ Basin with prescribed solution at temperature ordered
4. Bring equipment to bedside.
5. Expose only the area to be treated.
6. Protect bed and patient's clothing with bed protector (Chux®), Figure 25–7A.

PROCEDURES

COLOR PHOTOS AND DRAWINGS

Numerous color photos and illustrations, including more than 100 new photos, are provided to clarify the technical content and to show essential steps of the clinical procedures. Full-color anatomy drawings help students learn the names and locations of the major body organs.

COMPREHENSIVE PROCEDURES

The text contains 150 clinical procedures (including nine new procedures) in step-by-step format with illustrations and photos. Several icons are used to highlight appropriate procedures:

The OBRA icon identifies essential OBRA procedures that students must master for certification

The glove icon identifies procedures requiring universal precautions with the use of disposable gloves

The video icon identifies procedures appearing in *Delmar's Nursing Assistant Procedures Video Series*

The bar code identifies procedures contained in *Delmar's Nursing Assistant Laser Discs*. The bar codes are also the access keys to the video segments on the laser discs.

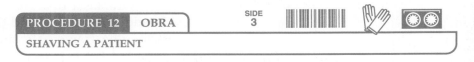

PROCEDURE 12   OBRA   SIDE 3

SHAVING A PATIENT

Each procedure, as appropriate, contains an equipment list to guide students in preparing to carry out the procedure. Special safety cautions are included as needed to protect the client and nursing assistant during the procedure.

UNIT SUMMARIES

At the end of each unit the key information is summarized, providing a useful tool in preparing for tests.

UNIT REVIEWS

A variety of review questions test student understanding of the unit objectives. For additional exercises, refer to the Student Workbook to reinforce learning. Answers to the text unit reviews and Student Workbook exercises appear in the Instructor's Guide.

SECTION REVIEWS

Provide an opportunity for students to integrate the content learned in several units. Answers to the Section Reviews appear in the Instructor's Guide.

STUDENT LEARNING TOOLS

This interactive package, including the Nursing Assistant textbook, Student Workbook, video series and/or laser discs, provides a comprehensive learning system. Repeatedly class tested, this system has proved to be successful in preparing nursing assistants to take their places in the health care workforce.

In addition to the bar codes placed throughout the textbook, we have included six generic bar codes to help you get the most from the laser disk. These generic bar codes enable you to control the laser discs quickly and easily. Some laser disc players and bar code readers come equipped with these or similar functions, but in case yours doesn't include these handy features, we've added them for you. Each bar code is described below.

	Play	Starts the laser disc from where it was last parked
	Pause	Stops the video and sound and shows a blank blue screen on the monitor.
	Step Forward	Stops the laser disc and freezes the still frame on the monitor. Sound is turned off and the user is able to move the video forward one frame at a time with each swipe of the bar code reader.
	Step Reverse	Same as Step Forward, but the video moves one frame at a time backwards.
	Slow Forward	Video plays at one-quarter speed with sound turned off.
	Start	Starts the laser disc from the beginning of the disc.

You may want to make a high-quality copy of this page so that you can have these generic bar codes handy. After repeated use you may find that the copy is more difficult to "read"; simply make a new copy and keep this original intact in the book so that you always know where it is.

We recommend that you familiarize yourself with these bar codes to get an idea of how useful they can be as you view the procedures throughout the text. To "read" these (and all other) bar codes, hold the bar code reader perpendicular to and to one side of the bar code. (Interestingly enough, the bar code reader can be swiped from left to right or from right to left, whichever you prefer.) Swipe the light over the bar code with a firm, steady movement. It may take a little while to get the feel for your particular bar code reader, but with a little practice you will be a pro in no time.

Study Skills

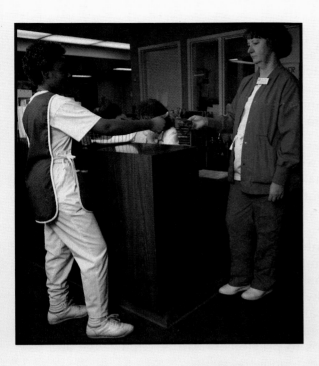

OBJECTIVES

After studying this unit, you will be able to:

- Spell and define terms.
- Describe the effect of study skills on successful learning.
- Write the steps involved in active listening.
- List interferences to effective listening.
- Use two techniques of notetaking.
- Name ways to improve study habits.
- Effectively use the textbook.

VOCABULARY

Learn the meaning and the correct spelling of the following words:

active listening   objectives
end unit materials   process
glossary   vocabulary

You are beginning a special time in your life. This is a period of training that will give you new information and skills. The information and skills will enable you to make a meaningful contribution to the well-being of others and to yourself.

The Learning Process

Students may feel anxious about the learning process. However, learning really can be pleasurable and rewarding if you have an open mind, a desire to succeed, and a willingness to follow some simple steps.

You already have won half the battle because you have entered a training program. This shows your desire to accomplish a real life goal: to become a nursing assistant.

Steps to Learning

There are three basic steps to learning:
- Active listening
- Effective studying
- Careful practicing

Active Listening

Listening actively is not easy, natural, or passive. It is, however, a skill that can be learned. Good listeners are not born, they are made. Studies show the average listening efficiency in this culture is only about 25 percent. That means that although you may hear (a passive action) all that is being said, you actually listen to and process only about one-quarter of the material. Effective listening requires a conscious effort by listeners. The most neglected communication skill is listening.

An important part of your work as a nursing assistant involves active listening to patients and coworkers. To learn this skill properly you must begin to listen actively to your instructor or supervisor. Hearing but not processing information puts you and your patient in jeopardy.

Active listening is listening with personal involvement. There are three actions in active listening:
- Hearing what is said (passive action)
- Processing the information (active action)
- Using the information (active action)

Hearing what is said. People speak at an average rate of 125 words per minute. You must pay close attention to the speaker to hear what is said. This is not a difficult task if you do not let other thoughts and sounds interfere with your thinking. If you sit up straight and lean forward in the classroom or stand erect in the clinical area, your whole body is more receptive. Position yourself where you can adequately see or hear and keep your attention focused on the speaker. Make eye contact if possible and remain alert.

Many distractions can break your concentration unless you take action to prevent them from doing so. For example, distractions may be:
- Interruptions such as other activities in the classroom or in the patient's unit that catch your attention or create noise
- Daydreaming and thinking about personal activities or problems
- Physical fatigue; sleep and rest are powerful influences on the ability to concentrate

- Lack of interest because you cannot immediately see the importance of the information

To be an effective listener, you must actively work at eliminating these distractions. You must put energy into staying focused.

Processing the information. Remember that hearing the words is not enough. You must actively process (make sense of) the words in your brain. You must put meaning to them, and that takes effort. There are things you can do to help the process. These include:
- Interact with the speaker with eye contact, smiles, and nods.
- Ask meaningful questions. Contribute your own comments if it is a discussion.
- Take notes.

These actions allow your memory to establish relationships to previously learned knowledge and to make new connections.

Taking notes gives you another way to imprint what you are processing. You are not only hearing the sounds of the words but can see the important ones on paper. Notetaking helps you recall points that you may have forgotten.

Notetaking is a skill that can be learned and, if used, will improve the learning process, Figure 1. You may

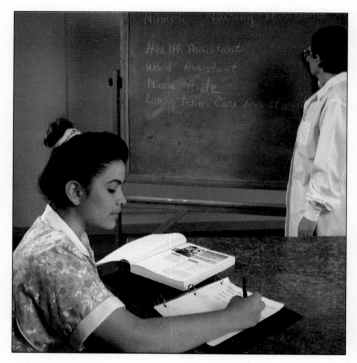

FIGURE 1. Taking good notes can be of great value to the learning process.

I. Textbook Organization
  A. Title
    1. Gives topic
    2. Sets frame of reference
  B. Objectives
    1. Direct learning
    2. Read before and after studying
  C. Vocabulary
    1. Explained in lesson
    2. Phonetically written in glossary
    3. Defined in glossary
  D. Body of text
    1. Simple language
    2. Explains important concepts
    3. Explains procedures
  E. End unit materials
    1. Test learning
    2. Provide practice

FIGURE 2. In this form of outlining, letters and numbers are used to show important points.

need to take notes in class, during demonstrations, and when your supervisor or instructor gives you a clinical assignment. Here are some hints to make developing this skill easier.

- Come prepared with a pencil and paper.
- Don't try to write down every word.
- Write down only the important points or key words.
- Learn to take notes in an outline form.
- Listen with particular care to the beginning sentence. It usually reveals the primary purpose.
- Pay special attention to the final statement. It is often a summary.

Outlines include the important points summarized in a meaningful way. Be sure to leave room so that you may add material.

There are different ways of outlining. One way is to use letters and numbers to designate important points, Figure 2. Another is to draw a pattern of lines to show relationships, Figure 3. Use either way or one of your own design, but be consistent. Practice helps you master the skill of outlining.

As you make notes of material that is not clear, add a star or some other mark next to the material. When the speaker asks for questions, you can quickly find yours.

If the speaker stresses a point, be sure to mark your outline by underlining the information. This will call special attention to the points when you use the outline for study.

After class you can reorganize your notes and compare them to your text readings.

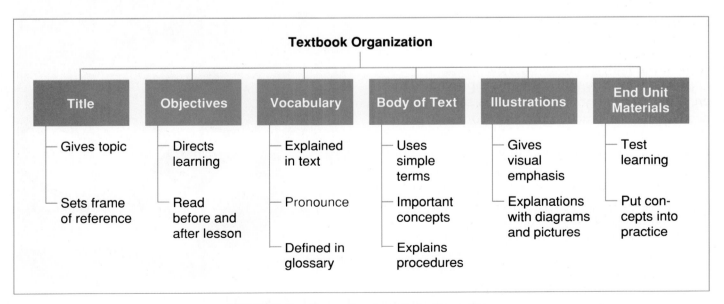

FIGURE 3. Example of a schematic outline

Effective Studying

Being a knowledgeable, skilled nursing assistant will require study, hands-on practice, and a lifetime of continuous learning. At this early time in your career, you should begin to develop study habits you can use the rest of your life.

Studying effectively requires planning and discipline. Here is how to start:

- Make a schedule of classes, study time, home responsibilities, and leisure activities. Follow it as much as possible.
- Have a special study area at home.
- Come to class expecting to learn.
- Review the behavioral objectives and read the related assignment before each class or clinical experience.
- Observe and listen carefully to the teacher's explanations and demonstrations. Use your teacher and supervisor as role models and follow their example.
- Keep a pad and pencil handy to jot down notes and questions to ask.
- Write down assignments. It's easy to forget.
- Following class, reread your text and reorganize your notes. Use a highlighter pen to draw attention to important information.
- Use the glossary in the text to learn the meaning of new terms. Practice using them.
- After you have studied independently, you may find it useful to review materials with classmates.

Careful Practicing

Being responsible for assisting in the nursing care of others means performing your skills in a safe, approved way. You will see many approved "hands-on skills." To carry out these skills safely you will need to practice, practice, practice. Your instructor or clinical supervisor will plan guided laboratory and clinical experiences for you, but you have a responsibility to:

- Seek experiences and skills that you have been taught in the laboratory and classroom when in the clinical area. Inform your instructor of skills you lack or in which you need additional practice.
- Practice new skills under supervision until you and your teacher feel confident in your ability and safety, and the instructor evaluates and assesses your performance of the skills.

The Textbook

The authors have prepared some tools to assist you to master the learning process. These tools include:

- The textbook
- A workbook
- Basic procedure videos

The textbook is the foundation for all other tools. Knowing how to use your text effectively can be of great advantage to you in your study.

Textbook Organization

First take some time to look through your text. Notice how it is organized, Figure 4. It has been prepared carefully to assist your learning process. You will find the following in each unit:

- A unit title tells you the topic of the unit and sets the frame of reference.
- Objectives (outcomes) direct your learning. Objectives are the things you should know and understand when you have completed the unit. Read these before you read the text and before your instructor explains the material. Reread them after studying the unit. Be sure

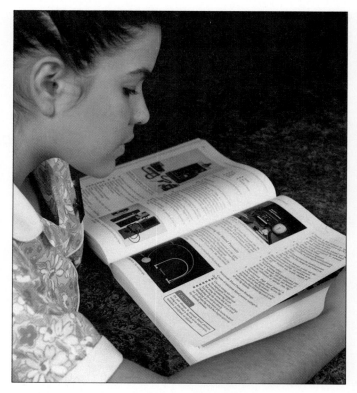

FIGURE 4. Carefully review the text to determine how it is organized.

you have achieved each one before going to the next lesson. If in doubt, ask your teacher for help or go back and reread your text or notes.

■ A list of **vocabulary** words. Try saying each word out loud so you become familiar with how they sound. You will then be able to recognize them when your instructor uses them. Look up their meanings and pronunciations in the glossary at the back of the text. This is an important step to help you understand each word as you discover it in the lesson. Be sure you can spell each term properly. You will be using them and other terms as you legally document the care you give. Finally, each new word is explained in the text. When the word is explained, it appears in color. This makes it easy for you to learn and to find the new words.

■ The body of the text is written in a logical manner using simple terminology. The text is designed to explain important and interesting information that you will need as a nursing assistant. Related procedures are explained step by step to guide you. Look for special indicators. These are letters or symbols that give special information about a procedure. For example:

■ OBRA   These letters represent a procedure that all nursing assistants must master for certification.

■   These procedures require the use of disposable gloves to conform to universal precautions.

■ 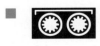   This symbol indicates that the procedure can be viewed on videotape.

■   A bar code indicates that the procedure can be viewed on a laser disc. Access to the procedure on the laser disc is achieved by "reading" the bar code using a special electronic device.

■ Illustrations enhance the written words. It has been said that a single picture is worth a thousand words. The pictures in each lesson were selected with this in mind. Look at them carefully, read the captions, and relate them to the lesson.

■ **End unit materials** have been written to give you an opportunity to test your learning. They put into immediate action the knowledge you have learned in the unit.

Helpful References

Now turn to the end of the book where you will find helpful reference materials. You will locate:

■ A **glossary** (listing of words and their definitions) of all the words introduced in the text. Note that each word has a phonetic pronunciation so that you can learn how to pronounce it correctly.

■ A checklist of procedures and other skills the nursing assistant needs. Procedures are step-by-step explanations of how to carry out care. The stars indicate the skill or procedure competencies required for certification under established regulations. Your instructor can record your level of skill in the spaces provided. You can use it as a guide to know which additional experiences you need.

■ A subject index, which lists the topics alphabetically to make location of a subject easier.

■ An alphabetized procedure index for rapid location of a particular procedure. Knowing where to look for information is a valuable asset to your learning process. It will save time and energy.

SUMMARY

Developing effective study habits can be important to a lifetime of learning. A few simple steps can make the process easier.

■ Be familiar with your text. It will save time in locating information.

■ Practice the steps to learning by being an active listener.

■ Take notes for reference and study.

■ Plan study times and practice in ways that promote learning.

UNIT REVIEW

A. True/False. Answer the following statements true or false by circling T or F.

T   F   1. Good study habits improve the learning process.

T   F   2. Objectives need to be read only if you have difficulty understanding the information in the chapter.

T   F   3. Vocabulary words are found only in the glossary.

T   F   4. End unit materials give you an opportunity to test your new knowledge and put it into practice.

T   F   5. The easiest way to find a procedure you want to review is to look it up in the subject index.

T   F   6. Active listening is a skill that can be developed.

T   F   7. Active listening requires effort.

T   F   8. Body posture can influence your ability to listen actively.

T   F   9. Taking notes is not important if you pay attention in class.

T   F   10. When taking notes, write down every word you hear.

B. Completion. Complete the following statements in the space provided.

11. Three basic steps to learning are:
    a. _____
    b. _____
    c. _____

12. Three actions of an active listener are:
    a. _____
    b. _____
    c. _____

13. Four distractions to effective listening include:
    a. _____
    b. _____
    c. _____
    d. _____

14. Five things you can do to develop better study habits are:
    a. _____
    b. _____
    c. _____
    d. _____
    e. _____

15. Outline this chapter using numbers and letters or with diagrammatic lines.

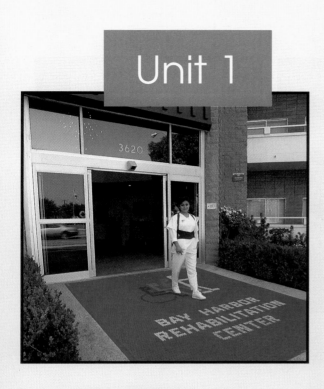

Unit 1

Community Health Care Facilities

SIDE
1

OBJECTIVES

As a result of this unit, you will be able to:

- Spell and define terms.
- List community settings that employ nursing assistants.
- Explain the health responsibilities of community agencies.
- Discuss the interrelationships between agencies from the local level to the international level.
- Describe the various types of health care facilities and the types of patients admitted to each.
- List and describe major departments in the hospital organization.

VOCABULARY

Learn the meaning and the correct spelling of the following words:

acute care	logo
agency	long-term care facility
ancillary	nursing home
client	ombudsman
community	orthopedic hospital
extended care	patient
health-related facility	psychiatric hospital
hospice	rehabilitative hospital
hospital	resident
facility	

Nursing assistants are health care assistants who play an important role in the care of people who are ill or who cannot fully take care of themselves. The care you will give to these persons will be under the direction and supervision of licensed, professional health care workers, such as doctors and nurses. As a nursing assistant, you will carry out this care in a variety of **community** settings, Figure 1–1, such as:

- Hospitals for acute care
- Facilities for rehabilitation
- Facilities for long-term care
- Homes for the chronically ill or infirm
- Facilities for the mentally ill

7

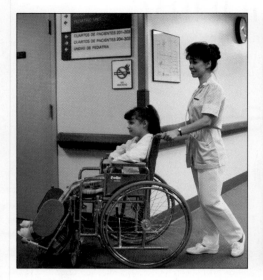

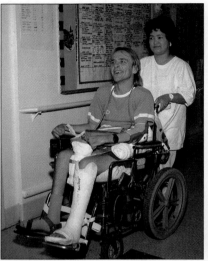

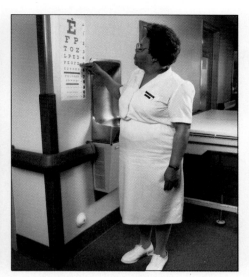

A. Acute care hospital   **B.** Long-term care   **C.** Clinic setting.

FIGURE 1–1.   Facilities in which nursing assistants are employed

- Physicians' offices
- Clinics of various kinds
- Hospices for the care of the terminally ill
- Home health agencies

The health care facilities that will employ you have five basic functions and purposes, which include:

1. Providing for the ill and injured
2. Preventing disease
3. Promoting individual and community health
4. Providing facilities for the education of health workers
5. Promoting research in the science of medicine and nursing

Needs of the Community

Citizens who live in a common area and share common health needs form a community. Provisions for disposal of wastes, assurance of safe drinking water, healthful foods, protection from disease, and health care are important to every person within a community. Safe drinking water, disposal of wastes, and food control are mandated by public health laws and enforced by government agencies.

Health care is provided by specially trained workers at home, in long-term care facilities, clinics, doctors' offices, homes for the aged, and hospitals. Nursing assistants help provide this care mainly in acute care hospitals and extended care facilities.

When illness or accidents strike, when a baby is born, or when people get older and are unable to care for their own everyday personal needs, workers in some type of community agency provide care for them. This care may be short-term or long-term. It can include:

- Emergency care, which may save a life
- Surgery to repair an injured body or remove a diseased organ
- Routine checkups to identify and treat minor problems before they become serious
- Long-term maintenance and support, such as that provided for a chronically or emotionally ill client, or for those requiring assistance in performing the activities of daily living

Community Agencies

Since you will be part of the health care team, you should have an understanding of the different types of health care agencies.

There are three broad categories of community agencies:

- Private (for profit)
- Governmental or tax supported
- Nonprofit, which receive support through voluntary contributions

These three types of community agencies provide the numerous services both required and desired by the citizens.

Private (for Profit) Agencies

Private health care agencies are operated for profit. These agencies are licensed and regulated by the federal and/or state governments. The patient and/or another party such as an insurance company or public health fund pays for the service provided. Services offered by these agencies include:

■ Emergency care
■ General hospital care for acute illness
■ Home health care
■ Long-term care

These agencies employ many nursing assistants to help provide the needed care.

Governmental Agencies

Governmental agencies set standards, collect statistics, and are organized on the local, state, national, and international levels. The national health-related agency in the United States is called the United States Public Health Service. Its international counterpart is called the World Health Organization, Figure 1–2.

Records and statistics are gathered by agencies on the local level. They are compiled and compared at the state and national levels. From this information, patterns of disease and other health problems are charted. These statistics provide vital information that helps health care providers at all levels address the specific health needs of either a community, a nation, or the world.

Information and regulations for control of these health problems then move from the national level back down to the local level, where they are put into action. The county health department is an example of a governmental agency that is responsible for meeting local health needs. The types of programs conducted depend on the needs of the community.

Some services provided by the local health department are:

■ Immunizations
■ Sanitation inspections
■ Maternal and child health services
■ Chest X-rays, blood pressure screening
■ Statistical services, such as collecting data

These are but a few of the many services that the health department can offer to the citizens.

The World Health Organization (WHO) is an international organization that is concerned with world health problems. It was founded in 1948 and meets annually in Geneva, Switzerland, its home office. Its concerns are world-wide and include compiling statistics, publishing health information, investigating serious health problems, and providing medical consultants whenever the need arises. Through the work of the WHO, smallpox, once a dreaded, world-wide disease, has been completely eliminated throughout the world.

Nonprofit Agencies

Many nonprofit agencies provide services similar to those offered by private agencies. Others engage in research and educational services. Examples of nonprofit agencies are:

■ The American Heart Association
■ The National Multiple Sclerosis Society
■ Hospitals such as Veterans Administration facilities

Many of the agencies have logos or symbols that help to identify them, Figure 1–3. They use their resources to conduct research into the causes and care of specific conditions. They receive support through voluntary contributions.

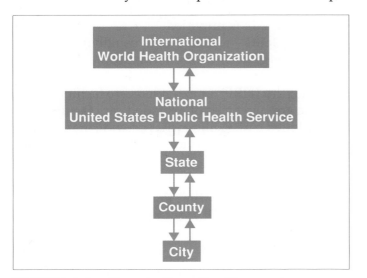

FIGURE 1–2. Organization of health agencies

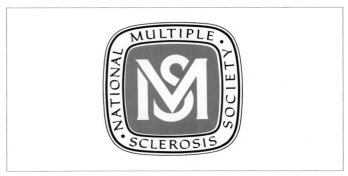

FIGURE 1–3. Logo of the National Multiple Sclerosis Society *(Courtesy National Multiple Sclerosis Society)*

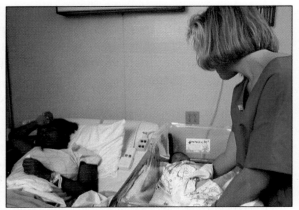

A. Infants and their mothers

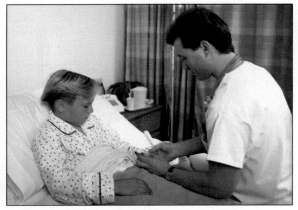

B. Children

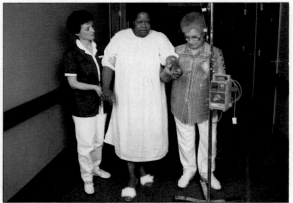

C. Adults

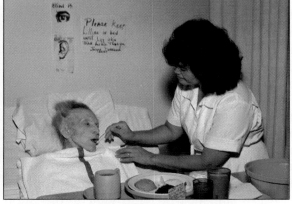

D. Older adults

FIGURE 1–4.   People needing care

Through the work and efforts of some of these agencies, many of the causes of disease have been identified and cures or preventive techniques have been developed. For example, the National Foundation of the March of Dimes was once dedicated primarily to the control and elimination of poliomyelitis, a severe, crippling, viral disease. Now that this disease has been successfully brought under control by immunization, this agency has turned its attention to understanding, preventing, and correcting birth defects.

Health Care Facilities

Patient care facilities are also called health care agencies. These facilities include:

- Acute care for immediate, short-term health care. These facilities include acute care hospitals and emergicenters.
- Extended care for longer term health care. This group of facilities includes private homes, board and care homes, adult day care, and nursing homes.

The health care field calls persons needing health care, Figure 1–4:

- Patients—a term that is generally used in acute care facilities.
- Clients—a term that is usually used when home care is provided.
- Residents—a term that is usually used when care is given in a long-term care facility such as a rest home, nursing home health-related facility (HRF), or extended care facility (ECF).

There are two types of extended care facilities:

- Skilled care facilities that provide many of the same nursing services provided in an acute care facility.
- Intermediate care facilities, often referred to as nursing homes, that provide supportive and rehabilitative care.

Hospitals

Some hospitals are small, serving the needs of an individual community. Other hospitals are extremely large, operating as part of a complex medical center. In some large facilities, highly sophisticated machinery and treatments are available, while other hospitals focus largely on research or teaching.

Some hospitals only take care of patients with special conditions or care for special age groups or special groups of people. Examples of these hospitals are:

■ Psychiatric hospitals—provide care for people who are mentally ill.

■ Orthopedic hospitals—provide care to persons with bone, joint, or muscle disease or injury.

■ Pediatric or children's hospitals—provide care to infants and children up through the teen years.

■ Rehabilitative hospitals—provide services to patients after an acute illness or trauma injury. The rehabilitative hospital helps the patient achieve as high a level of self-care as possible.

■ Government hospitals—provide care for government service personnel and their dependents. These are owned and operated by the federal government.

The entire care of a patient may be provided within one facility. In some cases, patients requiring specialized care may be transferred by ambulance or helicopter from one facility to another.

Most hospitals, however, whether they are privately or governmentally owned, small or large, specialized or providing care for patients of all ages with varied health problems, have the common denominator of needing trained health care providers at all levels.

Hospital Organizations. Hospitals are organized in ways that provide the most efficient delivery of service. Major departments are established within each facility to meet the needs of patients with specific conditions, Figure 1–5, or to provide particular support services. For example, the

■ Medical department—cares for patients with medical conditions.

■ Surgical department—cares for patients undergoing surgery.

■ Pediatric department—cares for sick or injured children.

■ Obstetrical department—cares for maternity patients and the newborn.

■ Emergency department—cares for trauma victims or victims of natural disasters or medical emergencies.

Special units within departments offer specialized care. For example, within the obstetrical department, there usually is a

■ Labor and delivery unit—caring for mothers before and during birth.

■ Postpartum unit—caring for mothers after delivery.

■ Nursery—caring for the newborn infant.

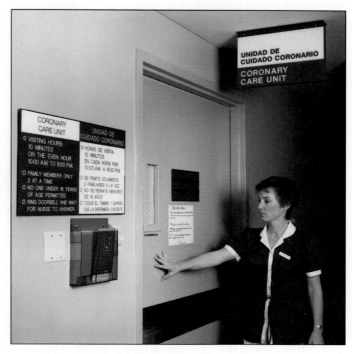

FIGURE 1–5. The coronary care unit is an example of a specialized unit that provides care for persons who have special needs, such as a person who has had a heart attack.

Patients may be transferred from one unit to another within a facility. For example, a patient with a female condition might be admitted to the gynecological unit (GYN unit) within the surgical department, then may be moved to the operating room (OR) for surgery. She then usually spends some time in the post anesthesia room (PAR) before being returned to the original unit.

Many ancillary, or supportive, departments are needed to help provide the service needed in the patient care units. These ancillary or support departments include the

■ Nursing department—provides nursing service and nursing education.

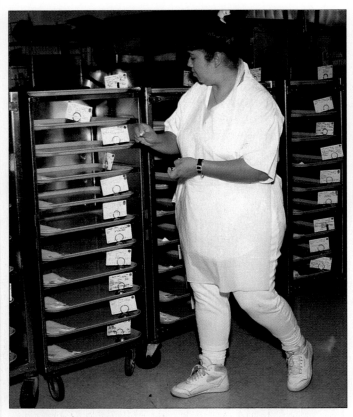

FIGURE 1–6A. The dietary department prepares meals for patients.

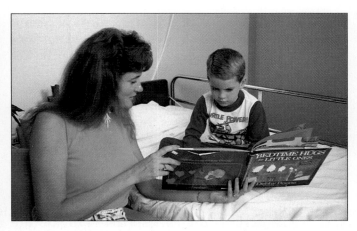

FIGURE 1–6B. Volunteers contribute important support services.

- Physical therapy department—assists patients regain control of their skeletal muscles.
- Speech therapy department—helps patients regain the ability to speak and communicate more effectively.
- Occupational therapy department—helps patients regain control of small muscle action; for example, in the use of the hands.

- Dietary department—provides meals for patients and staff (sometimes), Figure 1–6A.
- Housekeeping department—cares for the overall cleaning of the hospital.
- Maintenance department—cares for and repairs equipment.
- Business services—takes care of billing and other financial matters.
- Volunteer department—provides special services free of charge, Figure 1–6B, such as delivering mail and flowers, escorting patients to therapy areas or other departments, writing letters for patients, cheering and supporting patients and their families, providing reading materials and puzzles, and running gift shops and bazaars with the proceeds going toward the health care facility.
- Social services department—provides counseling for patients and their families, helps families in need obtain financial assistance, plans for patient discharge, and arranges for transfers from one facility to another, Figure 1–7.

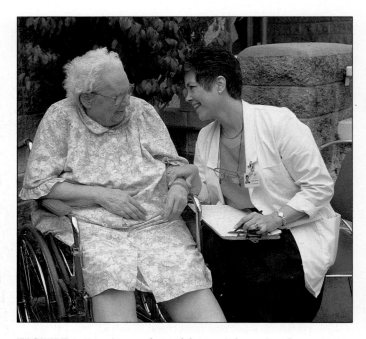

FIGURE 1–7. A member of the social service department assists patients in solving personal and financial problems.

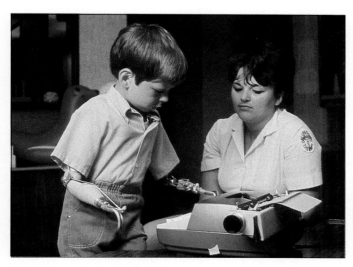

FIGURE 1–8. The rehabilitation department helps people reach maximum levels of self-care in activities of daily living. *(Courtesy March of Dimes—Birth Defects Foundation)*

Still other departments help identify patients' conditions and provide treatment, Figure 1–8. For example, these departments provide the following services:

- Radiology (X-ray)—takes X-rays and uses other imaging equipment to diagnose and treat disease conditions.
- Pathology—examines body tissues and fluids and carries out laboratory tests.
- Pharmacy—prepares and dispenses medications.

Very large medical centers have many different departments and units. Smaller hospitals have fewer departments and support services, but each plays an important role in meeting the community's health needs, Figure 1–9.

You will become familiar with the locations and functions of all the different departments and units within your health care agency as you proceed with your education.

Extended (Long-term) Care Facilities

In the United States, the growing size of the aging population has resulted in an increase in the number of long-term care facilities. Nursing assistants provide a major portion of this care, Figure 1–10.

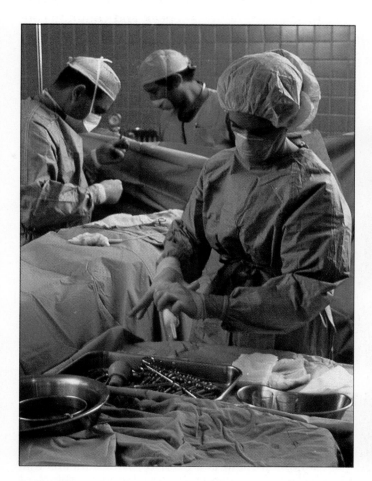

FIGURE 1–9. The operating room of each hospital contains high-technology equipment and is staffed with specially trained and skilled workers. *(Photo courtesy of the U.S. Army)*

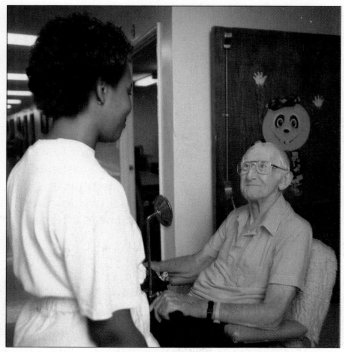

FIGURE 1–10. There is an increasing need for the services provided in a long-term care facility.

The Omnibus Budget Reconciliation Act of 1987 required the training and certification of nursing assistants in all states for employment in long-term care facilities. This law mandated that nursing assistants pass a competency test effective January 1989 and October 1990. The growing numbers of long-term care facilities with their increasing need for nursing assistants required this form of regulation to ensure standards of care.

Long-term care facilities are custodial care units providing for the basic physical and life needs of the residents in their care. The care and services they provide focus on maintaining a positive quality of life and promoting maximum restoration. All have nursing dietary departments and recreational services. In some, rehabilitation services are available. Although equipment for medical treatments is available, much of the supplies are disposables so that central service departments usually are not needed. In-service education and training are provided for their personnel.

An ombudsman is a nurse, social worker, or trained volunteer who functions as patient advocate and works for the social service needs of the resident.

The best extended care facilities make an effort to create an atmosphere that is home-like. For many residents, the facility becomes their home.

Trained and certified nursing assistants are employed in the community health facilities described in this unit. In many states, certification as a nursing assistant and/or home health aide is done through the Department of Health.

Career Opportunities

Nursing assistants carry out important functions in various health agencies. The nursing assistant is a skilled and valuable worker in the community. You can become that person as you practice the activities taught in your health care assistant class and perfect the procedures.

Other Health Care Facilities

Meeting the health needs of the nation involves more than the direct care given in the facilities already described. Care and service are given through:
- Blood banks
- Hospices
- Boarding homes
- Physicians' offices

- Emergicenters
- Clinics
- Home health care agencies

Nursing assistants are employed in each of these areas.

The hospice supports the terminally ill and their families, sometimes in the person's own home and sometimes in a separate facility. Hospice nursing assistants give direct supervised care to patients in this group.

In physicians' offices and clinics, nursing assistants may make appointments, prepare supplies, and assist the physicians and nurses in preparing patients for examination and treatment.

In blood banks, the nurses draw the blood, but nursing assistants may assist in maintaining supplies, monitoring donors, and checking vital signs.

In the home, the nursing assistant combines her/his health care skills with basic homemaking activities in the care of the elderly or homebound clients.

Financing Health Care

The cost of health care today is very high. It is met through:
- Out-of-pocket expenditures by the consumer for prescriptions, doctor's visits, and over-the-counter (OTC) medications and health aids.
- Private insurance plans paid for by the individual. These may only pay a percentage of the total costs.
- Group insurance plans that are sometimes paid for as a fringe benefit to employees by their employers, or may be paid entirely by the beneficiary. Some of these programs allow individual or group members to select a physician and services from a list of approved providers. Others use a prepaid health maintenance organization (HMO) to provide health care services.
- Government programs such as Medicare and Medicaid that help provide for the costs of those who are on Social Security, disabled, or indigent.
- Charitable and public agencies that contribute to the cost of treating those in special circumstances.

Cost containment is a priority, which means that the maximum benefit of health care must be achieved for every dollar spent. Each care provider must do everything possible to avoid waste and to keep the levels of expenditures down.

SUMMARY

Government and private agencies work together to provide for individual and community health needs by:
- Compiling statistics regarding health problems and health needs

- Formulating plans to meet the health needs of the nation and communities
- Providing direct health care

Health care agencies employ professional and assistant workers to give care.

UNIT REVIEW

A. True/False. Answer the following true or false by circling T or F.

T F   1. Citizens who live in a common area and share common health needs form a community.

T F   2. Psychiatric hospitals provide care for people who are mentally ill.

T F   3. The U.S. Public Health Service provides direct care to patients.

T F   4. Records regarding health problems are compiled at the local level and are then transmitted to the state and then the national level.

T F   5. WHO stands for women's health occupations.

T F   6. The American Diabetes Association is an example of a "for profit" organization.

T F   7. The National Foundation of the March of Dimes gives support to patients with respiratory diseases.

T F   8. Patients are people who receive health care in an acute care setting.

T F   9. An orthopedic hospital offers care to persons with diseases of the muscles, bones, and joints.

T F 10. A government hospital provides care for government service personnel and their dependents.

T F 11. The gynecological unit of the hospital provides care for heart patients.

T F 12. The maintenance department is one of the ancillary departments of the health care facility.

T F 13. The ombudsman is a nurse who gives direct nursing care to the patient.

T F 14. The hospice provides care for the terminally ill.

T F 15. Nursing assistants work in a variety of health care settings.

B. Matching. Match the department with its function.

_____ 16. Emergency

_____ 17. Surgical

_____ 18. Obstetrical

_____ 19. Pathology

_____ 20. Housekeeping

a. Provides care for pregnant women and newborns
b. Provides care for trauma victims
c. Provides for patients by maintaining the overall cleanliness of the facility
d. Provides care for patients requiring surgery
e. Provides support for patients by identifying conditions

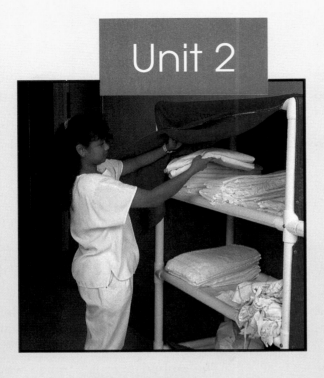

Unit 2

Role of the Nursing Assistant

OBJECTIVES

As a result of this unit, you will be able to:

- ■ Identify the members of the nursing team.
- ■ List the job responsibilities of the nursing assistant.
- ■ Make a chart showing the lines of authority an assistant follows.
- ■ List the rules of personal hygiene and explain the importance of a healthy mental attitude.
- ■ Describe the appropriate dress for the job.
- ■ Describe the importance of good human relationships.
- ■ List the ways to build productive working relationships with staff members.

VOCABULARY

Learn the meaning and the correct spelling of the following words and abbreviations:

attitude
burnout
interpersonal
 relationships
licensed practical
 nurse (LPN)
licensed vocational
 nurse (LVN)

Nurse Aide Compe-
 tency Evaluation
 Program (NACEP)
nursing assistant
nursing team
Omnibus Budget
 Reconciliation Act
 (OBRA)
registered nurse (RN)
scope of practice

Throughout recorded history, ill people have been helped to regain health through nursing care. In ancient Egypt, the lady of the house directed this care, assisted by helpers. These helpers were the first nursing assistants.

Today, registered nurses plan and direct the nursing care of patients in cooperation with the doctor's orders, Figure 2–1. To provide nursing care, the professional registered nurse has the assistance of other registered nurses, licensed vocational or licensed practical nurses, and nursing assistants. This group of health care providers is called the **nursing team**

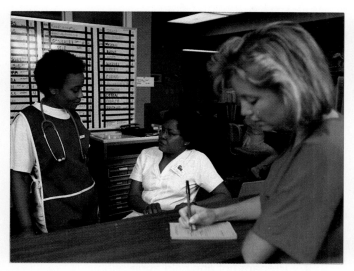

FIGURE 2–1. The members of the nursing team are under the direction of the registered nurse.

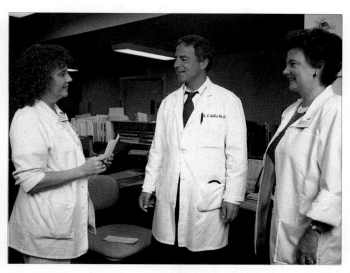

FIGURE 2–2. Each member of the team has special skills. For example, the physician (center) writes orders for medical care; the registered nurse (left) plans and coordinates the nursing care; and the social worker (right) helps the patient find ways to manage social and financial problems.

The Nursing Team

The Registered Nurse

The **registered nurse** (RN) has passed a federally required examination given by each state to become registered. The nurse has a four-year college education with a baccalaureate degree, or an associate in applied science degree from a community college or technical school, or a diploma from a hospital school of nursing. Because they have taken and successfully passed a licensing examination and are registered, all of these nurses use the initials RN after their names.

Registered nurses have been educated to assess, plan for, evaluate, and coordinate the many aspects of patient care, Figure 2–2. Registered nurses teach patients and their families about good health practices and provide nursing care and supervise those duties they delegate to others.

The Licensed Practical/Vocational Nurse

The **licensed vocational** or **licensed practical nurse** has generally completed a 1-year to 18-month training program and has passed a licensure examination administered by the state. She/he is identified by the initials LVN or LPN. This nurse works under the supervision of the registered nurse, a physician, or a dentist. The LPN is able to provide most of the care when the nursing needs are not complex and assists the RN in more complicated situations.

Nursing Assistant

The **nursing assistant** is trained to assist with the care of patients under either an RN's or LPN's supervision. Because the assistant's responsibilities and skills are not as complex as those of the RN or LPN/LVN, the basic training period is shorter. However, growth and learning will continue throughout your career as a care giver. In the health care facility, the assistant is called by one of the following names:

- Patient care attendant
- Nurse's aide
- Home health aide
- Nursing assistant
- Health care assistant
- Ward attendant
- Orderly
- Patient care technician

Role of the Nursing Assistant

The assistant works directly with the patient, giving physical care and emotional support. The nursing assistant is an important person who can contribute much to the comfort of the patient. Important observations made during the delivery of care are reported to the nurse and are recorded on the patient's chart. Remember that although this care is always given under the direction of a registered nurse, not all health care facilities assign the same tasks to the assistant, Figure 2–3.

The nursing assistant plays a vital role in carrying

Nursing assistants commonly participate in the nursing process by carrying out the following activities:

1. **Assist with patient assessment and care planning.**
   a. Check and record vital signs
   b. Measure height and weight
   c. Measure intake and output
   d. Collect specimens
   e. Test urine and feces
   f. Observe patient response to care given
   g. Report and record observations

2. **Assist patients in meeting nutritional and elimination needs.**
   a. Check food trays
   b. Pass food trays
   c. Feed patients
   d. Provide fresh drinking water and nourishments
   e. Assist with bedpans, urinals, and commodes
   f. Empty urine collection bags
   g. Assist with colostomy care
   h. Give enemas
   i. Observe feces

3. **Assist patients with mobility.**
   a. Turn and position
   b. Provide range-of-motion exercises
   c. Transfer to wheelchair or stretcher
   d. Assist with ambulation

4. **Assist patients with personal hygiene and grooming.**
   a. Bathe patients
   b. Provide nail and hair care
   c. Give oral hygiene
   d. Provide denture care
   e. Shave male patients
   f. Assist with dressing and undressing

5. **Assist with patient comfort and anxiety relief.**
   a. Protect patient privacy and maintain confidentiality
   b. Keep call bell within patient's reach
   c. Answer call bells promptly
   d. Provide orientation to the room or unit and to other patients and visitors
   e. Assist patients with communications
   f. Protect personal possessions
   g. Provide diversional activities
   h. Give back rubs
   i. Prepare hot and cold applications
   j. Use universal precautions while providing care

6. **Assist in promoting patient safety and environmental cleanliness.**
   a. Use side rails and restraints appropriately
   b. Keep patient unit clean and clutter-free
   c. Make beds
   d. Clean and care for equipment
   e. Carry out isolation precautions
   f. Observe oxygen precautions
   g. Assist in keeping recreational and non-patient areas clean and free of hazards
   h. Participate in fire drills and patient evacuation procedures

7. **Assist with unit management and efficiency.**
   a. Transport patients
   b. Take specimens to lab
   c. Assist with special procedures
   d. Do errands as required
   e. Assist with cost containment measures

FIGURE 2–3. Typical job description for a nursing assistant *(Courtesy of Eileen Cowart, Director of Education, International Career Institute, Panama City, FL)*

out the plan of care developed for the patient. By observing the patient, the nursing assistant contributes information to the nurse's initial assessment and evaluation of the patient's condition and needs. Once the nursing care plan is developed, the nursing assistant helps to implement the plan by providing specific care. The nursing assistant also observes and reports the patient's response and progress. This information is vital to the success of the nursing care plan.

Nursing care is organized in three ways:

- Primary nursing
- Functional nursing
- Team nursing

The nursing assistant has a functional role in each.

Primary Nursing

In primary nursing, care is given by a registered nurse. This nurse is responsible for an assigned patient's care for his/her entire hospitalization. Licensed staff and assistants help with the care during the hours that the RN is not actually on duty. The nurse plans the nursing care, does teaching, carries out treatments, gives direct nursing care, and plans for the patient's discharge. Patients appreciate primary nursing since it enables them to relate directly to one specific nurse. The RN is assigned responsibility for six to eight patients in the primary nursing situation.

Functional Nursing

Functional nursing is a task oriented type of service organization. It is an older method that is once more being utilized. In this service organization, the charge nurse is the one person responsible for all patients. All other staff members are assigned specific tasks such as giving medications, administering treatments, or providing hygienic care.

Patients may find this type of nursing confusing since many people are involved in their care. However, some facilities feel that this method utilizes available, qualified personnel to the best advantage.

Team Nursing

This is one of the most common methods of delivering nursing care. In this system, a registered nurse team leader determines the nursing needs of all the patients assigned to the team for care. Team members receive instructions and assignments from and report back to the team leader.

Federal/State Regulations

Nursing assistants must understand the scope of the specific tasks they will be expected to carry out. They should also know the state regulations that govern their clinical practice. Federal regulations for the training and certification of nursing assistants require that all states spell out the duties and responsibilities of the assistant, as well as the basic education and level of competency required for practice.

In 1987 a federal law was passed that regulates the education and certification of nurse aides. The law was called the Omnibus Budget Reconciliation Act (OBRA). OBRA comprised statements from the Department of Health and Human Services, Health Care Financing Administration, that established the minimum requirements for nurse aide competency evaluation programs.

Effective October 1, 1990, all persons working as nurse aides had to complete a competency evaluation program or approved course. The actual training and education of nursing assistants is under individual state

jurisdiction, guided by federal regulations.

The National Council of State Boards of Nursing, Inc. then developed the Nurse Aide Competency Evaluation Program (NACEP) NACEP meets the requirements of OBRA. NACEP is a guide for individual programs to register and credential nurse aides. NACEP specifies the minimum skills to be achieved. Programs may exceed these minimums.

Nursing assistants who wish to be certified must complete a minimum of 75 hours of theory and practice. Some states require a minimum of 80 to 120 program hours in written or oral and clinical skills in several areas. These areas include:

- Basic nursing skills
- Basic restorative services
- Mental health and social service needs
- Personal care skills
- Resident rights
- Safety and emergency care

Other regulations that guide nursing assistant practice include:

- Completion of a competency evaluation program by October 1, 1990, of all persons working as nurse aides prior to July 1989
- At least three opportunities for noncertified nurse aides to meet requirements
- Completion of a new training and competency program by those persons wishing to work as aides but who have not performed nursing or nurse-related services for pay for a continuous 24-month period after completing a training and competency evaluation program
- Continuing education (12–48 hours per year in some states)

The OBRA regulations are important because they:

- Give nursing assistants recognition through registration
- Help define the scope of nursing assistant practice
- Assure better uniformity of care provided by nursing assistants
- Promote educational standards for nursing assistants

Be sure you are familiar with any specific state regulations or legislation that relate to your role as an assistant.

Lines of Authority

Nursing assistants receive their assignments from the team leader or charge nurse, nurse manager, or unit manager. Upon completion of their assignment, they report to this same person. This represents the assist-

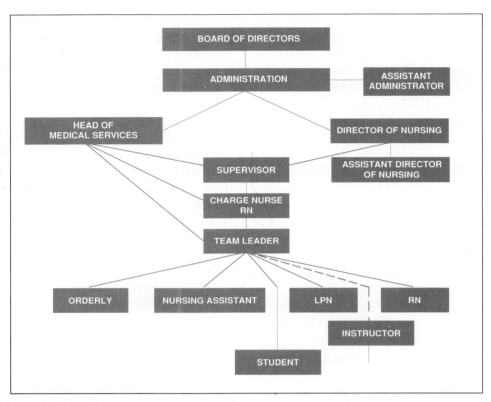

FIGURE 2–4.   Lines of authority for patient care (one typical model; there are others)

ant's immediate line of authority and communication.

If the hospital is a large one, the assistant may function on a team whose leader is a licensed practical nurse or a registered nurse. In this case, the assistant's immediate superior is the team leader. The team leaders receive their instructions from the charge nurse. The charge nurse is responsible for the total care of a certain number of patients. Sometimes this includes all the patients on a wing, a unit, or a floor of the facility. Supervisors are responsible for several charge nurse units. They receive their authority and direction from the director of nursing. Health care facilities vary in the complexity of their staffing.

Assistants should learn the lines of authority in their health care facility, as shown in Figure 2–4. As a student, your immediate authority is your teacher or someone designated as your supervisor.

The physician directs the patient's medical care. The registered nurse carries out the physician's orders and plans the patient's nursing care. The authority for nursing care passes from the registered nurse supervisor to the charge nurse or team leader and then to the nursing assistant. When you accept the responsibility for an assignment, you must fully understand the assignment and be capable of handling it. *If there is any doubt, you should discuss it with the team leader or charge nurse, Figure 2–5.*

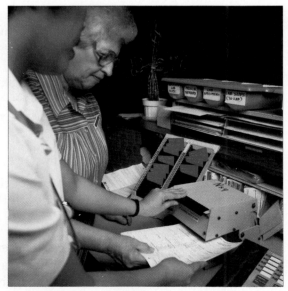

FIGURE 2–5.   Always ask for clarification if you are unsure how to proceed.

Guidelines for the Nursing Assistant SIDE 1

Only perform tasks you have been trained to do. If you feel unsure of carrying out a procedure that was part of your training program, inform the nurse. Do not feel embarrassed. It is better to ask for clarification and supervision than to make an error and injure a patient.

Seeking Higher Authority

Sometimes a report you make to your immediate supervisor is not taken seriously. It seems to fall on "deaf ears." Make very sure of your facts and try again to make your supervisor understand. If you fail and your information is very important, you can move up the chain of command.

For example, if you report that a person is being harmed by inattention by a coworker, but your supervisor doesn't listen to your report of the situation, for your patient's safety you must try again. If the second attempt also fails, the next step is to bring the problem to the attention of the next level of authority. This is a situation that should not occur often if there are good staff relations, but it can happen.

Scope of practice consists of the skills the nursing assistant is legally permitted to perform by state regulations. If another health care worker asks you to perform a task that is clearly out of your scope of training, such as giving medications, be prepared to refuse. Explain in a courteous manner that this is a task for which you have not been technically or legally prepared. Report the incident to your charge nurse so that your scope of duties can be clearly understood by all staff members.

For the same reason, nursing assistants do not take orders from doctors or tell families about the contents of patient care plans or records because these actions are not within the scope of nursing assistant functions.

On the other hand, be willing to learn new skills under the close supervision of your nurse. If the new skill is within the scope of nursing assistant practice, this will increase your ability to provide good, safe nursing care. If, for example, your nurse suggests a new way to lift a patient that is different from that which you have learned in your program, listen and watch carefully as the instruction is given. Seek supervision as you practice the new technique until both you and your supervisor feel you can do it safely on your own.

Not everyone can be a nursing assistant. Nursing assistants are special people: they are interested in others, they take pride in themselves, and they are willing to learn the skills necessary to care for those who are ill.

This interest in and caring for people can be a valuable asset to the entire nursing team. You are the person who that patient sees most often. In that capacity, you have the chance to observe and hear many things which the other team members will not. By transmitting these observations to your charge nurse, you are likely to give the other team members a valuable insight into the patient's illness and attitude toward that illness. For example, you will observe that the patient's attitude toward the attending doctor or nurse is much less relaxed than it is with you, the nursing assistant. For that same reason, the patient is far more likely to tell you of "minor complaints" that may not be minor at all. Competent, caring nursing assistants make a valuable contribution to the comfort and safety of the patients.

Personal Health and Hygiene

Good personal grooming is essential since the assistant is in close contact with patients. Because the work of the assistant, although rewarding, is not physically easy, it is particularly important that all body odors be controlled. The nursing assistant is often the last one to know that he or she has bad breath or body odor. A daily bath and the use of an antiperspirant/deodorant are essential. The mouth and teeth must be kept clean. The nursing assistant should also recognize that strong perfumes, aftershave lotions, and cigarette odors are often offensive to patients.

Hair and fingernails should be kept short and clean. If nail polish is used by female assistants, it should be clear, not colored.

Stockings and socks should be freshly laundered. Shoes and shoelaces should be cleaned daily. Fatigue will be lessened if shoes give proper support to the feet and are well-fitted.

Jewelry is not part of the nursing assistant's uniform, as it is a ready medium for bacteria to grow. There is also the possibility of jewelry causing injury to the patient or to the assistant, especially if the patient is confused or is a young child. Long dangling earrings can be especially dangerous to the assistant if caught in linen or pulled out by a combative patient. Most health care agencies do permit the members of the nursing staff to wear wedding rings, small earrings, and watches with second hands. The watch is used in monitoring the condition of patients and to measure vital signs.

Uniforms

Some hospitals today allow health care workers great leeway in selecting the type and style of their uniforms. Traditionally, patients were able to identify the various types of health care workers by their uniforms, including caps. Today, it is often very difficult to distinguish between a physical therapist, registered nurse, physician, or social worker. It is no wonder that newly admitted patients are often confused as to whom they should approach for information or help. To help avoid this confusion, some states and many health care facilities require personnel to wear a name badge or photo identification tag at all times while on the job.

If your health care facility requires that you wear a uniform, it should only be worn while on duty. If your health care agency does not provide facilities for changing your uniform before and after going on duty, be sure to wear a cover-up as you travel to and from work so you will not spread germs. Upon arriving home, remove your uniform, fold it inside out, and put it into the laundry. This helps keep the dirtiest part of your uniform away from the other clothes in the laundry. Wearing a fresh uniform every day should become a habit. It should be clean and in good condition. Torn hems and missing buttons should be repaired and replaced.

Above all, remember that your patients' safety and comfort are your main concerns. Try to keep in mind their needs and feelings. After all, would you feel confident if you were ill and the assistant caring for you had long fingernails that could scratch you, or that could collect dirt and possibly infect your surgical incision? Or, how would you feel if the assistant who was preparing you for surgery kept having to push the hair out of his eyes? Or if the assistant assigned to give you a backrub wore clanking bracelets on her wrists?

Remember, too, that how you look reflects the pride that you have in yourself and in your work. Well-groomed nursing assistants who pay attention to the details of their person and appearance show others, especially their patients and coworkers, that they are likely to have the same pride and caring attitude in their work, Figure 2–6. If you are well groomed and have good personal habits, patients will feel more secure and confident, and other staff members will regard you as mature and reliable. As you develop good health habits, you become a role model for your family, friends, and coworkers.

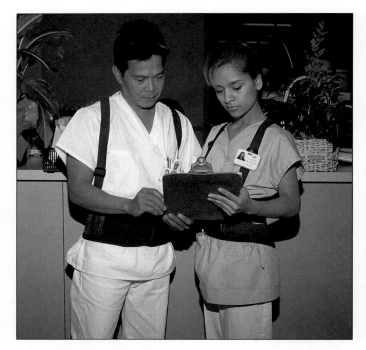

FIGURE 2–6. Nursing assistants who are well groomed reflect pride in themselves and in their careers.

Personal and Vocational Adjustments

There is a certain amount of personal adjustment that you will have to make to your new work situation. Health care facility rules and orders from supervisors must be obeyed promptly even if you do not agree with them. Rules are written for the protection and welfare of the patient and the health care provider. You must also learn to accept constructive criticism and profit by it. It means you are willing to learn and grow.

How mature you are shows in many other ways. You demonstrate:

- Dependability and accuracy by reporting for duty on time, Figure 2–7, and completing your assignment carefully.
- Respect for your coworkers and the place you share together on the nursing team when you are ready to help.
- Understanding of human relationships by being empathetic, patient, and tactful with others.

Interpersonal relationships simply mean interactions between people. You develop interpersonal relationships with everyone you know. Some are deep and lasting, and some are only casual. But to some degree, you react to others and they react to you. Friendship is a good example of an interpersonal

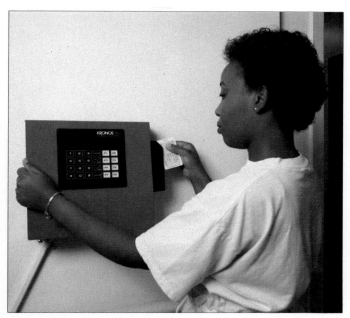

FIGURE 2–7. Reporting for duty on time demonstrates dependability.

relationship that is satisfactory to two people.

Much of the satisfaction that an assistant gets from work is due to the quality of the relationships that are developed with other staff members and patients. Some people call this the ability to "get along" with others.

Similarly, good relationships with others begin with your own personality and attitudes. If you are a warm and accepting person with positive attitudes, others will respond in the same way. If you walk down the street and someone smiles at you, without thinking, your reaction is to smile back. Most human relationships are like this.

It is not necessary for you personally to like someone else to be pleasant and cooperative with them as you carry out your duties.

Attitude

Perhaps the most important single characteristic that you bring to your job is your attitude. Your attitude is developed throughout your lifetime. It reflects the experiences you have had. Some people think an "attitude" means to be negative in your response, but all people demonstrate attitude in their behavior. Sometimes the attitude demonstrated is good and sometimes it is poor.

All the other characteristics described are an outer reflection of your inner feelings—of your attitude toward yourself and others.

Your attitude should reflect:
■ Courtesy
■ Cooperation
■ Emotional control
■ Empathy (understanding)
■ Tact
■ Sympathy

Patients have the right and need to be cared for in a calm, unhurried atmosphere by people with a caring attitude.

Patient Relationships

Patients come in all sizes and shapes and ages: young, old, and in between. Some have major, complicated illnesses. Others have physical problems that may be helped with rest and medication. Some patients are in the health facility to begin their lives. Others will end their lives there. A good nursing assistant shows empathy for the patient by being eager to serve and by using a gentle touch.

Every patient entering a health care facility presents a unique set of problems and concerns to the staff. These problems and concerns are important. As you compare the conditions of many patients in your own mind, however, it might seem that one has more serious problems than another. Since patients do not share your knowledge, they will not know this. Never forget that, to the patient, her/his problems are the most important.

Meeting the Patient's Needs

Patients' personalities are made up of their life experiences, which are now complicated with illness. Their social, spiritual, and physical needs must continue to be met even though they are in a different, more confined setting. The restrictions imposed by illness limit, to some degree, their ability to satisfy these needs through the normal channels. This is naturally frustrating and puts great strain on the patient's ability to establish and maintain good interpersonal relationships.

Some patients become irritable, complaining, and uncooperative because of:
■ Fears about their diagnosis, disfigurement, disability, and death
■ Pain
■ Unrealistic perceptions of activities around them
■ Uncertainties about the future
■ Worries about family
■ The loss or lack of social support systems
■ Dependence on others
■ Financial concerns

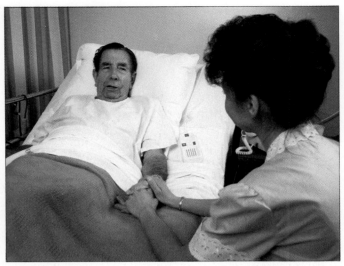

FIGURE 2–8. The worried patient responds to a gentle touch.

Offer emotional support, Figure 2–8, listen carefully, and report these concerns to the nurse.

Meeting the Family's Needs

Families and friends are very concerned when one of their loved ones is in a health care facility and, indeed, may have a life-threatening illness. This puts stress in their lives too. They need to be reassured. Their anxiety sometimes makes them demanding and uncooperative.

The nursing assistant who understands human behavior makes allowances for these stresses and realizes that ill people, coworkers, and families under stress are sensitive and not always on their best behavior. This is why sensitivity and awareness of the needs of others are most important at this time, Figure 2–9. It is in these situations that patience and tact are most needed. Sometimes just quietly listening to another or rephrasing your words and sentences can change an entire interaction. Try to be aware not only of the words used but of the body language. Look for clues such as the tone of a voice or the movement of hands that reveal, as with words, much about the inner feelings of another. Always keep in mind that people are three dimensional. They are physical beings, emotional beings, and social beings.

Staff Relationships

You are part of the staff of a health care facility. All of you share a single goal: to help the patient. This single purpose welds you together into a unit which must work smoothly if your goal is to be accomplished. Good interpersonal relationships will make

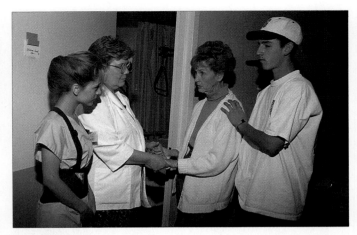

FIGURE 2–9. Concerned family members need the support of the staff.

your working hours satisfying and productive. Good relationships can be formed if you:

- Remember that each of you has a specific role to fulfill and jobs to carry out.
- Do not overstep your authority or criticize others.
- Listen to instructions from your supervisor carefully and phrase questions about your assignment in such a way that your supervisor knows you are looking for clarification—not challenging authority.
- Remember that your tone of voice and body language can often change the message that you are trying to convey.
- Are prompt in carrying out orders and report any work you are unable to finish.
- Are ready to offer help to others and accept help when you need it. Coworkers can often help one another when a task is particularly difficult or physically taxing. For example, lifting a heavy patient, moving equipment, or simply being available when another member of the team gets behind in his/her work.
- Have a cheerful, positive attitude. This is as important for staff members' relationships as it is in establishing rapport (sympathetic understanding) with patients, Figure 2–10.
- Extend the same dignity and courtesy to every staff member that you would to patients.
- Always keep your common goal in mind. Recognize coworkers as important members of the total team.

Reducing Stress

Your work as a nursing assistant is physically and emotionally demanding because you must give so

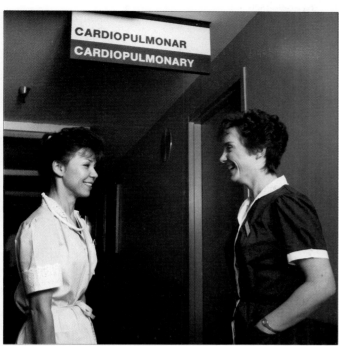

FIGURE 2–10. Keeping a positive attitude makes the workplace more pleasant.

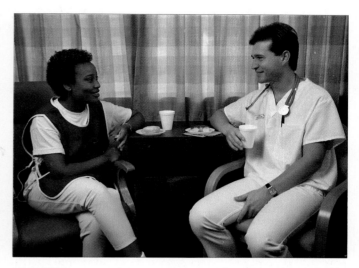

FIGURE 2–11. A quiet moment relaxing with a friend is a good way to reduce stress.

much of yourself to those in your care. To stay healthy and do your best, you will need:

- Sufficient rest
- Good nutrition
- Satisfying leisure activities
- Ways to reduce stress

Burnout is total mental, emotional, and sometimes physical exhaustion. Burnout is common among those working in health care facilities. You can reduce the stress that leads to burnout by balancing your work with rest and recreation, Figure 2–11. You can also learn stress-reducing techniques to help you. Food, alcohol, or other drugs are used by some people to reduce stress, but these substances can cause serious health problems. For example, some people use chemicals or drugs to reduce stress. This is dangerous since chemicals or drugs alter the body's chemistry, causing serious changes to thought and behavior. In some cases, drug use becomes addictive and can cause death.

There are better and safer ways to prevent burnout and relieve stress. To reduce stress:

- Talk to your supervisor; a team conference may help.
- Try sitting for a few moments with your feet up.
- Shut your eyes and take some deep breaths.
- With your eyes shut, picture a special place you like and, in your mind, take yourself there.

- Take a warm, relaxing bath.
- Listen to some quiet music.
- Carry out a specific relaxation exercise.
- Make yourself a cup of herbal tea and drink it slowly.
- Exercise.
- Devote time to hobbies such as sewing, painting, woodworking, or playing a musical instrument.
- Go for a walk.

The Career Ladder

Graduation from a nursing assistant program can lead to a lifetime of learning and productive work. It can also start you on the steps of a career ladder in nursing.

In some parts of the country, the training you receive as a nursing assistant can be counted toward earning a certificate of completion in a Licensed Vocational or Licensed Practical Nurse program. Then, your education and license as a practical or vocational nurse can be applied to the Registered Nursing program requirements.

Whether or not you use your knowledge to advance to other nursing responsibilities, you will want to continue to increase your skills in your chosen vocation.

SUMMARY

The nursing assistant:

- Has specific responsibilities that vary within different agencies but must always function within the scope of nursing assistant practice.

- Must follow established procedures and policies.
- Represents herself or himself and the agency. Good grooming is essential.
- Is ultimately responsible for his or her own actions.
- Must develop good interpersonal relationships with patients, visitors, and coworkers.

This will help the nursing assistant to be more effective.
- Will find that personal adjustment is made easier by understanding and obeying hospital policies and procedures. Also, that patients, coworkers, and visitors must be treated with dignity.
- Must take a written or oral, and clinical skills test to be certified.

UNIT REVIEW

A. True/False. Answer the following statements true or false by circling T or F.

T F 1. The registered nurse plans and directs the nursing care of patients.

T F 2. The doctor's orders are the basis of the medical care that is given.

T F 3. Health care providers act as a team.

T F 4. Registered nurses use the initials LVN after their name.

T F 5. The LVN has completed a 4-year college-based program.

T F 6. The nursing assistant is part of the nursing team.

T F 7. The nursing assistant gives physical care and emotional support to the patients under the direction of the registered nurse.

T F 8. The nursing assistant is an important member of the nursing team.

T F 9. Patients enjoy primary nursing because it allows them to relate directly to one specific registered nurse.

T F 10. Team nursing is a common way of providing for patient care.

T F 11. If there is any doubt about an assignment, the nursing assistant should check directly with the doctor.

T F 12. All nursing assistants will have the same duties in all health care facilities.

T F 13. It is alright to perform a task even if you feel unsure.

T F 14. Nursing assistants are special people.

T F 15. Nursing assistants should be willing to learn and practice new skills under the supervision of the nurse.

T F 16. Caring for people is a valuable asset for a nursing assistant.

T F 17. It is not important for the nursing assistant to be well groomed.

T F 18. Patients may find strong perfumes or after shaves offensive.

T F 19. Hair and fingernails should be kept short and clean.

T F 20. It is alright to wear your uniform when you go food shopping.

T F 21. How you look reflects the pride you feel in yourself.

T F 22. Patient safety and comfort are main concerns for all care givers.

T F 23. Being a nursing assistant can be very stressful.

T F 24. Smoking and eating are the best ways to reduce stress.

T F 25. One of the most important characteristics you bring to your job is a positive attitude.

B. Completion. Complete the following statement in the space provided.

26. The benefits of a nurse aide certification are:
    a. _____
    b. _____
    c. _____
    d. _____

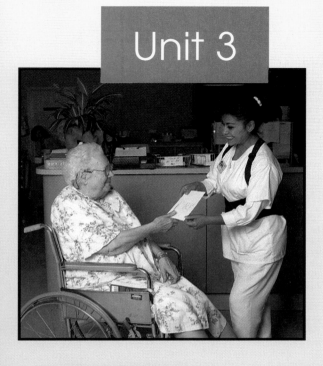

Ethical and Legal Issues Affecting the Nursing Assistant

OBJECTIVES

As a result of this unit, you will be able to:

- Spell and define terms.
- Identify key items in the Patient's Bill of Rights.
- Discuss ethical and legal situations in health care.
- Describe the ethical responsibilities of the nursing assistant concerning patient information.
- Describe tactful ways to refuse a tip offered by a patient.
- Describe the legal responsibilities of a nursing assistant.
- Describe how to protect the patient's right to privacy.
- List the guidelines for the use of restraints.

VOCABULARY

Learn the meaning and the correct spelling of the following words and phrases:

abuse
aiding and abetting
assault
battery
confidential
defamation
ethical standards
false imprisonment
informed consent
invasion of privacy

legal laws
liable
libel
negligence
Patient's Bill of Rights
physical abuse
psychological abuse
slander
verbal abuse

Even though they are in health care facilities, people continue to have certain basic rights. These rights are guarded by a staff that follows established ethical standards and federal or state laws.

Patient's Rights   SIDE 1

The American Hospital Association has developed a Patient's Bill of Rights, Figure 3–1. In some facilities, this document is presented to the patient at admission. In others, it is clearly posted in every unit. The Patient's Bill of Rights spells out the patient's basic rights in simple language. Among these rights are the right to:

- Know that orders will be followed accurately and procedures will be carried out efficiently.

AHA **Policy**   A Patient's Bill of Rights   **American Hospital Association**

This policy document presents the official position of the American Hospital Association as approved by the Board of Trustees and House of Delegates.

The American Hospital Association presents a Patient's Bill of Rights with the expectation that observance of these rights will contribute to more effective patient care and greater satisfaction for the patient, his physician, and the hospital organization. Further, the Association presents these rights in the expectation that they will be supported by the hospital on behalf of its patients, as an integral part of the healing process. It is recognized that a personal relationship between the physician and the patient is essential for the provision of proper medical care. The traditional physician-patient relationship takes on a new dimension when care is rendered within an organizational structure. Legal precedent has established that the institution itself also has a responsibility to the patient. It is in recognition of these factors that these rights are affirmed.

1. The patient has the right to considerate and respectful care.

2. The patient has the right to obtain from his physician complete current information concerning his diagnosis, treatment, and prognosis in terms the patient can be reasonably expected to understand. When it is not medically advisable to give such information to the patient, the information should be made available to an appropriate person in his behalf. He has the right to know, by name, the physician responsible for coordinating his care.

3. The patient has the right to receive from his physician information necessary to give informed consent prior to the start of any procedure and/or treatment. Except in emergencies, such information for informed consent should include but not necessarily be limited to the specific procedure and/or treatment, the medically significant risks involved, and the probable duration of incapacitation. Where medically significant alternatives for care or treatment exist, or when the patient requests information concerning medical alternatives, the patient has the right to such information. The patient also has the right to know the name of the person responsible for the procedures and/or treatment.

4. The patient has the right to refuse treatment to the extent permitted by law and to be informed of the medical consequences of his action.

5. The patient has the right to every consideration of his privacy concerning his own medical care program. Case discussion, consultation, examination, and treatment are confidential and should be conducted discreetly. Those not directly involved in his care must have the permission of the patient to be present.

6. The patient has the right to expect that all communications and records pertaining to his care should be treated as confidential.

7. The patient has the right to expect that within its capacity a hospital must make reasonable response to the request of a patient for services. The hosptial must provide evaluation, service, and/or referral as indicated by the urgency of the case. When medically permissible, a patient may be transferred to another facility only after he has received complete information and explanation concerning the needs for and alternatives to such a transfer. The institution to which the patient is to be transferred must first have accepted the patient for transfer.

8. The patient has the right to obtain information as to any relationship of his hospital to other health care and educational institutions insofar as his care is concerned. The patient has the right to obtain information as to the existence of any professional relationships among individuals, by name, who are treating him.

9. The patient has the right to be advised if the hospital proposes to engage in or perform human experimentation affecting his care or treatment. The patient has the right to refuse to participate in such research projects.

10. The patient has the right to expect reasonable continuity of care. He has the right to know in advance what appointment times and physicians are available and where. The patient has the right to expect that the hospital will provide a mechanism whereby he is informed by his physician or a delegate of the physician of the patient's continuing health care requirements following discharge.

11. The patient has the right to examine and receive an explanation of his bill regardless of source of payment.

12. The patient has the right to know what hospital rules and regulations apply to his conduct as a patient.

No catalog of rights can guarantee for the patient the kind of treatment he has a right to expect. A hospital has many functions to perform, including the prevention and treatment of disease, the education of both health professionals and patients, and the conduct of clinical research. All these activities must be conducted with an overriding concern for the patient, and, above all, the recognition of his dignity as a human being. Success in achieving this recognition assures success in the defense of the rights of the patient.

FIGURE 3–1.   A Patient's Bill of Rights *(Reprinted with permission of the American Hospital Association, copyright 1975.)*

■ Know that they will be properly identified so that treatments and medications intended for them will be carried out or given, Figure 3–2.

■ Feel secure that their needs will be recognized and given prompt attention; that you will recognize them as persons—not by condition—but by name. Mrs. Robinson is not "the gallbladder in Room 228." She is Mrs. Robinson!

Note: The Resident's Bill of Rights can be found in Unit 29 on Long-term Care.

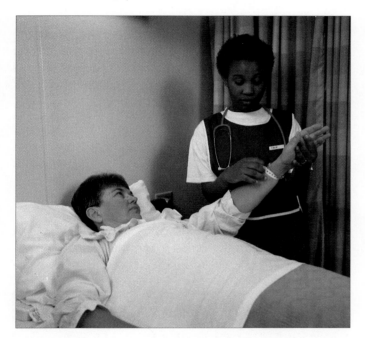

FIGURE 3–2. Checking the patient's arm band assures that the right patient receives the proper care.

Ethical/Legal Standards

Each day as you carry out your work and relate to patients, coworkers, families, and others from the community, you will be faced with decisions to make about your actions. Some of these decisions involve the moral right or wrong of an action. Other decisions involve the legality of your behavior.

Two sets of rules help govern these moral and legal actions you will take. They are:

1. **Ethical standards**: These are guides to moral behavior. People who give health care voluntarily agree to live up to these standards. When these rules are not followed, the nursing assistant fails to live up to the promise to give safe, correct care and do no harm.

2. **Legal laws**: These are guides to lawful behavior. When these laws are not obeyed, the nursing assistant may be **liable** (held responsible) for legal prosecution. Legal guilt can result in the payment of fines or imprisonment.

The ethical standards and legal laws are established to assure that only safe, quality care will be given. Following them also protects the care giver. Sometimes, the rules that govern moral actions and the laws that govern legal actions cover the same area.

Ethical Questions

Probably at no other time in history have the questions of medical ethics been under such scrutiny. Questions health care providers ask include:

■ When is life gone from a person on life support systems?

■ How much heroic effort should be given in situations of terminal illness?

■ How valid are "living wills" and Durable Powers of Attorney?

■ When does life actually begin?

■ How much assistance should be given to the conception process?

■ Should the body organs of a brain-dead person be harvested for transplants for the living?

■ Does an unborn baby have rights?

■ Is assisting a patient during or after an abortion right or wrong?

■ Do patients with HIV infection deserve the same care as other patients?

■ Is euthanasia (assisted death) ever justified?

■ Should animals be used in research of potential value to human life?

■ Should food and water be withheld to speed death when the patient has expressed the desire to have this action performed?

■ Who makes decisions about removing life support systems when there is no direct expression of the patient's wishes or there is conflict within the family?

■ How will a choice be made when two or more people could benefit from a kidney transplant but only one kidney is available?

■ How should limited money be spent when many serious disease conditions need to be researched?

■ Who has the final authority over whether a woman will carry a pregnancy to term?

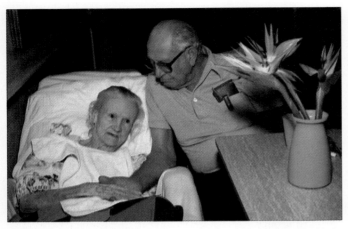

FIGURE 3–3. Promoting health and the quality of life is a primary goal.

Many facilities have ethics committees that serve in an advisory capacity to the staff on ethical matters. The members of the ethics committees often include staff, clergy, interested community members, and advocates for the sick and elderly.

The committee usually does not make recommendations for specific cases. Instead, the committee reviews the ethical problems and principles involved to help guide the staff and family.

Respect for patients and their wishes is the primary concern. Part of this respect for life is shown by having patients actively involved in deciding about their care and future.

As a nursing assistant, you will take directions from the legal and ethical guidelines established by your facility.

Respect for Life

One of the most basic rules of ethics is that life is precious. Everyone involved in the care of patients has the promotion of health and the quality of life as primary goals, Figure 3–3. Death, however, is a natural progression of life. When death is certain, the objective is to keep the person comfortable. Today, there is a greater appreciation of individual wishes and the quality of life expected. One fact remains clear—the major role of medicine and all members of the health care team is to maintain quality of life when possible and make comfortable those whose lives may not last much longer.

Respect for the Individual

Respect for each patient as a unique individual is another ethical principle. This uniqueness is demonstrated by differences in:

- Age
- Race
- Religion
- Culture
- Attitudes
- Background
- Response to illness

At times, you may find the differences that make the patient so special also make dealing with the patient challenging or difficult. If you respect each patient as a valuable person, you can learn to accept and work with each one in the best possible way.

Patient Information

The ethical code asserts that information about patients is privileged and must not be shared with others, Figure 3–4.

1. Discuss patient information only in appropriate places.
   a. It is unwise to discuss a patient's condition while in the patient's room, even if the patient is unresponsive. The patient may be

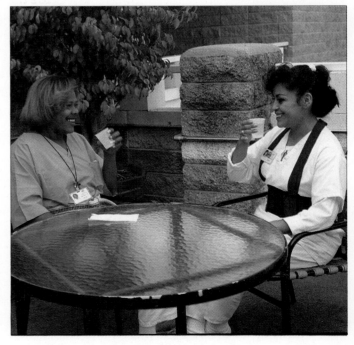

FIGURE 3–4. Information about patients is confidential and must not be discussed casually with others.

able to hear everything that is said. This could cause the patient unnecessary worry.
   b. Never discuss the patients in your care with your family or in the community.
   c. Never discuss the patients during lunch or coffee breaks, even with your coworkers.
2. Discuss information only with the proper people.
   a. At times you will be approached by others requesting information about a patient. For example, you may be asked for such information by:
      ■ Other patients
      ■ Family members
      ■ Members of the public, such as news-people
   b. Discuss patients and their personal concerns only with your supervisor during conference or report. Make sure you will not be overheard by visitors or other patients.
   c. You will learn to evade inquiries tactfully by:
      ■ Stating that you do not know all the details of the treatment or patient's condition.
      ■ Redirecting inquirers to the proper authority.
      ■ Firmly, but politely, indicating that you do not have the authority to provide the answers they seek.
3. Refer patient requests for information to the nurse or doctor. Interpreting laboratory findings or evaluating a patient's condition requires a professional level of education.
4. Let the nurse or doctor relay information about a patient's death. Never give information concerning the death of a patient to the patient's family. Treated with tact, a refusal of this kind is rarely resented by the family.
5. Follow the ethical code to ensure respect of the patient's personal religious beliefs. People of all faiths or beliefs and those with no proclaimed faith are admitted for care. These differences must be respected. You show your respect when you:
   a. Inform the nurse of requests for clergy visits.
   b. Know correct information about the type of chaplain services available in your facility.
   c. Know if a chapel is open for use by patients and families.

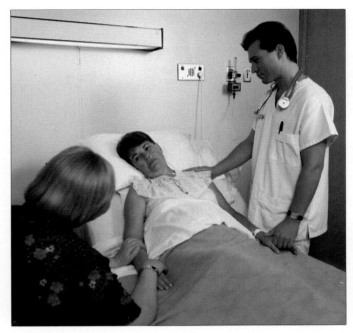

FIGURE 3–5. A visit from clergy or other members of the religious community can be reassuring and helpful to the patient.

   d. Respectfully treat religious articles of the patient such as a Bible, crucifix, Koran, or holy pictures.
   When the clergy visits, Figure 3–5, you should:
   a. Be helpful and courteous.
   b. Escort the clergy to the patient's bedside.
   c. Draw the curtains or close the door for privacy.
   d. Leave the room.

Tipping

Following the ethical code, the service you give will depend on need. It will not depend upon the patient's race, creed, color, or ability to pay. There is no place for tipping within the health care system, Figure 3–6.

Patients are charged for the services they receive while in the hospital. The salary you are paid is included in that charge.

Sometimes patients offer a "little something" to you. A firm but courteous refusal of the money is usually all that is necessary to assure the patient of your meaning.

As you can see, the ethical code assures that the patient is treated with dignity and respect in ways that always promote safe care.

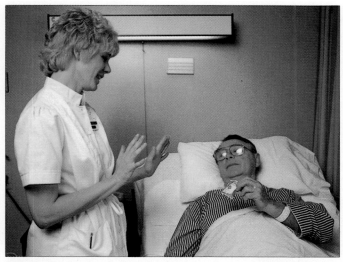

FIGURE 3–6.   Tips must be courteously refused.

Legal Issues

Laws are passed by governmental bodies and are to be obeyed by citizens. Anyone who fails to obey a law may be **liable** (responsible) for fines or imprisonment.

You need not fear breaking these laws if you are careful to:

- Do only those things that you have been taught and that are within the scope of your training.
- Keep your skills and knowledge up to date.
- Act in ways that keep the safety and well-being of the patient always foremost in your mind.
- Make sure you thoroughly understand directions for the care you are to give.
- Perform your job according to facility policy.
- Stay within OBRA guidelines.
- Maintain inservice requirements of OBRA.
- Do no harm to the patient.
- Respect the patient's belongings (property).

Here are some situations you will wish to avoid.

Negligence

Nursing assistants are trained care providers and are expected to perform in certain ways. When a nursing assistant fails to give care that is expected or required by the job, that assistant is guilty of negligence.

You would be guilty of negligence if you injured a patient by:

- Not performing your work as taught. For example, a patient is burned by an enema solution that was prepared by you and was too hot.
- Not carrying out your job in a conscientious manner. For example, though your facility has a policy that bed rails must be up at night, in your hurry you fail to secure the bed rails and the patient falls and is injured.

Theft

Taking anything that doesn't belong to you makes you guilty of stealing. If you are caught, you will be liable. The article taken need not be expensive to be considered stolen.

If you see someone stealing something and do not report it, you are guilty of **aiding and abetting** the crime, Figure 3–7.

Because of the nature of their work, people working in facilities must be honest and dependable. Despite careful screening, dishonest people are sometimes hired and things do disappear. These range from washcloths, money, and patient's personal belongings to drugs.

Sometimes workers are reluctant to report things that they see other people doing. Remember, however, that you are responsible for your own actions and must take the proper actions. As a nursing assis-

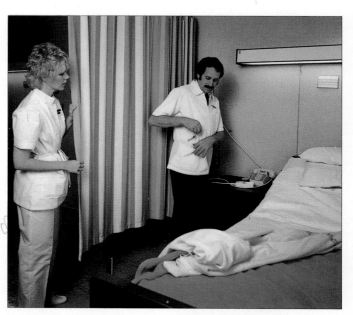

FIGURE 3–7.   Failing to report a dishonest act that you observe makes you guilty of aiding and abetting.

tant, the opportunities for poor practice, illegal activities, and neglect are ever present. Resist the temptation to lower your standards. Honesty and integrity are the hallmarks of the sincere and conscientious nursing assistant.

Defamation

If you make false statements about someone to a third person and the character of the first person is injured, you are guilty of defamation. This is true if you make the statement verbally (slander) or in writing (libel). For example, if you inaccurately tell a coworker that a patient has AIDS, you have slandered that individual. If you write the same untrue information in a note, you are guilty of libel.

False Imprisonment

Restraining a person's movements or actions without proper authorization constitutes unlawful or false imprisonment. For example, patients have the right to leave the hospital *with* or *without* the physician's permission. You may not interfere with this right. If you do interfere, you will be guilty of false imprisonment.

If you learn of a patient's intention to leave the hospital without permission, inform your supervisor. The supervisor will handle the situation.

Using physical restraints or even threatening to do so in order to make a patient cooperate can also constitute false imprisonment. It is sometimes necessary to support and restrain the movement of patients. Whenever used, supports and restraints must always be applied in accordance with a physician's order. The physician's order indicates the extent of restraint or support to be used and the reason for it.

Assault and Battery

Assault and battery are serious legal matters. Assault means intentionally attempting to touch the body of another or even threatening to do so. Battery means actually touching another without that person's permission.

The care we give is given with the patient's permission or informed consent. This means the patient must know and agree to what we plan to do before we start. Consent may be withdrawn at any time, Figure 3–8. For example, you are assigned to give a patient a warm foot soak. Despite your explanation of the reasons for the order, the patient refuses. You may not force the patient to submit. To do so would make you

guilty of battery. To threaten the patient by telling her/him that you will get others to assist you if she/he refuses is to be guilty of assault.

Either situation could make you liable for legal charges. You can avoid this legal pitfall by:

- Informing the patient of what you plan to do.
- Making sure the patient understands.
- Pausing before starting to give the patient an opportunity to refuse.
- Reporting refusal of care to supervisor and documenting the facts.
- Never carrying out a treatment on your own against the patient's wishes.

Invasion of Privacy

Patients have a right to have their person and personal affairs kept confidential. To do otherwise is an invasion of privacy. Invading the privacy of another is against the law.

You can protect the patient's privacy by:

- Protecting the patient from exposure of body parts.
- Knocking and pausing before entering a room.
- Drawing curtains when carrying out care.
- Leaving while visitors are with the patient.
- Not listening as patients make telephone calls.
- Abiding by the rules of confidentiality.
- Not trying to force a patient to accept your personal beliefs or views.

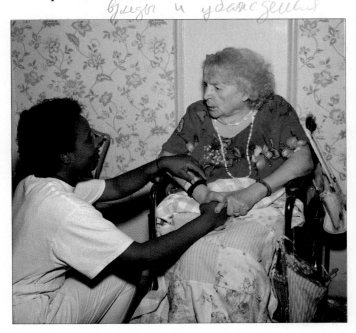

FIGURE 3–8. Patients have the right to refuse treatment.

Abuse

Abuse of (doing harm to) a patient violates ethical principles and makes you liable for legal prosecution. Ethical standards require that you do no harm to patients. Legal standards enforce this by applying laws with subsequent penalties if you are guilty.

Abuse can occur in several forms including physical abuse, verbal abuse, and psychological abuse. **Physical abuse** does actual physical harm to the patient. This could occur if you:

- Handle a patient too roughly.
- Perform the wrong treatment on the patient.
- Hit or push or pinch the patient.
- Neglect to turn the patient, causing circulation to be impaired.
- Do not carry out proper exercises and the patient experiences pain when unused joints are finally moved.
- Fail to see that the patient has food or water.
- Fail to carry out proper patient hygiene.

Verbal abuse may be directed toward the patient or may be expressed about the patient. You would be guilty of verbally abusing a patient if you:

- Used profanity in dealing with the patient.
- Raised your voice in anger at the patient.
- Called the patient unpleasant names.
- Teased the patient unkindly.
- Used threatening gestures.
- Made written threats or abusive statements.

Psychological abuse occurs when you:

- Make the patient fearful of you.
- Threaten the patient with harm.
- Threaten to tell something to others that the patient doesn't want known.
- Make fun of or belittle the patient in any way.

You must never abuse any patient in any way. If you suspect that a person in your care is being abused by others, you should discuss the matter with your supervisor. Laws *require* that a health care provider who suspects abuse report the situation so the patient can be protected. In some states the person *not* reporting the abuse is held as guilty as the abusing person.

Anyone can be abused, but the old and young are the most vulnerable. Usually, it is the care giver or a family member who is responsible for the abuse.

It may be difficult to understand why anyone would abuse another who is weak or infirm, but it happens. A few people may take satisfaction out of feeling they have control of others. Most abuse, however, probably originates in feelings of frustration or fatigue.

If you feel your own tolerance level is being tested, you need to find ways to safeguard the patient and release your own stress. You might:

- Try to identify the exact cause of your irritation.
- Talk with your supervisor about your feelings.
- Consider asking to be temporarily assigned to another patient.
- Try to reduce your overall stress and fatigue so you bring a more positive, patient attitude to your job.

Abuse is discussed in Units 29 and 31.

Safety Devices and Restraints

Safety devices or restraints may be jackets, belts, vests, or straps. When used to restrain the patient's activities, either for the patient's protection or the protection of others, there are guidelines that must be followed.

A restraint is any technique or device that is attached or next to the patient's body that the patient cannot easily remove and that restricts freedom of movement or normal access to one's body. The inappropriate and/or incorrect use of restraints can cause serious injury or death to the patient.

1. Alternatives to safeguard the resident should be implemented before resorting to restraints.
2. A physician's order must be obtained by the nurse before applying restraints. The order must indicate the type of restraint to use and the reason for its use.
3. Even if the patient does not seem to understand, always explain what you are doing.
4. Use the right type and size of restraint. All restraints **must** be applied according to manufacturer's directions. Check the device before use—do not use if it is frayed, torn, has parts missing, or is soiled. Restraints are put on over clothing, never next to bare skin.
5. After application, check the fit of the device. You should be able to slip the width of two fingers between the restraint and the patient's body. The device should never restrict breathing.
6. The patient must have access to a call light and drinking water while restrained.
7. Check every 15 minutes for the patient's comfort and safety. Make changes as needed.

8. The restraint must be released at least every 2 hours to:
- Check for irritation or poor circulation
- Change the patient's position
- Exercise—ambulate the patient or do passive range of motion exercises
- Take the patient to the bathroom
- Change incontinent patients and cleanse their skin
- Provide fluid or nourishment
- Attend to any other needs

9. When restraints are used in chairs, the patient should always be in good body alignment.

10. Use a quick-release tie for restraints so that they may be released quickly by pulling on one strap.

11. When restraints are used in bed:
- There must be full side rails on the bed, in the up position.
- The patient should always be positioned in the middle of the mattress.
- Always secure restraint to the movable part of the bed frame.

12. Do not use restraints in moving vehicles or on toilets unless you are sure it is a device that is intended for that use by the manufacturer. (Make sure you know the facility policies for the use of restraints in these situations.)

Whenever postural supports or restraints are used, extra nursing care and supervision are required to prevent harm to the patient, Figure 3–9.

SUMMARY

All persons giving health care voluntarily adhere to a set of ethical standards. They agree to:
- Protect life
- Promote health
- Keep personal information confidential
- Respect personal death beliefs
- Give care based on need, not gratuities (tips)
- Provide safety

Nursing assistants have legal responsibilities. Legal situations the nursing assistant wants to avoid include:
- Negligence
- Assault and battery
- Theft
- Invasion of privacy
- Abuse

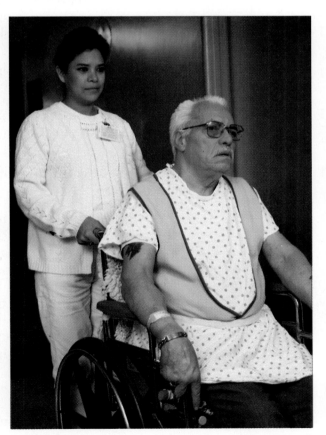

FIGURE 3–9. When postural restraints are used, extra nursing care and supervision are needed.

UNIT REVIEW

True/False. Answer the following statements true or false by circling T or F.

T F 1. A patient may not refuse any treatment prescribed by his/her physician.

T F 2. You may learn much about a patient's personal life as you provide care.

T F 3. Lunchtime is the best time to discuss your patients with others.

T F 4. When a person dies, you should call and inform the family.

T F 5. In accepting a tip, you are guilty of abuse.

T F 6. Your patient has an order to encourage fluid intake, and you fail to do this. You are guilty of negligence.

T F 7. You forget to put side rails up at night, and a patient falls. You are negligent in the action.

T F 8. Failure to report your observation of an illegal act makes you guilty of aiding and abetting the action.

T F 9. Leaving a patient unnecessarily exposed is an invasion of the patient's privacy.

T F 10. Jackets, belts, vests, or straps can be safety devices.

T F 11. Ethics relates to moral rights and wrongs of behavior.

T F 12. Anxiety can sometimes make a person very demanding.

T F 13. It is not always easy to keep the basic rule of ethics in mind when you witness a patient suffering.

T F 14. People give up their right to privacy when they are admitted to health care facilities.

T F 15. You add to a patient's sense of security when you use terms of endearment like "Honey."

T F 16. Your primary purpose is to help the patient by assisting the nursing staff.

T F 17. If an error occurs as you give care, it is important to report it immediately.

T F 18. Patients should not question the cost of care.

T F 19. Every patient has the right to considerate, respectful care.

T F 20. You should knock and pause before entering a patient's room.

T F 21. It is alright for you to give your evaluation of the patient's condition to the patient himself.

T F 22. Honesty and integrity are the hallmarks of a conscientious nursing assistant.

T F 23. You should report all requests for clergy visits to the doctor.

T F 24. If a patient resists you, you may apply restraints to make sure the treatment is given.

T F 25. Patients may not be subjected to either verbal or physical abuse.

SELF-EVALUATION   Section 1

A. Choose the phrase that best completes each of the following sentences by circling the proper letter.

1. An example of a tax-supported agency is the
   a. American Heart Association.
   b. Association for the Blind.
   c. health department.
   d. Tuberculosis Association.

2. The official international health agency is called the
   a. International Health Association.
   b. World Health Organization.
   c. World Health Service.
   d. International Health Service.

3. Your daily assignment is usually given to you by the
   a. assistant.
   b. director of nursing.
   c. team leader.
   d. physician.

4. The Patient's Bill of Rights includes the right to know that
   a. orders will be properly carried out.
   b. privacy will be preserved.
   c. needs will be recognized and met.
   d. All of the above.

5. One of the following is *not* part of your job.
   a. Starting IVs
   b. Collecting specimens
   c. Assisting patients to ambulate
   d. Giving enemas

6. Personal information about patients
   a. may be discussed during coffee break.
   b. must never be discussed outside the hospital.
   c. may be discussed with other patients.
   d. may be used for your personal advantage.

7. When a patient offers you a tip for your services, you should
   a. refuse in a firm, courteous manner.
   b. accept the tip and share it with the other team members.

   c. refuse and act shocked that the offer was ever made.
   d. accept and then return the tip to a member of the patient's family.

8. A case of negligence would arise if a patient
   a. who has bathroom privileges falls when the nursing assistant is out of the room.
   b. falls because water on the floor was not wiped up.
   c. develops an infection when the nursing assistant performs a procedure that had not been taught.
   d. develops an important symptom that he does not report to the nursing team.

9. A case of negligence would arise if a patient were injured because you
   a. forgot to follow the hospital policy to put up side rails at night.
   b. carried out a special procedure in which you had not been instructed.
   c. wiped up some water on the floor.
   d. reported a defective electrical wire.

10. When caring for a patient with different religious beliefs from your own, you are obliged to
    a. help the patient understand your faith.
    b. show the patient how wrong her faith is.
    c. respect his religious beliefs.
    d. arrange to have your clergyman make a visit.

11. Important characteristics for the nursing assistant include
    a. interest in others.
    b. willingness to learn.
    c. good personal grooming.
    d. All of the above.

12. Part of good grooming includes
    a. cleaning shoes every week.
    b. keeping fingernails long and polished.
    c. taking a bath daily.
    d. wearing expensive jewelry.

13. Lines of authority are important. Your immediate line of authority is
    a. another nursing assistant.
    b. a staff LVN/LPN or registered nurse.
    c. the administrator.
    d. the physician.

14. You protect the patient's privacy by
    a. exposing the patient.
    b. knocking before entering a patient's room.
    c. always staying when visitors are present.
    d. listening to personal telephone calls.

15. You learn something personal about a patient from her chart. You should
    a. keep quiet about the information.
    b. share it with other patients.
    c. share it with coworkers during coffee break.
    d. let the patient know what you have learned.

16. You observe a coworker stealing supplies and fail to report it. You are guilty of
    a. malpractice.
    b. aiding and abetting.
    c. gossip.
    d. loyalty.

17. A patient tells you he is worried about being able to pay his bill. You should
    a. talk to his wife about the problem.
    b. report to your team leader/registered nurse/supervisor.
    c. share the information with a coworker.
    d. call the physician.

18. When the patient's clergyperson comes for a visit, you should
    a. move other patients out of the room.
    b. draw the curtains for privacy.
    c. ask the patient's visitor to remain.
    d. stay with the patient.

19. Nursing assistants function as health care providers in
    a. acute hospitals.
    b. long-term care facilities.
    c. homes.
    d. All of the above.

20. The service that you give to a patient is determined by the patient's
    a. race.
    b. need.
    c. color.
    d. creed.

B. Match Column I with Column II.

Column I	Column II
_____ 21. medical department	a. cares for pregnant women and newborns
_____ 22. surgical department	b. cares for children
_____ 23. pediatric department	c. cares for trauma victims
_____ 24. obstetrical unit	d. cares for patients with medical conditions
_____ 25. emergency department	e. cares for patients with surgical conditions

C. Answer the following statements true or false by circling T or F.

T F 26. Patients have the right to considerate and respectful care.

T F 27. Patients must participate in any treatment their physician feels is necessary.

T F 28. It is alright to discuss patients' treatment in front of visitors.

T F 29. Patients have the right to refuse to participate in research programs that might help them.

T F 30. Information about patients' bills are not discussed with patients since they are sent to the insurance company.

T F 31. Alternatives to the use of restraints should always be tried first.

T F 32. One finger width should be able to be inserted between the restraint and the patient's body.

T F 33. The patient must always have access to a call light and drinking water when restrained.

T F 34. Patients who are restrained must be checked about once each hour.

T F 35. A quick-release tie must be used to secure restraints.

36. List five actions you can take to ensure your practice remains within legal guidelines.

Unit 4

Basic Anatomy and Physiology

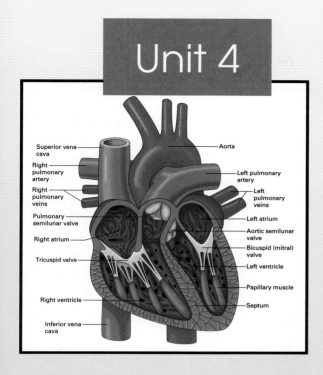

Superior vena cava
Right pulmonary artery
Right pulmonary veins
Pulmonary semilunar valve
Right atrium
Tricuspid valve
Right ventricle
Inferior vena cava
Aorta
Left pulmonary artery
Left pulmonary veins
Left atrium
Aortic semilunar valve
Bicuspid (mitral) valve
Left ventricle
Papillary muscle
Septum

OBJECTIVES

As a result of this unit, you will be able to:

- Spell and define terms.

- Describe the simple to complex organization of the body.

- State the structure of a cell and its relationship to the formation of tissues, organs, and systems.

- Name the four types of tissues and their characteristics.

- Use the correct terms to identify body parts.

- List the systems of the body and their functions.

- Properly locate major organs as parts of body systems.

- Describe the effects of the aging process on each system.

VOCABULARY

Learn the meaning and the correct spelling of the following words:

abduction
adduction
adrenal glands
anatomic position
anatomy
anterior
artery
atrium
axon
bolus
bones
Bowman's
    capsule
bursae
capillary
cardiac cycle
cardiac muscle
caudal
cell
chromosomes
chyme
connective tissue
cornea
coronal
cortex
cranial
cytoplasm
defecation
dendrite
deoxyribonucleic
    acid (DNA)
dermis
diastole
disease

distal
dorsal
endocrine glands
epidermis
epithelial tissue
erythrocytes
estrogen
eustachian tube
exocrine glands
extension
flexion
genes
genitalia
glomerulus
gonads
health
hormones
inferior
insertion
involuntary
    (or visceral)
    muscles
iris
islets of
    Langerhans
joints
labia majora
labia minora
lateral
leukocytes
ligaments
lymph
medial
medulla

melanin
membranes
menarche
meninges
menstruation
mitosis
mucous
mucus
muscular tissue
nephron
nerve
nervous tissue
neuron
nucleus
organs
origin
ossicles
ovary
ovulation
ovum
parietal
pelvis
pepsin
pericardium
peristalsis
peritoneum
physiology
pituitary gland
planes
plasma
pleura
posterior
progesterone
proximal

pyloric sphincter
quadrants
respiration
retention
rotation
sagittal
scrotum
sebaceous
    glands
secretions
serous fluid
sperm
stimulus
sudoriferous
    glands
superior
suppression
synapse
system
systole
tendons
testis
testosterone
thrombocytes
tissues
tympanic
    membrane
umbilicus
vein
ventral
ventricle
visceral
voluntary
    muscles

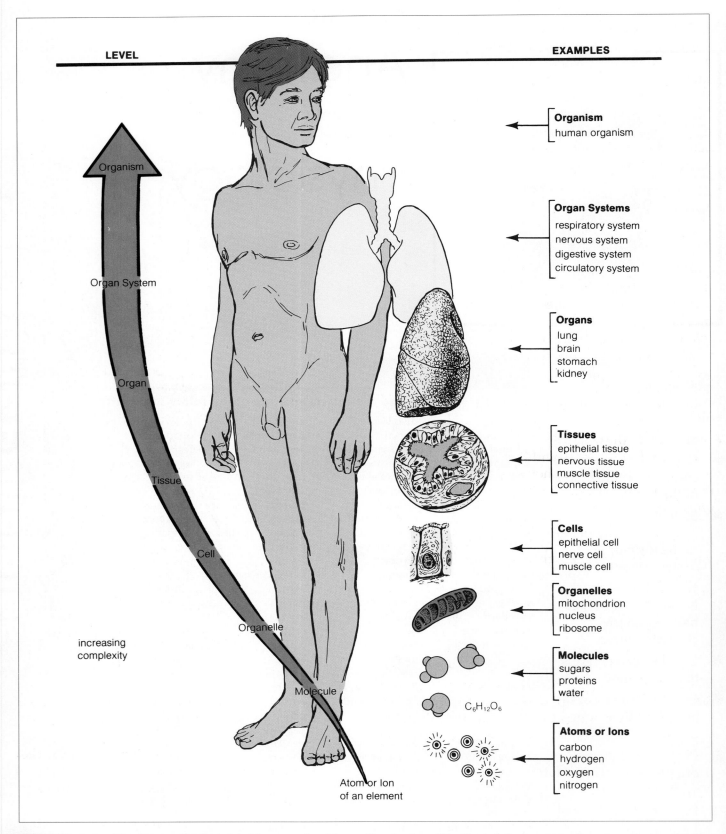

LEVEL

Organism

Organ System

Organ

Tissue

Cell

Organelle

Molecule

increasing
complexity

Atom or Ion
of an element

EXAMPLES

Organism
human organism

Organ Systems
respiratory system
nervous system
digestive system
circulatory system

Organs
lung
brain
stomach
kidney

Tissues
epithelial tissue
nervous tissue
muscle tissue
connective tissue

Cells
epithelial cell
nerve cell
muscle cell

Organelles
mitochondrion
nucleus
ribosome

Molecules
sugars
proteins
water

$C_6H_{12}O_6$

Atoms or Ions
carbon
hydrogen
oxygen
nitrogen

FIGURE 4–1. The human body is highly organized from the single cell to the total organism. *(From Fong, Ferris, and Skelley,*
Body Structures and Functions, *7th Edition, 1989, Delmar Publishers Inc.)*

All nursing care is directed toward helping patients reach optimum health and independence. Health is a state of well-being where all parts of the body and mind are functioning properly. Disease is any change from the healthy state. Disease takes many forms. Medical science is the study of disease and its effects on the human body. These effects are easier to understand when you have a clear picture in your mind of a normal and properly functioning body, Figure 4–1.

Basic Anatomy and Related Terminology

The anatomy (structure) and physiology (function) of the body are most easily understood and learned if they are studied in a systematic, orderly manner. Special terms can be used to describe the relationship of one body part to another.

Whenever we describe the relationship of the body parts, keep in mind the anatomic position, Figure 4–2, which is:

■ Standing erect with feet together or slightly separated
■ Facing the observer
■ Arms at the sides with the palms forward

In our own minds, we should always position the body in this way before describing any body part or area. This gives everyone the same frame of reference.

Notice as you look at a patient's body or the pictures in the book that you are seeing a mirror image of yourself. The patient's right side is opposite to your left and your left is opposite to the right of the patient or the picture.

Planes

Imaginary lines or planes, Figure 4–3, can be used to divide the body in order to better learn and describe the relationships of its parts. The planes are:

■ Transverse—lines drawn from side to side
　— Superior (cranial)—body parts above the line
　— Inferior (caudal)—body parts below the line
■ Median (sagittal)—line drawn through the center of the body from head to floor. It divides the body into two equal sides.

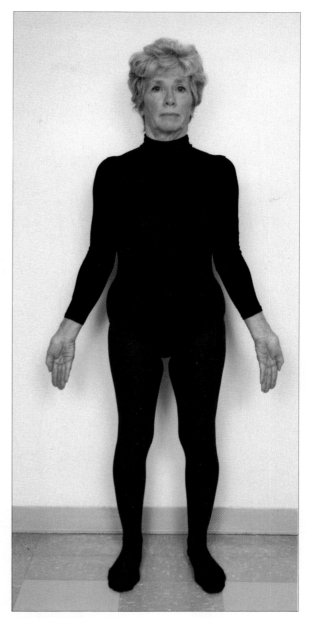

FIGURE 4–2. All references to body parts are made in relationship to the anatomic position.

　— Medial—body parts close to the midline
　— Lateral—body parts away from the midline
■ Frontal (coronal)—line drawn to divide the body into back and front
　— Anterior (ventral)—body parts in front of the line
　— Posterior (dorsal)—body parts behind the line

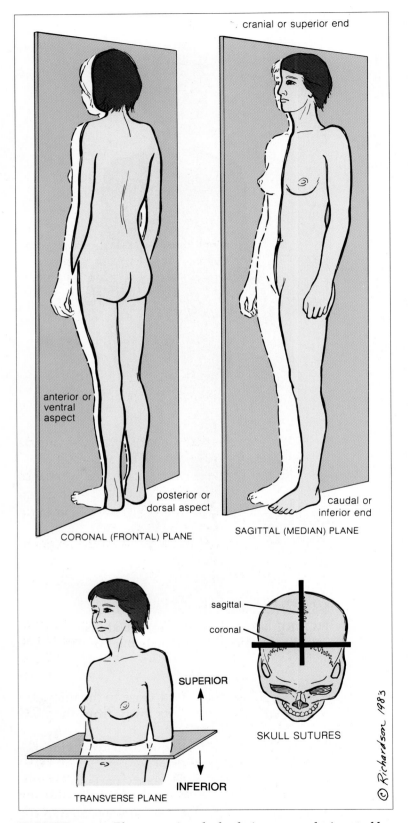

FIGURE 4–3. Planes section the body into areas designated by special terminology. *(From Fong, Ferris, and Skelley,* Body Structures and Functions, *7th Edition, 1989, Delmar Publishers Inc.)*

The entire body may also be divided into two major groups:

1. Torso—composed of the head, neck, and trunk
2. Appendages—composed of the upper and lower extremities
   a. The upper extremities include the:
      ■ fingers
      ■ hands
      ■ wrists
      ■ forearms
      ■ upper arms
   b. The lower extremities include the:
      ■ toes
      ■ feet
      ■ ankles
      ■ lower leg
      ■ thigh
   c. The thigh attaches the lower extremities to the torso at the hip.

Two terms can be used to describe the relationship of one part of an extremity to another part and to the point of attachment. The terms are:

1. **Proximal**: This term is used to describe the part being compared that is closest to the point of attachment. For example, the elbow is *proximal* to the wrist. This means that the elbow is closest to the point of attachment of the arm at the shoulder. The knee is proximal to the ankle.
2. **Distal**: This term is used to describe the part being compared that is farthest away from the point of attachment. For example, the wrist could be described as being *distal* to the elbow since it is farthest away from the shoulder. The toes would be described as distal to the ankles.

Cavities

There are spaces within the solid-looking body called cavities, Figure 4–4. The cavities are lined with membranes and usually contain the body organs such as the heart, liver, and brain. The dorsal cavity is divided into the cranial cavity and the vertebral cavity.

The large ventral cavity is divided by a dome-shaped muscle, the diaphragm, into the thoracic cavity and the abdominopelvic cavity. Figure 4–5 lists the cavities and locates the organs within them.

Membranes

There are two types of membranes in the body:
1. **Mucous** membranes:
   a. Line body cavities that open to the outside, such as the nose, digestive tract, and reproductive tract
   b. Secrete a whitish fluid called **mucus**, which keeps these passages always moist
2. Serous membranes:
   a. Produce a clear yellowish fluid called **serous fluid**

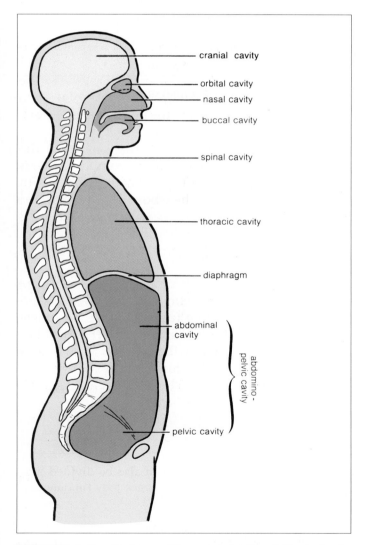

FIGURE 4–4. Body cavities contain the delicate body parts. *(From Fong, Ferris, and Skelley,* Body Structures and Functions, *7th Edition, 1989, Delmar Publishers Inc.)*

CAVITY	ORGANS
Cranial	Brain, pineal body, pituitary gland
Spinal	Nerves, spinal cord
Thoracic	Lungs, heart, great blood vessels, thymus gland
Abdominal	
Peritoneal	Stomach, small intestine, most of large intestine, liver, gallbladder, pancreas, spleen
Pelvic	*Male* — Seminal vesicles, prostate gland, ejaculatory ducts, urinary bladder, urethra, rectum *Female* — Uterus, oviducts, ovaries, urinary bladder, urethra, rectum
Retroperitoneal Space	Kidneys, adrenal glands, ureters

FIGURE 4–5. Organ placement in body cavities

b. Line cavities that do not open to the outside such as the cranial and thoracic cavities
c. Subdivide large cavities into smaller spaces
d. Are composed of two layers. The **parietal** (outer) layer lines the cavity and the **visceral** (inner) layer covers the organs.
e. Secrete enough fluid between the layers to prevent friction
f. Have special names

Names of Serous Membranes

The **meninges** line the cranial cavity and spinal cavity. They cover the brain and spinal cord. The **pleura** lines the thoracic cavity, covers the lungs, and divides the lungs into lobes. The **pericardium** separates the pericardial cavity from the mediastinum and pleural cavities. It covers the heart. The visceral layer also serves as epicardium.

The **peritoneum** lines the abdominal cavity. It covers the organs of digestion such as the stomach, small and large intestines, liver, gallbladder, pancreas, and spleen. It separates the abdominal cavity into the peritoneal cavity, which is surrounded by the peritoneum. The retroperitoneal space is the part of the abdominal cavity behind the peritoneum. The pelvic cavity is the part below the peritoneum.

Abdominal Regions

The abdomen is divided into four quadrants, with the umbilicus (navel) at the central point, Figure 4–6A. The abdomen can also be divided into nine regions, Figure 4–6B. Knowing these regions will be important as you report and document your observations.

Body Organization

The body is formed in a highly organized manner. The basic unit is the cell. Cells are organized into tissues. Tissues are organized into organs, and organs are organized into a body system. Each component has a job to perform, which contributes to the structures and functions of the body.

Cells

Cells are the microscopic basic units of life, Figure 4–7. The entire body is composed of these tiny units. On a small scale, the living cell carries out the same functions as the body. These functions include:

- Respiration
- Energy production
- Nutrition
- Reproduction
- Elimination

The structure of cells varies, but it always includes three main parts:

1. Nucleus—directs the activities of the cell and plays an important role in reproduction. The nucleus is the command center. It controls:
   a. Cellular division—which permits cells to reproduce themselves.
   b. Cellular activity—which allows the cell to contribute to the well-being of the body as a whole.
2. Cytoplasm—a jelly-like substance which carries out the activities of the cell.
3. Cell membrane—controls passage of materials that enter and leave the cell.

Cellular Division (Mitosis). Cellular division, Figure 4–8, is a complex process that involves a special protein called deoxyribonucleic acid (DNA) The DNA forms chromosomes, which contain the information of heredity, or genes. During cellular division, the 46 chromosomes of DNA arrange themselves in the center of the cell:

- Each chromosome duplicates itself.
- Half of the chromosomes move to opposite sides of the cell.

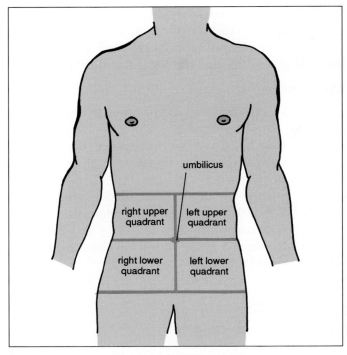

FIGURE 4–6A.   The abdominal quadrants

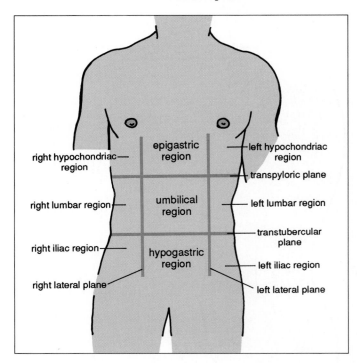

FIGURE 4–6B.   The abdomen can also be divided into nine regions. *(From Fong, Ferris, and Skelley,* Body Structures and Functions, *7th Edition, 1989, Delmar Publishers Inc.)*

- The cell divides.
- The cytoplasm increases.
- The cell separates into two equal cells.

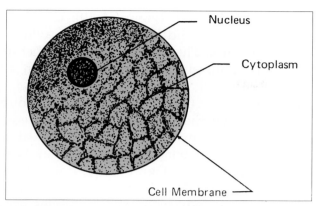

FIGURE 4–7. Animal cell structure

DNA	Deoxyribonucleic acid
RNA	Ribonucleic acid
mRNA	Messenger RNA
tRNA	Transfer RNA
Ribosomal RNA	Found in cytoplasm

FIGURE 4–9. Nucleic acids

Cellular Activity. Cellular activity also depends upon the direction of the DNA code. For example, a cell has the job of producing a protein hormone. The directions for how to make that hormone are found like a recipe in the DNA of the nucleus. Four different proteins are involved in this process, Figure 4–9.

The function of each nucleic acid is:

DNA	contains the code	like a recipe
mRNA	takes a picture of the code and carries it into the cytoplasm	like a foreman who carries the plans from the office into the factory

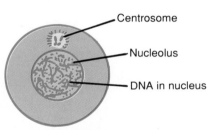

A. DNA molecules duplicate themselves

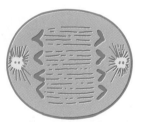

D. Chromosomes separate

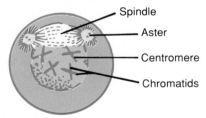

B. Centrosomes separate and a spindle forms between them

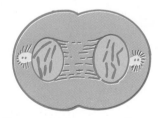

E. Two nuclei form as cell separates

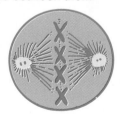

C. Duplicated chromosomes line up along center of spindle

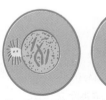

F. Each new cell has the full number of chromosomes

FIGURE 4–8. Cellular reproduction

Ribosomal RNA	mRNA attaches to the ribosomal RNA in the cytoplasm	like the foreman placing the plans on a workbench
tRNA	brings the necessary components from the cytoplasm and matches them to the mRNA; ribosomal RNA combination	like workers gathering the materials to match the directions and make the product
Separation of the final product	the final ribosome base forms the hormone	like the foreman picking the product up and taking it to the salesperson

Tissues

Tissues are special groups of cells that carry on particular activities. There are four basic tissue types:

1. **Epithelial tissue** (Figure 4–10): Covers the body as skin and lines the body cavities as membranes. The cells are close together and are specialized for absorption, secretion, and protection.
2. **Connective tissue** (Figure 4–11): Found throughout the body. It holds other tissues together. The many forms of connective tissue include blood, bone, fibrous and elastic types.
3. **Muscular tissue** (Figure 4–12): Has cells that have the special ability to shorten (contract) and to lengthen (relax). When muscles are attached to bones, they enable the body to move. Some muscles help to form the walls of organs. The heart is a highly specialized form of muscle tissue.
4. **Nervous tissue** (Figure 4–13): Extends from the brain and spinal cord throughout the body.

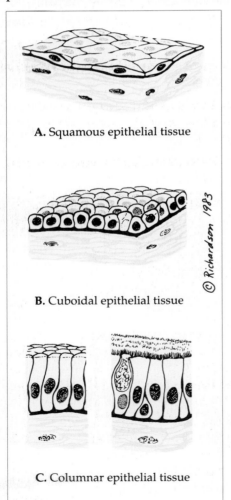

FIGURE 4–10. Epithelial tissue (*From Fong, Ferris, and Skelley,* Body Structures and Functions, *7th Edition, 1989, Delmar Publishers Inc.*)

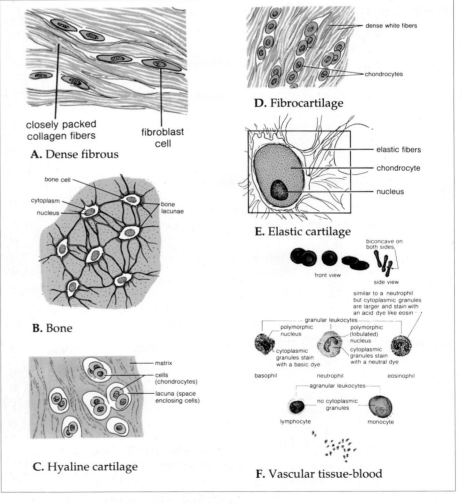

FIGURE 4–11. Connective tissue (*From Fong, Ferris, and Skelley,* Body Structures and Functions, *7th Edition, 1989, Delmar Publishers Inc.*)

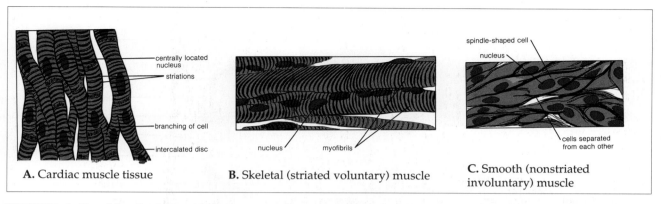

FIGURE 4–12. Muscle tissue *(From Fong, Ferris, and Skelley,* Body Structures and Functions, *7th Edition, 1989, Delmar Publishers Inc.)*

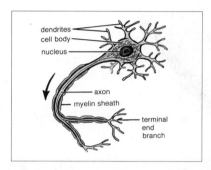

FIGURE 4–13. Nerve tissue *(From Fong, Ferris, and Skelley, Body Structures and Functions, 7th Edition, 1989, Delmar Publishers Inc.)*

This tissue carries messages and regulates body functions.

Sheets of tissues form the **membranes** of the body.

Organs

Groups of different tissues acting together to carry out a specific function are called **organs**, Figure 4–14. For example, the stomach is an organ that aids in digestion. It is made up of nervous, connective, muscular, and epithelial tissues.

Some organs are found in pairs. It is peculiar to this group that if one of the organs is surgically removed, the other will operate alone to perform the necessary functions. Even when the organ is singular, like the stomach, from one-third to one-half can be removed without interfering with its routine function.

Systems

When several organs combine to perform a special function, they are called a **system**. The digestive system, for instance, includes the:

- Mouth
- Tongue
- Pharynx
- Esophagus
- Salivary glands
- Intestines

- Liver
- Gallbladder
- Stomach
- Pancreas

Figure 4–15, page 49, provides a list of the names of the body systems and the organs included in each. Notice that some organs function in more than one system.

The Integumentary System

Structure and Function

The integumentary system includes:
- Skin
- Hair
- Nails
- Sweat glands
- Nerves
- Oil glands

The hair, nails, and glands are called skin appendages. The skin covers the body. It is composed of two functionally separated but anatomically fixed layers of tissue. These layers of tissue are attached to the subcutaneous fat and muscles below the skin, Figure 4–16 (page 50).

- The **epidermis** is the outer layer of skin. It is made up of many layers of cells. The deepest layer of cells produces new cells. The new cells are constantly being pushed to the surface of the skin and are shed. Melanin is found in this bottom layer. **Melanin** is a substance that gives color to the skin.

- The **dermis** lies beneath the epidermis. It is solidly attached to the epidermis. It is full of nerves and blood vessels. The hair and glands are found here. They extend upward through the epidermis to the surface of the body.

- The nails are horny cell structures found on the dorsal, distal surfaces of the fingers and toes. They protect the sensitive fingers and toes.

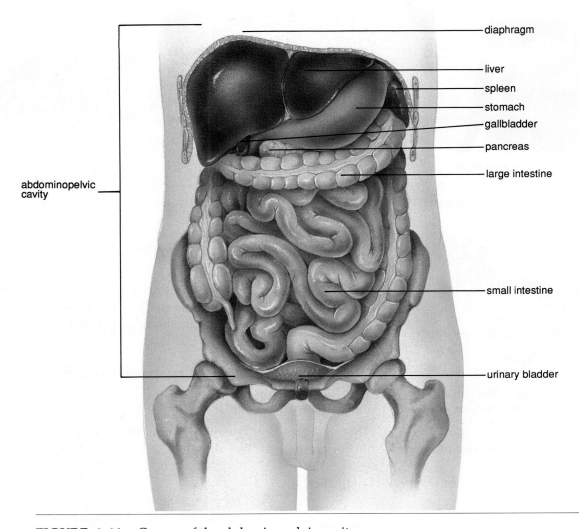

FIGURE 4–14. Organs of the abdominopelvic cavity

The nerves in the skin form sense organs. The sense organs receive information about the environment such as:

- Pressure
- Heat
- Cold
- Pain

Glands

Glands are special body structures made of complex epithelial tissue. They produce substances called secretions. Some glands have ducts that carry the substances to the body surfaces. These glands are called exocrine glands.

The exocrine glands of the skin are of two types:

1. Sudoriferous (sweat) glands. These produce perspiration. The perspiration forms on the surface of the body, carrying heat out of the body. Perspiring is a major mechanism for heat management. When the weather is cold, less perspiration is formed and less heat is lost from the body.
2. Sebaceous (oil) glands. These pour an oily substance (sebum) into the hair follicles. The sebum acts as a lubrication for the hair.

The hair is a slender thread-like structure that develops in hair follicles in the dermis. Hair is found all over the body, except for the soles of the feet and the palms of the hands.

The function of the skin includes:

- Protection: The intact skin is a mechanical barrier to injury and disease.
- Heat regulation: Many small blood vessels are present in the deeper part of the skin, the dermis. When they dilate with blood, heat is

SYSTEM	FUNCTION	ORGANS
Circulatory	Transports materials around the body. Carries oxygen and nutrients to the cells and carries waste products away	Heart, arteries, capillaries, veins, spleen, lymph nodes, lymphatic vessels, blood, lymph
Endocrine	Produces hormones that regulate body processes	Pituitary gland, thyroid gland, parathyroid gland, thymus gland, adrenal gland, testes, ovaries, pineal body, islets of Langerhans in pancreas
Gastrointestinal	Digests, transports food, absorbs nutrients, and eliminates wastes	Mouth, esophagus, pharynx, stomach, small intestines, large intestines, salivary glands, teeth, tongue, liver, gallbladder, pancreas
Integumentary	Protects the body against infection, regulates body temperature, eliminates some wastes	Skin, hair, nails, sweat and oil glands
Musculoskeletal	Supports and protects body parts; allows the body to move	Muscles, bone, joints, ligaments, tendons
Nervous	Coordinates body functions	Brain, spinal cord, spinal nerves, cranial nerves, special sense organs such as eyes and ears
Respiratory	Brings in oxygen and eliminates carbon dioxide	Sinuses, nose, pharynx, larynx, trachea, bronchi, lungs
Urinary	Manages fluids and electrolytes of body, eliminates liquid wastes	Kidneys, ureters, urinary bladder, urethra
Reproductive	Reproduces the species, fulfills sexual needs, develops sexual identity	*Male:* Testes, epididymis, urethra, seminal vesicles, ejaculatory duct, prostate gland, bulbourethral glands, penis, spermatic cord *Female:* Breasts, ovaries, oviducts, uterus, vagina, Bartholin glands, vulva

FIGURE 4–15. Systems of the body

brought to the surface where it escapes from the body. When heat needs to be conserved, these vessels constrict (become narrow by squeezing together). Heat is thereby kept within the body. This mechanism operates with the perspiration glands.

■ Storage: Energy in the form of fat as well as some vitamins is stored in this vital area.

■ Elimination: Some waste products as well as excess water are cast off (excreted) as perspiration through the activities of the sweat glands.

■ Sensory perception: The many nerve endings found in the skin tell us much about our environment. This is called our sense of touch or tactile sense.

Aging Changes

As a person ages, changes become evident in the skin and its appendages. These changes include:
■ Glands that are less active
■ Decreased circulation
■ Dryness, thinning, and scaling
■ Thickening of finger and toe nails
■ Loss of fat and elasticity
■ Loss of hair color
■ Development of skin irregularities such as skin tabs, moles, and warts

The Respiratory System

The respiratory system, Figure 4–17 (page 51), is sometimes called the lifeline of the body. It extends from the nose to the tiny air sacs or alveoli which make up the bulk of the lungs.

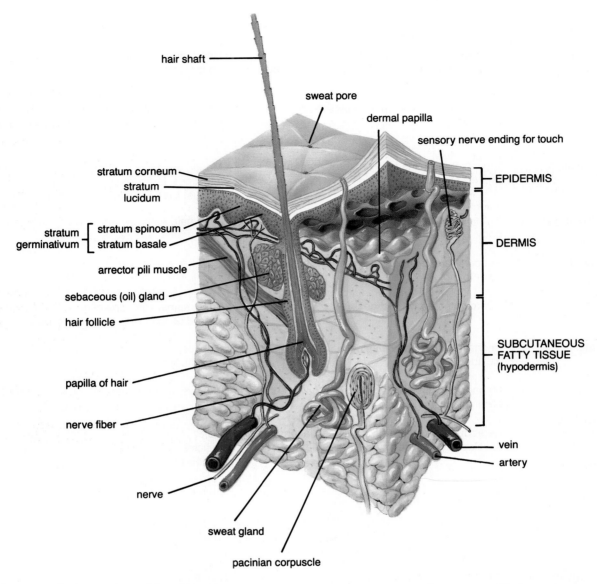

hair shaft

sweat pore

dermal papilla

sensory nerve ending for touch

EPIDERMIS

stratum corneum

stratum lucidum

stratum germinativum { stratum spinosum / stratum basale

DERMIS

arrector pili muscle

sebaceous (oil) gland

hair follicle

SUBCUTANEOUS FATTY TISSUE (hypodermis)

papilla of hair

nerve fiber

vein

artery

nerve

sweat gland

pacinian corpuscle

FIGURE 4–16.   Cross section of the skin *(From Anatomy and Physiology Plates, copyright 1992 by Delmar Publishers Inc.)*

Structure and Function

The organs of the respiratory system include the:

■ Nose
■ Pharynx (throat)
■ Larynx (voice box)
■ Trachea (windpipe)
■ Bronchi
■ Lungs

The sinuses, diaphragm, and intercostal muscles between the ribs are called auxiliary structures.

Air is warmed, moistened, and filtered as it passes through the nasal cavities, which are separated by the nasal septum. The air passes through the pharynx, a common passageway for air and food, into the larynx, trachea, bronchi, and alveoli. It is at the level of the alveoli that the exchange of gases takes place.

The purpose of this system is to bring oxygen (O_2) into the body to meet cellular needs and to expel carbon dioxide (CO_2). Carbon dioxide is a gaseous, metabolic waste produced by the cells. It also functions in voice production (phonation).

Each cell in the body must have a constant supply of oxygen. The oxygen is used to produce the energy for cellular activity.

Nutrients + oxygen → energy + water + CO_2

This reaction is known as cellular respiration. Blood transports the oxygen from the lungs to the cells and carbon dioxide from the cells back to the lungs.

The carbon dioxide is brought to the lungs by the pulmonary artery. It passes through tiny capillaries which surround the alveoli. The carbon dioxide escapes through the walls of the alveoli and is exhaled. The oxygen absorbed by the blood is carried back to the heart by the pulmonary vein. It is then pumped through the general circulation.

The center for respiratory control is in an area of the brain called the medulla. The need for oxygen is sensed by the cells of this special area. The medulla then transmits the message through nerves to the muscles of respiration. The respiratory nerves are the phrenic to the diaphragm and the intercostals to the intercostal muscles.

The respiratory cycle (one respiration) consists of two phases:

1. Inspiration (inhalation): When they are stimulated by the phrenic and intercostal nerves, the diaphragm and intercostal muscles contract. This creates a vacuum in the thoracic cavity, causing air to rush into the lungs.
2. Expiration (exhalation): The messages from the nerves stop and these same muscles relax. The thorax becomes smaller. This makes the space within the lungs smaller and forces the air out.

The lungs are:

- Found in the thoracic cavity.
- Covered by the double-walled pleura (membrane). A small amount of fluid between the layers prevents friction. The pleura is attached to the chest wall and diaphragm.
- Pointed at the top (apex).
- Broad at the bottom (base).
- Composed of all the tiny air sacs (alveoli) that are surrounded by the capillaries.
- Divided into lobes. The left lung has two lobes and the right lung has three lobes.

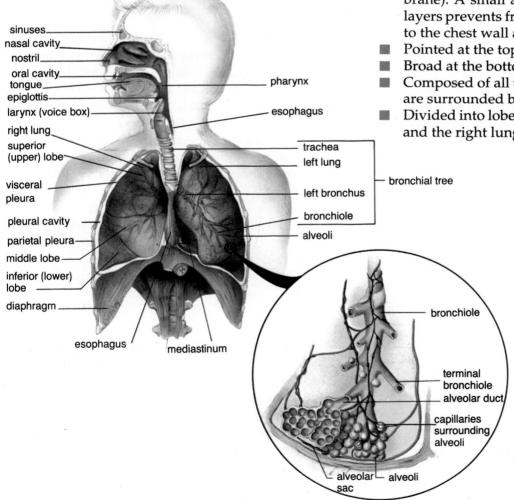

FIGURE 4–17. Respiratory system *(From Anatomy and Physiology Plates, copyright 1992 by Delmar Publishers Inc.)*

Voice Production

Expiration rids the body of excess carbon dioxide. As exhaled air passes through the larynx, it may also be used to produce sound. Two folds of tissue, known as the vocal cords, extend across the inside of the larynx. Changes in the length of these folds and the opening (glottis) between them, as air passes outward, produce the sounds we use to speak. These sounds are further changed by being bounced against the walls of the sinuses (cavities in the head) and being shaped by the tongue and lips. When you have a cold, the sinuses often become filled with mucus and cannot function properly. The changes in your voice are easy to detect.

Aging Changes

Changes in the respiratory system due to aging include:
- Reduced elasticity of the lungs
- Changes in the larynx
- Enlarged alveoli
- Diminished breathing capacity
- Fibrotic changes in the diaphragm
- Decreased functioning of the respiratory muscles

The Circulatory (Cardiovascular) System

The circulatory system may be thought of as a transportation system. It takes nourishment and oxygen to the cells and carries away waste products. The closed system is kept in motion by the force of the heartbeat. Diseases that attack any part of this system interfere with the overall function.

Structure and Function

The organs of the circulatory system include:
1. Heart—a central pumping station
2. Vessels
   a. **Arteries** are tubes that carry blood away from the heart. They
      - have muscular, elastic walls with smooth linings
      - branch to form arterioles with thinner walls. Arterioles then become capillaries where walls are one cell thick
      - carry blood with high concentration of nutrients and oxygen to the body cells
   b. **Veins** are tubes that carry blood toward the heart. They
      - have thinner muscular walls
      - carry blood back to the heart
      - carry blood with lower concentration of oxygen, more carbon dioxide, and more waste products
      - have cup-like valves that help move the blood
   c. **Capillaries** are tubes that connect arteries and veins. They
      - have walls only one cell thick
      - are the site of exchange of nutrients and oxygen from the blood to the cells and carbon dioxide and waste products from the cells to the blood
3. Lymphatic vessels—tubes that carry lymph or tissue fluid to the bloodstream. Fluid from the bloodstream passes into the tissue spaces where it is called tissue fluid. Some of the tissue fluid returns to the bloodstream by way of the capillaries. Some of it is first drawn off into the lymphatic vessels where it is called **lymph**. Eventually the lymph is returned to general circulation and becomes once more part of the blood.
4. Lymph nodes—masses of lymphatic tissue along the pathway of the lymph. They filter the lymph.
5. Spleen—a lymphatic organ. The spleen produces some of the blood cells and helps destroy worn out blood cells. It acts as a blood reservoir or blood bank.
6. Blood—a connective tissue made up of a liquid (**plasma**) and cellular elements.

The Blood

Blood is a red body fluid composed of plasma and cellular elements, Figure 4–18. The body contains 4–6 quarts (liters) of blood. Fifty-five percent of the blood is formed of the liquid plasma. Plasma is a watery solution containing:
- Antibodies (gamma globulin)—chemicals to fight infection
- Nutrients—such as glucose, amino acids, fats, salts
- Gases—such as oxygen and carbon dioxide
- Waste products—such as urea and creatinine

The blood cells are produced in the bone marrow and lymphatic tissues of the body. The bone marrow, liver, and spleen destroy worn out blood cells.

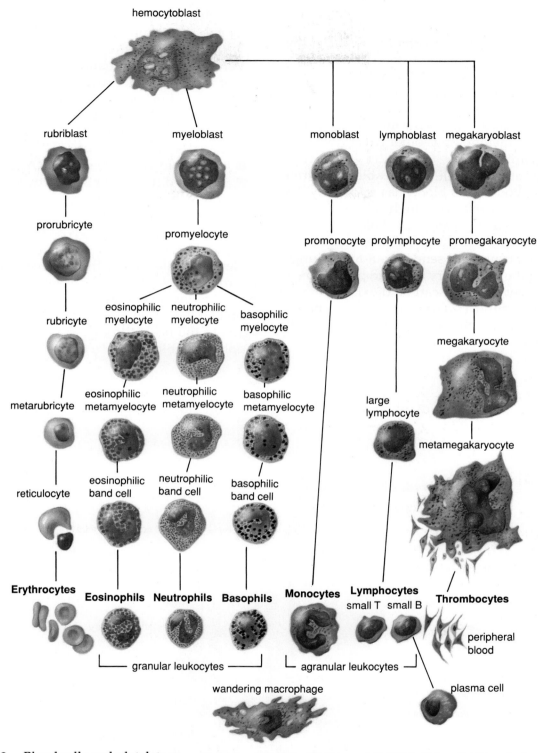

FIGURE 4–18. Blood cells and platelets *(From Anatomy and Physiology Plates, copyright 1992 by Delmar Publishers Inc.)*

- Red blood cells (RBC)—erythrocytes—carry most of the oxygen and small amounts of carbon dioxide. There are 4.5–5 million/mm³.
- White blood cells (WBC)—leukocytes—fight infection. There are 7,000–8,000 WBC/mm³.

- Thrombocytes—platelets that are not whole cells but only parts of cells. They seal small leaks in the walls of blood vessels and initiate blood clotting. There are 200,000–400,000 thrombocytes/mm³.

The Heart

The heart is a hollow, muscular organ about the size of a fist, Figures 4–19A and B. It is divided into a right and left side by a muscular wall called the septum and into four chambers. There are three layers to the heart wall. The endocardium lines the heart chambers. The myocardium is the muscle layer. The pericardium is a membranous outer covering.

The four chambers are:

1. The right atrium (RA)—receives blood from all over the body. This blood has a low oxygen content and a relatively high carbon dioxide level. It is called deoxygenated blood.
2. The right ventricle (RV)—receives blood from the right atrium and sends it out to the lungs through the pulmonary artery to pick up oxygen and get rid of the carbon dioxide.
3. The left atrium (LA)—receives oxygenated blood from the lungs and sends it to the left ventricle.
4. The left ventricle (LV)—receives blood from the left atrium and sends it out through the aorta to the entire body.

Valves separate the chambers. They also guard the exit of the pulmonary artery and aorta to prevent back flow and maintain a constant forward motion. The pulmonary artery carries blood to the lungs. The aorta is the largest blood vessel in the body. The valves are located as follows:

- Tricuspid valve—between RA and RV
- Bicuspid (mitral) valve—between LA and LV
- Pulmonary semilunar valves—between RV and pulmonary artery
- Aortic semilunar valve—between LV and aorta

Nerve impulses make the heart contract regularly according to body needs. For example, when you run, the body cells need more oxygen. The cells signal the brain that they need more oxygen. The brain sends a signal to the heart through the nerves that it must supply more blood. These nerve impulses cause the

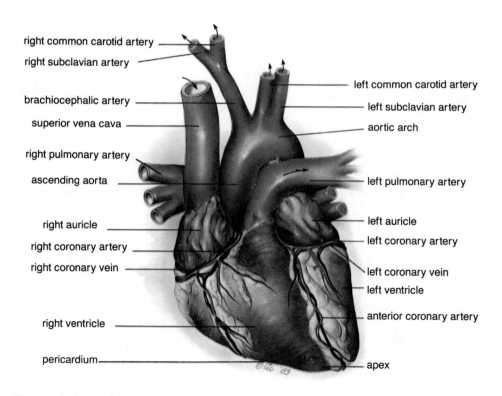

FIGURE 4–19A.   External view of the heart *(From Anatomy and Physiology Plates, copyright 1992 by Delmar Publishers Inc.)*

heart to beat faster. Thus, more oxygenated blood is pumped to the body cells to supply the oxygen required. These impulses cause the heart to beat faster.

The Cardiac Cycle

The heart pumps blood through the body by a series of movements known as the **cardiac cycle** First, the upper chambers of the heart, called atria, relax and fill with blood as the lower chambers contract, forcing blood out of the heart through the aorta and pulmonary arteries. Next, the lower chambers relax, allowing blood to flow into them from the contracting upper chambers. Then the cycle is repeated. Each cycle lasts about 0.8 second. This happens about 70–80 times per minute.

The rate and rhythm of the cardiac cycle are regulated by the conduction system. The conduction system is composed of special neuromuscular tissue that sends out impulses. The impulses eventually reach the myocardial cells, which respond by contracting.

- The impulses begin at the S-A node in the right atrium and spread across the two atria, Figure 4–20.
- The atria contract.
- Impulses from the S-A node reach the A-V node in the right atrium.
- Messages from the A-V node then spread through the bundle of His in the septum. From there they go through the Purkinje fibers to the walls of the ventricles.
- The ventricles contract, forcing the blood forward.

Blood Vessels

Many large arteries and veins take their names from the bones they are near or from the part of the body they serve. For example, the femoral artery and vein run close to the femur (thigh bone). The subclavian arteries and veins are found under the clavicle. And, the axillary arteries and veins are found in the axillary (armpit) area. Figure 4–21A shows the arterial system that distributes blood from the heart. Figure 4–21B (page 58) shows the venous system that returns blood to the heart.

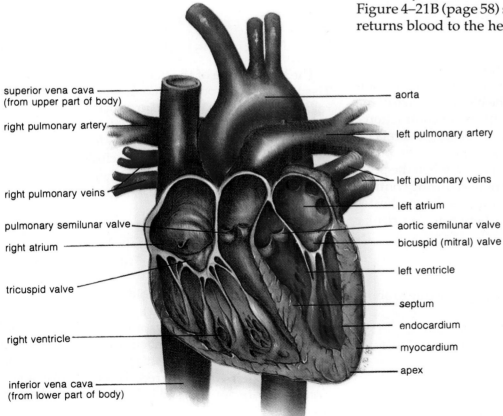

superior vena cava
(from upper part of body)

right pulmonary artery

right pulmonary veins

pulmonary semilunar valve

right atrium

tricuspid valve

right ventricle

inferior vena cava
(from lower part of body)

aorta

left pulmonary artery

left pulmonary veins

left atrium

aortic semilunar valve

bicuspid (mitral) valve

left ventricle

septum

endocardium

myocardium

apex

FIGURE 4–19B.   Internal view of the heart *(From Fong, Ferris, and Skelley,* Body Structures and Functions, *7th Edition, 1989, Delmar Publishers Inc.)*

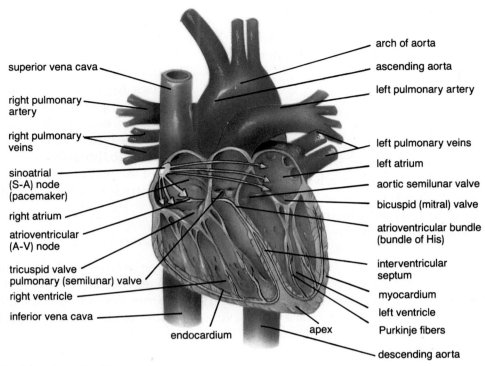

superior vena cava

right pulmonary artery

right pulmonary veins

sinoatrial (S-A) node (pacemaker)

right atrium

atrioventricular (A-V) node

tricuspid valve
pulmonary (semilunar) valve

right ventricle

inferior vena cava

endocardium

arch of aorta

ascending aorta

left pulmonary artery

left pulmonary veins

left atrium

aortic semilunar valve

bicuspid (mitral) valve

atrioventricular bundle (bundle of His)

interventricular septum

myocardium

left ventricle

Purkinje fibers

apex

descending aorta

FIGURE 4–20. Conduction system *(From Anatomy and Physiology Plates, copyright 1992 by Delmar Publishers Inc.)*

Blood Pressure

The blood pressure is the force the blood exerts against the walls of the blood vessels. It is the combined effect of the volume of the blood, the size of the blood vessels, and the force of the heart contractions. Pressure varies with contraction (systole) and relaxation (diastole) of the ventricles. The systolic blood pressure reading indicates the period when the pressure within the arteries is the greatest during contractions of the ventricles. The diastolic reading indicates the lowest point of pressure between ventricular contractions.

Aging Changes

Changes in the cardiovascular system due to aging include:
- Vascular walls become less flexible
- Vascular lumen (space within the vessel) narrows
- Blood pressure increases
- Cardiac output decreases
- Blood chemistry is less efficient
- Capillaries become more fragile
- Heart rate decreases

The Musculoskeletal System

The bony frame of the body is called the skeleton. Tissue that is composed of contractile (contracts and relaxes) fibers or cells that produce movement are called muscles. Together, the skeleton and muscles are termed the musculoskeletal system.

The musculoskeletal system includes:
- Skeletal muscles
- Bones
- Joints
- Tendons
- Ligaments

The system functions to:
- Give shape and form to the body
- Protect and support delicate body parts
- Permit movement
- Produce some blood cells
- Store calcium and phosphorus

When muscles, bones, or joints have been injured, a long period of rest and inactivity may be required for the part to heal. During this period, it is important that all other moving parts receive sufficient exercise. Bones that are not stressed lose calcium and become less functional.

Structure and Function

Bones. It will be helpful for you to learn the names and general location of the bones of the body. To learn

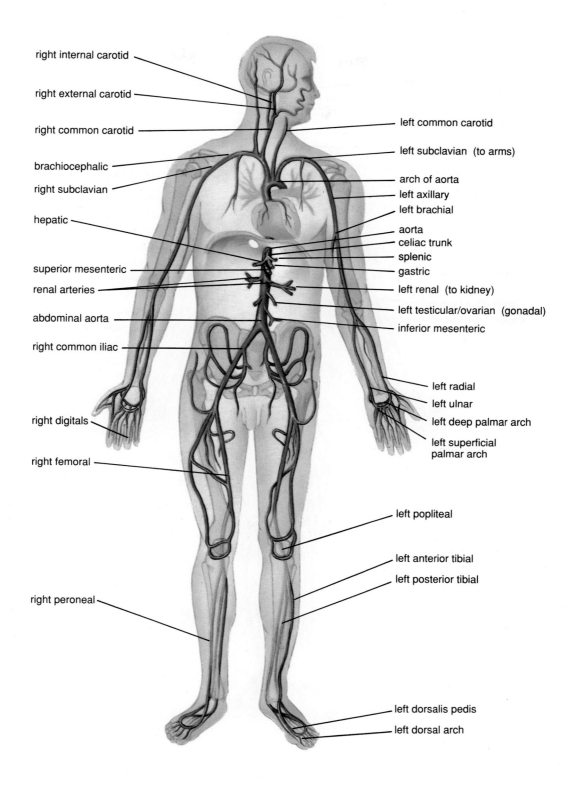

FIGURE 4–21A. Arterial distribution *(From Anatomy and Physiology Plates, copyright 1992 by Delmar Publishers Inc.)*

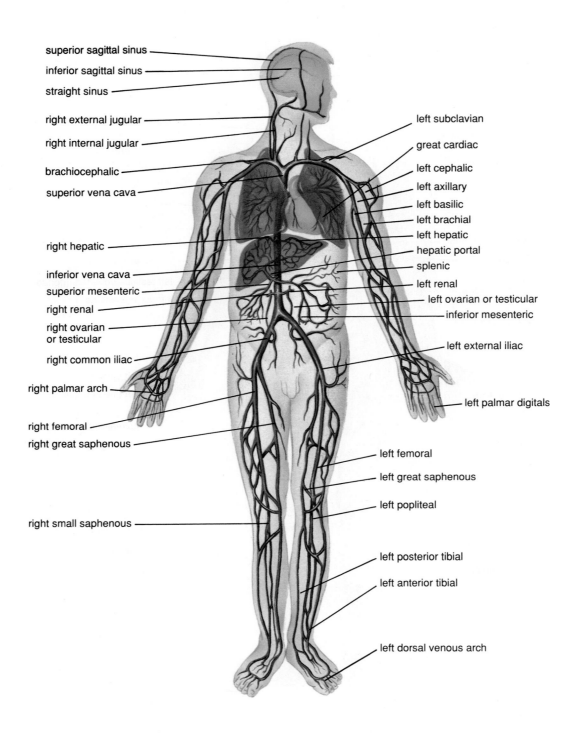

FIGURE 4–21B. Venous distribution *(From Anatomy and Physiology Plates, copyright 1992 by Delmar Publishers Inc.)*

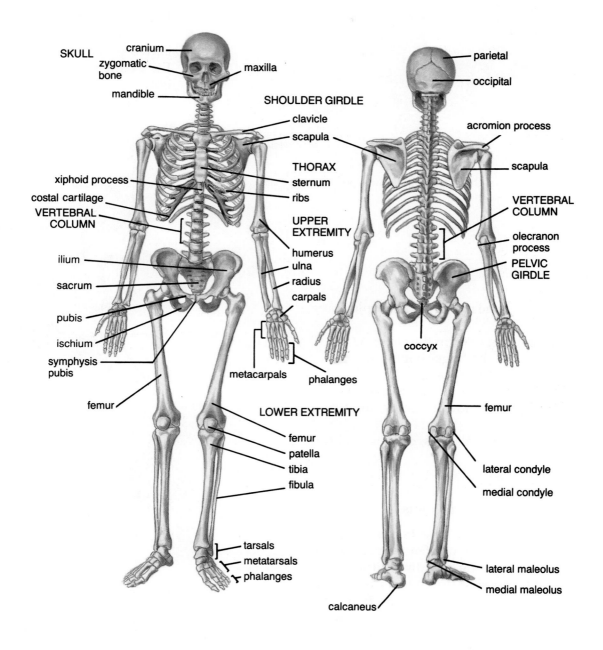

FIGURE 4–22A. Bones of the skeleton *(From Anatomy and Physiology Plates, copyright 1992 by Delmar Publishers Inc.)*

the names, study the skeleton in Figure 4–22A and the skull in Figure 4–22B. Note that the same number and kinds of bones are found on one side of the midline as on the other.

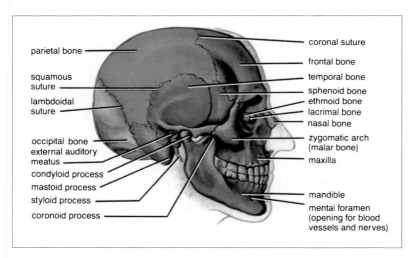

FIGURE 4–22B. Bones of the skull *(From Anatomy and Physiology Plates, copyright 1992 by Delmar Publishers Inc.)*

The bones:
■ Number 206.
■ May share the same name. For example, there are:
— 24 ribs helping to form the chest
— 56 phalanges, the finger bones
— 2 femurs, the thigh bones.
■ Are of different shapes and sizes, such as
— long, like the femur, humerus, ulna, and radius
— short, like the phalanges, carpals, and tarsals
— flat, like the scapula and cranial bones
— irregular, like the vertebrae and mandible.
■ Meet one another to form joints.

Joints. Joints are points where bones come together and there is the possibility of movement. Without movable joints, walking, bending, lifting, and sitting would not be possible. **Ligaments** are strong bands of fibrous tissues which hold the bones together and support the joints. **Bursae** are small sacs of synovial fluid which are located around joints and help reduce friction.

There are three kinds of joint unions:
1. Synarthrotic—nonmovable joints such as those of the skull bones
2. Amphiarthrotic—slightly movable joints such as the bodies of the vertebrae
3. Diarthrotic—freely movable joints such as the shoulder, hip, elbow, knee, and wrist, Figure 4–23.

Special terms are used to describe the different movements in a diarthrotic joint.
■ **Flexion:** Decreasing the angle between two bones, Figure 4–24A. For example, bending the elbow.
■ **Extension:** Increasing the angle between two bones, Figure 4–24B. For example, straightening the elbow.

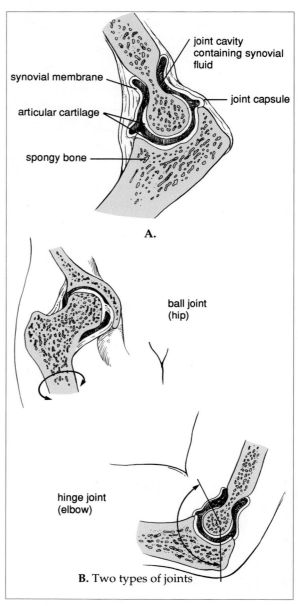

A.

B. Two types of joints

FIGURE 4–23. Diarthrotic joints

- **Rotation**: Circular motion in a ball-and-socket joint, Figure 4–24C. For example, the shoulder and hip joints which can move in all directions.
- **Abduction**: Moving away from the midline, Figure 4–24D.
- **Adduction**: Moving toward the midline, Figure 4–24E.

Muscles. There are more than 500 muscles in the body, Figures 4–25A and B. The muscles work in groups. There are three kinds of muscles:

1. **Cardiac muscle** forms the wall of the heart.
2. **Voluntary muscles** are skeletal muscles that are attached to bones. When we wish to pick up something, we can make our muscles contract and perform the necessary movements.
3. **Involuntary** or **visceral muscles** form the walls of organs. These muscles operate without our conscious control.

Muscles receive their names in three ways:

1. Their location. For example, rectus femoris—near the femur
2. Their shape. For example, trapezius—trapezoidal shape
3. Their action. For example, flexors—bring about flexion

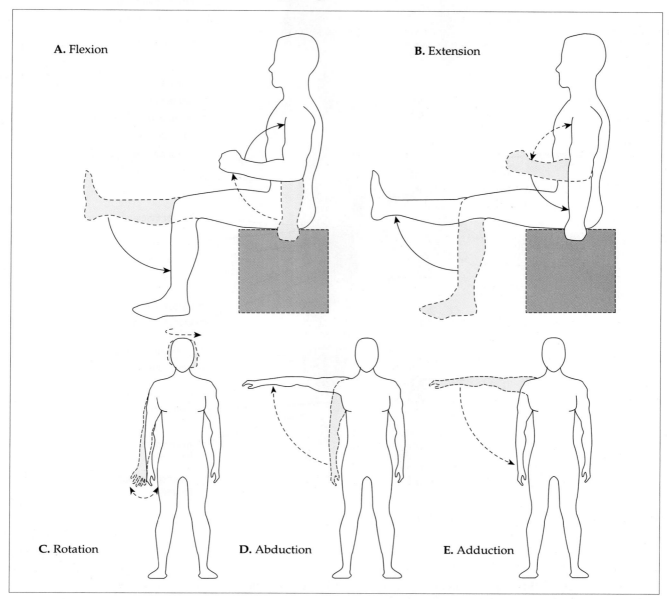

A. Flexion **B.** Extension **C.** Rotation **D.** Abduction **E.** Adduction

FIGURE 4–24. Joint movements

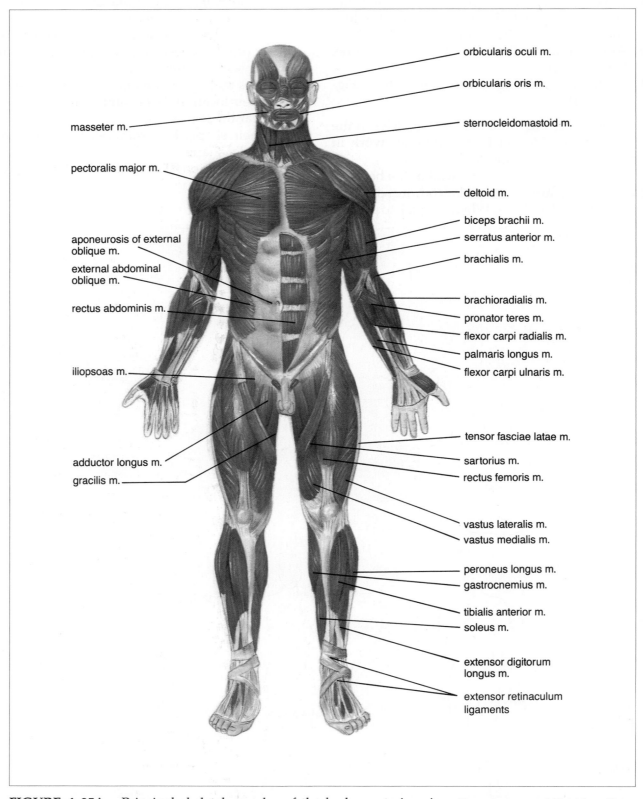

FIGURE 4–25A. Principal skeletal muscles of the body—anterior view *(From Anatomy and Physiology Plates, copyright 1992 by Delmar Publishers Inc.)*

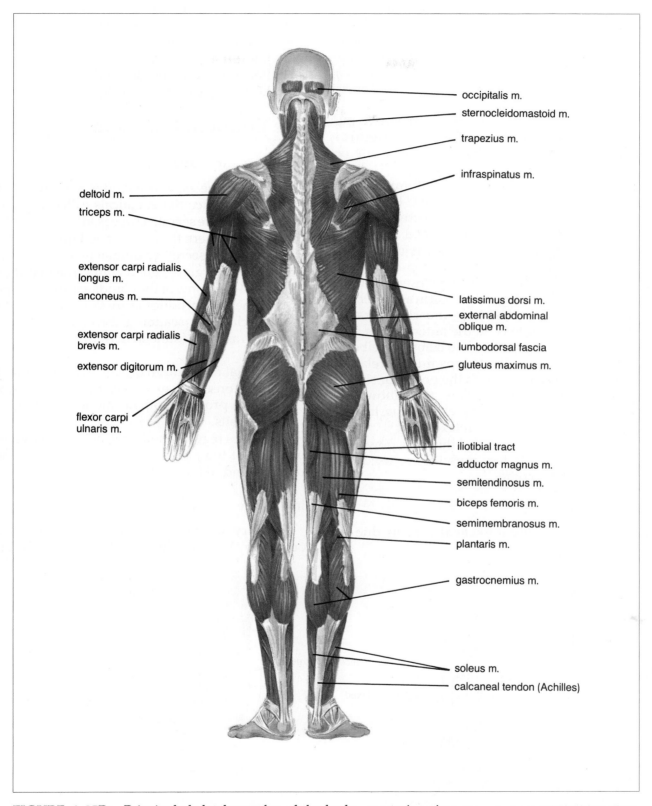

FIGURE 4–25B. Principal skeletal muscles of the body—posterior view *(From Anatomy and Physiology Plates, copyright 1992 by Delmar Publishers Inc.)*

You can easily locate the major muscle groups responsible for an activity if you remember that:

- Muscles can only shorten (contract) and lengthen (relax), Figure 4–26. Contraction occurs when nerves bring the message (**stimulus**) to the muscle cells. Muscles relax when there is no stimulus.
- Muscles have two points of attachment to the bone. As they stretch from one point (**origin**) to the other (**insertion**), they cross over one or more joints.
- Muscles are not inserted directly into bones. Rather, they are connected to the bone by a strong, fibrous band of connective tissues called **tendons** that attach skeletal muscle to bone. Ligaments support bones at joints.
- As muscles contract, they shorten, pulling their points of origin and insertion closer together. For example, bending the forearm at the elbow takes place when the biceps muscle contracts. The biceps muscle is on the anterior arm and extends from the shoulder to below the elbow. At the same time, the triceps muscle relaxes. This muscle is attached to the posterior shoulder and to the arm below the elbow. To straighten the arm at the elbow, the triceps contracts and the biceps relaxes.
- The more muscles are used the more powerful they become. The less muscles are used the weaker they become.

Aging Changes

Changes in the musculoskeletal system due to aging include:

- Loss of muscle strength, size, and tone
- Slower muscle/nerve interaction
- Postural changes
- Joints are less flexible
- Bones are more porous and brittle
- Loss of height

The Endocrine System

Structure and Function

The endocrine system includes special secretory units that produce the chemicals called **hormones**. The hormones are secreted (released) directly into the bloodstream where they are carried quickly all over the body. These secretory units may be:

- Distinct organs, called **endocrine glands**, Figure 4–27. Some of the glands are found in pairs. Some may produce more than one hormone.
- Special cells scattered throughout the body, such as those found in the kidney and intestinal tract.
- Special cells within organs that carry on other functions. For example, the female ovaries which produce both hormones and reproductive cells.

Hormones regulate and control body activities. A summary of the glands and the hormones they secrete is found in Figure 4–28.

Endocrine Glands

Pituitary Gland. The pituitary gland is surrounded by bone. It is located at the base of the brain.

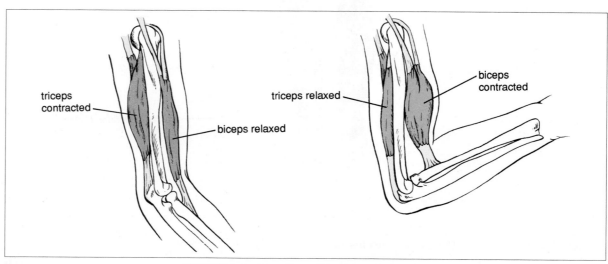

FIGURE 4–26. Coordination of muscles

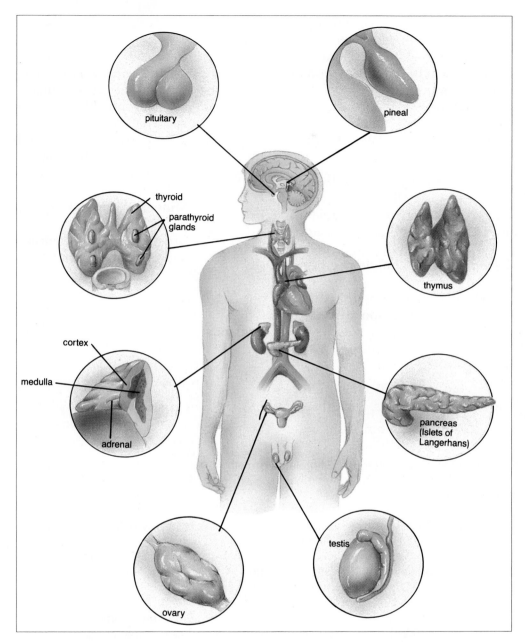

FIGURE 4–27. Location of the endocrine glands *(From Anatomy and Physiology Plates, copyright 1992 by Delmar Publishers Inc.)*

Because it controls most of the other glands, the pituitary gland is called the master gland.

The pituitary gland has two portions called lobes. Each of the lobes secretes more than one hormone.

1. The anterior lobe secretes:
   a. STH (somatotropic hormone)—a growth hormone that stimulates the growth of long bones
   b. TSH (thyroid-stimulating hormone)—stimulates the thyroid gland
   c. FSH (follicle-stimulating hormone)—promotes growth of the ovarian follicle in which the egg develops during the menstrual cycle
   d. ACTH (adrenocorticotropic hormone)—stimulates production of the adrenal gland
   e. LH (luteinizing hormone)—in females helps stimulate ovulation during the menstrual cycle

f. ICSH (interstitial cell-stimulating hormone)—stimulates the male testes

g. Lactogenic hormone (LTH)—stimulates milk production in the pregnant woman

2. The posterior lobe secretes:

a. ADH (antidiuretic hormone)—acts on kidneys to prevent excess water loss

b. Pitocin (oxytocin)—stimulates uterine contractions during childbirth

Pineal Body. This is a small gland also located in the skull beneath the brain. Very little is known about this gland. It is thought to be somehow related to sexual growth since it tends to get smaller at maturity. It produces:

- Glomerulotropin—which influences the adrenal gland
- Serotonin—which acts in the brain
- Melatonin—which inhibits too early sexual maturity

Adrenal Glands

There are two adrenal glands. Each gland is located on top of one of the two kidneys. Each gland has two distinct portions which secrete separate hormones.

1. The adrenal medulla (inside) produces norepinephrine (noradrenalin) and epinephrine (adrenalin), which stimulate the body to produce energy quickly during an emergency.

2. The adrenal cortex (outside) produces:

a. Glucocorticoids—elevate blood sugar levels and control the response of the body to stress and inflammation. They also depress inflammation.

b. Mineral corticoids—manage sodium and potassium levels

c. Gonadocorticoids—influence both male and female sex hormones

Gonads

The term gonads refers to the male and female sex glands. The female gonads (two ovaries):

1. Are located within the pelvic cavity on either side of the uterus.

2. Produce two hormones, estrogen and progesterone. These hormones are responsible for

GLAND	HORMONE	ACTION	HYPERSECRETION	HYPOSECRETION
Pituitary (Anterior Lobe)	Somatotropic Hormone (STH)	Stimulates growth of long bones	Giantism in youth. Acromegaly in adulthood	Dwarfism
	Thyroid Stimulating Hormone (TSH)	Stimulates thyroid gland	Hyperthyroidism	Hypothyroidism
	Adrenocorticotropic Hormone (ACTH)	Stimulates the adrenal gland	Hyperadrenalism	Hypoadrenalism
	Follicular Stimulating Hormone (FSH)	Stimulates sex cell development in ♂ and ♀. Promotes ♀ sex characteristics	Early development of ♀ sex characteristics	♀ Lack of sexual development. Sterility in both sexes
	Interstitial Cell Stimulating Hormone (ICSH) (♂)	Stimulates production of testosterone	Premature sexual development in males	Sterility
	Luteinizing Hormone (LH) (♀)	Promotes egg development and ovulation		Sterility
	Lactogenic Hormone (LTH)	Stimulates production of milk	Nonpregnant ♀ produces milk	Inadequate milk production

FIGURE 4–28. Endocrine glands and the hormones they secrete

GLAND	HORMONE	ACTION	HYPERSECRETION	HYPOSECRETION
Pituitary (Posterior Lobe)	Pitocin	Stimulates contractions of pregnant uterus	Unknown	Unknown
	Antidiuretic Hormone (ADH)	Increases return of water from kidneys to bloodstream	Water retention	Diabetes insipidus
Thyroid	Thyroxin	Stimulates and regulates cellular activity	Graves' disease (Exophthalmic goiter)	Newborns—cretinism Adults—myxedema
Parathyroids	Parathyrine (Parathormone)	Regulates levels of blood calcium and phosphates	Hypercalcemia with loss of bone calcium	Hypocalcemia, severe muscle spasm (tetany)
Pancreas (beta cells)	Insulin	Decreases blood sugar level	Hypoglycemia (insulin shock)	Hyperglycemia (diabetes mellitus)
(alpha cells)	Glucagon	Increases blood sugar level	Hyperglycemia	—
Ovaries (female)	Estrogen	Promotes ♀ sex characteristics	Early development of sex characteristics	Delayed sexual maturity
	Progesterone	Pregnancy maintaining hormone	—	Sterility
Testes (male)	Testosterone	Promotes ♂ sex characteristics	Premature sexual development	Delayed maturity
Adrenal (Cortex)	Glucocorticoids	Elevate blood sugar; depress inflammation; aid in coping with stress	Cushing's syndrome	Less resistance to stress
	Mineral corticoids	Manage sodium and potassium electrolytes	Aldosteronism	Addison's disease
	Androgenic	Complement hormones of ovaries and testes	Premature sexual development ♂; Masculinization of ♀	—
Adrenal (Medulla)	Epinephrine (Adrenalin) Norepinephrine (Noradrenalin)	Prepares body for emergencies; acts with nervous system	Hypertension	—

Key: ♂ male
      ♀ female
      — unknown

FIGURE 4–28.   Endocrine glands and the hormones they secrete (cont.)

the development of female characteristics such as:

a. Breast development
b. Pubic and axillary hair
c. Onset and regulation of menstruation
d. Pregnancy

The male gonads (two **testes**):

1. Are located outside of the body in a pouch called the **scrotum**.
2. Produce the hormone **testosterone**. This hormone is responsible for secondary male characteristics such as:
   a. Muscular development
   b. Deepening voice
   c. Hair growth

The male and female gonads also produce the special cells—in the female, the **ovum** and in the male, the **sperm**. These cells unite to form a new human being during fertilization.

Thyroid Gland

This gland has two lobes and is found in the neck, anterior to the larynx. Hormones secreted by this gland are thyroxine and thyrocalcitonin. Thyroxine regulates metabolism. Iodine is an important component of this hormone. Thyrocalcitonin regulates calcium and phosphorus levels.

Parathyroids

These are tiny glands embedded in the posterior thyroid gland. The hormone they manufacture is called parathormone. Parathormone helps control the utilization of two minerals, calcium and phosphorus, by the body. Insufficient amounts of calcium result in severe muscle spasms or tetany. Untreated tetany can lead to death.

Islets of Langerhans

The **islets of Langerhans** are small groups of cells found within the pancreas. These cells produce two hormones: insulin and glucagon. Insulin lowers blood sugar. Glucagon elevates blood sugar.

Aging Changes

Changes in the endocrine system due to aging include:

■ Decreased glucose tolerance
■ Increase in the levels of TSH and parathormone
■ Decrease in vaginal secretions

The Nervous System

Structure and Function

The nervous system controls and coordinates all body activities, even the production of hormones. Special parts of the nervous system are concerned with maintaining normal day-to-day functions. Other parts act during emergency situations. Still others control voluntary activities. Neurological conditions require highly specialized nursing care. You will assist with the less technical aspects of that care.

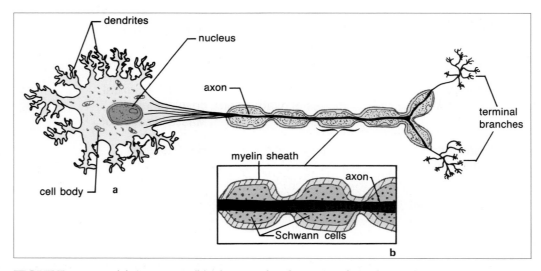

FIGURE 4–29. (a) A neuron; (b) a longitudinal section of myelinated axon *(From Fong, Ferris, and Skelley,* Body Structures and Functions, *7th Edition, 1989, Delmar Publishers Inc.)*

Neurons

Cells of the nervous system are called neurons Figure 4–29. They are specialized to conduct electric-like impulses. The neuron has extensions called axons and dendrites. Impulses enter the neuron only through the dendrites and leave only through the axon.

Although neurons do not actually touch each other, the axon of one neuron lies close to the dendrites of many other neurons. In this way, impulses may follow many different routes. The space between the axon of one cell and the dendrites of others is called a synapse. Axons and dendrites in the periphery are covered with myelin, which acts as insulation.

Nerves

Some axons and dendrites are long. Others are short. Axons and dendrites of many neurons are found in bundles. The bundles are held together by connective tissue. These bundles resemble telephone cables and are called nerves. The cell bodies of the axons and dendrites in these nerves may be found far from the ends of the nerves in clusters called ganglia.

Sensory nerves are made up of dendrites. They carry sensations to the brain and spinal cord from the various body parts. Feeling is lost when these nerve impulses are interrupted. Motor nerves carry impulses from the brain and spinal cord to muscles that cause body activity. Paralysis or loss of function occurs when these nerves are damaged.

For easier study, the nervous system can be divided into two parts: the central nervous system (CNS) and the peripheral nervous system (PNS). The CNS is composed of the brain and spinal cord, Figure 4–30. The PNS is composed of the 12 pairs of cranial nerves and 31 pairs of spinal nerves that reach throughout the body, Figure 4–31. Remember, though, that the nervous system is one interwoven system, a complex of millions of neurons.

The Central Nervous System

The brain and spinal cord are:
- Surrounded by bone
- Protected by the membrane called meninges
- Cushioned by cerebrospinal fluid (CSF)

The brain and spinal cord are a continuous structure found within the skull and spinal canal. The spinal cord is about 17 inches long. It ends just above the small of the back. Nerves extend from the brain and the spinal cord.

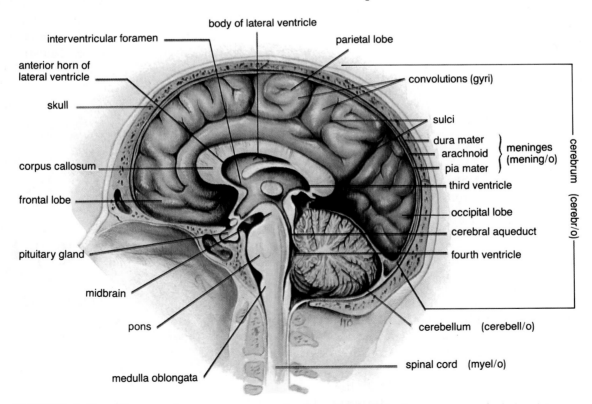

FIGURE 4–30. The central nervous system—brain and spinal cord *(From Anatomy and Physiology Plates, copyright 1992 by Delmar Publishers Inc.)*

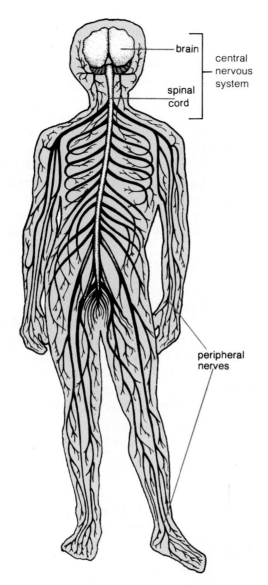

FIGURE 4–31. The peripheral nervous system connects the central nervous system to the various structures of the body. Messages are relayed from these structures back to the brain through the spinal cord. *(Courtesy of CPR, Teaneck, NJ)*

The Brain

The brain (encephalon) is a large, soft mass of nerve tissue contained within the cranium. It is composed of gray matter and white matter. Gray matter consists principally of nerve-cell bodies. White matter consists of nerve cells which form connections between various parts of the brain.

The brain can be further subdivided into the:
1. Cerebrum: The largest portion of the brain. The outer portion is formed in folds known as

convolutions and separated into lobes. The lobes take their name from the skull bones that surround them, Figure 4–30.
  a. The outer portion, the cerebral cortex, is composed of cell bodies and appears gray.
  b. The inner portion is composed of axons and dendrites and so appears white.
  c. All mental activities—thinking, voluntary movements, interpreting sensations and emotions—are carried out by cerebral cells, Figure 4–32. Certain activities are centered in each lobe.
  d. In general, the right side of the cerebrum interprets for and controls the left side of the body and vice versa.
2. Cerebellum: Found beneath the occipital lobe of the cerebrum. It, too, has an outer layer of gray cell bodies. This portion of the brain coordinates muscular activities and balance.
3. The brain stem: The midbrain, pons, and medulla are in the brain stem. They are composed mainly of axons and dendrites. These fibers serve as connecting pathways between the control centers in the cerebrum and cerebellum and the spinal cord. Control centers are found within the brain stem for involuntary movements of such vital organs as the:
  a. Heart   d. Stomach
  b. Blood vessels   e. Intestines
  c. Lungs

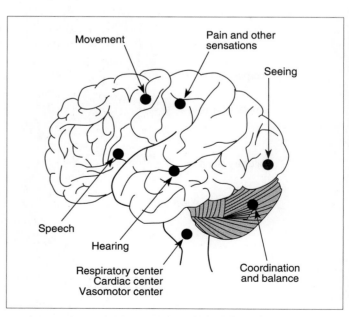

FIGURE 4–32. Functional areas of the brain

The Spinal Cord

The spinal cord, Figure 4–33, extends from the medulla to the second lumbar vertebra in the spinal canal, which is above the small of the back, a distance of about 17 inches. Nerves entering and leaving the spinal cord carry impulses to and from the control centers. Certain reflex activities performed without

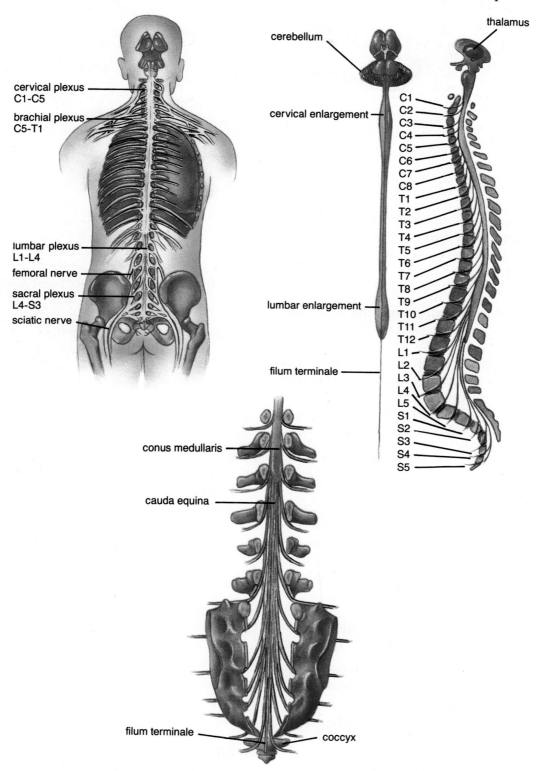

FIGURE 4–33. Spinal cord and nerves *(From Anatomy and Physiology Plates, copyright 1992 by Delmar Publishers Inc.)*

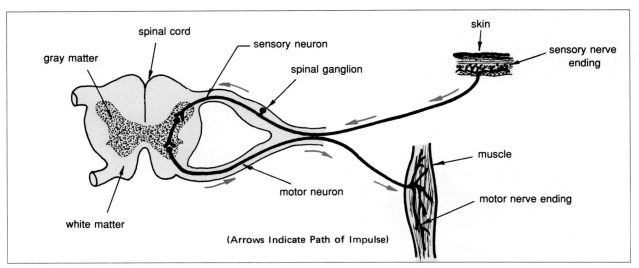

FIGURE 4–34.   The reflex arc

conscious thought are controlled within the cord. Pulling your hand away from something hot is an example of this type of reflex activity, Figure 4–34.

The Meninges

Three membranes surround both the brain and spinal cord. They are the dura mater, the arachnoid mater, and the pia mater.

The dura mater is the tough outer covering. The arachnoid mater is the middle, loosely structured layer. It is filled with cerebrospinal fluid. The pia mater is the innermost, delicate layer. It is very vascular and clings to the brain, spinal cord, and nerve roots.

Cerebrospinal Fluid (CSF)

Ventricles are cavities within the cerebrum that are lined with highly vascular tissue. These tissues produce cerebrospinal fluid, which flows around the brain and the spinal cord. The cerebrospinal fluid bathes the central nervous system as tissue fluid and cushions it against shock and possible injury.

Special Relationships: The Autonomic Nervous System (ANS)

The autonomic nervous system (ANS) refers to special pathways that travel in cranial and spinal nerves, Figure 4–35. The control center is in the brain stem. The pathways begin in the CNS and reach out to the glands, smooth muscle walls of organs, and heart.

The autonomic nervous system consists of two parts: sympathetic fibers and parasympathetic fibers.

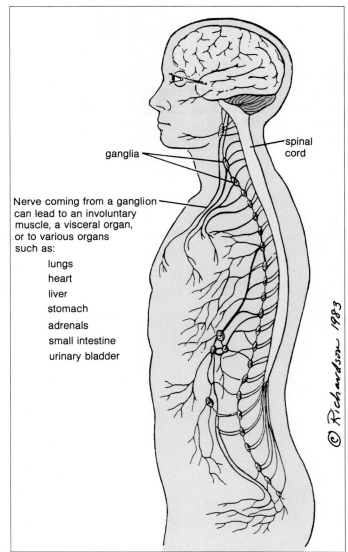

FIGURE 4–35.   The autonomic nervous system (*From Fong, Ferris, and Skelley, Body Structures and Functions, 7th Edition, 1989, Delmar Publishers Inc.*)

Sympathetic fibers stimulate activities that prepare the body to deal with emergency situations. It is called the mechanism of "fight or flight." Parasympathetic fibers control the usual functions of moderate heartbeat, digestion, elimination, respiration, and glandular activity.

Sensory Receptors

The ends of the dendrites carrying sensations to the central nervous system are found throughout the body.

- Some begin in joints and bring information about body positions to the brain.
- Others in the skin carry sensations of pain, heat, pressure, and cold.
- Those in the nose carry the sense of smell.
- The dendrites in the tongue carry the sense of taste.

Sensory dendrites also receive stimulation through two very special end organs, the eye and the ear. All of these structures are called sensory receptors because they carry information about the outside world to the brain. The brain interprets and processes the information.

The Eye

The eye, Figure 4–36, is a hollow ball filled with two liquids called the *aqueous humor* and the *vitreous humor*. The wall of the eye is made up of three layers:

- The sclera: A tough, white outer coat that is protective. The cornea is the transparent portion in the front. Light rays pass through the cornea into the eye.
- The choroid: The nutritive layer that is found beneath the sclera. The choroid nourishes the eye tissues through its large number of blood vessels.

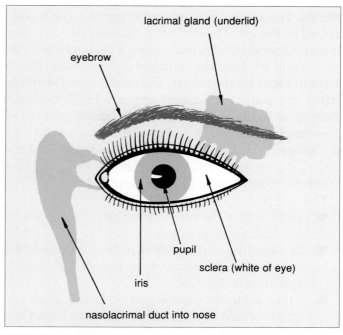

FIGURE 4–36A. External view of the eye

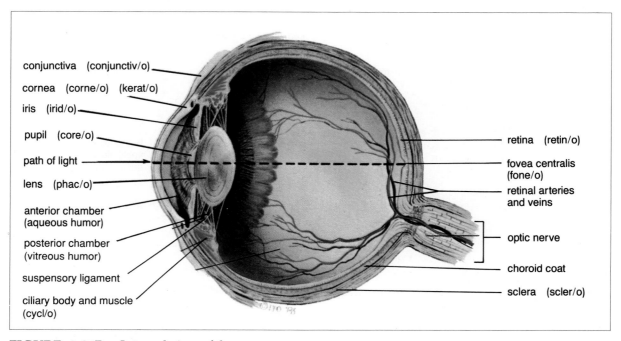

FIGURE 4–36B. Internal view of the eye *(From Anatomy and Physiology Plates, copyright 1992 by Delmar Publishers Inc.)*

■ The retina: The innermost layer is made up of neurons which are sensitive to light. The neurons join together and their axons leave the eye as the optic nerve. The two nerves cross beneath the brain and carry their impulses to the occipital lobe of the cerebrum to let us know what we are seeing.

Seeing. We see as light enters the eye through the cornea. The amount of light entering the eye is controlled by the iris. The **iris** is the colored portion of the eye. It is found behind the cornea. Fluid between the cornea and iris helps to bend the light rays and bring them to focus on the retina. The opening in the iris is called the pupil. The pupil appears black because there is no light behind it. Directly behind the iris is the lens. Small muscles pull on either side of the lens to change its shape. The changing shape of the lens makes it possible for us to adjust the range of our vision from far to near or from near to far.

The eye is:

■ Held within the bony socket by muscles which can change its position.

■ Covered by a mucous membrane, called the conjunctiva. The conjunctiva lines the eyelids and covers the eye.

■ Protected by the eyelids and eyelashes. Tears are manufactured by the lacrimal glands found beneath the lateral side of the upper lid. Tears protect the eye as they wash across the eye, keeping it moist, and then drain into the nasal cavity.

The Ear

Just as the eye is sensitive to light, the ear is sensitive to sound, Figure 4–37. The ear functions in hearing and equilibrium (balance). The ear has three parts: the outer ear, the middle ear, and the inner ear. The outer ear consists of the visible external structure known as the pinna and a canal, which directs sound waves toward the middle ear. At the end of the canal is the eardrum, or **tympanic membrane**. Sound waves cause the eardrum to vibrate.

The middle ear is made up of three tiny bones called **ossicles**. The ossicles form a chain across the middle ear from the tympanic membrane to an opening in the inner ear. These bones are known as the:

■ Incus or anvil

■ Malleus or hammer

■ Stapes or stirrup

Small tubes, called the **eustachian tubes**, lead from the nasopharynx into the middle ear to equalize pressure on either side of the eardrum. Sound waves pushing against the tympanic membrane cause the ossicles to vibrate and push against the opening of the inner ear. This motion starts fluid moving in the inner ear.

The inner ear is a very complex structure. It has two main parts: the cochlea and three semicircular canals. The cochlea looks somewhat like a coiled snail shell. Within the cochlea are the tiny dendrites of the hearing or auditory nerve. Fluid covers the dendrites. When the fluid is set in motion by the vibration of the middle ear bones, it stimulates the dendrites with

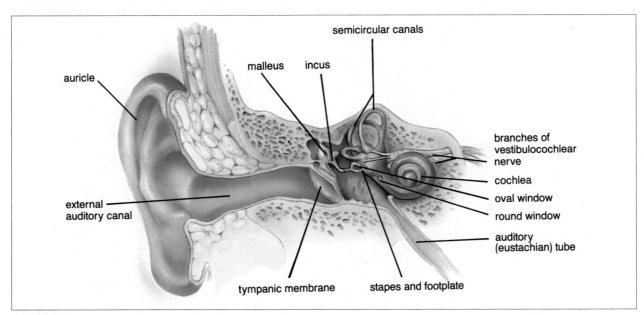

FIGURE 4–37. Internal view of the ear *(From Anatomy and Physiology Plates, copyright 1992 by Delmar Publishers Inc.)*

sound sensations. The auditory nerve, one from each ear, carries the sensations to the temporal lobe of the cerebrum to let us know what we are hearing.

The three semicircular canals also contain liquid and nerve endings. When these nerve endings are stimulated, impulses about the position of the head are sent to the brain. This helps us keep our balance.

Aging Changes

Aging changes in the nervous system include:
- Loss of nerve cells
- Increase in reaction time
- Receptors become less sensitive, so require greater stimuli for response
- Changes in memory
- Decrease in response of the special senses such as seeing, hearing, and taste.

The Gastrointestinal System

Structure and Function

The gastrointestinal system (alimentary tract) is also called the GI or digestive tract. It extends from the mouth to the anus and is lined with mucous membrane, Figure 4–38. The organs along the length of this system change food into simple forms able to pass through the walls of the small intestine and into the circulatory system. The circulatory system then carries the nutrients to the body cells. The gastrointestinal system includes the:
- Mouth, teeth, tongue, salivary glands
- Pharynx
- Esophagus (gullet)
- Stomach
- Small intestine
- Liver, gallbladder, pancreas
- Large intestine

In the digestive system:
- Proteins are changed to amino acids.
- Carbohydrates are changed to simple sugars like glucose.
- Fats are changed to fatty acids and glycerol.

These changes are brought about by mechanical action and chemicals called enzymes. The nondigestible portions of what we eat are moved along the intestines, and are finally excreted from the body as feces. Several organs contribute to the digestive process and many disease conditions affect them.

Mouth

In the mouth, Figure 4–39, food is chewed so it can be swallowed easily. The digestive process begins with the help of the:
- Tongue—a skeletal muscle that is covered by taste buds. The tongue pushes the food between the teeth to be broken up. It assists in mastication (chewing). It propels the food backward toward the pharynx to assist in swallowing. It also aids in speech formation.
- Salivary glands—secrete saliva containing a digestive enzyme, salivary amylase.
  — Salivary amylase begins carbohydrate digestion
  — 1-1/2 quarts of saliva are secreted daily
  — Saliva-moistened food helps in swallowing
- Teeth—mechanically break up the food into smaller particles, forming a bolus of food. The bolus is then swallowed. There are two natural sets of teeth. The first set (deciduous or temporary) numbers 20. The second set (permanent) numbers 32 and gradually replaces the deciduous set.
- Pharynx—serves for the passage of both food and air. Leads to the esophagus.
- Esophagus—a tube 10–12 inches long that carries the food to the stomach. Strong muscular contractions called peristaltic waves move the food along the tract. They begin in the esophagus and continue throughout the intestinal tract.

Figure 4–40 lists the enzymes that aid in digestion.

The Stomach

The stomach
- Is a hollow, muscular, J-shaped organ
- Is found in the peritoneal cavity
- Is two-thirds to the left of the midline
- Is just below the diaphragm
- Has circular muscles at either end that hold the food while it is thoroughly mixed with digestive enzymes
- Begins the chemical process of digestion
- Holds the food between 3–4 hours

The stomach has three parts:
1. Fundus—the area above the entrance of the esophagus
2. Body—holds the food

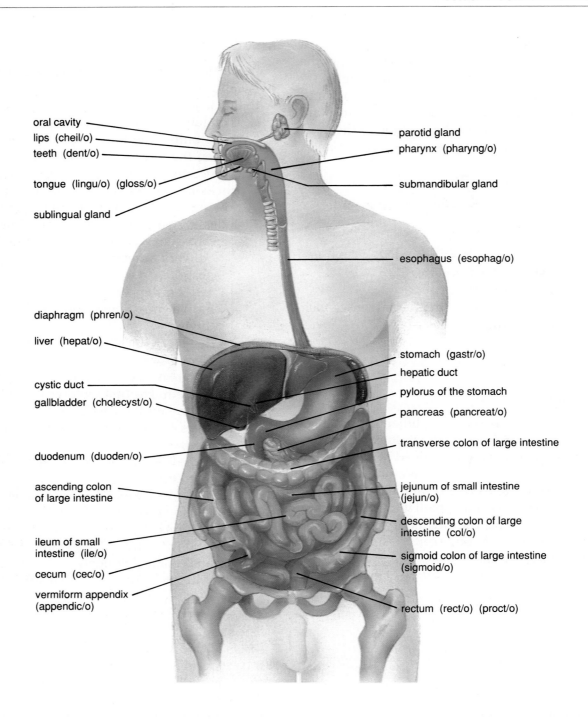

FIGURE 4–38. The gastrointestinal tract *(From Anatomy and Physiology Plates, copyright 1992 by Delmar Publishers Inc.)*

3. Pylorus—the long, narrowly tapered distal end which connects with the small intestines. The muscle guarding this exit point is called the **pyloric sphincter**. Sometimes in babies the muscle is so tight (pyloric stenosis) that milk cannot get through and the muscle must be cut surgically.

The stomach cells produce gastric juice which contains:

■ Proteolytic enzyme (**pepsin**)—begins protein breakdown

■ Hydrochloric acid (HCl)

■ Intrinsic factor—needed for the absorption of vitamin B_{12}

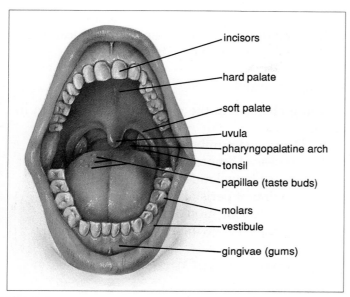

incisors

hard palate

soft palate

uvula

pharyngopalatine arch

tonsil

papillae (taste buds)

molars

vestibule

gingivae (gums)

FIGURE 4–39.   The mouth

The Intestines

When food leaves the stomach, it is in a semiliquid form called chyme. Chyme enters the small intestine where any undigested nutrients are broken down by intestinal and pancreatic enzymes and bile from the liver.

Materials continue to be moved through the intestines by waves of peristalsis. Food digestion is completed in the small intestine. Most of the nutrients and food the body needs is absorbed into the bloodstream through the walls of the small intestine. Figure

ORGAN	IMPORTANT ENZYMES	FOOD ACTED UPON
Salivary glands	Amylase	Starches
Stomach	Pepsin Lipase	Proteins Fats
Pancreas	Lipase Amylase Trypsin	Fats Starches Proteins
Small intestine	Lactase Sucrase Maltase Peptidase	Lactose (sugar) Sucrose (sugar) Maltose (sugar) Protein

FIGURE 4–40.   Digestive enzymes

4–40 gives the digestive enzymes, their sources, and the foods they act on.

The small intestine is about 20 feet long. It coils within the peritoneum. There are three main portions:

1. The duodenum—about 12 inches long. Has an opening in the back to receive the bile and pancreatic secretions.
2. The jejunum—about 8 feet long.
3. The ileum—the last 12–13 feet. Terminates in the ileocecal valve and is connected to the large intestine. The ileocecal valve prevents food from traveling backward into the small intestine.

The large intestine (colon) is 4-1/2 feet long. It is divided into several sections:

- Cecum
- Ascending colon
- Transverse colon
- Descending colon
- Sigmoid colon
- Rectum
- Anus

No digestive enzymes are secreted in the colon. The colon is the place where:

- Some vitamins are absorbed into the circulatory system.
- More complex carbohydrates are acted upon by bacteria.
- Much of the remaining water is absorbed through the walls of the large intestine, changing wastes to a more solid form. In this way, the large intestine helps to maintain the water balance of the body.

Peristalsis continues to move waste through the large intestine until it reaches the rectum. When a certain amount has been collected in the rectum, it is eliminated as feces through the anus. This process is called defecation.

The Appendix

The appendix is located in the lower, right quadrant, attached to the cecum. Its function is not known. When it becomes inflamed, the condition is called appendicitis.

Liver and Gallbladder

The liver is a large gland that has four lobes. It is located just beneath the right diaphragm. It carries on numerous metabolic functions. For example, the liver helps control the amount of protein and sugar in the blood by changing and storing excess amounts. It produces blood proteins such as prothrombin and fibrinogen, which are important factors in the blood clotting process. The liver also produces bile, which is carried directly to the small intestine for use in digestion or to the gallbladder for storage. Bile prepares (emulsifies) fats for digestion.

The gallbladder is a small hollow sac that is attached to the underside of the liver. It holds about two ounces of bile that it receives from the liver. It releases bile into the small intestine to help digest a fatty meal. The presence of bile in the digestive tract gives solid wastes the usual brown color.

The Pancreas

The pancreas is a glandular organ that produces both exocrine secretions (digestive enzymes) and endocrine secretions (insulin and glucagon). It extends from behind the stomach into the curve of the duodenum. It manufactures pancreatic juice. The pancreatic juice is sent into the duodenum to aid in the digestion of foods. The pancreas also produces insulin and glucagon. Both insulin and glucagon are sent directly into the bloodstream.

Aging Changes

Aging changes in the gastrointestinal system include:

■ Decreased number of taste buds
■ Decreased amount of digestive enzymes
■ Loss of bowel muscle tone
■ Slowing of peristalsis
■ Slower absorption of nutrients
■ Decreased chewing capacity

The Urinary System

Structure and Function

The urinary system is also referred to as the excretory system, Figure 4–41. As the name implies, the organs of this system produce urine—liquid waste—which is excreted from the body. The urinary system also helps to control the vital water and salt balance of the body. Inability to secrete urine by the kidneys is known as **suppression**. Inability to excrete urine that has been produced by the kidneys is called **retention** The organs of this system include:

■ Kidneys: Organs that produce the urine, Figure 4–42.
■ Ureters: The tubes that carry the urine from the kidneys to the urinary bladder. These tubes are 10–12 inches long and about 1/4 inch wide.
■ Urinary bladder: Holds the urine until expelled. The urge to urinate (micturate or void) occurs when 200–300 ml of urine is in the bladder. The bladder is capable of holding more urine than this amount.
■ Urethra: The tube that carries the urine to the outside. The female urethra is about 1-1/2 inches long. The male urethra is about 8 inches long. The opening to the outside is called the external urinary meatus. The meatus is guarded by a round sphincter muscle that relaxes to release the urine.

The Kidneys

The two bean-shaped kidneys are located behind the peritoneum. They are held in place by capsules of fat. Each weighs about 5 ounces. The outer portion of the kidney is called the **cortex**. It is in this area that the

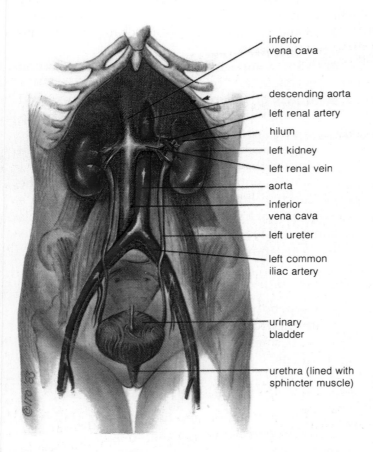

inferior
vena cava

descending aorta

left renal artery

hilum

left kidney

left renal vein

aorta

inferior
vena cava

left ureter

left common
iliac artery

urinary
bladder

urethra (lined with
sphincter muscle)

FIGURE 4–41. The urinary system *(From Fong, Ferris, and Skelley, Body Structures and Functions, 7th Edition, 1989, Delmar Publishers Inc.)*

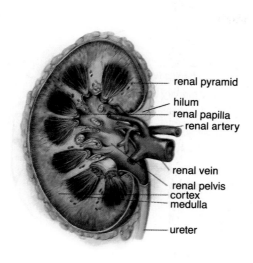

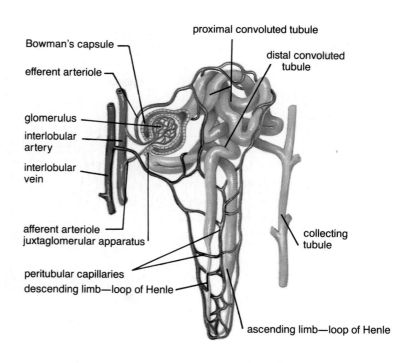

FIGURE 4–42. Cross section of the kidney *(From Anatomy and Physiology Plates, copyright 1992 by Delmar Publishers Inc.)*

FIGURE 4–43. The nephron is the functional unit of the kidney that produces urine. One million of these structures are found in the cortex of each kidney. *(From Anatomy and Physiology Plates, copyright 1992 by Delmar Publishers Inc.)*

urine is produced. The middle area is known as the medulla. It is a series of tubes that drain the urine from the cortex. The pelvis of the kidney receives the urine and directs it to the ureter.

Urine Production. The renal arteries carry blood to each kidney. Their many branches pass through the medulla to the cortex. In the cortex, urine is produced in units called nephrons, Figure 4–43. In each nephron:

- Blood vessels branch to form balls of capillaries called glomeruli. There are approximately one million glomeruli in each kidney.
- Each glomerulus is surrounded by a blind tube, the end of which resembles a cup. This is called Bowman's capsule.
- The tube twists and coils within the cortex, and dips down into the medulla. It eventually drains urine through the structures of the medulla into the pelvis of the kidney and then into the ureter.
- Waste products in large amounts of water are passed from the glomerulus to Bowman's capsule.

- Much of the water is reabsorbed back into the bloodstream as the branches of the capillaries encircle the twisted tubule in the cortex. The blood vessels then merge to leave the kidney as the renal vein.

Waste products excreted in urine include urea, creatinine, uric acid, and various salts. The average urine output is 1,000–1,500 ml every 24 hours. The amount is influenced by the hormones ADH and aldosterone, and the total fluid intake.

Urine. Urine is a liquid waste product. Its color is pale yellow to white. It has an acid reaction. Urine should not contain glucose, albumin, blood, pus, or acetone. Any of these substances indicate disease, trauma, or infection.

Aging Changes

Changes in the urinary system due to aging include:

- Decreased kidney size
- Loss of smooth muscle tone
- Diminished blood flow

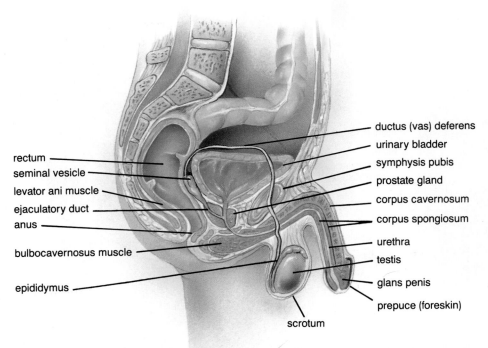

FIGURE 4–44. The male reproductive organs *(From Anatomy and Physiology Plates, copyright 1992 by Delmar Publishers Inc.)*

■ Less ability of kidneys to concentrate urine
■ Difficulty emptying the urinary bladder
■ Less efficient elimination
■ Decreased bladder capacity

The Reproductive System

Both the male and female reproductive organs have dual functions. They:
1. Produce reproductive cells. The male produces sperm. The female produces the ovum.
2. Produce hormones which are responsible for sex characteristics.
   a. Males produce testosterone.
   b. Females produce estrogen and progesterone.

In the reproductive process the:
■ Male and female engage in sexual intercourse.
■ Male ejaculates (propels) the sperm and the seminal fluid in which they swim into the female vagina.
■ Sperm and egg meet in the female fallopian tube. One sperm penetrates the egg and conception takes place.
■ Baby (fetus) develops in the uterus until birth.
■ Female breasts (mammary glands) produce milk to nourish the newborn.

The Male Reproductive Organs

Structure and Function

The male organs, Figure 4–44, include the:
■ Testes: Two glandular organs located in the scrotum. The testes produce sperm and the hormone testosterone.
■ Epididymis: A 20-foot coiled tube located on the top and back of each testes. The epididymis stores the sperm and allows them to mature.
■ Vas deferens: A tube that leads from the epididymis. It carries the sperm upward into the pelvic cavity to the seminal vesicles during ejaculation. The vas deferens is accompanied by nerves and blood vessels. Together, they form the spermatic cord.
■ Seminal vesicles: Located behind the bladder. They receive and store the sperm from the vas deferens. They contribute nutrients to the seminal fluid. The small ejaculator duct leads from the seminal vesicles to the urethra just below the prostate gland.
■ Prostate gland: Found just below the urinary bladder surrounding the urethra. It secretes a fluid that increases the ability of the sperm to move in the seminal fluid. Enlargement of the prostate gland may prevent urine from passing

through the urethra. This is a fairly common occurrence in older men.

- Penis: Composed of special tissue that can become filled with blood, making the organ enlarge and become stiffened so that it may enter the vagina to deposit seminal fluid. Loose-fitting skin covers the penis (the prepuce or foreskin).

The Female Reproductive Organs

Structure and Function

The external female structures (**genitalia**), Figure 4–45, include the:

- Vulva: Made up of two liplike structures, the **labia majora** and **labia minora**. When the labia are separated, other external structures may be seen.
- Clitoris: A highly erotic structure found just behind the juncture of the labia minora.
- Urinary meatus: The opening of the urethra to the outside.
- Vaginal meatus: The opening to the vagina or birth canal.

The Internal Female Structures

The internal female reproductive organs, Figures 4–46 and 4–47, include the following structures.

- Ovaries: Two small glands, found on either side of the uterus, at the ends of the oviducts (fallopian tubes) in the pelvis. They produce two hormones: estrogen and progesterone, and the egg (ovum). The eggs are contained in many little sacs called follicles. About once each month, a follicle matures and releases an ovum. The ovum makes its way into one of the 4-inch oviducts. This process is called **ovulation**. The cells of the follicles that are left produce progesterone. The progesterone causes changes within the uterus, readying it for the possibility of receiving a fertilized ovum.
- Fallopian tubes (oviducts): Two tubes, approximately 4 inches long, that serve as a pathway between the ovary and uterus. The sperm and egg meet in the tubes. Fertilization takes place here.
- Uterus: A hollow, pear-shaped organ. Its walls are made up of involuntary muscles. It is lined with special tissue called endometrium. The uterus has three main parts: the fundus, body, and cervix. The body and the fundus can stretch enough to hold a fetus, the amniotic sac, and the afterbirth (placenta). The cervix extends into the vagina. During labor, the cervix opens up to allow the baby to be delivered.

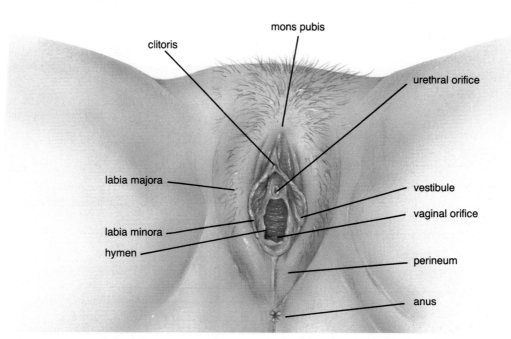

FIGURE 4–45. Female external reproductive organs (*From Anatomy and Physiology Plates, copyright 1992 by Delmar Publishers Inc.*)

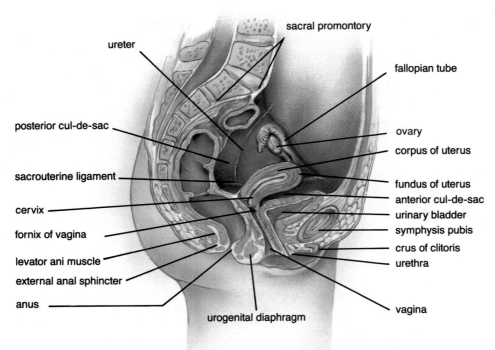

FIGURE 4–46. Lateral view of the female internal reproductive organs *(From Anatomy and Physiology Plates, copyright 1992 by Delmar Publishers Inc.)*

■ Vagina: Found between the urinary bladder and rectum. Its muscular walls are capable of much stretching. It is lined with mucous membrane. Two glands known as Bartholin's glands are found on either side of the external vaginal opening. They provide lubrication.

Menstruation and Ovulation

Menstruation is the loss of an unneeded part of the uterine lining (endometrium). It occurs for approximately three to five days each month.

At the end of each menstrual period, an ovum begins to mature in a follicle in one of the ovaries. As the follicle and its ovum grow, it produces the hormone estrogen. Estrogen causes the endometrium to develop new blood vessels and tissues. Ovulation usually takes place about 12 to 14 days after the first day of the last menstrual period. When ovulation occurs, the follicle secretes progesterone. Progesterone is a hormone that causes the endometrium to become somewhat soft and sticky in preparation for pregnancy.

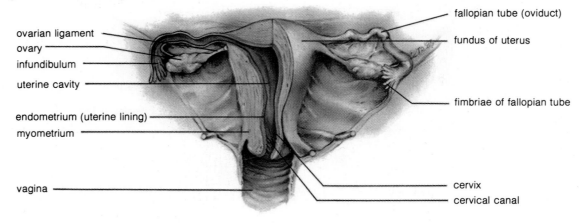

FIGURE 4–47. Female internal reproductive organs *(From Fong, Ferris, and Skelley,* Body Structures and Functions, *7th Edition, 1989, Delmar Publishers Inc.)*

Sperm are capable of moving by means of a flagellum so that they can travel from the vagina, through the uterus, to the oviduct. If the ovum unites with a sperm in the oviduct, it begins to divide into many cells and journeys to the uterus. In the uterus, it attaches to the uterine wall, grows, and develops into a fetus. If the ovum does not meet a sperm as it passes through the oviduct, it is expelled from the body. It is too small, however, to be seen.

If pregnancy does not occur after ovulation, the production of progesterone decreases after 12 days. Shortly thereafter the unneeded, newly built-up portion of the endometrium is shed as menstrual flow. The processes of ovulation and menstruation are known as the menstrual cycle. It occurs from puberty (sexual maturity) to menopause (about 50 years of age). The first menstrual cycle (period) occurs usually between ages 11–15. It is called **menarche**

Terms used in discussing menstruation include:
- Dysmenorrhea—painful menstruation
- Amenorrhea—without menstruation
- Menorrhagia—excessive bleeding

The Breasts

The breasts are two glands located on the anterior chest wall. They develop at puberty, but they do not produce milk until pregnancy occurs. Ducts from the glandular cells drain into a central duct which opens into the nipple. Surrounding the nipple is tissue that is slightly darker in color. This tissue is called the areola.

Aging Changes

Changes in the male reproductive system due to aging include:
- Decrease in size of testes
- Decreased production of sperm
- Ejaculation delayed or not as forceful
- Slower sexual response

Changes in the female reproductive system due to aging include:
- Breasts sag
- Menopause—loss of reproductive function
- Tissues of vulva and vaginal lining thin
- Vaginal secretions scantier

SUMMARY

The human body is highly organized into:
- Various kinds of cells
- Four basic tissue types
- Multiple organs
- Nine systems

Each contributes in a special way to the total structure and physiology of the body. A careful study of the healthy body and its organization provides a foundation for learning about your own body and the bodies of your patients. An understanding of the normal body will assist your study of the changes disease causes. It will also give you the ability to more accurately report and document your observations.

UNIT REVIEW

A. Multiple Choice. Select the one best answer.

1. When describing the relationship of the hand to the elbow, you should refer to it as being
   a. proximal   c. distal
   b. posterior   d. anterior

2. The appendix is located in which quadrant of the abdomen?
   a. URQ   c. ULQ
   b. LRQ   d. LLQ

3. Which membrane covers the lungs?
   a. pleura   c. peritoneum
   b. pericardium   d. meninges

4. Which organs are located in the dorsal cavity?
   a. heart and liver
   b. kidney and spleen
   c. brain and spinal cord
   d. uterus and testes

5. Which organ pumps blood throughout the body?
   a. lungs   c. liver
   b. heart   d. adrenal glands

6. Which organ is part of the skeletal system?
   a. ureters   c. gallbladder
   b. sternum   d. testes

7. Which gland produces testosterone?
   a. ovary   c. adrenal
   b. thymus   d. testes

8. The voice box is located in the
   a. larynx   c. trachea
   b. thymus   d. bronchi

9. The breasts are part of which system?
   - a. muscular
   - b. urinary
   - c. cardiovascular
   - d. reproductive

10. The organ that produces bile is the
    - a. gallbladder
    - b. stomach
    - c. liver
    - d. pancreas

11. Food is absorbed through the walls of the
    - a. pancreas
    - b. stomach
    - c. small intestine
    - d. large intestine

12. Thyroxine is a hormone produced by the
    - a. parathyroid gland
    - b. thyroid gland
    - c. thymus
    - d. pineal body

13. The gland known as the master gland is the
    - a. pineal body
    - b. pituitary
    - c. adrenal
    - d. thyroid

14. How many teeth are there in the adult permanent set?
    - a. 18
    - b. 20
    - c. 32
    - d. 38

15. Solid wastes eliminated through the digestive tract are called
    - a. saliva
    - b. feces
    - c. urine
    - d. sputum

16. Membranes that line body cavities that open to the outside are called
    - a. mucous membranes
    - b. mucus membranes
    - c. serous membranes
    - d. fibrous membranes

17. The heart has how many chambers?
    - a. 2
    - b. 3
    - c. 4
    - d. 5

18. The air sacs that make up the lungs are called
    - a. nephrons
    - b. alveoli
    - c. neurons
    - d. islet cells

19. Urine is formed in which part of the kidney?
    - a. cortex
    - b. pelvis
    - c. medulla
    - d. ureter

20. The conducting cell of the nervous tissue is the
    - a. osteocyte
    - b. fibrocyte
    - c. astrocyte
    - d. neuron

21. The long bone of the upper leg is the
    - a. tibia
    - b. ulna
    - c. femur
    - d. humerus

22. Bones of the wrist are called
    - a. carpals
    - b. tarsals
    - c. metacarpals
    - d. phalanges

23. The cavities within the brain that are filled with fluid are called
    - a. atria
    - b. ventricles
    - c. sinuses
    - d. cavities

24. The eye and ear are part of which system?
    - a. endocrine
    - b. nervous
    - c. cardiovascular
    - d. digestive

25. Decreasing the angle between two bones is called
    - a. flexion
    - b. extension
    - c. abduction
    - d. adduction

B. True/False. Answer the following statements true or false by circling T or F.

T F 26. The urinary bladder and gallbladder are the same structures.

T F 27. The outer layer of the skin is called the epidermis.

T F 28. Sweat glands secrete perspiration.

T F 29. Neurotransmitters allow passage of the nerve impulses between neurons.

T F 30. The largest part of the brain is the cerebellum.

T F 31. Motor control is handled in the frontal lobe of the cerebrum.

T F 32. The female reproductive cell is called the sperm.

T F 33. The pancreas functions in both the digestive and endocrine systems.

T F 34. The male urethra is much longer than the female urethra.

T F 35. DNA holds the master genetic code and is found in the nucleus.

C. Completion. Complete the following statement in the space provided.

36. The differences between the sudoriferous glands and the adrenal glands include:
    - a. _____
    - b. _____
    - c. _____

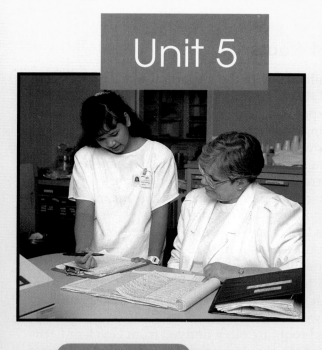

Medical Terminology

As a result of this unit, you will be able to:

- Spell and define terms.
- Identify the meanings of common medical root words.
- Write the abbreviations commonly used in health care facilities.
- Recognize the meanings of the most common prefixes and suffixes.
- Build medical terms from word parts.
- Analyze and define medical terms.

Learn the meaning and the correct spelling of the following words and phrases:

abbreviation   suffix
combining form   word root
prefix

Medicine has its own special language, called terminology. In this language, the terms are formed by building on common word parts, Figure 5–1. The language is developed by combining:

- Word roots—the foundation of a medical term. Word roots usually, but not always, refer to the part of the body or condition that is being treated, studied, or named by the term.
- Combining forms—to make it easier to form medical words, a vowel may be added to the end of the word root. This combination of the word root and vowel is called a combining form.
- Prefixes—terms added to the beginning of a word to change or add to its meaning.
- Suffixes—added to the end of a word to change or add to its meaning.
- Abbreviations—shortened forms of words (often letters). You are already familiar with abbreviations such as RN (registered nurse) and LPN (licensed practical nurse). You will soon become familiar with additional abbreviations that are common to the world of medicine.

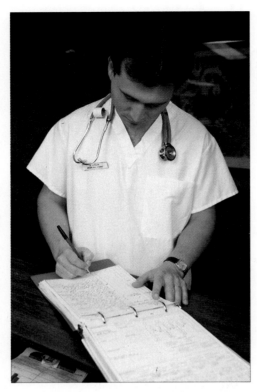

FIGURE 5–1. A knowledge of medical terminology will help make charting and record keeping easier.

Each hospital also has special abbreviations that it uses. You will need to learn those abbreviations. Check with the procedure policy of your facility to determine which abbreviations have been approved for use. A good medical dictionary is also a very helpful tool.

Word Roots

Familiarity with the important word parts will be gained through study and repeated usage. You will gain experience with the word parts as your practice reporting and charting, and by communicating with your coworkers.

A single medical word root can sometimes be placed in different parts of a word and still have a specific meaning. For example, the root *cyte* means cell:

- *cyt*ology—the study of cells
- a leuko*cyte*—a white blood cell
- poly*cyt*osis—an illness in which there are too many red and white blood cells

No matter where the form *cyte* occurs in a medical word, it refers to cells. It may be a prefix, a suffix, or a root word.

Word roots are often derived from Greek or Latin. For example, the stem or root word *nephro* is derived from the word for kidney. This root may be used to form a variety of medical terms. For example:

- Nephroma—a tumor of the kidney
- Nephrectomy—surgical excision of the kidney
- Nephroptosis—a kidney dropped out of place

Give special attention to the exercises and activities in this unit. Learning the new words and parts of words in this unit will make it easier for you to recognize meanings of medical terms.

Medical Word Parts

Following are word roots pertaining to body parts.

Combining Form	Meaning	Example	Meaning
abdomin (o)	abdomen	abdominal	portion of body between the thorax and pelvis *cepęžuna veubota (x)*
aden (o)	gland	adenoma	a glandular tumor
adren (o)	adrenal gland	adrenocortical hormone	one of the steroids produced by the adrenal cortex
angi (o)	vessel	angiogram	an X-ray of a blood vessel
arteri (o)	artery	arteriogram	a tracing of the arterial pulse
arthr (o)	joint	arthritis	inflammation of a joint
bronch (i) (o)	bronchus bronchi	bronchiectasis	one of the larger passages conveying air to and within the lungs becomes abnormally enlarged

Combining Form	Meaning	Example	Meaning
cardi (o)	heart	cardialgia	pain in the region of the heart
cephal (o)	head	cephaloma	soft or encephaloid tumor
cerébr (o)	brain	cerebrovascular accident	another name for a stroke
chol (e)	bile	cholecystitis	inflammation of the gallbladder
chondr (o)	cartilage	chondrocyte	mature cartilage-producing cell
col (o)	colon, large intestine	colectomy	excision of the colon
cost (o)	rib	intercostal	between two ribs
crani (o)	skull	craniotomy	opening of the skull
cyst (o)	bladder, cyst	cystitis	inflammation of the bladder
cyt (o)	cell	cytology	study of cells
dent (i) (o)	tooth	dentist	person licensed to practice dentistry
dermat (o)	skin	dermatitis	inflammation of the skin
encephal (o)	brain	pneumo-encephalogram	film produced by pneumoencephalography
enter (o)	small intestine	enteritis	inflammation of the intestines
erythr (o)	red	erythrocyte	red blood cell
gastr (o)	stomach	gastritis	inflammation of the lining of the stomach
geront (o)	old age	gerontology	study of the aged
gloss (o)	tongue	glossitis	inflammation of the tongue
hem (o), hemat (o)	blood	hematuria	discharge of blood in urine
hepat (o)	liver	hepatitis	inflammation of the liver
hyster (o)	uterus	hysterectomy	surgical removal of the uterus
ile (o)	ileum	ileitis	inflammation of the ileus
lapar (o)	abdomen, loin, flank	laparotomy	incision of the abdominal wall
laryng (o)	larynx	laryngectomy	partial or total removal of the larynx by surgery
mamm (o)	breast	mammary gland	secretes milk for nourishment of the young
mast (o)	breast	mastitis	inflammation of the breast
men (o)	menstruation	menstrual	pertaining to menstruation
my (o)	muscle	myalgia	muscular pain
myel (o)	spinal cord, bone marrow	myelogram	an X-ray of the spinal cord after injection of a contrast medium

Combining Form	Meaning	Example	Meaning
nephr (o)	kidney	nephrolithiasis	presence of renal calculi
neur (o)	nerve	neuropathy	any disease of the nervous system
ocul (o)	eye	ocular	pertaining to the eye
oophor (o)	ovary	oophorectomy	excision of an ovary
ophthalm (o)	eye	ophthalmologist	person licensed to practice ophthamology
oste (o)	bone	periosteum	specialized connective tissue covering all bones of the body
ot (o)	ear	otitis media	inflammation of the middle ear
pharyng (o)	throat, pharynx	pharyngitis	inflammation of the pharynx
phleb (o)	vein	phlebitis	inflammation of a vein
pneum (o)	lung, air, gas	pneumonectomy	resection of lung tissue
proct (o)	rectum	proctoscopy	rectal exam with a proctoscope
psych (o)	mind	psychology	study of human behavior
pulm (o)	lung	pulmonary	pertaining to the lungs
rect (o)	rectum	rectocele	hernial protrusion of part of the rectum into the vagina
rhin (o)	nose	rhinitis	inflammation of the mucous membrane of the nose
salping (o)	auditory (eustachian) tube, uterine (fallopian) tube	salpingitis	inflammation of a fallopian tube
splen (o)	spleen	splenectomy	excision of the spleen
stern (o)	sternum	substernal	below the sternum
stomat (o)	mouth	stomatitis	inflammation of the mucosa of the mouth
thorac (o)	chest	thoracotomy	opening of the chest
thym (o)	thymus	thymectomy	excision of the thymus
thyr (o)	thyroid	thyroidectomy	excision of the thyroid
trache (i) (o)	trachea	tracheotomy	incision of the trachea for exploration
ur (o)	urine, urinary tract, urination	urinalysis	analysis of the urine
urethr (o)	urethra	urethritis	inflammation of the urethra
urin (o)	urine	urinometer	an instrument for determining the specific gravity of urine
uter (i) (o)	uterus	uterine	pertaining to the uterus
ven (o)	vein	venipuncture	puncture of a vein for therapeutic purposes

Other common combining forms are:

Combining Form	Meaning	Example	Meaning
fibr (o)	fiber	fibroma	tumor composed mainly of fibrous or fully developed connective tissue
glyc (o)	sugar	glycemia	sugar in the blood
gynec (o)	woman, female	gynecology	branch of medicine dealing with diseases of the reproductive organs in women
hydr (o)	water	hydrocephalus	enlargement of the cranium caused by abnormal accumulation of fluid
lith (o)	stone	lithiasis	formation of stones in any hollow structure of the body
ped (o)	child	pediatric	pertaining to diseases of children
py (o)	pus	pyogenic	producing pus
thromb (o)	clot	thrombosis	formation of blood clots inside a blood vessel
tox (o), toxic (o)	poison	toxemia	presence in the blood of toxic (harmful) products

Prefixes

Many of the words have common beginnings (prefixes) or common endings (suffixes). By learning some of the more common prefixes and suffixes it is possible to put together many new words.

Prefix	Meaning	Example	Meaning
a-	without	asepsis	without infection
ante-	before	antepartum	before birth
anti-	against, counteracting	antidote	substance that counteracts the effects of a poison
bio-	life	biopsy	inspection of living organism (tissue)
brady-	slow	bradycardia	slow heart rate
contra-	against, opposed	contraindicate	against the usual treatment
dys-	pain or difficulty	dysuria	painful urination
hyper-	above, excessive	hypertension	high blood pressure
hypo-	low, deficient	hypotension	low blood pressure
inter-	between	intercellular	between the cells
intra-	within	intravenous	within a vein
neo-	new	neoplasm	any new growth or formation
pan-	all	pandemic	widespread epidemic

Prefix	Meaning	Example	Meaning
peri-	around	pericardium	membrane that covers the heart
poly-	many	polyuria	excessive urine
pre-	before	premenstrual	before the menses
pseudo-	false	pseudopregnancy	false pregnancy
tachy-	fast	tachycardia	pulse rate above normal

Suffixes

Suffix	Meaning	Example	Meaning
-ectomy	removal of	appendectomy	removal of the appendix
-itis	inflammation of	hepatitis	inflammation of the liver
-gram	record	electrocardiogram	record produced by electrocardiography
-logy	study of	hematology	study of blood
-lysis	destruction	hemolysis	rupture of erythrocytes with release of hemoglobin into the blood
-megaly	enlargement	acromegaly	abnormal enlargement of facial features, hands, feet; resulting from overproduction of pituitary gland
-otomy	incision – in to	tracheotomy	incision of trachea
-pathy	disease	adenopathy	any disease of the glands
-penia	lack, deficiency	thrombocytopenia	decrease in the number of platelets in circulating blood
-plegia	paralysis	hemiplegia	paralysis of one side of the body
-pnea	breathing, respiration	apnea	temporary cessation of breathing
-ptosis	falling, sagging, dropping down	nephroptosis	downward displacement of a kidney
-rrhagia	excessive flow	menorrhagia	excessive menstruation
-rrhea	profuse flow, discharge	leukorrhea	vaginal discharge, usually white or yellowish in color
-scope	examination instrument	otoscope	instrument for inspecting or auscultating the ear
-scopy	examination using a scope	proctoscopy	rectal exam with a proctoscope
-stasis	maintaining a constant level	hemostasis	stopping the escape of blood by either natural or artificial means

Common Abbreviations

Lists of abbreviations and their meanings follow. They have been grouped according to most common usage for easier learning. Other abbreviations will be presented in following units where they find their greatest application.

Body Parts

abd —abdomen
AD —right ear
AS —left ear
AU —both ears
bld —blood
BK —below knee
cx —cervix
GB —gallbladder
GI —gastrointestinal
GU —genitourinary
H & L —heart and lungs
jt —joint
KLS —kidney, liver, spleen
lt —left
OD —right eye
OS —left eye
os —mouth
OU —both eyes
sh —shoulder
umb —umbilicus
vag —vagina, vaginal

Diagnosis

ab —antibody
ABE —acute bacterial endo-carditis
ac —acute
ACVD —acute cardiovascular disease
AFB —acid fast bacillus
Ag —antigen
AgNO$_3$ —silver nitrate
AIDS —acquired immune deficiency syndrome
AKA —above knee amputation

AMI —acute myocardial infarction
ARC —AIDS related complex
ARDS —adult respiratory distress syndrome
ARF —acute respiratory failure
ASCVD —arteriosclerotic cardiovascular disease
ASHD —arteriosclerotic heart disease
BKA —below knee amputation
BPH —benign prostatic hypertrophy
c̄ —with
CA —cancer
CAD —coronary artery disease
CBC —complete blood count
CHD —coronary heart disease
CHF —congestive heart failure
CO —coronary occlusion
COLD —chronic obstructive lung disease
COPD —chronic obstructive pulmonary disease
CRD —chronic respiratory disease
CVA —cerebrovascular accident; stroke
DJD —degenerative joint disease
DM —diabetes mellitus
DOA —dead on arrival
FB —foreign body
FTND —full term normal delivery
FUO —fever of unknown origin
Fx —fracture
GSW —gunshot wound
HCVD —hypertensive cardio-vascular disease
IH —infectious hepatitis
IHD —ischemic heart disease
Ig —immunoglobulin
KS —Kaposi's sarcoma

LBP —low back pain
LBW —low birth weight
MI —myocardial infarction: refers to the death of tissues due to loss of blood supply
MS —multiple sclerosis
NB —newborn
NGU —nongonococcal ure-thritis
NSU —nonspecific urethritis
OBS —organic brain syndrome
OJD —osteoarthritic joint disease
PID —pelvic inflammatory disease
PUD —peptic ulcer disease
PVD —peripheral vascular disease
RF —renal failure
RHD —rheumatic heart disease
SDAT —senile dementia of Alzheimer's type
SIDS —sudden infant death syndrome
STD —sexually transmitted disease
TIA —transient ischemic attack
TUR —transurethral resection
URI —upper respiratory infection
UTI —urinary tract infection

Patient Orders and Charting

aa —of each
ADL —activities of daily living
ad lib. —as desired
adm —admission
ADT —admission, discharge, transfer
amb —ambulate, ambulatory
AMA —against medical advice
aq —aqueous
ASA —aspirin

ASAP	—as soon as possible	NG	—nasogastric	
as tol	—as tolerated	NPO	—nothing by mouth	
ausc	—auscultation, auscultate	N/S	—normal saline	
		N & V	—nausea and vomiting	
B.M., bm	—bowel movement	NVD	—nausea, vomiting, diarrhea	
B.R.	—bed rest	O₂	—Oxygen — 2 норма	
BRP	—bathroom privileges	OOB	—out of bed	
c̄	—with	per	—by	
cath	—catheterize	pH	—acidity/alkalinity	
CBR	—complete bed rest	p.o. (per os)	—by mouth	
cib	—food			
ck	—check	PO	—postoperative	
cl liq	—clear liquid	preop	—preoperative	
DAT	—diet as tolerated	prep	—prepare	
DC,D/C	—discontinue	p.r.n.	—whenever necessary	
disch	—discharge	pt	—patient; pint (500 ml)	
DNI	—do not intubate	Px	—prognosis (prog)	
DNR	—do not resuscitate	q.s.	—sufficient quantity	
DOB	—date of birth	qt	—quiet	
DR	—doctor	rehab	—rehabilitation	
dr	—dressing	resp	—respiration	
D/S	—dextrose and saline	rt	—right, routine	
DSD	—dry, sterile dressing	Rx	—treatment	
DW	—distilled water	s̄	—without	
D/W	—dextrose and water	s̄s̄	—one-half	
Dx	—diagnosis	semi	—half	
E	—enema	sm	—small	
EBL	—estimated blood loss	sos	—if necessary	
et	—and	spec	—specimen	
FM	—flow meter	SSE	—soap suds enema	
FU	—follow-up	stat	—at once	
gtt	—drops	Surg	—surgery	
HO	—hyperbaric oxygen	Sx	—symptoms	
HOB	—head of bed	tinct	—tincture	
ht	—height	TKO	—to keep open	
Hx	—history	top	—topically	
irrig	—irrigation	TPN	—total parenteral nutrition	
isol	—isolation			
IV	—intravenous	TWE	—tap water enema	
L	—liter (1,000 ml, quart)	Tx	—traction	
lap	—laparotomy	ung.	—ointment (oint)	
lb	—pound	ur	—urine	
L & D	—labor and delivery	w/c	—wheelchair	
lg	—large	wt	—weight	
liq	—liquid	YOB	—year of birth	
L/min	—liters per minute	U/C	—urine culture	
Na	—sodium	U/A	—urine analysis	
N/C	—no complaints			
neg	—negative			

Physical and History

DOB	—date of birth
FH	—family history
LMP	—last menstrual period
L & W	—living and well
M & F	—mother and father
MH	—marital history
NB	—newborn
PI	—present illness
PMH	—past medical history
PVD	—peripheral vascular disease
R/O	—rule out
UCD	—usual childhood diseases
UK	—unknown
WDWN	—well-developed, well-nourished
WNL	—within normal limits
YOB	—year of birth

Tests

ABC	—aspiration, biopsy, cytology
ABG	—arterial blood gas study
BUN	—blood urea nitrogen
CBC	—complete blood count
FBS	—fasting blood sugar
FPG	—fasting plasma glucose
GA	—gastric analysis
Hb	—hemoglobin
MRI	—magnetic resonance imaging
Myel	—myelogram
S & A	—sugar and acetone
UA	—urinalysis

Places or Departments

CS	—central supply
DR	—delivery room
EENT	—eye, ear, nose, throat
ED/ER	—emergency department or emergency room
GI	—gastrointestinal
GU	—genitourinary
Gyn	—gynecology

ICCU	—intensive coronary care unit	alt noct	—alternate nights
ICU	—intensive care unit	AM	—morning
Lab	—laboratory	b.i.d.	—twice a day
L & D	—labor and delivery	BIN	—twice a night
MRD	—medical record department	h	—hour
		h.s.	—hour of sleep (bedtime)
Nsy	—nursery	noc, noct	—night
OB	—obstetrics		
OPD	—outpatient depart- ment	p	—after
		p.c.	—after meals
OR	—operating room	PM	—evening or afternoon
OT	—occupational therapy	preop	—preoperative
PAR	—post anesthesia room	q	—every
Peds	—pediatrics	qd	—every day
PT	—physical therapy	qh	—every hour
RR	—recovery room	q2h	—every two hours
SICU	—surgical intensive care unit	q.i.d.	—four times a day
		qm (qAM)	—every morning

Time Abbreviations

a.c.	—before meals
alt dieb	—alternate days, every other day
alt hor	—alternate hours

qn	—every night
qod	—every other day
t.i.d.	—three times a day
WA	—while awake

Roman Numerals

I	—1	VI	—6
II	—2	VII	—7
III	—3	VIII	—8
IV	—4	IX	—9
V	—5	X	—10

Measurements and Volume

oz	—ounce
dr	—dram
c	—centimeter
cc	—cubic centimeter
ml	—milliliter
L	—liter

Weight/Height

kg	—kilogram
lb	—pounds
in	—inches

Temperature

F	—Fahrenheit
C	—Celsius
°	—degree

SUMMARY

Medical terminology is developed by arranging and combining word parts. It is a language used by health personnel in health care facilities. The words are formed of:
- Word roots
- Prefixes at the beginning of words
- Suffixes at the end of words
- Combining forms referring to body parts and medical actions
- Abbreviations—usually letters

Learning medical terminology will improve your understanding and will help you communicate more effectively in the health care setting.

UNIT REVIEW

A. Matching. Match the abbreviations in Column I with their meanings in Column II.

Column I	Column II
_____ 1. a.c.	a. three times a day
_____ 2. b.i.d.	b. whenever necessary
_____ 3. OR	c. night
_____ 4. p.r.n.	d. before meals
_____ 5. p.o.	e. operating room
_____ 6. stat	f. by mouth
_____ 7. noct	g. after meals
_____ 8. c̄	h. without
_____ 9. ung.	i. twice a day
_____ 10. s̄	j. at once
	k. ointment
	l. with

B. Matching. Match the prefixes in Column I with their meanings in Column II.

Column I   Column II

_____ 11. angi (o)   a. bile
_____ 12. cardi (o)   b. tongue
_____ 13. chol (e)   c. lung
_____ 14. dermat (o)   d. vessel
_____ 15. gastr (o)   e. muscle
_____ 16. gloss (o)   f. pharynx
_____ 17. lapar (o)   g. stomach
_____ 18. pneum (o)   h. larynx
_____ 19. my (o)   i. heart
_____ 20. pharyng (o)   j. abdomen
                             k. chest
                             l. skin

C. Define the following medical terms. Then circle the prefix or suffix that you have learned.

21. erythrocyte _____
22. dysuria _____
23. pneumonitis _____
24. adenopathy _____
25. craniotomy _____

D. Define the following medical terms. Then circle the prefix that you have learned.

26. asepsis _____
27. antidote _____
28. contraindicated _____
29. hypertension _____
30. tachycardia _____

E. Define the following medical terms. Then circle the suffix that you have learned.

31. neuralgia _____
32. erthrocyte _____
33. appendectomy _____
34. hematology _____
35. thrombocytopenia _____

F. Write the medical term that means the following.

36. dropped kidney _____
37. examination of the rectum using an instrument

    _____

38. procedure to remove fluid from the thorax____

    _____

39. inflammation of the stomach _____
40. meaning a lack of white blood cells _____

G. In each of the following, circle the prefix and underline the suffix.

41. anemia
42. stomatitis
43. glossitis
44. costal
45. tracheotomy

H. Print the Roman numerals for each of the following.

46. 2 _____   49. 9 _____
47. 5 _____   50. 10 _____
48. 6 _____

I. Define each medical term and abbreviation used on the sample Kardex.

1.	Patient Name	Bruce Tratt	Age 47	Rel Prot	#876–3291–7
2.	Physician	R. Morgan M.D.	Dx Splenomegaly—Diabetes Mellitus		
3.		**Orders**			
4.	**Preop orders**	3/18	on call for OR @ 8 am 3/19		
5.	Stat CBC, ABG, FBS				
6.	UA				
7.	NG Tube @ 6 am 3/19				
8.	Foley cath this pm.				
9.	Surg Prep.				
10.	NPO p`midnight				
11.	SSE @ HS.				
12.	Amb ad Lib. this pm.				
13.					
14.	Anesthesiologist will call preop medication orders.				
15.					

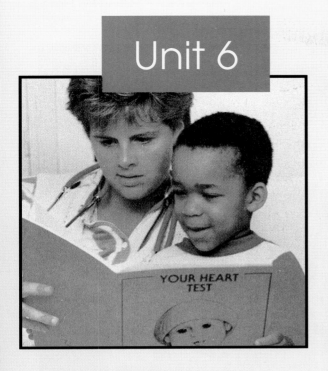

Unit 6

Classification of Disease

Learn the meaning and the correct spelling of the following words and phrases:

acute disease
antibodies
autoimmune
benign
cachexia
carcinogens
carcinoma
chronic disease
complication
congenital
direct cause
etiology
genetic
hypersensitivity
infection
inflammation
invasive
ischemia

malignant
medical diagnosis
metastasize
neoplasm
noninvasive
objective observation
obstruction
pathology
predisposing cause
prognosis
protocol
sarcoma
signs
subjective complaint
symptoms
therapy
trauma
tumor

OBJECTIVES

As a result of this unit, you will be able to:

- Spell and define terms.
- Define disease and list some possible causes.
- Identify disease-related terms.
- Distinguish between signs and symptoms.
- List ways in which a diagnosis is made.
- List four modes of therapy.
- List six major health problems.

The nurse values your observations when making evaluations and planning the nursing care for patients as part of the nursing process. The better you understand the basic principles of disease, the more accurate information you can provide.

Disease is any change from a healthy state. The disease (pathology) may be a change in structure or function, or it may be the failure of a part of the body to develop properly. Each illness has a/an

- Etiology—cause of the illness or abnormality
- Usual set of indications that the illness is in progress. These are called signs and symptoms
- Usual course or disease progression
- Prognosis or probable outcome of the process

95

Causes of Disease

Many factors may contribute to the development of disease, illness, or injury in the body.

1. The exciting cause (etiology) is the immediate or direct cause. For example, an injury (trauma) from a fall may cause a bone to break, Figure 6–1. The blow of the fall is the exciting cause of the injury.
2. Exogenous etiologies—originate outside the person's body. These include:
   a. traumas
   b. radiation
   c. microorganisms
   d. electric shock
   e. chemical agents
   f. extremes of temperature
   g. unusual pressure
3. Endogenous etiologies—originate within the person's body. These include:
   a. metabolic disorders
   b. congenital abnormalities, Figure 6–2
   c. tumors
4. Predisposing cause (etiology)—factors that contribute to the development of illness, Figure 6–3. These factors include:
   a. age
   b. malnutrition
   c. certain occupations
   d. heredity
   e. previous illness

A young child who is malnourished and underweight is much more apt to develop an infection

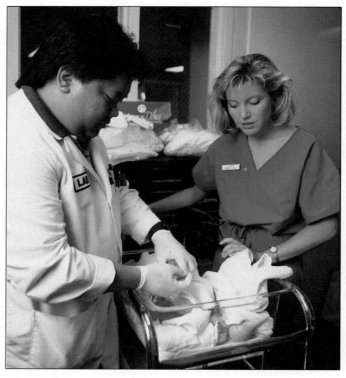

FIGURE 6–2. The laboratory technician has taken a sample of blood from the heel of this newborn. A test will be performed to determine if the baby has a congenital condition called phenylketonuria (PKU).

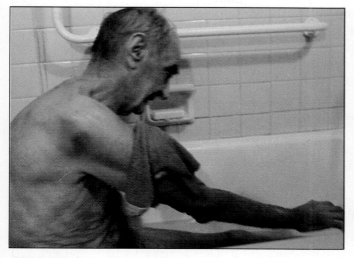

FIGURE 6–1. Note the bruise on the person's shoulder—evidence of a trauma resulting from a fall

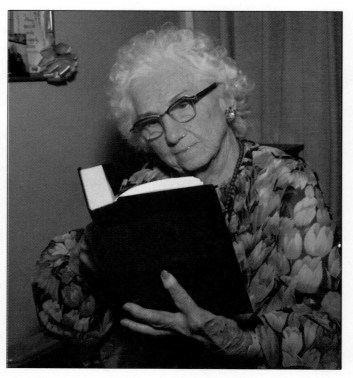

FIGURE 6–3. Advanced age is a predisposing factor to the development of some illnesses.

than one who is well-nourished. The germs causing the infection are the exciting cause of the illness, but the age and nutritional state of the child contribute to the development of the infectious process.

Signs and Symptoms

Signs and symptoms are evidence of disease processes going on within the body, Figure 6–4. **Signs** of a disease are objective: they can be seen by others. The color or condition of the skin is an example of a sign of disease, Figure 6–5. **Symptoms** are subjective: they are felt by the patient, who tells us about them. Pain is a symptom common to many pathological conditions, Figure 6–6.

Describing Signs and Symptoms

Your observations of signs and symptoms will need to be reported and recorded. You must be very

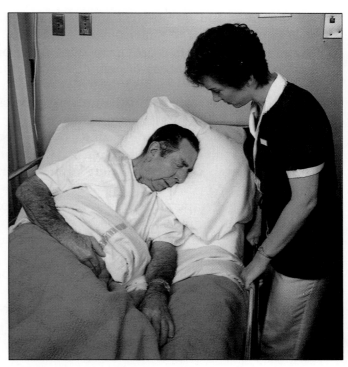

FIGURE 6–6. Sometimes the patient experiencing the symptom of pain reveals this information by his body language.

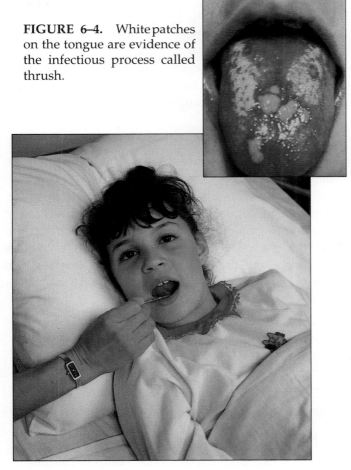

FIGURE 6–4. White patches on the tongue are evidence of the infectious process called thrush.

FIGURE 6–5. The flushed skin of this child may indicate an elevated body temperature (pyrexia).

careful to distinguish between **objective observations** which you make and **subjective complaints** which the patient experiences and tells you about. For example, if you pick up a tray of food that is only partially eaten, you should report this as "one-half of lunch eaten." This is an objective observation. It would be incorrect to report "the patient only ate half his food—guess he must not have been hungry." This is a subjective statement on your part. It may be a fact that the patient wasn't hungry, but it might have been that the:

- Food was cold
- Patient was nauseated
- Patient had pain
- Meal was interrupted
- Patient found feeding herself/himself too difficult

Complaints of pain provide good clues to the type of pathology going on in the body. It is not enough for the nursing assistant to simply note that the patient has pain. It is important to learn from the patient the:

- Kind (character) of the pain. For example, "sharp," "burning," "stabbing," "dull"
- Exact location of the pain. For example, LLQ, epigastrium, right posterior superior chest

■ Intensity and duration of the pain. For example, "constant," "intermittent"

Report this information promptly to the nurse or team leader. All observations of signs and symptoms must be noted and reported because they are valuable to the assessment step of the nursing process and they help to determine proper treatment.

Specific signs and symptoms that must be reported are described with each system to make correlation easier. In general, you must be alert to and report changes in:

■ Skin color, temperature or texture, presence of eruptions, Figure 6–7

■ Rate, rhythm, or character of pulse and respirations

■ Character or amount of fluid intake and/or output

■ Unusual behavior

■ Speech, responsiveness, or movement

■ Bodily discharge of any kind

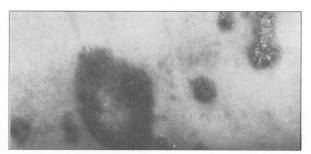

FIGURE 6–7. This person shows the characteristic lesions of ringworm. *(Photo courtesy of the Centers for Disease Control, Atlanta, GA)*

The Course (Pattern) of Disease

The development and course of different illnesses vary greatly. Acute conditions progress rapidly, last a predictable period, and then the person recovers. For example, the signs and symptoms of an infected finger may develop rapidly and last a relatively short period. Then, as the body controls the process, recovery is seen. This type of disease process is classified as an **acute disease**. Rubeola, another example of acute disease, is shown in Figure 6–8.

Chronic conditions are prolonged illnesses. **Chronic disease** states often have periods when the patient experiences the signs and symptoms and periods when evidence of the disease is less pronounced or disappears altogether. Rheumatoid arthritis is such a disease. At times the affected joints are red, hot to

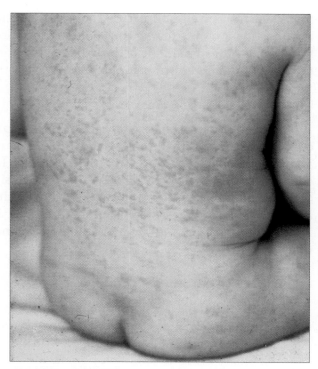

FIGURE 6–8. Note the maculopapular rash which is characteristic of the lesions of measles (rubeola). *(Photo courtesy of the Centers for Disease Control, Atlanta, GA)*

touch, swollen, and painful. At other times, the signs and symptoms seem to go away. Figure 6–9 shows some common signs and symptoms.

Complications

Diseases such as measles or mumps—which are usually acute and follow a rather predictable course—are sometimes made more serious by the development of pneumonia (a serious lung condition). The pneumonia makes the original process more harmful and is regarded as a **complication**. As you learn more about patients and their illnesses, you will begin to associate specific signs and symptoms with a particular disease state.

SIGNS (OBJECTIVE INDICATIONS)	SYMPTOMS (SUBJECTIVE INDICATIONS)
Skin color	Nausea
Rapid pulse (Tachycardia)	Dizziness
High blood pressure (Hypertension)	Pain
Vomiting	Anxiety

FIGURE 6–9.

The Disease Process

The body is like a complex chemical factory that depends upon delivery of needed supplies to run efficiently. It is subject to both external and internal stress which threatens its ability to keep functioning. Like any well-run factory, when one area is under threat, the other parts compensate to keep the factory running.

Some of the major conditions or illnesses that can affect the body's functional ability are:

■ Ischemia: This is the lack of adequate blood supply to a body tissue, which prevents the delivery of the essential oxygen and nutrients. As a result, the normal chemistry of cells cannot be carried out. Ischemias usually originate from factors within the body. For example, a blood clot (thrombus) that has formed within the blood vessel wall can block a blood vessel. The ischemia would be an endogenous cause of disease since without blood and the vital oxygen that it carries, cells cannot function, become diseased, and die.

■ Congenital abnormalities: These are abnormalities that are present at birth, Figure 6–10. Some are developmental, occurring during the time the baby is growing in the mother's uterus. Examples of developmental abnormalities include:

— Spina bifida—a defect in the formation of the vertebral column
— Cleft lip—an imperfection in the formation of the upper lip
— Agenesis of a kidney—one kidney fails to develop so that the baby is born with only one kidney
— Talipes (club foot)—the child's foot is turned or twisted out of its normal position

Some are genetic abnormalities that are due to defects in the genetic information passed on from the parents to the child. Examples of genetic congenital abnormalities include:

— Sickle cell anemia—the red blood cells are improperly formed so they do not maintain their normal disc shape
— Color blindness—the person is unable to distinguish between certain colors
— Hemophilia—there is a lack of an important blood component needed for proper blood clotting

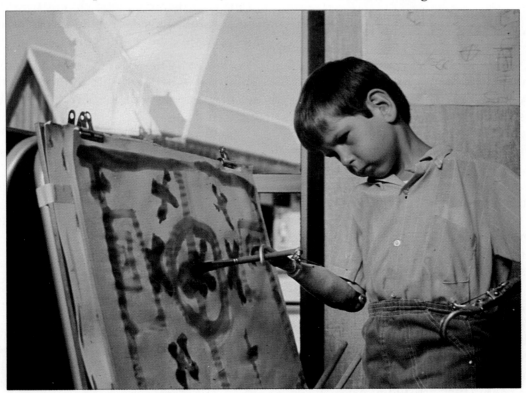

FIGURE 6–10. This child with phocomelia has no hands because a drug taken by his mother during early pregnancy interfered with limb development. *(Photo courtesy of the March of Dimes—Birth Defects Foundation)*

■ **Infection**: These are disease processes caused by infectious organisms or their products. They include pneumonias, scarlet fever, and abscesses. **Inflammation** usually is part of the infectious process.

■ Inflammations that develop for reasons other than infection include:
  — **Autoimmune** reactions: These are situations where the mechanisms that are designed to protect the body turn against the body and cause damage, such as rheumatoid arthritis (RA), systemic lupus erythematosus (SLE), and multiple sclerosis (MS).
  — **Hypersensitivity** reactions: These are allergic types of reactions such as hay fever, skin rashes, and asthma.
  — Irritations: These could be caused by seeds in the intestinal tract or stones in the gallbladder or kidney.

■ Metabolic imbalances: These include conditions of fluid and electrolyte imbalance. They include malnutrition, edema, scurvy, alcoholism, and diabetes mellitus.

■ **Obstruction**: Tubes throughout the body carry a variety of materials that must continue to flow. Obstructions impede the flow. Examples of obstructions include blood clots in blood vessels, stones in the bile ducts or in the kidneys, and obstructions that occur when the tube structures become twisted, as in an intestinal obstruction.

■ **Trauma**: Injuries that can cause tissue damage such as those that might develop from a blow to the body or an auto accident. Exposure to unusual pressure or extremes of temperature also causes traumas. A fractured bone can be due to trauma when someone is thrown from a motorcycle and strikes his leg against a curbstone.

■ Neoplasm: The word **neoplasm** means new growth. It is another term for **tumor**. Neoplasms are an important kind of disease. There are two types of neoplasms: benign or nonmalignant tumors and malignant tumors. Sometimes benign tumors can change and become malignant. People with a malignant tumor or a malignancy are said to have cancer.

Neoplasms

Each type of neoplasm has its own characteristics.
■ **Benign** or nonmalignant tumors:
  — Usually grow slowly
  — Do not spread
  — Do not cause death unless located in a vital area such as the brain
  — Can be dangerous if they put pressure on vital organs
  — Are usually named by stating the part of the body involved and adding the suffix *oma*. For example, *osteoma* names a benign bone tumor
  — May have special names such as some "polyps"

■ **Malignant** tumors or cancerous growths:
  — Grow more rapidly
  — Spread to other body parts (**metastasize**)
  — May have special names; for example, "leukemia"
  — If untreated, cause death

Different types of tumors are more common among some groups. Children have more tumors of the nervous system, urinary system, and hematopoietic (blood forming) system. Adults have more tumors of the reproductive organs, lungs, and colon.

Etiology. The etiology of malignancies is not known. It is believed that a complex interaction of several factors probably plays a role. These factors include:
■ Viruses—tiny infective agents
■ **Carcinogens**—chemicals that cause abnormal cellular changes
■ Exposure to radiation
■ Heredity (abnormal genes)
■ Exhaustion of the basic immune response
■ Chronic irritation

Naming Malignancies. In naming malignant tumors, the terms **sarcoma** and **carcinoma** are often used. Some tumors have special names.
  1. Sarcomas are:
    a. Derived from connective tissues
    b. Spread principally via the bloodstream
    c. Frequently metastasize to the liver, lungs, and bone
    d. Seen more commonly in persons under 40 years of age

2. Carcinomas are:
   a. Derived from epithelial tissues
   b. Spread principally via the lymphatics
   c. Spread to the lymph nodes
   d. Found more commonly in persons over 40 years of age

Early Detection. Early detection of cancer can often result in total cure. The earlier the cancer is found, the higher the rate of cure. Pain is not usually an early symptom. Early signs and symptoms of malignancies include:

- Change in bowel or bladder habits
- A sore that does not heal
- Unusual bleeding or discharge
- Thickening or lump in breast or elsewhere
- Indigestion or difficulty in swallowing
- Obvious change in wart or mole
- Nagging cough or hoarseness

Note the first letters of these early signs and symptoms spell CAUTION

Late Signs and Symptoms. Late signs and symptoms may include:

- Cachexia or general wasting of the body tissues with loss of weight
- Fever of unknown origin
- Anemia
- Pain due to pressure, obstruction, and ischemia
- Hormonal irregularities
- Inflammations of the skin

Diagnosis

Before the physician can prescribe the proper treatment for the patient, the disease process must be determined. Naming the disease process is known as establishing a medical diagnosis. In order to do this, the patient is examined, a history of previous illness is taken and reviewed, and various laboratory tests are performed, Figures 6–11A and B.

The doctor then compiles all the information, matches it to possible diseases, and then names the process.

Diagnostic Studies

Laboratory tests and diagnostic studies give the physician valuable information for planning the proper treatment for the patient. The nursing staff prepares the patient for the ordered tests and cares for the patient after the tests are completed. The nursing assistant helps in this process. The nursing assistant also may be assigned to collect certain specimens.

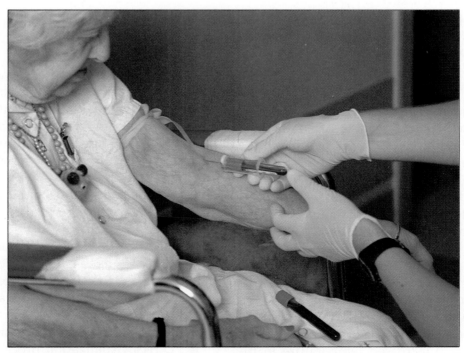

FIGURE 6–11A. Blood tests reveal much about the chemistry of the body and contribute to making a correct medical diagnosis.

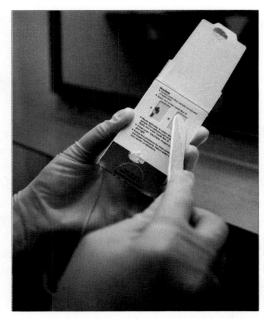

FIGURE 6–11B. Stool specimens may be taken and examined for occult (hidden) blood.

Protocols are standards of procedure and care developed for the preparation and care of the patient for each test or study. Protocols must be followed carefully to achieve satisfactory results. Improper patient preparation can result in:

- Inability to perform the test
- Inaccurate test results
- Delayed diagnosis
- Increased costs
- Increased patient anxiety

Noninvasive Tests

Tests and studies may be noninvasive. This means the techniques used do not break the skin or damage body tissues. For example, X-rays do not break the skin but do give information about internal body structures.

Commonly ordered noninvasive tests include:

- Ultrasound—Sound waves are bounced against the body to measure variations in tissue density. For example, the Doppler ultrasound probe measures the blood flow in blood vessels. Sonograms of the pregnant uterus give information about the growing fetus.
- Thermography—measures the temperature in different body tissues. Thermograms of the breast indicate increased temperature in tumorous tissue.

- X-ray and fluoroscopy—uses short-wavelength electromagnetic radiation to examine internal tissues. X-ray techniques are sophisticated. One of the newest techniques is computerized axial tomography (CT scan or CAT scan). This procedure provides a three-dimensional view of the internal structures of the body. A computer records and provides a printout of information.
- Magnetic resonance imaging (MRI)—is an imaging technique that provides excellent pictures (images) with minimal risk to the patient. The body is placed in a strong magnetic field. Radio frequency pulses cause certain chemicals (ions) in body tissues to change position. When the radiowaves are discontinued the ions assume the original position. As they return to normal, energy given off can be recorded. All of this occurs without sensations being felt by the patient.
- Recording of the electrical activity occurring in different body organs. A recording of this activity is made on paper or on a screen for viewing. Such examinations include:
  — Electrocardiogram (EKG or ECG) to record electrical activity of the cardiac cycle
  — Electroencephalogram (EEG) to record electrical activity of the brain
  — Electromyogram (EMG) to record electrical activity of muscles

Invasive Tests

Invasive tests and studies invade or actually penetrate body surfaces. Examples of invasive tests include taking tissue samples, introducing contrast media, and probing deeply into body cavities.

A sternal puncture is a procedure in which a needle pierces the sternum to draw a sample of blood-producing cells. For some invasive examinations, iodine dyes, barium compounds, or air may be introduced into a body cavity to produce contrast when making recordings and pictures.

Most of these invasive techniques are carried out in special areas, such as laboratories, that are specifically designed for this purpose. Also, samples of patient specimens usually are examined in the laboratories.

Some special invasive procedures include:

- Direct visualization procedures—to examine body parts with instruments (scopes) introduced into the body. For example, the procto-scope, inserted in the anus, allows direct observation of the interior rectum. Other direct visualization procedures are:

— Cystoscopy to observe the bladder
— Laryngoscopy to observe the larynx
— Sigmoidoscopy to observe the colon

■ Dye studies—dyes are introduced into the body to outline body parts so X-rays can be taken. Some examples are:

— Upper GI series (barium swallow)—the patient swallows a barium solution and then X-rays or fluoroscopy show the structures highlighted
— Lower GI series (barium enema)—the patient is given the barium rectally. The patient holds the solution while X-rays are taken
— Myelogram—dye is introduced into the spinal canal and then X-rays are taken.

■ Cardiac catheterization—a catheter (small sterile tube) is introduced into the vascular system and delivers a dye. As the catheter is moved through the blood vessels and heart chambers, a monitor shows the dye flowing through this system.

Other Techniques

Chemical and microscopic studies examine various body tissue and secretion samples. Some samples require invasive procedures. Some samples require noninvasive procedures. The most common samples are:

■ Blood
■ Urine
■ Sputum from the lungs
■ Cultures from infected tissues
■ Gastric secretions
■ Feces

Nursing Assistant Responsibilities

The responsibilities of the nursing assistant in caring for patients having diagnostic procedures include:

■ Providing emotional support
■ Correctly preparing the patient according to instructions
■ Carefully collecting and handling specimens
■ Promptly delivering specimens

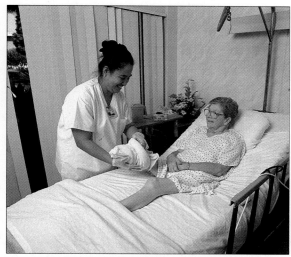

FIGURE 6–12. This patient's leg was amputated because of peripheral vascular disease.

■ Documenting procedures
■ Performing aftercare according to directions
■ Completing a checklist for accuracy

These actions correctly done contribute to implementing the nursing process.

Therapy

Once the medical diagnosis is confirmed, it is possible to predict the course of the disease and a probable prognosis (likely outcome or course of the disease process). Then the most appropriate therapy (treatment) is determined.

There are four basic approaches to therapy. They may be used singularly or in differing combinations.

1. Surgery: This form of therapy may remove unhealthy tissue, Figure 6–12, replace unhealthy parts, or repair injured, malformed, or congenitally defective areas. Prostatectomies remove unhealthy prostate glands. Coronary bypasses replace blocked arteries with other arteries. Herniorrhaphies repair weakened muscle walls.

2. Chemotherapy: This form of therapy uses drugs and chemicals to promote and improve body functions and to control pain, Figure 6–13. For example, the patient with a fever is given an antipyretic such as aspirin to reduce the temperature. When applied to cancer therapy, chemotherapy often refers to special combinations of drugs that interfere with the growth of cancer cells.

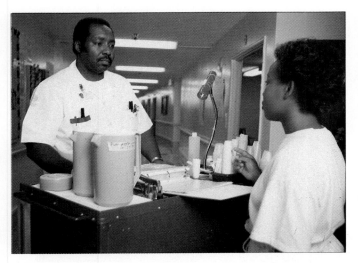

FIGURE 6–13. The nursing assistant reports the patient's complaint of pain to the registered medication nurse who will administer the ordered pain reliever.

3. Radiation: This form of therapy uses controlled radioactivity to destroy tumor cells.
4. Supportive (palliative) care: This form of therapy is designed to support the patient's body in its attempt to stay healthy, Figure 6–14. For example, positioning a person in an upright position makes it easier for him to breath when he is having an asthmatic attack. Pain control, rest, proper nutrition, fluid intake, and good hygiene all aid the body's own attempt to control the effects of the illness.

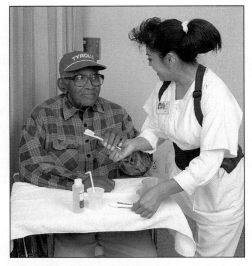

FIGURE 6–14. Supportive care includes rest, good nutrition, and proper hygiene.

Body Defenses

The body has a natural line of defense against disease. These defenses include:

- Unbroken skin and mucous membranes, which serve as mechanical barriers
- Mucus, which traps foreign particles, and cilia, which propel them out of the body
- The acidity of certain body secretions such as perspiration, saliva, and stomach juices, which slows the growth of microorganisms
- White blood cells, which surround and destroy anything foreign that enters the body
- Special body cells that produce chemicals, called **antibodies**, that protect the body against specific infections
- Inflammation

Inflammation

The process of inflammation, which we often associate with infections such as boils and abscesses, is really an important part of the body's natural defenses. When anything foreign enters the body, small blood vessels (capillaries) in the area get bigger (dilate), bringing more blood to the infected part. In the blood are white blood cells and other protective substances. Fluid (serum) and white blood cells pass through the capillary walls into the area and a wall is gradually built up around the foreign object. As the white blood cells try to destroy the invader, pressure builds up to force the material to the surface of the body. The inflammatory process takes place to some extent in the body whenever injury occurs. The signs and symptoms of acute inflammation are:

- Redness
- Swelling
- Heat
- Loss of function

Medical Specialties

The field of medicine has expanded so rapidly that many physicians have limited their practice to one area. These physicians are called specialists, Figure 6–15. The area of medicine in which they work is known as a medical specialty. Some of the major specialties are further subdivided. Figure 6–16 lists some of the medical specialties and describes the kind of care provided.

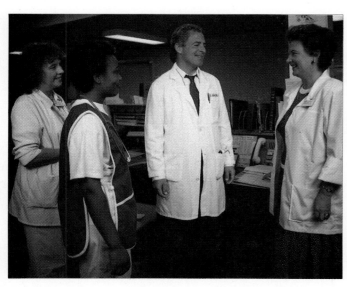

FIGURE 6–15. The internist is a specialist. Here he expresses pleasure to the staff about the patient's progress.

Nursing Specialties

Nurses are also practicing in specialty fields. Some common nursing specialties include:

- Maternal and child health
- Anesthesiology
- Gerontology
- Oncology
- Administration
- Public health
- Teaching
- Telemetry
- Surgery
- Home care
- Cardiac care
- Independent practice (nurse practitioner)
- Research

SPECIALTY	PHYSICIAN	TYPE OF CARE
Allergy	Allergist	Diagnoses and treats patients with hypersensitivities
Cardiovascular diseases	Cardiologist	Diagnoses and treats patients with diseases of the heart and blood vessels
Dermatology	Dermatologist	Diagnoses and treats patients with disorders of the skin
Gastroenterology	Gastroenterologist	Diagnoses and treats patients with conditions of the digestive system
Gerontology	Gerontologist	Specializes in diagnosing and treating conditions of the aging person
Hematology	Hematologist	Diagnoses and treats patients with diseases of the blood and blood-forming organs
Internal medicine	Internist	Diagnoses and treats patients with diseases and disorders of the internal organs
Neurology	Neurologist	Diagnoses and treats patients with diseases and disorders of the nervous system
Obstetrics	Obstetrician	Specializes in providing care to women during pregnancy, childbirth, and immediately thereafter
Oncology	Oncologist	Diagnoses and treats people with tumors
Ophthalmology	Ophthalmologist	Diagnoses and treats diseases and disorders of the eyes
Pediatrics	Pediatrician	Diagnoses, treats, and prevents disorders and diseases of children
Radiology	Radiologist	Diagnoses and treats disorders with X-rays and other forms of radiant energy

FIGURE 6–16. Medical specialties

SUMMARY

Disease has many forms and causes. Signs and symptoms are important indications of the presence of disease and must be carefully observed, reported, and recorded. Major disease conditions include:

- Congenital disorders
- Traumas
- Chemical imbalances
- Infections
- Ischemias
- Neoplasms

Once the diagnosis has been made, the therapy is prescribed. It may include:

- Surgery
- Chemotherapy
- Radiation
- Supportive care

The nursing assistant makes a valuable contribution to the nursing care process by accurately reporting pertinent observations.

UNIT REVIEW

A. Matching. Match the etiology with the type of cause of illness by matching Column I with Column II.

Column I	Column II
_____ 1. being elderly	a. specific cause
_____ 2. being under-nourished	b. predisposing cause
_____ 3. infectious micro-organisms	
_____ 4. blow from a broken branch	
_____ 5. electric shock	

B. Matching. Indicate which of the items in Column I is a sign and which is a symptom by matching Column I with Column II.

Column I	Column II
_____ 6. dry, flushed skin	a. sign
_____ 7. nausea	b. symptom
_____ 8. dizziness	
_____ 9. rapid pulse	
_____ 10. elevated temperature	

C. Matching. Match the abnormality with its classification by matching Column I with Column II.

Column I	Column II
_____ 11. abscessed tooth	a. ischemia
_____ 12. adenosarcoma	b. congenital
_____ 13. renal stones	c. infectious
_____ 14. thrombosis	d. inflammation
_____ 15. scarlet fever	e. metabolic imbalances
_____ 16. frostbite	f. traumas
_____ 17. osteoma	g. neoplasm
_____ 18. rheumatoid arthritis	h. obstruction
_____ 19. spina bifida	
_____ 20. sickle cell anemia	

D. Completion. Write out early signs of possible malignancies.

21. C _____

22. A _____

23. U _____

24. T _____

25. I _____

26. O _____

27. N _____

E. Matching. Match each diagnostic test in Column I with one word in Column II.

	Column I	Column II
_____	28. magnetic resonance imaging	a. invasive
_____	29. ultrasound	b. noninvasive
_____	30. lower GI series	
_____	31. X-ray	
_____	32. electromyogram	
_____	33. laryngoscopy	
_____	34. sigmoidoscopy	
_____	35. sonogram	
_____	36. upper GI series	
_____	37. myelogram	
_____	38. thermography	
_____	39. fluoroscopy	
_____	40. cystoscopy	
_____	41. electrocardiogram	
_____	42. sternal puncture	
_____	43. cardiac catheterization	
_____	44. electroencephalogram	
_____	45. tissue biopsy	

SELF-EVALUATION Section 2

A. Define the following words.

1. a cell _____

2. an organ _____

3. a system _____

4. neoplasm _____

5. etiology _____

B. Match Column I with Column II on planes and relationships.

Column I	Column II
_____ 6. above	a. midline
_____ 7. back	b. transverse
_____ 8. structure	c. frontal
_____ 9. divides the body into right and left sides	d. posterior
	e. anterior
	f. inferior
_____ 10. away from the midline	g. superior
_____ 11. front	h. anatomy
_____ 12. divides the body into upper and lower parts	i. physiology
	j. lateral
	k. medial
_____ 13. divides the body into back and front	l. dorsal

C. Choose the phrase that best completes each of the following sentences by circling the proper letter.

14. The tissue that carries messages is called
    a. epithelial.   c. muscular.
    b. connective.   d. nervous.
15. The tissue that protects, secretes, and absorbs is called
    a. epithelial.   c. muscular.
    b. connective.   d. nervous.

16. Included in the gastrointestinal system is/are
    a. stomach.   c. testes.
    b. ovaries.   d. adrenals.
17. Included in the respiratory system is/are
    a. lungs.   c. ovaries.
    b. stomach.   d. liver.
18. Included in the urinary system is/are
    a. gallbladder.   c. spinal cord.
    b. kidneys.   d. uterus.
19. Included in the nervous system is/are
    a. oil glands.   c. joints.
    b. larynx.   d. brain.
20. The small intestine is found in the
    a. peritoneal cavity.   c. spinal cavity.
    b. pelvic cavity.   d. thoracic cavity.

D. Match Column I with Column II.

Column I	Column II
_____ 21. an inadequate blood flow to an area	a. chronic
	b. acute
_____ 22. an abnormal condition that is present at birth	c. complication
	d. congenital
_____ 23. a condition that progresses rapidly and lasts a relatively short period	e. ischemia
_____ 24. a condition that persists over a long time	
_____ 25. a condition made more serious by another already existing condition	

E. **Complete the following statements correctly.**

26. Ultrasound is frequently performed on the uterus to give information about _____.

27. When a patient undergoes MRI, he will experience _____.

28. The examiner directly observes the _____ by using a proctoscope.

29. During a barium swallow, the patient swallows a barium solution while _____ are being taken.

30. Besides providing emotional support for patients during diagnostic procedures, the nursing assistant should:

   a. _____

   b. _____

   c. _____

F. **Select the correct spelling by circling the word.**

31. vane   vein   vien   vene

32. lateral   leteral   laterale   laterel

33. retenshion   retinshin   retenshon   retention

34. cardiak   cardiac   kardiac   kardiak

35. abdamen   abdomine   abdamin   abdomen

36. disurea   disuria   dysuria   dysurea

37. neoplasm   nioplasm   neoplasme   neoplasem

38. cachachia   cachaxia   cachoxya   cachexia

39. troma   trauma   tromma   traumer

40. protosols   protachols   protocols   protokols

G. **For each term in section F, write a definition.**

41. _____

42. _____

43. _____

44. _____

45. _____

46. _____

47. _____

48. _____

49. _____

50. _____

H. **Select five specialty fields of nursing practice.**

maternal and child health	anesthesiology
teaching	gerontology
administration	surgery
telemetry	public health
home care	independent practice
cardiac care	research

51. _____

52. _____

53. _____

54. _____

55. _____

I. **Match the physician and the type of care provided.**

____ 56. Allergist

____ 57. Gerontologist

____ 58. Obstetrician

____ 59. Ophthalmologist

____ 60. Radiologist

a. diagnoses and treats aged persons

b. diagnoses and treats disorders of the eye.

c. diagnoses and treats disorders through forms of radiant energy.

d. provides care for women during pregnancy and childbirth.

e. diagnoses and treats persons with hypersensitivities.

Principles of Observation and Communication

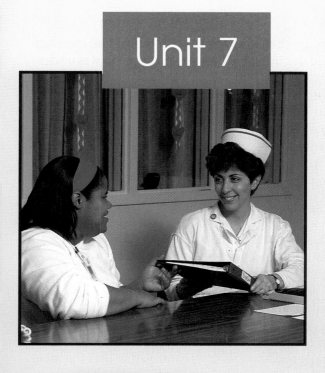

Yes

OBJECTIVES

As a result of this unit, you will be able to:

- Spell and define terms.

- Explain why observation is an important part of the nursing assistant's responsibilities.

- Explain the types of verbal and nonverbal communication.

- List the barriers to effective communication.

- Describe and demonstrate how to answer the telephone while on duty.

- Properly answer the patient's call bell.

- Describe and demonstrate an oral report about a patient to the team leader.

- Identify the steps in the nursing process.

- Explain the nursing assistant actions in relation to the nursing process.

- Name the components of the patient chart.

- Chart patient information appropriately (if facility policy permits).

VOCABULARY

Learn the meaning and the correct spelling of the following words and phrases:

assessment
body language
communication
charting
disk
DRG
evaluation
files
flow sheet
graphic chart
icon
implementation
Kardex
keyboard

menu
nonverbal communication
nursing care plan
nursing process
objective observation
observation
oral report
problem-oriented medical record (POMR)
SOAPIE
subjective statement
verbal communication

Communication is a two-way process. It is the way that information—whether it is facts or feelings—is shared. In order for communication to happen, both a "sender" and a "receiver" of the information are needed. Information can be sent orally, in writing, and through body language.

111

Nursing assistants communicate with their patients, Figure 7–1, with their coworkers, and with their supervisors when they are working. As a nursing assistant, you will need to receive and send information about your:

- Observations and care of patients
- Interactions with patients and visitors
- Patients' feelings

As a nursing assistant, you are a member of a nursing team. It is important that you communicate with the other members of the team. You must write down what you see. You must tell your coworkers and supervisors your thoughts and feelings as clearly as you can. Remember that it is very hard and possibly dangerous to work with someone who does not or cannot communicate well and effectively.

Communication Skills

Communication between staff members must be effective if the patient is to receive the safest and best care. Communication with your patients and their visitors is also important. You and your patients must understand each other. Visitors must know what you

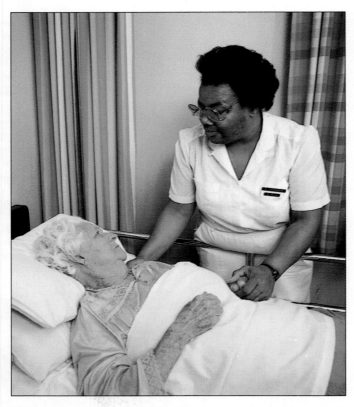

FIGURE 7–1. When you talk to your patients about their care, you will choose your words carefully.

are saying when you speak with them. The message you send out must be the same message that is understood.

There are three things needed for successful communication. They are (1) a sender, (2) a clear message, and (3) a receiver.

Information is communicated or made known to others in a variety of ways.

Verbal Communications

Verbal communication uses words. They may be spoken or written. You will use words to explain to patients what you plan to do in carrying out a procedure and how they can help. Your nurse or team leader will use words to explain your assignment. You will use words to report your observations, Figure 7–2. Visitors will use words to ask about visiting hours. You will use words to give them this information. Choose words carefully so that the message is clear. Did you recognize the fact that the nurse stressed that one of your patients must be given care early before going for tests?

Tone of voice, choice of words, and hand and facial movements give clues to the real meaning of the message. Listen carefully to the message in directions and assignments that are given to you. It is your responsibility to ask the team leader to explain something if it is unclear. Listen to the words that patients and others say.

Nonverbal Communication

Nonverbal communication is a message that is sent through the use of one's body, rather than through speech or writing. This kind of communication, called body language, can tell you a great deal. Often, nonverbal messages send even stronger signals than verbal messages. A patient who is in pain may protect the affected area. Tears or an unwillingness to make eye contact with you may be a sign of depression. Some of the other ways your patients may "talk" to you through their body language include:

- Posture
- Hand/body movements
- Activity level
- Facial expressions
- Overall appearance
- Body position

For example, does the patient say she feels well but is repeatedly rubbing her forehead?

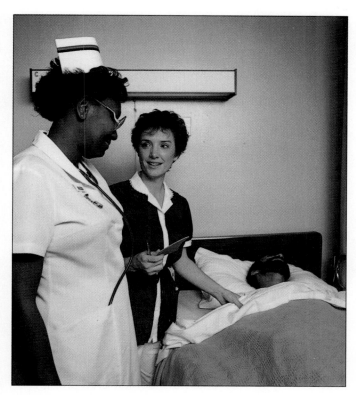

FIGURE 7–2. You will use correct terms to report your observations to the nurse.

Be sure your own language is accurate so that you will not confuse the listener by the message you send. Your body language also has meaning for your patient and coworkers, Figure 7–3. When you are in a hurry and your patient wants to talk with you, do you glance at your watch frequently? When your patient seems to take a long time to change his hospital gown, do you roll your eyes or tap your foot impatiently? Do you avoid eye contact with the patient who is dying? Do you draw pictures as your nurse explains your assignment? Do you look out the window as a visitor asks about her loved one? All of these nonverbal signals tell your patients, coworkers, and visitors how you really feel.

Barriers to Effective Communications

Special communication skills may be needed in some circumstances. For example, special skill may be needed when the:

- Patient is confused or speaks a different language. This patient may have trouble understanding anything but the simplest words or directions.
- Patient is hearing impaired. This patient may not be able to understand your words. You may need to use sign messages or written messages.
- Patient is blind. This patient will not be able to see your facial expressions. Your words and tone of voice will be even more important.
- Patient has aphasia and is not able to comprehend or communicate thoughts and ideas effectively.

Your attitude can also affect how well you understand and send messages. For example, when you are angry or anxious, you are apt to miss some of the key words. This is also true of patients who are angry or anxious. However, if you are open and willing to listen to what someone is saying, you hear more.

Improving Communications

Some things that you can do to improve communications are:

- Listen.
- Try to stay centered on the conversation. Do not, however, force the patient to continue if he/she becomes anxious or seems to wish to change the subject.

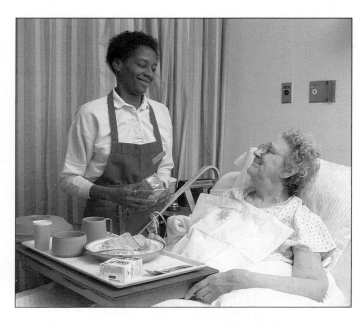

FIGURE 7–3. The warmth and rapport between the nursing assistant and the patient are clearly seen in their facial expressions.

- Use body language that indicates your interest and concern. Touch the patient, if it seems appropriate. Lean forward, listen intently, and maintain eye contact.
- Offer factual information. Do not insert your personal opinion into the conversation.
- Try to reflect the feelings and thoughts the patient is expressing by rewording questions.
- Give your coworkers your full attention.
- Ask questions to clarify unclear messages.
- Do not interrupt until the sender has completed the message.
- Provide a quiet environment without distractions.

Communicating with Patients

There are several points to keep in mind when communicating with patients. The first point is that you are there to provide care and support to the patient. Be open and gracious in all your interactions. Answer call bells promptly. Also:

- Make sure you have the patient's attention.
- Use words that are nonthreatening. For example, "This is what I would like to help you with," rather than "This is what I am going to do to you." "I am going to count your pulse," rather than "I am going to take your pulse."
- Speak clearly, courteously, and pleasantly.
- Respect another's space by not standing too closely.
- Use body language that is appropriate.
- Be alert to the patient's needs to communicate with you. Allow time for answers to your requests and to answer patient questions.

Answering the Call Bell

Each patient will have a call bell or signal light to communicate a need for assistance. Always answer call bells promptly, Figure 7–4. Because of age or weakness, some patients may find it difficult to use these devices. Be sure you pay extra attention to these patients. Make extra visits to their rooms. Stay alert for cries for help. When patients press the signal, it will show as a:

- Lighted room number at the nurse's station
- Light over the door of the room
- Light over the bed in the room

Answer call bells in the following manner:

- Locate the room and identify the patient.

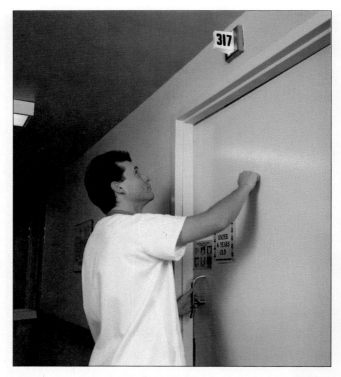

FIGURE 7–4. Call bells must be answered promptly. Knock before entering the patient's room.

- Turn off the signal so other staff members will know the light has been answered.
- If necessary, signal for assistance.
- Listen to the patient and respond to the request. If you are unsure of the safety or correctness of the request, tell the patient you will check with the nurse and return with an answer.
- Place the signal within easy reach of the patient before leaving.
- Before leaving, check the safety of the patient. For example, if the patient is in bed, the bed should be left at the lowest horizontal level. If the patient is in a wheelchair, the wheels should be locked.
- Report and, if appropriate, document your actions and the patient's response.

Communicating with Visitors

Visitors should be treated with the same good manners you would use if they were guests in your home. Remember that they are concerned and often very anxious about the loved one in your care. You represent the facility and staff to these people, Figure 7–5. Never get involved in fights between the patient and visitors. You should know:

- The proper visiting hours for your unit.

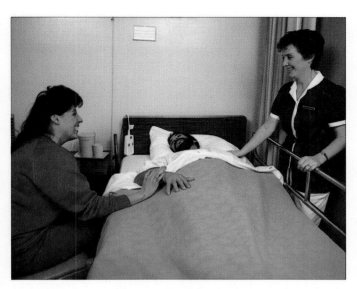

FIGURE 7–5. Remember when talking to visitors that you represent the facility to them.

- Restrictions to visitors. For example, people visiting a particular patient may be allowed to stay only for a certain length of time.
- That visitors are not allowed to bring food to the patient except under special circumstances.
- That stressful or tiring visits should be reported to the nurse.
- That requests for information about the patient's condition should be referred to the nurse.
- That information given to you by visitors or family members about the patient that might affect care should be reported to the team leader.
- How to make a proper report about visitor concerns or complaints to the team leader.

Answering the Phone

At some time while you are on duty, you may have to answer the unit phone, Figure 7–6. Your answer should be made in the following manner:

- Identify the unit.
- Identify yourself and your title.
- Ask the caller's name and ask her to wait while you get the person asked for, or
- Take a message, noting the date, time, caller's name, and telephone number.
- Sign the message with your name.

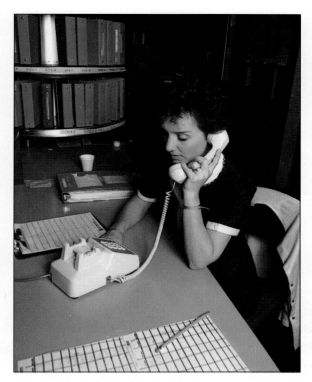

FIGURE 7–6. Identify yourself, your title, and the location of the unit when answering the telephone.

For example, if you are in the west wing on the fifth floor of the hospital and your name is Mrs. Brown, you might answer in this way: "5-west, Mrs. Brown, nursing assistant, speaking." Answering the telephone in this way lets callers know immediately if this is the unit they want and if you are an appropriate person to take their call. This is especially important in health care settings, since misspent minutes can mean endangering a life. For the same reason, a nursing assistant should never use the facility's telephone to make personal calls. Each facility has pay telephones for this purpose.

Communicating with Other Staff Members

Communications with other staff members take three forms, Figure 7–7:

1. Oral communications or reporting
2. Written communications in the form of:
   a. Nursing care plans
   b. Flowcharts
   c. Charting or documentation
   d. Assignments
3. Body language

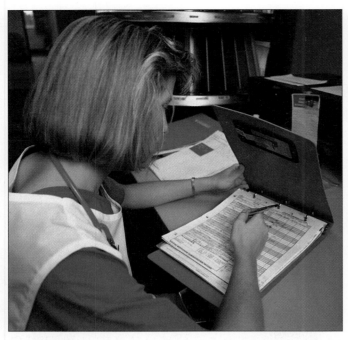

FIGURE 7–7. Information is made available to all staff members by recording it on the patient's chart.

Report

The **oral report** is used to make sure that all members of the health care team fully understand the nursing care that has been planned for each patient, Figure 7–8. The health care team on the oncoming shift takes the report from those who have cared for the patients during the previous shift.

From the report, you should learn the following information regarding each of your patients:

■ Name and location
■ Diagnosis (name of the patient's condition) and doctor
■ Special instructions for patient care
■ Update on patient's status or condition

If there is any doubt with regard to your assignment, clarify it with your charge nurse or team leader before you start to work.

You will usually make a report about your patient to the nurse just before the end of your shift. When it is necessary, you should report to the nurse at other times during your shift. You should report information on only one person at a time. Include in your report:

■ The identification and location of each patient
■ A discussion of the care you gave and anything you left undone
■ The patient's reaction and the observations you have made

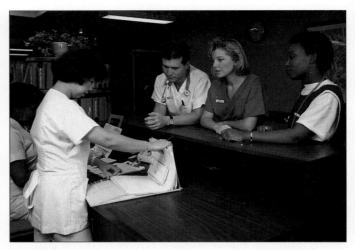

FIGURE 7–8. You should learn about any special care instructions during the oral report. The nurse uses the Kardex to review each patient's care plan.

■ Accurate, brief, but complete information
■ What the patient told you

Reporting in this way contributes to the evaluation step of the nursing process.

If, for some reason, you are unable to complete your assignment, make sure that the nurse knows exactly what remains to be done. You should never leave your assigned location without giving a report to your team leader. This is important whether you are going on a break or leaving for the day.

Observation

Observing patients is an important part of your job as a nursing assistant. An **observation** is an accurate, timely, and objective report, verbal or written, of a patient's condition. Observing means more than just looking at a person. To observe your patients properly, you must use all your senses. Note anything unusual or out of the ordinary. Report what you have observed to the nurse or team leader.

Observation of Normal Values

The nursing assistant must know the range of normal observations so that you will recognize that which is not normal. For example, the normal range of respirations is 16–20 breaths per minute in an adult. Respirations of 8 per minute should be reported to the nurse because the respirations are not within the normal range. The normal blood pressure in an adult is in the range of 120 mm Hg/80 mm Hg. A sudden change to 160 mm Hg/100 mm Hg should be reported.

Your eyes are a major asset when making patient observations. Be careful and consistent when making visual observations. With practice, you will develop the skill to quickly identify unusual situations and responses. Your other senses will also provide valuable information. For instance, you might note a change in skin color, a faster respiration, or the slowing of a pulse. You might smell a strange odor, hear a moan, or feel an unusual lump in the skin.

Observations by Body System

Try to establish a routine way of observing. Keep in mind the age, sex, and known illness of your patient. You might review each body system, noting the following:

- Integumentary system (skin, teeth, nails)— color; temperature; flexibility; dryness; clarity; moisture; areas of redness; any sores or bruises, swellings, scars, rashes, or other abnormalities
- Musculoskeletal system (muscles, bones joints)—deformities; ability to walk, sit or move; any pain associated with movement; posture, twitching, or abnormal movements
- Circulatory system (heart, blood vessels, blood)—skin color; heart rate; character of pulse; blood pressure, color of nails and lower extremities
- Respiratory system (upper respiratory tract and lungs)—any difficulty in breathing; cough; blueness of skin (cyanosis); shortness of breath on exertion or while still; rate of respirations; noisy respirations; crackles, wheezing, productive cough and type of mucus
- Nervous system (brain, spinal cord, nerves, sense organs)—response to questions (articulation and words); paralysis; orientation as to time or place; conditions of eyes and ears; level of consciousness
- Urinary system (kidneys, ureters, bladder, urethra)—frequency, amount and character of urination; inability to hold urine; drainage, if present; color of urine; blood, if present in urine, dysuria (pain on urination)
- Digestive system (true digestive organs and ancillary structures)—appetite; tolerance to foods; elimination problems such as diarrhea, constipation, gas, or incontinence; difficulty chewing or swallowing; color and consistency of stool, nausea and vomiting

Some patients have conditions that make special observations of particular importance. For example, a patient with pneumonia (a respiratory condition) should have respirations, temperature, cough, nature and amount of secretions, and skin color closely monitored. A patient with nephritis (a renal condition) should have intake and output volumes measured. He should also be checked carefully for fluid retention.

It is important for you to have some understanding of the condition and disease process. You will use what you know to detect important clues to the patient's status and disease progression.

Be objective in your observations. Report only facts. For example, you might report that the patient is complaining of pain in his stomach (an objective observation). You would not report that you guess he must have eaten something that did not agree with him.

Observations of Equipment and Environment

Observing the patient is a very important part of your job. You must also observe the environment and equipment that are used in patient care and treatment. For example, your patient is receiving fluids into a vein (IV infusion), Figure 7–9. In addition to your other duties and observations, you must check the:

- Level of fluid in the infusion container
- Rate of drops flowing

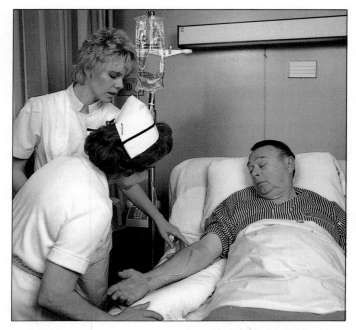

FIGURE 7–9.   The signs of inflammation and infiltration around the infusion site must be reported immediately.

- Lines (tubes) carrying the fluid into the patient's vein; lines must not be obstructed or twisted
- Point where the fluid enters the body (infusion site)
- Pumps in use are on and cycling

You must report the following observations:
- Inaccurate flow rates
- Blood in the lines
- Redness or swelling at the infusion site
- Containers before they are empty
- Sounding pump alarms

For example, if your patient is on urinary drainage, you must check and report:
- The amount of drainage
- The character of drainage
- Any changes in the amount or character of drainage
- Blockage of the drainage tubing

Equipment such as Aquamatic K® pads, traction, or oxygen sources must be checked for power source and proper function.

Always be on the lookout for safety factors. Equipment that is out of place, water on the floor, or frayed straps must be attended to if accidents and injury are to be avoided.

With practice you will be able to quickly recognize unusual situations and changes in your patient's condition. As you become more experienced, you will make many observations automatically as you enter any patient unit. For example, you will quickly note:
- Equipment failure
- Drainage and infusion rates
- Body position
- Changes in the patient's condition
- General appearance of the unit

You may be able to sense a problem or change before you actually discover its nature. Communicate your observations effectively, accurately, and objectively to the nurse.

The Nursing Process

The registered nurse coordinates the activities of all the care givers. The nurse ensures continuity of care, plans, evaluates, and assesses the patient to determine if common goals and expectations are achieved.

This framework for nursing action is called the nursing process. You can make a valuable contribution to this process by:
- Carrying out assignments carefully and accurately
- Being observant
- Reporting changes in condition promptly

The nursing process is developed in four basic steps. The nursing assistant contributes to and supports each action.

Steps of the Nursing Process

Nursing Action

Step 1: Assessment. Involves learning about the patient, his present problem and past history, Figures 7–10A and B. The nurse will interview the patient and complete a nursing physical and history. The information gained is then sorted and organized. Goals are stated. A nursing diagnosis is made. The diagnosis identifies the patient's problems and suggests a cause. For example, the nursing diagnosis may be "alteration in fluid volume related to decreased intake." The cause may be a sore mouth which limits intake of fluids.

Nursing Assistant Action

- Observe carefully during the admission procedure.
- Listen carefully to what the patient and his family say.

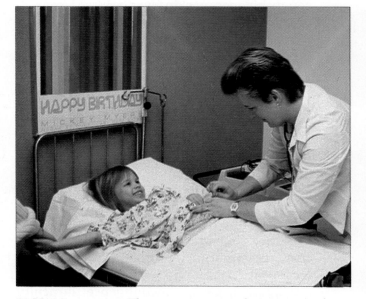

FIGURE 7–10A. The nurse assesses the patient's physical condition as part of the first step in the nursing process. *(Photo courtesy of Henrietta Egleston Hospital for Children, Atlanta, GA. Photograph by Ginger Lovering)*

PATIENT PREFERS TO BE ADDRESSED AS:

Carl

FROM: ☐ E.R. ☐ E.C.F. ☑ HOME ☐ M.D.'S OFFICE

COMMUNICATES IN ENGLISH: ☑ WELL ☐ MINIMAL ☐ NOT AT ALL

☐ INTERPRETER (NAME PERSON) ☐ NONE

MODE OF TRANSPORTATION:
☑ AMBULATORY ☐ OTHER **SMOKER:** Y ☐ N ☐
☐ WHEELCHAIR
☐ STRETCHER
☐ OTHER LANGUAGE (SPECIFY) _Spanish_
HOME TELEPHONE NO. (842) 7806
WORK TELEPHONE NO. (614) 7707

ORIENTATION TO ENVIRONMENT:
☑ ARMBAND CHECKED   ☑ CALL LIGHT
☑ BED CONTROL   ☑ PHONE
☑ TV CONTROL   ☑ SIDE RAIL POLICY
☑ BATH ROOM   ☑ VISITATION POLICY
☑ PERSONAL PROPERTY POLICY ☑ SMOKING POLICY

PERSONAL BELONGINGS: (CHECK AND DESCRIBE)
☐ CLOTHING _pajamas, Bathrobe, slippers_
☐ JEWELRY _1 plain yellow band_
☐ MONEY _$200_
☐ WALKER
☐ WHEELCHAIR
☐ CANE
☐ OTHER

DENTURES: ☑ UPPER ☐ PARTIAL ☐ LOWER ☐ NONE
CONTACT LENSES: ☐ HARD ☐ LT ☐ RT ☐ SOFT
GLASSES: ☑ Y ☐ N **HEARING AID:** ☐ Y ☑ N
PROSTHESIS: ☐ Y ☑ N
(DESCRIBE)

DISPOSITION OF VALUABLES:
☐ PATIENT
☑ HOME GIVEN TO: _R. Garcia_ RELATIONSHIP: _wife_
☐ PLACED IN SAFE _____ (CLAIM NO.)

IN CASE OF EMERGENCY NOTIFY:
NAME: _Rosa Garcia_
RELATIONSHIP: _wife_
HOME TELEPHONE NO. (842) 7806
WORK TELEPHONE NO. ( )

VITAL SIGNS
TEMP: 98.4 ☑ ORAL ☐ RECTAL ☐ AXILLARY
PULSE: 76 ☑ RADIAL ☐ APICAL RESPIRATORY RATE ____
B/P: 176/114 ☐ RT ☑ LT ☐ STANDING ☐ SITTING ☑ LYING
HEIGHT: 5'10" WEIGHT: 210 lbs ☐ BEDSIDE ☑ STANDING

ALLERGIES:
MEDICATIONS: ☐ NONE KNOWN FOOD: ☐ NONE KNOWN (SHELLFISH, EGGS, MILK, ETC.)
☐ PENICILLIN ☐ TAPE
☐ SULFA ☐ OTHER (LIST) _milk_
☐ IODINE
☑ ASPIRIN
☐ MORPHINE
☐ DEMEROL

MEDICATIONS: (PRESCRIPTIVE/NON PRESCRIPTIVE) DOSE/FREQUENCY LAST DOSE (DATE/TIME)
1. 2. 3. 4. 5. 6.

DISPOSITION OF MEDICATIONS:
☑ NONE BROUGHT TO HOSPITAL
☐ SENT HOME ____ WITH ____
☐ TO PHARMACY: (LIST)

ADMITTING DIAGNOSIS: _Hypertension_
NURSE'S SIGNATURE _B. Rodriguez L.N._ RN/LVN DATE ____ TIME 8 30/p

CHARTER SUBURBAN HOSPITAL
16453 SOUTH COLORADO AVENUE
PARAMOUNT, CALIFORNIA 90723
(213) 531-3110

NURSING ADMISSION ASSESSMENT PAGE 1 of 6

FIGURE 7–10B. The nurse records the patient's history in the assessment record. *(Courtesy Charter Suburban Hospital, Paramount, CA)*

PATIENT ASSESSMENT

PATIENTS STATED
REASON FOR ADMISSION: *un controlled hypertension.*

PRESENTING SYMPTOMS: *headache, flushed face, elevated B/P.*

D
E
T
O
X

O
N
L
Y

WHAT IS YOUR DRUG OF CHOICE? HOW MUCH HAVE YOU BEEN USING?
OVER WHAT PERIOD OF TIME, AND THE LAST TIME YOU USED? _____

HAVE YOU EVER HAD CONVULSIONS, HALLUCINATIONS OR MEMORY LAPSES?   ☐ Y ☒ N
HAVE YOU EVER BEEN IN ANY HOSPITAL OR FACILITY FOR: CHEMICAL DEPENDENCE OR ANY OTHER REASON?   ☐ Y ☒ N

PAST MEDICAL ILLNESSES:

☐ RESPIRATORY DISEASE   ☒ HYPERTENSION   DATE AND REASON FOR PREVIOUS HOSPITALIZATIONS:
  (COPD)
☐ CARDIAC DISEASE   ☐ OTHER (I.E. SURGERIES)
  (MI, ANGINA, CHF)
☐ DIABETES   *appendectomy   1977*   *acute appendicitis*

☐ CVA (STROKE)   *hemorrhoidectomy 1981* *external / internal hemorrhoids*

☐ CANCER

NEUROLOGICAL:

LOC: ORIENTATION:

☒ ALERT   ☒ RESPONDS TO VERBAL   ORIENTED TO: ☒ SELF ☒ PERSON ☒ PLACE ☒ TIME

☐ LETHARGIC   STIMULI   DISORIENTED TO: ☐ TIME ☐ PLACE ☐ PERSON ☐ SELF

☐ UNRESPONSIVE   ☐ RESPONDS TO PAIN ONLY

MOTOR ABILITY: ☒ FULL R.O.M.   ☐ LIMITED R.O.M (DESCRIBE) _____

AMBULATION: ☐ NEEDS ASSISTANCE   ☒ INDEPENDENT   ☐ TOTAL BEDREST

COMMUNICATION ABILITIES:

SPEECH: HEARING: VISION:

☒ ADEQUATE   ☒ ADEQUATE   ☒ ADEQUATE

☐ DEFICIENT   ☐ DEFICIENT   ☐ DEFICIENT

☐ UNABLE TO ASSESS   ☐ UNABLE TO ASSESS   ☐ UNABLE TO ASSESS
DESCRIBE   DESCRIBE   DESCRIBE
DEFICIENCIES: _____   DEFICIENCIES _____   DEFICIENCIES _____
                                                          Wears glasses

---

CARDIOVASCULAR/PULMONARY:

CHARACTERISTICS OF PERIPHERAL PULSES:

			LT	RT	
0 - ABSENT	4 - BOUNDING	CAROTID	✓	✓	☐ PERMANENT PACEMAKER
① PRESENT	⑤ STRONG	FEMORAL	✓	✓	NECKVIEN DISTENTION:
2 - WEAK	6 - REGULAR	RADIAL	✓	✓	☒ Y ☐ N
3 - THREADY	7 - IRREGULAR	PEDAL	✓	✓	☐ EDEMA ☐ NONE ☐ PITTING + ___

CHARACTERISTICS OF RESPIRATIONS:

☒ REGULAR   ☐ SHALLOW   ☐ ORTHOPNEA   ☐ DYSPNEA / S.O.B. ON EXERTION   ☐ KUSSMAUL

☐ IRREGULAR ☐ DEEP   ☐ DYSPNEA / S.O.B.   ☐ CHEYNE-STOKES

BREATH SOUNDS: ☒ AUDIBLE BILATERALLY

☐ CRACKLES (LOCATION)   ☐ RHONCHI (LOCATION)   ☐ WHEEZE (LOCATION)   ☐ DIMINISHED (DESCRIBE)

_____   _____   _____   _____

_____   _____   _____   _____

COUGH: ☐ Y   ☒ N   ☐ NON PRODUCTIVE   CONSISTENCY: _____
                    ☐ PRODUCTIVE   COLOR: _____

FIGURE 7–10B.   The nurse records the patient's history in the assessment record. (cont.)

INTEGUMENTARY:

COLOR: ☐ PALE ☑ FLUSHED ☐ CYANOTIC ☐ NORMAL ☐ OTHER _____

TEMP: ☑ WARM ☐ HOT ☐ COOL ☐ DRY/FLAKY ☐ DIAPHORETIC ☐ OTHER _____

INTEGRITY: ☑ INTACT

☐ WOUNDS/INCISIONS
(LOCATION/DESCRIBE)
_____
_____

☐ AMPUTATION
(DESCRIBE)
_____
_____

☑ SCARS
(LOCATION/DESCRIBE)
Rt. inguinal

☐ RASH
(LOCATION/DESCRIBE)
_____
_____

☐ ECCHYMOSIS
(LOCATION/DESCRIBE)

☐ LACERATIONS
(LOCATION/DESCRIBE)

☐ CONTRACTURE
(DESCRIBE)
_____
_____

☐ Other (GFT, AV Shunt, IV Access)
(LOCATION/DESCRIBE)
_____
_____

☐ PRESSURE AREAS
_____
_____
_____
_____
_____
_____
_____

LABEL FIGURE

W= WOUNDS   L= LACERATIONS
P= PRESSURE AREA   R= RASH
E= ECCHYMOSIS   S= SCARS

LEGEND: STAGES OF PRESSURE AREA

STAGE I: Reddened Area not Relieved by Local Circulatory Stimulation

STAGE II: Superficial Skin Break

STAGE III: Loss of Deep Skin, Drainage Present

STAGE IV: Full Thickness Loss of Skin, Invasion to Deeper Tissues, Necrosis Present

GASTROINTESTINAL:

ABDOMEN: ☑ SOFT ☐ HARD ☐ DISTENDED ☐ TENDER   BOWEL SOUNDS: ☑ PRESENT ☐ ABSENT ☐ HYPERACTIVE ☐ HYPOACTIVE

NUTRITION: SPECIAL DIET ☑ Y ☐ N IF YES, SPECIFY _Low salt_

PREFERENCES/DISLIKES _Dislikes Lamb_   NEEDS ASSISTANCE WITH FEEDING: ☐ Y   ☑ N

SPECIAL PROBLEMS (NO TEETH, LETHARGIC, DYSPHARGIA, NG TUBE, ETC.) _____
_____

GYN REPRODUCTION: ☐ N/A   DATE OF LMP _____

PROBLEMS (DESCRIBE) _____

BREAST/SELF-EXAM
☐ Y ☐ N

ELIMINATION: ☐ N/A

STOOL: ☑ VOLUNTARY ☐ INVOLUNTARY ☐ CONSTIPATION ☐ DIARRHEA ☑ REGULAR   DATE OF LAST B/M _3/8_

URINE: ☑ VOIDING ☐ INCONTINENT ☐ DYSURIA ☐ NOCTURIA ☐ FOLEY CATHETER ☐ EXTERNAL CATHETER INSERTED AT C.S.H: ☐ Y ☐ N

SPECIAL PROBLEMS _____

PSYCHOSOCIAL:

☐ APPROPRIATE	☐ DEPRESSED	☐ ANGRY	☐ SAD	☐ WITHDRAWN	☐ DEFENSIVE
☐ HAPPY	☐ ELATED	☐ CONVERSANT	☐ NON-CONVERSANT	☐ COOPERATIVE	☐ NON-COOPERATIVE
☐ APATHETIC	☐ FLAT AFFECT	☑ ANXIOUS	☐ CALM	☐ RESTLESS	☐ COMBATIVE

PATIENT LIVES: ☐ ALONE ☑ WITH SPOUSE ☑ WITH CHILDREN ☐ NURSING HOME (NAME) _____

☐ OTHER _____

VOCATION/AVOCATION: OCCUPATION _Fireman_

HOBBIES _Woodworking_   INTERESTS _Supports + is active in Boy Scouts_

FIGURE 7–10B. The nurse records the patient's history in the assessment record. (cont.)

CHARTER SUBURBAN HOSPITAL
PATIENT CARE PLAN

Bowen
827-654-82

Dr. Jajana

ADDRESSOGRAPH

DISCHARGE PLANS: _To extended Care facility when stable_

DATE	PROBLEMS/NEEDS/CONCERNS	EXPECTED OUTCOME/ SHORT TERM GOALS	APPROACHES/INTERVENTION	NURSES SIGNATURE
2/6	Fluid vol. deficit related to decrease fluid intake	Rehydrate/ Establish fluid balance	Force Fluid / I & O Continue IV.	J. Wilson, R.N
	Potential skin impairment related to immobility	Maintain skin integrity	Position qh ROM BID Heel protectors Check B/P q 4h	J. Wilson R.N.
	Potential for hypovolemia			

ROOM NO. _118 W_   NAME _BOWEN, JAMES_   RELIGION _PROT_   OCCUPATION _ACCOUNTANT Retired_

FORM NO. PGH-501

FIGURE 7–11A. The patient care plan *(Form courtesy of Charter Suburban Hospital, Paramount, CA)*

- Measure vital signs accurately.
- Report findings to the nurse.
- Report changes in the patient's condition, response, behavior.
- If permitted, chart or document according to facility procedure.

Nursing Action

Step 2: Planning. The nursing care plan is then prepared. It states the nursing actions to meet the specific patient needs, Figure 7–11A. The care plan is followed by all care givers. For example, the care plan for the dehydrated (fluid deficit) patient might include alternate ways to provide fluid.

Nursing Assistant Action

- Be informed of and follow the nursing care plan, Figure 7–11B.

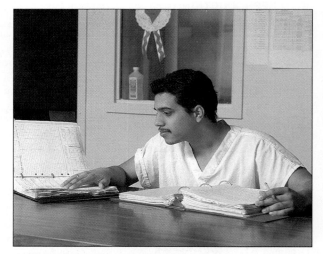

FIGURE 7–11B. Record your observations and actions on the nursing care plan or flow sheet.

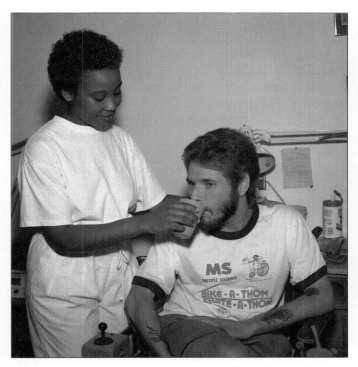

FIGURE 7–12. Following the care plan to improve hydration, you will encourage the patient to take fluids.

- If invited, participate in the planning conference.
- Question any part of your responsibility that is unclear.

Nursing Action

Step 3: Implementation. This step involves seeing that the care plan is followed, Figure 7–12. The efforts of all team members must be coordinated.

Nursing Assistant Action

- Carry out assignments correctly.
- Be willing to cooperate and help other team members.

Nursing Action

Step 4: Evaluation. The evaluation process determines how well the care goals have been met, Figure 7–13. Sometimes the nurse may make this determination alone. More often, however, the entire team discusses the patient's progress and contributes to additional planning.

Nursing Assistant Action

- Continue to report your observations.
- If invited, participate in the team conference.
- Review the new plans for care.

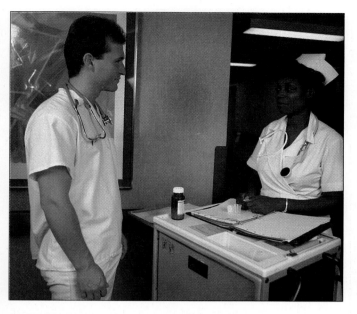

FIGURE 7–13. Report significant observations that can contribute to the ongoing evaluation of the patient's condition and progress.

Factors Influencing Care

Two factors influencing the delivery of care are the computer and diagnosis related groupings (DRGs).

Computers in Health Care

Management of information by computer is a way of life in many facilities. Computers will be more important in the future because of the increase in information to be processed, Figure 7–14.

All computers have a display screen and a keyboard. The keyboard is like the keyboard of a typewriter. The information typed appears on a screen. Computers use flat, square disks to store information. Some disks are flexible and others are hard. A disk has a menu that lists the types of information or files that can be opened, created, or edited on the disk. Icons are pictures or figures representing different functions. The various menu programs can be used by typing the proper codes.

If your facility uses computers to process information, you may be asked to use one for your documentation. You must learn how to use a computer correctly and be supervised until you become proficient.

The nursing process is helped by computers. They can:

- Maintain patient records. Care plans, physician's orders, and nursing assessments can be made instantly available.

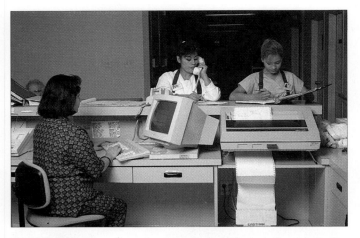

FIGURE 7–14. Computers are used in nursing to maintain records and serve as a valuable source of information and communication.

- Print protocols that can be individualized for each patient.
- Keep an inventory of supplies.
- Monitor the delivery of specific medications or treatments.
- Provide a bank of drug information.
- Schedule appointments.
- Help make more accurate diagnoses through computerized machines.

Computers provide an instant, current summary of data. Using this data, medical and nursing decisions can be made.

Diagnosis Related Grouping (DRGs)

In recent years, the cost of health care has increased steadily. The government has introduced a program to encourage hospitals to cut medical costs. There are 467 related diagnostic groupings or DRGs in this program. Hospitals are paid a specific amount of money for the care of an individual who has a particular condition or disease that is covered by a DRG.

If the hospital can provide the needed care and discharge the patient early, thereby saving costs, the hospital may then keep the difference. If, however, the person needs to be hospitalized for longer than expected and the costs are higher, the hospital absorbs the additional cost. These standards do not apply to private patients. They apply to those patients whose care is being paid for by the federal government, such as Medicare patients. Following hospitalization, many patients are discharged to long-term care facilities for additional rehabilitation or to home to finish recuperation.

The Nursing Care Plan

Written communications document observations, give directions for care to be given, and provide a record of the care that has been given and the patient's response. The general term for the process of recording this information is charting.

Nursing care plans are a required part of patients' records. Working from these plans, the nurse or team leader makes individual assignments to other health care providers for patient care. Nursing care plans are evaluated and revised periodically to reflect the patient's condition and progress.

Nursing care plans are often kept in a special place called the Kardex. The Kardex contains a separate card or form for each patient. The cards may be held in a folder or metal carrier. The nursing care plan developed for each patient is transferred to the Kardex so that it is readily available for reference by the staff.

In many facilities, nursing assistants are given directions for patient care activities on an assignment form. Special instructions or reminders may be put into the Kardex. Changes in the plan may be made as the patient's condition changes.

The Patient's Chart

Many members of the health care team, including nursing assistants, may be responsible for charting. The chart is a legal document. It may be called (subpoenaed) to court and read as evidence in legal actions.

It is important that each person know who is responsible for legal documentation. This responsibility varies from one type of facility to another and within a facility. The responsibility also varies from state to state.

Components of the Chart. Every patient has a chart, Figure 7–15. The chart usually consists of individual forms. These forms are filled with information about the patient. The following forms are usually included in the basic chart:

- Front sheet with information regarding sex, marital status, admission diagnosis, and employment
- Physical examination and a history record (maintained by the physician)
- Daily progress report (maintained by the physician)
- Graphic chart for recording temperature, pulse, and respiration rate

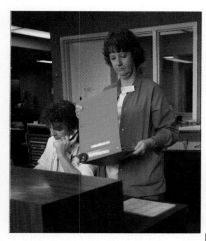

FIGURE 7–15. The charge nurse checks the progress and care in each patient's chart.

lating to temperature, pulse, and respiratory rates are marked along one side. Sometimes, blood pressure, voiding, and defecation are also charted on this sheet. Temperature, pulse, and respiration rates (TPRs) are plotted by placing solid dots on the lines that correspond to the readings and the time the readings were taken. For example, the graphic chart shows that on April 1 at 6 AM (0600), T=99.4, P=86, R=18; at 10 AM (1000), T=99.4, P=90, R=16.

Some health care facilities chart rectal temperatures in red. Others use red ink for all night charting (7 PM – 7 AM). An *R* should be placed above a rectal

■ Nurses' notes on which pertinent information regarding the patient is recorded by the nursing staff

Other record forms are added according to the patient's condition. All records are dated. They are identified with the patient's name, location, physician, and hospital number. Many health care facilities now use Addressograph cards which provide this information. If this is the policy at your facility, be sure every sheet is individually stamped. The two records that will be of most concern to you are the graphic chart and the nurses' notes. Sometimes the daily progress report and the nurses' notes are combined in one form. When this is the case, all personnel use the single form.

The Graphic Chart. The graphic chart varies in form, Figure 7–16, but it always has two basic markings. The time is marked in blocks across the top. Numbers re-

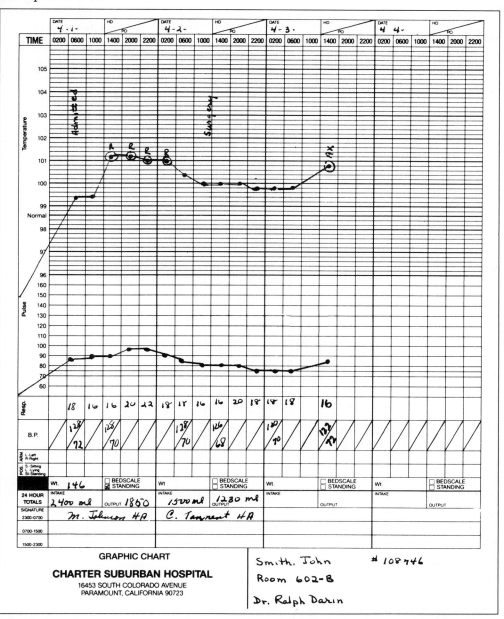

FIGURE 7–16. The graphic chart *(Chart courtesy of Charter Suburban Hospital, Paramount, CA)*

temperature reading (measured by placing the thermometer in the rectum). An *Ax* should be placed above an axillary temperature reading (measured in the axillary area).

Intake and output records of all liquids taken in or eliminated are kept on some patients, Figure 7–17. Totals are then computed for each shift and for 24-hour periods. A complete discussion of these records can be found in Unit 24 on recording intake and output. When more frequent recordings must be made, a special form called a *flow sheet* may be used.

Nurses' Notes

General Guidelines for Charting. Charting must be both accurate and easy to read.

- Print notations unless script writing is allowed by your facility.
- Use the color of ink that is correct for your service or time on duty. Some facilities state that all charting must be done in black ink. Black ink must be used when charts are to be microfilmed.

- Do not use the term *patient* since the entire chart concerns the patient.
- Use short, concise phrases.
- Always chart after the event.
- Always indicate the time of the event.
- Leave no blank lines.
- Sign each entry with your first initial and last name and title.
- Never erase or cross out an error. Draw a single line through the wrong entry. Print the word *error* and your initials.

Many health care facilities use computers to make recordkeeping easier. Charting in international time is becoming more common for use with computers. Using this system, time is not indicated as AM or PM. Twelve midnight (12 AM) is recorded as 2400, Figure 7–18. The new date starts at 2400 hours or 12:00 AM. For this reason, only the minutes are recorded for the first hour of the new day. For example, 12:10 AM is recorded as 0010. 12:10 PM is recorded as 1210. Also, 6:15 AM is recorded as 0615, and 1:20 PM is written as 1320.

Potterstown General Hospital
Fluid Intake and Output

Name Abrazzi, Cynthia #88-862-457   **Unit** 5-W **Rm** 118-B

Date	Time	Intake			Output			
		Method of Adm.	Solution	Amounts Rec'd.	Time	Urine Amount	Others	
							Kind	Amount
9/12	0700	P.O.	Water	6 z	0715	350 ml		
	0800	P.O.	Coffee Orange Juice	240 ml 120 ml				
	1030	P.O.	Sherbert	120 ml				
					1130	250 ml		
	1230	P.O.	Milk	240 ml				
	1400	P.O.	Water	150 ml				
Totals	1500			1050 ml		600 ml		

FIGURE 7–17. The intake/output chart

AM	INT'L. TIME
12 midnight	2400
1	0100
2	0200
3	0300
4	0400
5	0500
6	0600
7	0700
8	0800
9	0900
10	1000
11	1100
PM	
12 noon	1200
1	1300
2	1400
3	1500
4	1600
5	1700
6	1800
7	1900
8	2000
9	2100
10	2200
11	2300

FIGURE 7–18. International time

Charting Forms. How much routine care is to be charted depends on individual health care facility policy. However, anything out of the ordinary should always be charted. In other units of this text, specific patient procedures are introduced. These procedures and their effects need to be charted. This is done by noting that they have been done on the patient's chart. An example of nurses' notes can be seen in Figure 7–19.

POMR. Some health care facilities are taking a special approach to charting. All health team members use the same record to record observations and pertinent information about the patient. This record form is called a Problem-oriented Medical Record (POMR). Each recording is organized around a strength or problem of the patient. It includes a(n):

- Subjective statement. A subjective statement is a feeling expressed by the patient. An example is "I feel so hot."
- Objective observation. An objective observation is one made by a team member. An example is "Looks flushed and is sweating a great deal."
- Assessment. An assessment is a judgment about what was seen. An example is "Has temp 102°F orally."
- Plan. A plan is made for meeting the patient's needs. For example, "increase fluids, limit activity."
- Implementation. How the plan is put to work. "6 ounces H_2O P.O. Returned to bed."
- Evaluation. The patient is watched to see if the plan is working or should be changed.

Hospital __City General__   Case Number __108746__
                                          Doctor __W. Darin M.D.__
Name __Smith, Robert J.__   Room or Ward __602 – B__

Date	Time	Temp.	Pulse	Resp.	Urine	Stool	Treatment or Medication	Nourishment	Remarks
4-1-96	0730	99	84	20					65 yr. old male adm. to rm.
									602–B via wheelchair
							B/p 128/72		c/o "Cramp like abd. pains"
							wt. 146 lbs.		abd. distended
	0800				150 ml				to lab.
	0815						C B C		ordered
							Hinten		Dr. Darin notified
									J. Mathews, CNA
	0930						Darvon Comp. 65 mg.		P.O.
	1130							tea and dry toast	appetite good
	1200	99.4	88	18					c/o increased pain and
									abd. disten.
	1300						Harris Flush		given c̄ tap H_2O - 105°
									lg. amt. flatus expelled
									J. Mathews, CNA
	1600	99.4	88	22	150 ml		B/p 128/70		Coughing—had some diffi-
									culty holding thermometer
									in mouth
									R. Jones, CNA

FIGURE 7–19.   Sample nursing notes

The first letter of each concept spells SOAPIE. Some facilities add a final concept. This concept is

■ Revision. The plan is changed, if necessary.

This makes the form SOAPIER. You will be able to see that SOAP charting is a natural extension of the nursing process.

You will usually record only subjective and objective observations and report to the team leader. Figure 7–20 shows a sample charting using the SOAPIE approach. Notice that the date, the time, and the signature of the person recording are included for each recording. Each hospital may change these basic techniques of charting. Be sure you know which charting form is used at your facility.

Patient records:

■ Are private and confidential
■ Should be read only by authorized personnel

Be sure you know your facility's policy:

■ You are ethically bound never to reveal information about the patient to anyone.
■ Refer all questions to the nurse.

SUMMARY

Communication is a two-way process of sharing information. Communication must be clear between health care providers, patients, and those in authority. Communications are sent through oral or verbal language, body language, and written messages.

Information that is written on patient records is confidential and must be accurate, clean, concise, and legible. Documentation must be in the form that is accepted by your facility.

UNIT REVIEW

A. True/False. Answer the following statements true or false by circling T or F.

T F 1. Communication is a two-way process of sharing information.

T F 2. All senses should be used in making observations.

T F 3. When making an observation related to the digestive system, color of the skin should be considered.

T F 4. Verbal messages are those that are sent with words.

T F 5. Body and hand movements can sometimes send a message that is different from the words spoken.

T F 6. When answering a call bell, leave the call light lighted until you have helped the patient so other staff members will know you are in the room.

T F 7. Always identify your title when answering the facility phone.

T F 8. The name of the patient's condition is the prognosis.

T F 9. The framework for nursing action is called the nursing process.

T F 10. DRGs are related to the amount of money hospitals are reimbursed for the care of Medicare patients.

B. Completion. Record the following TPRs on the practice graphic chart provided.

	Day 1	Day 2	Day 3
0800	99.6—88—20	98.6—72—18 (axillary)	97.2—68—16
1200	99.4—84—18	98.4—72—16	97.6—64—16
1600	99.4—80—18	101.4—82—20	99—72—18
2000	101—92—20 (rectal)	101.6—88—22	99.8—74—18
2400	102.2—96—22 (rectal)	103—92—20	100—80—18

NURSING NOTES

DATE: Dec. 31	NOTES:
1500	PROBLEM: PAIN IN CHEST
	S: "I HAVE A TERRIBLE PAIN IN MY CHEST. I'M GOING TO DIE."
	O: GRASPS CHEST
	A: IN PAIN, EXPRESSING FEAR OF DEATH
	P: CHARGE NURSE NOTIFIED IMMEDIATELY B. LESLIE, N.A.
1505	S: "HURRY UP, I'M GOING TO DIE."
	O: LABORED BREATHING
	A: MEDICATION NEEDED TO RELIEVE PAIN
	P: NITROGLYCERINE 0.4MG SUBLING GIVEN
1525	E: MEDICATION RELIEVED CHEST PAIN AND BREATHING IS LESS LABORED P. RYDER, R.N.

Atlantic Hospital	Bruce James 123456 146-B S. White, M.D. Patient Record

FIGURE 7–20. A sample charting using the SOAPE approach

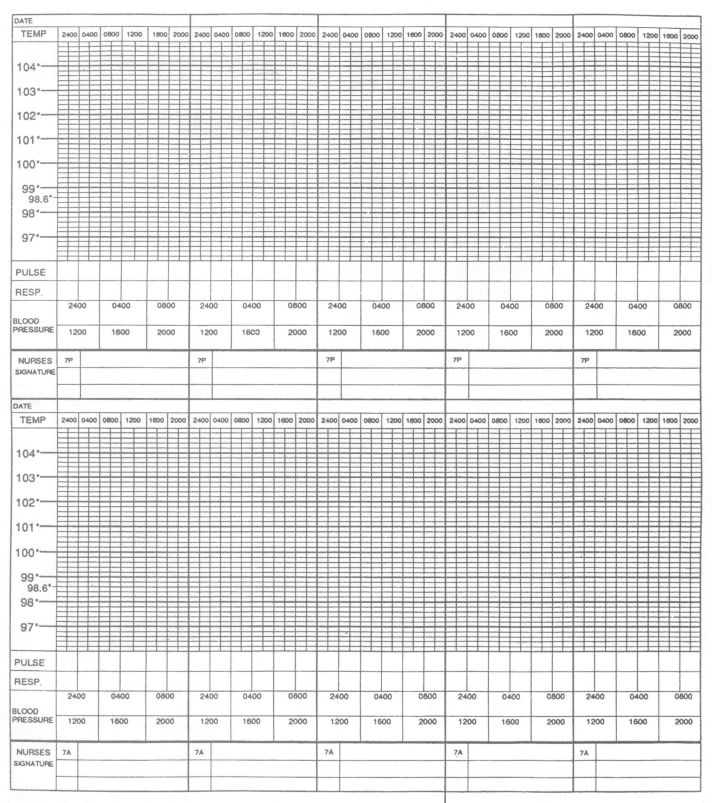

BAY HARBOR REHABILITATION CENTER
GRAPHIC CHART

02-6190-02   Rev. 6/92

(Courtesy of Bar Harbor Rehabilitation Center, Torrance, CA)

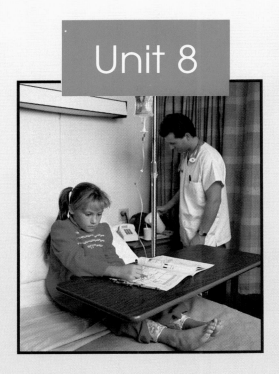

Meeting Basic Human Needs

OBJECTIVES

As a result of this unit, you will be able to:

■ Spell and define terms.

■ Describe the stages of human growth and development.

■ List some physical and emotional needs of patients.

■ List the main reasons patients have difficulty sleeping.

■ Define self-esteem.

■ Describe how the nursing assistant can meet the patient's emotional needs.

■ Discuss methods of dealing with the fearful patient.

■ List nursing assistant actions to ensure patients have the opportunity for intimacy.

■ List the guidelines to assist patients in meeting their spiritual needs.

VOCABULARY

Learn the meaning and the correct spelling of the following words and phrases:

adolescence
bisexuality
celibate
coitus
continuum
development
gavage
growth
heterosexuality
homosexuality
intimacy
intravenous infusion (IV)
masturbation

neonate
orthopneic
personality
preadolescence
reflex
self-esteem
self-identity
tasks
tasks of personality development
toddler
total parenteral nutrition (TPN)

Each of us has things that we need to live successfully. These are called "needs" simply because we cannot get along without them. When a patient is admitted to the hospital, these needs come too. The difference now is in the way these needs are expressed and fulfilled. Expression and fulfillment have to be different because of the hospital environment and the illness. Remember that the basic needs remain the same, regardless of how they are expressed or how they have to be met because of an individual's level of development or state of health.

Neonate	Birth to 1 month
Infancy	1 month to 2 years
Toddler	2 years to 3 years
Preschool	3 years to 5 years
School Age	5 years to 12 years
Preadolescent	12 years to 14 years
Adolescence	14 years to 20 years
Adulthood	20 years to 50 years
Middle Age	50 years to 65 years
Later Maturity	65 years to 75 years
Old Age	75 years and beyond

FIGURE 8–1. Stages of growth and development

Human Growth and Development

Human beings change as they age through the processes of growth and development. Growth involves the changes that take place in the body. It is usually measured in height and weight and degree of system maturation. Development involves the changes that take place on a social, emotional and psychological level. Developmental levels are shown in behavior and interpersonal skills.

People move from one level of development to the next, Figure 8–1. At each level, they change in both the way they look and in the way they think and act, Figure 8–2. Each level presents tasks that must be mastered before the person can move on to the next level.

The tasks to be mastered are those things that lead to healthy and satisfactory participation in society. The tasks are defined by the needs of the individual and the pressures of society.

Sometimes growth spurts occur and developmental skills must catch up. Both growth and development progress from simple to complex. Each is dependent upon the other to achieve the orderly progression. For example, the child cannot be toilet trained until the nerve pathways have matured.

Growth and development follow a set of basic principles of progression.

- There is a continuous movement from simple to more complex. For example, baby sounds progress to speech patterns.
- Development and growth move from head to feet and from torso to limbs. The infant's head is raised, followed by sitting, standing, and finally walking.

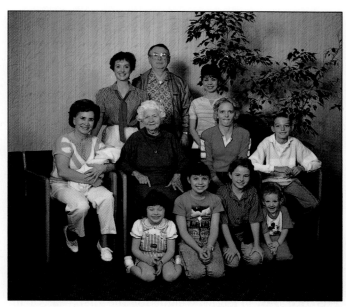

FIGURE 8–2. Continuum of life. The characteristics of the different age groups are reflected in this group picture.

- Each stage of development has a specific set of tasks that the person must master before successfully moving on to the next level. For example, the child learns to catch big balls before she can catch a baseball.
- Progression moves forward in an orderly manner, but the rate varies for each person. There are growth spurts in the preschool and teen years, but not all children grow to the same extent or at the same rate.
- Growth patterns progress at their own individual rate.

Neonatal and Infant Period (Birth to 2 years)

The neonatal and infant period extends through the first two years of life. It is a time of rapid physical growth and development, Figure 8–3. The infant gradually learns to:

- Sit
- Crawl
- Stand
- Take first steps

Other changes occur during this period:

- Emotional attachments move from self-awareness and parental or care-giver attachment to ties with other family members.
- Systems that are relatively immature at birth become more stabilized.
- Alertness and activity increase.
- Teeth appear (erupt).

AGE (Months)	HEIGHT (Inches)	WEIGHT (Pounds)
Birth	20	7–8
1 Month	21 1/4	7 1/2
2 Months	22 1/2	10
3 Months	23 3/4	11 1/2
4 Months	24 3/4	12 1/2
5 Months	25 1/2	14
6 Months	26	15
7 Months	26 3/4	16 3/4
8 Months	27 1/2	18
9 Months	28	19
10 Months	28 1/2	20
11 Months	29	20 3/4
12 Months	29 1/2	21 1/2
Remember that the figures are averages only.		

FIGURE 8–3. Height/weight for the first year of life (boys)

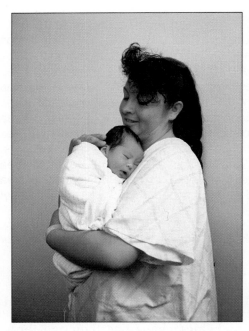

FIGURE 8–4. This newborn weighs 7 pounds 12 ounces and is 19-1/2 inches long.

■ Food intake progresses from milk to solid food.
■ Verbal skills begin to develop.

The mother or primary care giver of the infant is the central figure of emotional attachment. Growth and development progress so rapidly that changes can be seen each month.

The **neonate** (newborn), Figure 8–4:

■ Weighs 7–8 pounds
■ Is approximately 20–21 inches long
■ Has a head that seems disproportionately large compared to the body
■ Has skin that is wrinkled, thin, and red
■ Has an abdomen that seems to stick out (protrude)
■ Has dark blue eyes

In the newborn the:

■ Conversion of cartilage to bone (ossification) is not complete. This can be seen in the soft spots (fontanels) and suture lines (joints) of the skull.
■ Nervous system is not fully developed so muscular activities are uncoordinated.
■ Vision is not clear, but hearing and taste are developed. Certain **reflexes** (automatic responses) are also developed. They are the:
— Moro reflex—when a loud noise startles the infant, the arms are spread across the chest, the legs are extended, and the head is thrust back. This response is also called the startle reflex.

— Grasp reflex—touching the infant's palm causes the fingers to flex in a grasping motion.
— Rooting (sucking) reflex—stroking the cheek or side of the lips stimulates the infant to turn his head in the direction of the stroking. This is important in finding the nipple to suck the milk.

■ Diet is milk or milk substitute.
■ Routine is largely sleeping, eating, and eliminating.

The neonate is completely dependent on the care giver for all needs. The infant is unable to support her head so must be handled carefully and be well-supported when held.

The three-month-old infant:

■ Has gained enough muscular coordination to hold her head up and raise her shoulders.
■ Has lost the Moro, rooting, and grasp reflexes.
■ Produces real tears.
■ Can follow objects with his eyes.
■ Can smile and coo at the care giver.

The six-month-old infant:

■ Has learned to roll over.
■ Can sit for short periods of time.
■ Holds things with both hands and directs them toward his mouth.

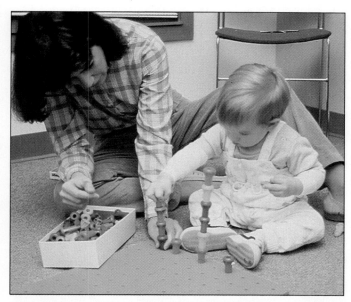

FIGURE 8–5. The toddler begins to develop gross manual skills. (*Photo courtesy of Henrietta Egleston Hospital for Children, Atlanta, GA. Photograph by Ginger Lovering*)

■ Responds with verbal sounds when care giver speaks.
■ Is beginning to cut front teeth.
■ Eats finger foods and strained fruits and vegetables.
■ Recognizes family members.
■ Develops fear of strangers.

The nine-month-old infant:
■ Crawls and may begin to stand when supported.
■ Has more teeth erupt.
■ Can respond to her name.
■ Says one- and two-syllable words such as "mama."
■ Shows a preference for right- or left-hand control.
■ Eats junior baby foods.

The one-year-old infant:
■ Understands simple commands such as "No."
■ Begins to take steps—supported at first, then independently.
■ Eats table foods and can hold her own cup.
■ Weighs three times what he weighed at birth (Refer to Figure 8–3).

Toddler Period (2 to 3 years)

The **toddler** period is a busy, active phase. It is a period in which exploration and investigation are the main activities. It is also a period in which motor abilities develop, Figure 8–5, and vocabulary and comprehension increase.

During this period, the toddler:
■ Learns to control elimination.
■ Begins to become aware of rights and wrongs.
■ Often reacts with frustration and negative responses to attempts at socialization and discipline as she becomes more aware of herself as a separate person.
■ Tolerates brief periods of separation from mother, but mother still remains the source of security and comfort.
■ May play in the company of other children but with no interaction. This age group is very possessive. "No" and "mine" are a major part of their vocabularies.

Reaching the end of this period, the toddler is able to:
■ Walk and run.
■ Display motor (manual) skills that include feeding and riding toys.
■ Put words together and speak more clearly. The average vocabulary of a 2-year-old is about 300 words.
■ Play near others, but is not able to interact in play with children of the same age (peers).

Preschool Years (3 to 5 years)

The 3- to 5-year-old, Figure 8–6, builds on the motor and verbal skills developed as a toddler.

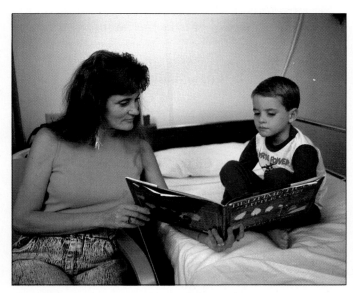

FIGURE 8–6. Growing less dependent upon mother, the preschooler expands his awareness of the world around him.

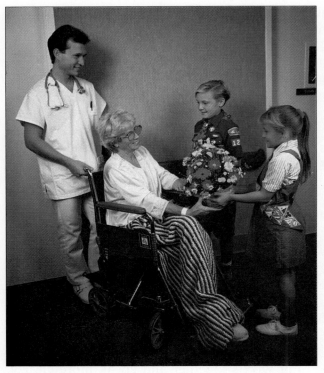

FIGURE 8–7. The school-age child joins groups like Scouts that help to identify the child as a person of a particular sex.

During this period, the preschooler:
■ Grows less reliant on mother. This age group begins to recognize its position as a member of the family unit and its uniqueness from other members.
■ Develops rivalries with siblings and develops greater attachments to the father or alternate care giver.
■ Gradually increases cooperative play.
■ Improves language skills and asks many questions.
■ Develops a more active imagination.
■ Becomes more sexually curious.

By the end of this period, children have become far more socialized than they were as toddlers. They are more cooperative. They seem almost eager to follow established rules within limits. They enjoy interacting with family members and peers.

School-age Children (6 to 12 years)

The school-age child, Figure 8–7:
■ Is able to communicate.
■ Has developed small motor skills. With these skills, the child is able to master tasks such as writing.

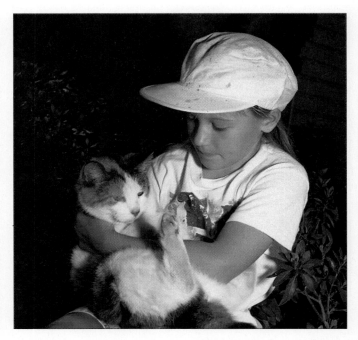

FIGURE 8–8. The young person develops motor skills and learns to reach out with concern for other living things.

■ Develops an increased sense of self.
■ Establishes peer relationships.
■ Reinforces proper social behavior through games, simple tasks, and play.
■ Chooses sex-differentiated friends.
■ Joins groups like Scouts. This serves to further identify the individual as a person of a particular sex.
■ Begins to show concern for other living things, Figure 8–8.

Preadolescent (12 to 14 years)

Preadolescence is a transitional stage, Figure 8–9. It is a period of great uncertainty.
During this period:
■ Hormonal changes stimulate the secondary sex characteristics.
■ The individual feels on the threshold of tremendous change, though not yet in a period of sexual functioning.
■ Mood swings and feelings of insecurity are common.
■ There is a growing awareness of and interest in the opposite sex.
■ Arms and legs seem out of proportion to the rest of the body.

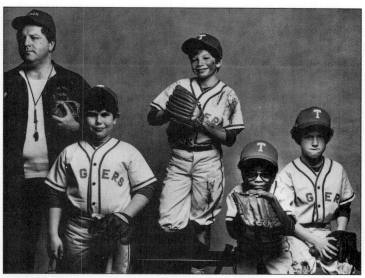

FIGURE 8–9. Peer relationships are important to the pre-adolescent who is developing awareness of himself as a sex-identified individual. *(Photo courtesy of Hollister Incorporated, Libertyville, IL)*

Adolescence (14 to 20 years)

Adolescence, Figure 8–10, is marked by:
■ The gradual development of sexual maturity.
■ A greater appreciation of the individual's own identity as a male or a female person.
■ Conflicting desires for the freedom of independence and the security of dependence. Because of these conflicting desires, this is often a troublesome period.

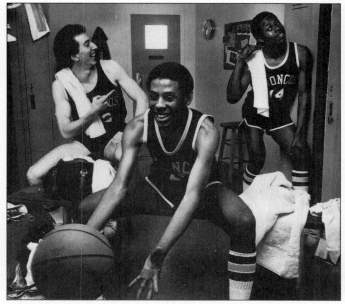

FIGURE 8–10. Adolescents are able to make independent judgments. *(Photo courtesy of Hollister Incorporated, Libertyville, IL)*

■ The establishment of personal coping systems and the ability to make independent judgments and decisions.
■ Gradual success in mastering the developmental tasks of the age. The adolescent is able to make comparisons between the values she has been taught and reality.

Adulthood (20 to 50 years)

Early adulthood, Figure 8–11, is marked by:
■ Independence and personal decision making
■ The choice of a mate
■ Establishment of a career and family life
■ Optimal health
■ The choice of friends to form a support group

Middle Age (50 to 65 years)

Middle age is frequently associated with:
■ Final career advancement, ending in retirement
■ Children who were reared during the period of adulthood leaving home to enter their own adult period

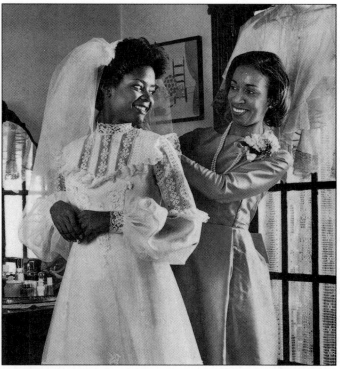

FIGURE 8–11. During adulthood, people establish families and careers. *(Photo courtesy of Hollister Incorporated, Libertyville, IL)*

- Health that is usually still at good levels, but some slowing may be seen
- Futures that are less certain, and more time that can be spent on leisure activities
- Financial pressures for those middle-aged persons who still have responsibilities for their own aging parents as well as for their children. The financial needs often complicate the planning of the individual's own retirement.

Later Maturity (65 to 75 years)

Later maturity is marked by:
- A gradual loss of vitality and stamina
- Physical changes that signal the aging process. For example, sight and hearing diminish
- Chronic conditions that develop and persist
- A period of gradual losses: loss of mate, friends, self-esteem, some independence
- Depression
- Examination of a lifetime

Support groups established in the adult and middle years can provide valuable help and social contacts. Persons in later maturity can function as important role models for younger age groups. The longer the person is independent, the more positive the changes during this period.

Old Age (75 years and beyond)

Old age is frequently characterized by:
- Failing physical health and growing dependency, Figure 8–12
- The need to deal with illness, loneliness, loss of friends and loved ones, and the realization of mortality

Success in this final period depends upon the mechanisms of coping which the older adult has developed over the years. The extent of available emotional and physical support is also important.

Basic Human Needs

Developmental skills and physical growth may vary during the life span. The basic human needs, however, are much the same for every individual.

Basic human needs are those activities required by all people to successfully and satisfactorily live their lives. The needs are the same for all people at all ages. Cultural backgrounds influence the way in which individuals express these basic needs. Culture refers to those customs and practices that are common to groups of people that become ingrained beliefs, habits, and responses. Culture embraces language, di-

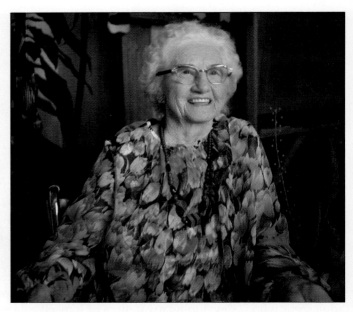

FIGURE 8–12. Physical status declines and dependency grows.

etary habits, health practices, expressions of spirituality, and ways of celebrating.

These cultural patterns are part of the uniqueness of each individual and must be considered when providing for the person's care.

Abraham Maslow and Erik Erikson are two leaders in the field of human behavior. They have helped us understand the basic needs and how people go about satisfying them.

Personality

Exactly how each person goes about satisfying personal psychological needs reflects his personality. Personality is the sum of ways we react to the events in our lives. It is gradually formed through experience and molded by cultural heritage.

Erikson suggested that our personalities are formed as we mature from infancy to old age. He believed that we pass through eight growing stages in search of who we really are (self-identity). During each stage, there are choices to be made before moving on to the next task. He called these the tasks of personality development, Figure 8–13.

Maslow dealt with human needs by describing them as physical, psychological, and sociological. He placed the needs on a continuum in which physical needs had to be satisfied first. The psychological or sociological needs could be met only after the physical needs had been satisfied, Figure 8–14. Note that the progression of needs also is called a hierarchy of needs.

Physical Stage	Year of Occurrence	Tasks to Be Mastered
Oral-sensory	Birth–1 year (Infant)	To learn to trust (Trust)
Muscular-anal	1–3 years (Toddler)	To recognize self as an independent being from mother (Autonomy)
Locomotor	3–5 years (Preschool years)	To recognize self as a family member (Initiative)
Latency	6–11 years (School-age years)	To demonstrate physical and mental skills abilities (Industry)
Adolescence	12–18 years	To develop a sense of individuality as a sexual human being (Identity)
Young Adulthood	19–35 years	To establish intimate personal relationships with a mate (Intimacy)
Adulthood	35–50 years	To live a satisfying and productive life
Maturity	50+ years	To review life's events and examine how they have influenced the development of a unique individual (Ego integrity)

FIGURE 8–13. Tasks of personality development according to the stages defined by Erikson.

Physical Needs

The most basic human needs are physical needs. They include:

- Nutrition
- Rest
- Oxygen
- Elimination
- Activity
- Sexuality

Illness at any age creates stresses that make meeting the needs a challenge for both patient and care givers.

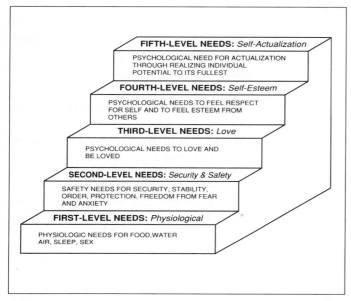

FIGURE 8–14. Maslow's hierarchy of needs

Meeting the Patient's Physical Needs

You will need to provide for the physical needs of your patients. They are the need to be sheltered, to breathe, to eat, to sleep, and to eliminate waste products.

Shelter. In the health care facility, the need to be sheltered is considered when the proper environment is maintained. Some examples include making sure that:

- The bed is comfortable and secure.
- Side rails are up when needed, Figure 8–15.
- Beds are left in the lowest, horizontal position.
- The patient is kept safe and warm.

These seem like simple requirements. By paying attention to safety details, however, you give the patient a real sense of security. Protection is the basis of this first physical need. Every patient has the right to feel cared for and safe.

Oxygen. Most of us take breathing for granted. We hardly give it more than a passing thought until it becomes difficult. There are many reasons that cause people to have difficulty in breathing. When they do have difficulty, though, the need is always the same. The body cannot live without oxygen, which is found in the air. It may be necessary, therefore, to supply the patient with an increased amount of oxygen and moisture to ensure that body tissues receive enough oxygen. Oxygen by cannula or mask may be used for

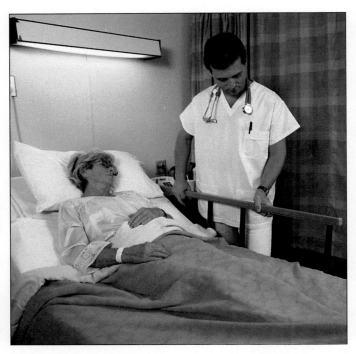

FIGURE 8–15. Side rails can contribute to a safe and secure environment.

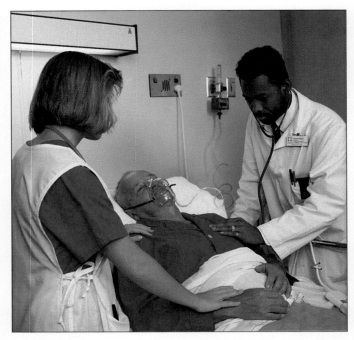

FIGURE 8–16. Oxygen may be delivered by a specially designed mask.

this purpose, Figure 8–16. Sometimes this need can be met by adjusting the over-bed table in such a way that the patient, supported by pillows, is able to lean on it. This position is called the orthopneic position.

Food. Patients are known to lose their appetites when they are in the hospital. Decreased appetite and intake of fluids may be due to:

- Inactivity
- Hospital odors
- Pain
- Fear and anxiety
- Types of food served
- Illness itself
- Age of the patient

Some patients have to be fed because of their condition. Some may be given only special foods. Some are unable to take food in the usual way. Some patients are given liquid nourishment through a tube that has been passed through the nose and into the stomach. Feeding through a tube is called gavage. Fluid replacement may also be given through a sterile tube into the veins. This process is known as intravenous infusion (IV). Nourishment may be provided through a major vessel, usually the subclavian vein. This process is known as Total Parenteral Nutrition, or TPN.

Since patients receive nourishment in such a variety of ways, you need to see to the special needs of each individual. There are, however, some general points to keep in mind:

- Appetites improve when food is served at the proper temperature in pleasant surroundings.
- Bathroom doors should be closed and room deodorants used for unpleasant odors.
- Unneeded equipment should be removed from sight.
- Cultural preferences should be considered.
- Patients should be prepared by allowing them to wash hands and face. Help them sit up in bed or get out of bed, if permitted.
- The tray should be offered in a calm, pleasant manner, even if the food is not what you like. Even a bland diet offered in this way is more acceptable.
- Patients should be allowed to do as much as they are able for themselves. Be available, however, to assist if needed.

Sleep. Noise and pain are the main reasons patients have difficulty sleeping. You should:

- Control noise whenever possible.
- Handle equipment carefully.
- Reduce the volume on television.
- Limit conversation with coworkers.
- Use a lowered voice.
- Keep the door to the patient's room closed.

To help the patient fall asleep, a few extra moments of your time is well spent in giving a soothing back rub, providing a change of position, and making the bed neat. Sometimes medication is needed to help the patient sleep. The patient is completely prepared for sleep before the nurse gives the medication. By doing this, the patient will not have to be disturbed after being medicated.

Worry also plays a role in a patient's sleeplessness. Patients worry about many things, such as:

- What the future will bring
- How much the hospitalization will cost
- Who is taking care of their home and work responsibilities

You will not have the answers to all these pressing concerns. You can listen, however. Share these concerns with the nurse. This is not gossiping. The nurse and the other members of the staff may be able to help the patient solve the problems. With worries reduced, the patient will rest easier.

Elimination. To stay healthy, the body must be able to rid itself of perspiration, urine, and feces properly. Elimination is promoted by:

- Bathing, which helps get rid of perspiration and keeps the skin healthy.
- Encouraging the patient to drink 6–8 glasses of fluids and, if possible, eat foods high in bulk.
- Providing additional help, if needed, to relieve the patient's body of waste. A sterile tube (catheter) is inserted into the urinary bladder and the urine is drained out. The sterile catheter may be left in the bladder to provide constant drainage. The tube is then attached to a bag which collects the urine. Enemas, laxatives, and suppositories help the bowels get rid of solid wastes in the form of feces.
- Helping patients who are unable to use the usual toilet facilities, by providing them with bedpans, urinals, and bedside commodes.

When you are helping the patient meet elimination needs, always remember the patient's right to privacy must be respected. Do this by:

- Keeping exposure to a minimum
- Screening the unit and leaving until the patient is finished, if the patient's condition permits
- Leaving a signal bell close at hand
- Providing a bedpan or urinal as soon as it is requested
- Being sure to check and remove the bedpan promptly

- Cleaning the patient, if necessary, in an efficient and tactful manner

Physical Activity. People, by nature, are active beings. When illness occurs, it often limits activity. Sometimes the patient must stay in bed for a long period of time. The staff must find ways to promote appropriate activity for these individuals. The capability of the patient and the goals of treatment must be kept in mind when the activity level of any patient is established.

Prolonged inactivity in bed is very dangerous for the patient. It has a negative effect on all body systems. There are, however, some actions that nursing assistants can carry out to diminish some of the negative effects.

Negative Effect of Immobility	Nursing Assistant Action
■ Loss of skeletal muscle tone and strength	Carry out range-of-motion activities as ordered
■ Formation of blood clots	Check for skin color, pain, temperature, and indication of inflammation; report all observations Do not massage legs Apply support hose (TED hose)
■ Development of contractures	Change position frequently (as ordered) Perform range-of-motion exercises Keep body aligned, and position with appropriate support
■ Fluid and electrolyte imbalance	Record intake and output Encourage fluids Report signs of edema, weakness, or slow response Report changes in vital signs Assist to upright position on bedpan to encourage complete emptying of the bladder

Negative Effect of Immobility	Nursing Assistant Action
◼ Poor cardiac and respiratory function	Check color and vital signs, and report Change position as ordered Encourage coughing and deep breathing
◼ An alteration in hormone levels	Collect urine samples as ordered
◼ Loss of calcium and bone mass with an increase in bone calcium and calcium excretion in the urine	Monitor input and output Report sediment in urine Use care in handling
◼ Infection	Report signs of infection such as elevated temperature, dyspnea, increased respiratory rate, cough
◼ Loss of appetite and constipation	Encourage food intake and fluids; record amounts Report amount and character of bowel movements; provide privacy
◼ Skin breakdown	Bathe skin and dry carefully Apply lotion Change position as ordered Report evidence of skin redness/breakdown
◼ Altered emotional response such as frustrated, angry outbursts	Be patient and understanding Do not take outbursts personally
◼ Diminished or inaccurate sensory interpretations	Listen carefully to patient's concerns Spend time talking with the patient Increase sensory stimuli as much as possible Keep room well lit

Activity promotes generally improved functioning of all systems. Circulation and respiration are increased. Muscles, bones, and joints function more adequately. The body, as a whole, responds in a positive way to activity.

When patients are unable to carry out activity, such as walking, getting in and out of bed, and using the bedpan or commode independently, you may have to help them, Figure 8–17. Be sure you are aware of the patient's limitations, as well as the degree and type of activity allowed. Do not allow patients to become either over-stressed or tired.

Emotional Needs

Emotional needs are the next level of Maslow's hierarchy of needs. The basic emotional needs are the same at any age. There is a need:

- ◼ To give love
- ◼ To feel love
- ◼ To be loved
- ◼ To be treated with respect and dignity
- ◼ To feel that self-esteem (our opinion of ourselves) is protected

All individuals—you, your coworkers, and your patients—have in their own minds an idea of how they appear and wish to appear to others. This idea is referred to as self-esteem. A person's self-esteem must be protected at all costs.

For example, a person might visualize and project to others the image of a very self-reliant person,

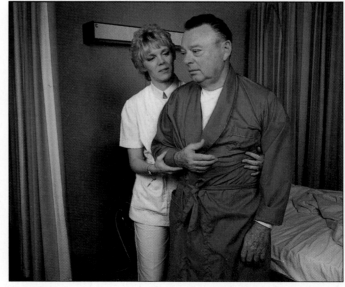

FIGURE 8–17. You may need to help the patient with physical activity to the degree permitted by the patient's condition.

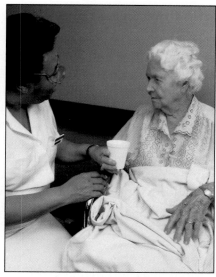

FIGURE 8–18. Much patience sometimes is needed to break through a wall of fear and frustration.

capable of making important decisions, and able to care for self and family. Suddenly that same person is scantily dressed in a hospital bed. A stranger is taking care of her most intimate physical functions. Even the times to eat and bathe are decided for her. This set of circumstances threatens even the most secure person's self-esteem.

How patients respond to this threat to their self-esteem depends on two things. First, it depends on how often each patient has had these feelings of helplessness before, and how well they have dealt with them. Second, it depends on you and your ability to appreciate those feelings.

One patient may feel frustrated and angry. She may not even know that it is out of fear. The patient may act out these feelings by complaining about the hospital, the staff, roommates, you, or the food. In fact, every aspect of the care may be cause for complaint. Be open and receptive to these actions, recognizing the underlying feelings.

Still another patient may react quite differently to the same emotional stress. That person may be quiet and withdrawn. She may be completely cooperative and noncomplaining, Figure 8–18. The behavior shown is a false front. It hides the patient's feelings of not being able to cope with the situation. The nursing assistant must be aware of these feelings and the need for caring support.

Intimacy Needs

Intimacy is a feeling of closeness with another human, Figure 8–19. It is a relationship marked by feelings of love. It is an integral part of human response.

Intimacy may be shared between friends or lovers. Also, a degree of intimacy is established when patient and care giver learn they can trust and have confidence in each other.

Intimate relationships may be sexual and expressed in different ways. Humans express sexual intimacy depending on orientation, preference, opportunity, and moral standards. Sexual behavior is a personal choice, but intimacy is an important aspect of the human sexual experience.

Each intimate relationship has an element of commitment. Sometimes this commitment includes a sexual aspect, and sometimes it does not. For example, a loving couple may choose not to have sexual intercourse. Despite remaining celibate (no sexual intercourse), they still share an intimacy and commitment that is natural and fulfilling.

It is important to recognize that not everyone has the same orientation, preference, opportunities, or moral standards. This does not mean that differences make one person wrong and another right. As a care giver, you must be understanding of others who may not share your personal views.

Some terms related to human sexual expression are:

■ **Heterosexuality**—sexual attraction between opposite sexes.

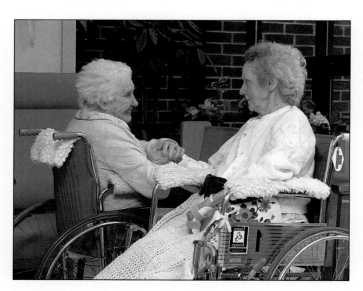

FIGURE 8–19. Intimacy is feeling close with another person.

- **Homosexuality**—sexual attraction between persons of the same sex. Female partners are called lesbians.
- **Bisexuality**—sexual attraction to members of both sexes.
- **Masturbation**—self-stimulation for sexual pleasure.

The range of expressing love is enormous. Genital and nongenital caressing, exchanging loving gestures, talking, and touching are all ways love is expressed between people. **Coitus** (intercourse), although an enjoyable part of many relationships, is not always necessary for satisfaction.

Opportunities for patients to meet sexual and intimate needs in a health care setting are not always easy. However, there are some actions that nursing assistants can do to help patients meet these needs:

- Respect patient's privacy. Always knock and wait before opening a closed door.
- Speak before opening curtains drawn around the bed.
- Do not judge behaviors and preferences that are different from yours as wrong.
- Do not discuss personal sexual information about a patient with others.
- Provide privacy if a patient is masturbating.
- Discourage patients who make sexual advances to you. State in a calm, matter-of-fact way that you are not interested and move on to other work. If a patient persists, report the matter to the nurse.
- Recognize that the need for intimacy is a basic human need that is expressed in many ways.

Human Touch

The need for human touch should not be overlooked. Pleasure and satisfaction are felt by a parent and child as they touch one another. The same human feelings are also experienced by adults.

As people grow older, they tend to reserve touching for intimate friends and family members. When circumstances change and opportunities for touching become fewer, people often feel deprived and lonely. This is especially true when one lives alone or is a resident in long-term care.

A friendly hug and smile, a pat on the shoulder, a clasp of a hand, and a back rub are ways nursing assistants can satisfy the patient's need for human contact. Never force your attentions on a patient, but be open to nonsexual touching. It can mean much to the lives of those in your care.

Dealing with the Fearful Patient

The experienced nursing assistant does not take remarks personally. The assistant realizes that the patient's complaints and refusal to cooperate may be a way of saying, "I need to be reassured and protected." Give the patient an opportunity to talk. Listen carefully to everything that is said, Figure 8–20. You may be able to convince the fearful patient to assume some personal care whenever possible. If help in feeding, shaving, elimination, or other such personal matters is needed, act in a very gentle, efficient manner and assure the patient's privacy at all times.

To handle these situations successfully, the nursing assistant must:

- Recognize that this patient is a person with individual likes and dislikes.
- Give the quality of care that considers these likes and dislikes.
- Help the patient find ways to occupy all the empty time while in the hospital, Figure 8–21. Boredom alone can lead to irritability. Some hospitals have volunteers who bring books and other activities directly to the bedside.

Patients in the hospital give up a good bit of control over their lives. They put their lives and well-being into the hands of care givers. In exchange, patients assume that certain of their rights will be assured. These rights include the right to privacy.

Patients must feel assured that their privacy will be protected. Even though you perform the most intimate procedures for them, you must do so in a way that neither exposes them unnecessarily nor embarrasses them.

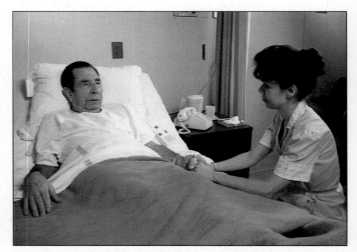

FIGURE 8–20. Successful communication is a two-way exchange.

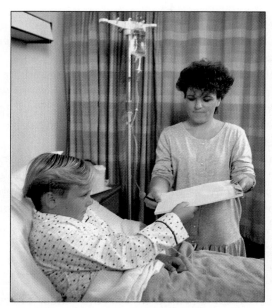

FIGURE 8–21. Activities help pass the time during convalescence.

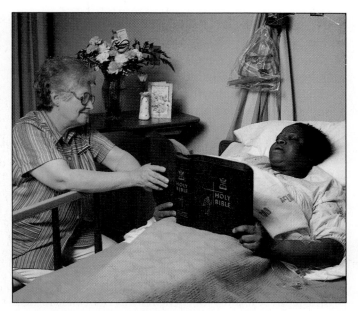

FIGURE 8–22. Spiritual needs are often greater when the patient is ill.

Privacy may be provided by means of:
- Curtains or screens, placed around the bed
- Knocking and saying the patient's name before entering a room
- Speaking to the patient before entering a screened area. Privacy must be provided for the patient who is:
  — Bathing
  — Using the bedpan
  — Receiving treatments
  — Being visited by clergy

Be prompt at other times to recognize a patient's need for privacy and to provide it.

Patients must also be secure in knowing that personal information they share with you will not be told to others. You add to the patients' sense of security if you always treat them with the courtesy you would extend to a guest in your home.

Understanding what patients are really trying to tell us is one of the most difficult parts of giving nursing care. When we are successful, it is probably the most rewarding. With this in mind, always remember to treat the patient as a unique individual.

Spiritual Needs

Spiritual beliefs are deeply held by some patients and disregarded by others. When beliefs are strongly held they are apt to guide a patient's actions and responses in direct ways such as praying, reading religious writings, and participating in ceremonies and celebrations. Some articles may have special religious significance and must be treated with respect.

The spiritual needs of the patient are often greater when fearful and ill, Figure 8–22. Be prepared to act on requests for clergy visits and spiritual support. Do not impose your beliefs on the patient.

There is always the temptation to share your personal religious faith with others. This is especially true when the patient directly asks your opinion. To appropriately handle such a situation is a challenge. Here are some guidelines to assist you.

- Remember that each person has a right to believe in any faith system or to deny the existence of any beliefs.
- You should listen to the patient's thoughts and keep them confidential.
- Your role is to reflect the patient's ideas. Do not try to convince the patient of your ideas. For example, if the patient asks you if you believe in God, reflect the patient's thinking with a statement such as "You have been thinking about God." or "Would you like to talk?"

The patient may want to visit with a familiar clergy member, or may ask about the chaplain or clergy service available at the health care facility.

Some health care facilities ask clergy from the community to make visits to patients who desire a visit, but who do not know a particular minister, priest, or rabbi. Larger facilities have chaplain educational residencies for people preparing for a clerical career. The residencies serve patients' spiritual needs while offering training for the chaplains.

Chapels are open in some facilities. Both visitors and ambulatory patients often find comfort in visiting them. Religious services are sometimes broadcast to patients' rooms from these chapels.

Get to know the services available to your patients. When asked, share this information, but do not recommend any particular service. Patients should be free to make their own choices. You should always be ready and willing to support the choice.

Social Needs

When primary physical, psychological, and spiritual needs are met, the person is free to pursue the third level of social needs and activities that are unique to the individual. These activities make one feel good as a person and increase self-esteem. They promote a sense of accomplishment. Sociological needs are met by interactions with others and opportunities for free personal expression.

One of the most basic needs of all people is the need to understand others and to be understood. We achieve this sense of understanding when we communicate successfully with others. We usually try to communicate verbally. Sometimes we do this also by the:

- Words we choose
- Way we say the words
- Tone of voice
- Facial expression
- Form of touch

Even the way we stand or reach out says a lot. We know it is not always easy to find the right words to express our thoughts and feelings. Thus, care givers must be constantly aware of the patient's need to communicate effectively, too.

Volunteers and visitors as well as television and reading can provide diversion for the patient who is confined. Try to find out about your patients' special interests. Look for ways to support them in these interests.

If all care providers are interested and unhurried in talking with their patients, they make it easier for patients to say what they need. This approach also makes it easier for the staff to find proper ways to fulfill these needs.

SUMMARY

Individuals develop at varying rates. There are, however, some well-defined developmental stages through which each person passes.

- Certain developmental skills are characteristically acquired at certain stages of life—from birth to death. A person's success in mastering these skills affects the progress of his development.
- Regardless of developmental level, people have common basic emotional and physical needs.
- The nursing staff must be sensitive to the influence of culture or the expression of individual needs.
- The way these needs are expressed varies, especially when a person is ill.
- The nursing staff must be sensitive to these individual needs. They must find ways of successfully providing for them.

UNIT REVIEW

A. Completion. Complete the following sentences.

1. Self-esteem means _____
   _____ .

2. The chief reasons patients have difficulty sleeping are _____
   _____ .

3. Waste products that need to be eliminated from the body are _____
   _____ .

4. Gavage is a technique used to _____
   _____ .

5. An experienced nursing assistant never takes a patient's remarks _____
   _____ .

B. Matching. Match the person with the appropriate chronologic age by matching Column I and Column II.

Column I	Column II
_____ 6. old age	a. 65 years old
_____ 7. adolescence	b. 16 years old
_____ 8. later maturity	c. 7 years old
_____ 9. school age	d. 35 years old
_____ 10. adulthood	e. 80 years old

C. Define the following terms.

11. Growth _____

_____ .

12. Development _____

_____ .

13. Developmental tasks _____

_____ .

D. True/False. Answer the following statements true or false by circling T or F.

T F 14. Growth and development progress from the simple to the complex.

T F 15. Body development proceeds from the head toward the feet.

T F 16. All individuals move through the stages of growth.

T F 17. Growth and development progression is interdependent.

T F 18. Ossification of bones is not complete at birth.

T F 19. The Moro reflex occurs when the infant's palm is touched.

T F 20. The sucking reflex occurs when the infant is startled.

T F 21. The three-month-old infant cries real tears.

T F 22. The six-month-old infant can walk if well-supported.

T F 23. First teeth begin to erupt about the sixth month of life.

T F 24. The one-year-old infant has progressed to eating table foods.

T F 25. The toddler period finds children interacting freely and playing well with one another.

T F 26. Between the ages of 3–5 years, the child seems to have an endless list of questions.

T F 27. The school-age child is interested in and chooses members of the same sex as close friends.

T F 28. One of the developmental tasks of old age is to learn to successfully deal with loss.

T F 29. Basic human needs are the same at all ages, but different ways must be found to satisfy them.

T F 30. Erikson believed that one of the developmental tasks of infancy is learning to trust.

T F 31. Erikson states that the developmental task of the middle years is to integrate life's experiences.

T F 32. Patients who are fearful often behave in angry or frustrated ways.

T F 33. Spiritual needs are part of basic human needs.

T F 34. Culture has no influence over how basic human needs are met.

SELF-EVALUATION Section 3

A. Match the observations in Column I with the systems in Column II. (Each may be used more than once.)

Column I	Column II
_____ 1. orientation to time and place	a. circulatory
_____ 2. shortness of breath	b. musculoskeletal
_____ 3. frequency	c. urinary
_____ 4. diarrhea	d. nervous
_____ 5. scars	e. respiratory
_____ 6. dryness	f. digestive
_____ 7. cough	g. integumentary
_____ 8. increased pulse rate	
_____ 9. inability to see	
_____ 10. wheezing	

B. Choose the phrase that best completes each of the following sentences by circling the proper letter.

11. Communications are transmitted in
    a. words.
    b. facial expression.
    c. body language.
    d. All of these.

12. A key to successful relationships is to remember
    a. all patients react to stress the same way.
    b. words alone communicate feelings and thought.
    c. people always say exactly what they mean.
    d. each person is unique.

13. The spiritual needs of people
    a. are less when they are sick.
    b. may be disregarded because physical needs come first.
    c. are usually greater when they are sick.
    d. do not change when they are sick.

14. If a patient expresses a desire for a visit from the clergy, you should
    a. call your rabbi.
    b. let the nurse know.
    c. tell the patient he is going to get better and doesn't really need a clergyperson.
    d. call the clergy.

15. Factors influencing patient appetites include
    a. inactivity.
    b. hospital odors.
    c. pain.
    d. All of these.

16. Breathing needs can be aided by
    a. keeping patients flat.
    b. positioning the patient properly.
    c. withholding oxygen.
    d. making the patient ambulate more.

17. Your patient is having trouble sleeping. You may help by
    a. giving medication for pain.
    b. allowing the patient to talk with you.
    c. disconnecting the IV.
    d. giving the patient a full meal.

18. Patients consider their problems
    a. less important than your own concerns.
    b. equally important to the problems of roommates.
    c. most important.
    d. less important than the concerns of other staff members.

C. Identify the age group with its characteristic by matching Column I and Column II. (Each may be used more than once.)

Column I

_____ 19. gradual loss of vitality and stamina

_____ 20. rapid growth and system stabilization

_____ 21. careers and families established

_____ 22. associated with final career advancement

_____ 23. desire for independence and security make this a turbulent period

_____ 24. period of beginning physical sexual changes

Column II

a. infancy
b. preschool
c. school age
d. preadolescent
e. adolescent
f. adulthood
g. middle age
h. later maturity
i. old age

D. Provide short answers to the following.

25. List three ways the nursing assistant can support the nurse for each of the steps of the nursing process.

Step of Nursing Process		Nursing Assistant Action
Assessment	a.	_____
	b.	_____
	c.	_____
Planning	a.	_____
	b.	_____
	c.	_____
Implementation	a.	_____
	b.	_____
	c.	_____
Evaluation	a.	_____
	b.	_____
	c.	_____

E. Complete the following statement correctly.

26. Write the appropriate nursing assistant actions that should be taken in each situation.

Negative Effects of Immobility	Nursing Assistant Actions
a. Loss of skeletal muscle tone	_____
	_____
	_____
	_____
b. Poorer cardiac and respiratory function	_____
	_____
	_____
c. Skin breakdown	_____
	_____
	_____
	_____
d. Diminished or inaccurate sensory interpretations	_____
	_____
	_____

F. Answer the following statements true or false by circling T or F.

T F 27. Intimacy is a feeling of closeness experienced with another human being.

T F 28. All intimate relationships are sexual in nature.

T F 29. Touching another person is a form of expressing intimacy.

T F 30. Skin contact is an important way of receiving and giving pleasure and satisfaction.

T F 31. Human intimate sexual expression may take many forms.

T F 32. Masturbation is self-stimulation for sexual pleasure and must not be permitted.

T F 33. The homosexual is sexually attracted to members of the opposite sex.

T F 34. Sexual preference is a personal matter and may or may not conform with the personal preference of the nursing assistant.

T F 35. Intimate relationships include an element of commitment between two persons.

T F 36. Standing too close to someone can be interpreted as invading personal space.

T F 37. Flow sheets are special record forms that are used when patients are progressing well and few notations need to be made.

T F 38. Printed nursing care protocols need to be individualized for each patient.

T F 39. All documentation is done exactly the same in every facility.

T F 40. Spiritual beliefs are often a strong guide to patient reactions and behaviors.

T F 41. Documentation must conform to the policy for each facility.

T F 42. Only authorized persons may read patient records.

T F 43. Questions about patients may be discussed with visitors.

T F 44. It is permissible to try to convince a patient that your personal beliefs are correct.

T F 45. Culture has no real influence over a patient's responses to illness and treatment.

46. Culture includes:

    a. _____

    b. _____

    c. _____

    d. _____

    e. _____

Unit 9

Basic Medical Asepsis

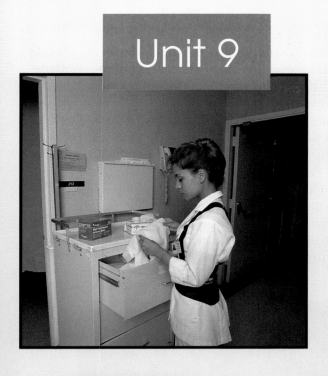

Contributed by Mary Jo Conaway, RN, MS
Nurse Epidemiologist
Mission Regional Medical Center
Mission Viejo, CA

OBJECTIVES

As a result of this unit, you will be able to:

- Spell and define terms.
- Identify the most common microbes and describe their shapes and characteristics.
- List the six components of the chain of infection.
- Name three specific microbes and the disease conditions they cause.
- List ways disease-producing microbes are transmitted and controlled.
- Demonstrate the procedure for handwashing.
- Demonstrate the procedure for removal of contaminated gloves.

VOCABULARY

Learn the meaning and the correct spelling of the following words:

aerobic
agent
allergies
anaerobic
antibodies
asepsis
autoclave
bacillus, bacilli
bacteria
bacteriocide
carrier
causative agent
chain of infection
clean technique
coccus, cocci
colony
contamination
culture
diplo-
disinfection
excreta
flora
fomites
fungus
host
hyperbaric chamber
infectious
immune response
immunization
medical asepsis
microbe

microorganism
mold
nonpathogen
nosocomial
organism
parasite
phagocyte
pathogen
portal of entry
portal of exit
protozoa
replication
reservoir
saprophytic
spirillum, spirilla
spore
staining
staphylo-
sterile field
sterile technique
sterilization
strepto-
surgical asepsis
susceptible host
toxins
transmission
universal precautions
vector
virus
yeast

Humans are surrounded by a world of tiny **organisms**, (living beings). These beings cannot be seen with the naked eye. They make their presence known only by their effect. This is much the same way that we are aware of the wind. We cannot see it either. We are aware of it because of its effect on the trees, which bend and sway.

These organisms can be seen only with a microscope, Figure 9–1. They are everywhere—in us, on us, and around us. They are:

- On our skin
- In our mouths
- Within our bodies
- In and on the food we eat
- On what we touch or handle

Micro means small. Because these organisms (**agents**) are so tiny, they are called **microorganisms** or **microbes**. The organisms live in relationship with us and with each other.

Many of these microbes are useful to us. They are called **nonpathogens** because they do not produce disease. They help in the

- Processing of cheese, beer, and yogurt
- Curing of leather
- Baking of bread

Other microbes are not useful. Microbes that cause disease in humans are called **pathogens** or pathogenic organisms.

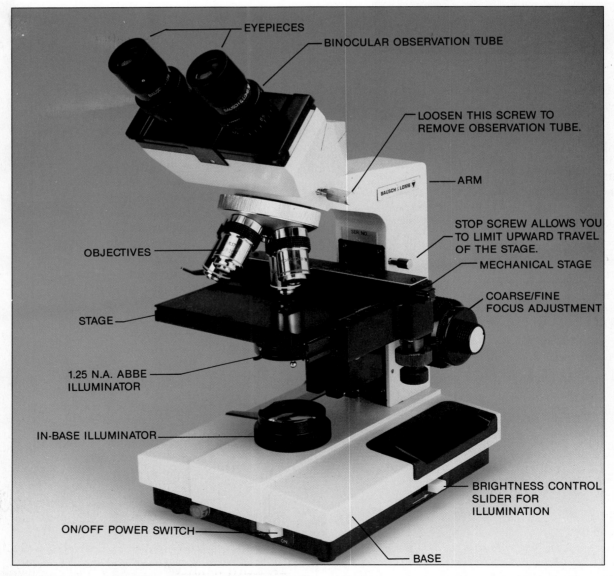

FIGURE 9–1. This binocular microscope magnifies microbes so that we can see them. *(Photo courtesy of Bausch & Lomb, Inc., Rochester, NY)*

Body Flora

Different microorganisms live in communities on our body surfaces. These microbes are normal body **flora**. The flora is not the same in all body areas. For example, the organisms making up the flora of the intestinal tract are different from those of the respiratory tract.

Healthy individuals live in harmony with the normal body flora. However, the balance may be disturbed by pathogenic microbes that cause disease. Some of the organisms that are normally found on the body surfaces can become pathogens or disease-producing microorganisms. Infection does not occur, however, until these pathogens gain entrance into the body.

Drugs such as antibiotics are given for an infection. As a result, the organisms causing the infection are often reduced. Other organisms, however, may flourish and cause a different kind of infection.

When the normal flora of one body system, such as the intestinal tract, remains within its normal environment, the body functions properly. However, when microbes from the intestines are transferred into the urinary tract, a serious urinary tract infection can result. Organisms that are natural inhabitants and nonpathogenic in one part of the body may become pathogenic when in another part of the body.

Characteristics of Microbes

Characteristics are special features. For example, the color of a person's hair is a characteristic. It helps to distinguish the person from other people. Microbes also have distinguishing characteristics, including:

- Their shape
- The way they grow in a special environment in the laboratory
- Special requirements they need to live and multiply

Microorganisms can be studied by:

- Growing (**culturing**) them on a nutrient material (culture media)
- Adding colored dyes (**staining**) to help certain characteristics show more clearly under a microscope

Understanding the characteristics of microbes and their growth requirements enables us to control their growth, reproduction, and spread (**transmission**).

Pathogenic microbes grow best:

- At body temperature
- Where light is limited
- Where there is moisture
- Where there is a simple food supply

Some microbes, however, exist at temperatures high or low enough to kill other plant or animal life. They have been found in hot sulfur springs and in the cold depths of the ocean. They are known to adapt to their environment even under the most difficult conditions for life.

Microbes are found everywhere. They are found on objects that we use in everyday living. We can come in contact with disease-producing microorganisms from objects used by others, such as items used in the delivery of health care. This is one way microbes may be transmitted from one source to another.

Classification of Microbes

There are several classifications of microbes: protozoa, bacteria, fungi, and viruses. In each classification, there are members that are pathogenic to human beings.

Protozoa

Protozoa are simple one-celled parasitic organisms. **Parasites** are organisms that live on living organic matter. They cause diseases such as:

- Malaria
- Toxoplasmosis
- African sleeping sickness
- Amebiasis

Some signs and symptoms associated with protozoan diseases include:

- Diarrhea
- Dysentery
- Inflammation of the brain (encephalitis)

Figure 9–2 shows the intestinal protozoa *Entamoeba coli*.

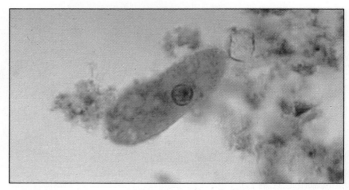

FIGURE 9–2. Intestinal protozoa *Entamoeba coli* (*Courtesy of the Centers for Disease Control, Atlanta, GA*)

Bacteria (Bacterium)

Bacteria are simple one-celled microbes. They are:

- Smaller than yeast
- Larger than a virus
- Named according to their shape and arrangement

Shapes. In the following list, the first term is the singular form of the word. The word in parentheses is the plural form.

- **Coccus** (**cocci**)—round or spherical, Figure 9–3
- **Bacillus** (**bacilli**)—straight rod, Figure 9–4
- **Spirillum** (**spirilla**)—spiral, corkscrew, or slightly curved, Figure 9–5

Arrangements. Bacteria grow in groups called **colonies**. If a small part of a colony is examined under a microscope, we see that the bacteria typically are arranged in pairs, clusters, or chains.

- Single (example: E. coli)
- Pairs (**diplo-**) (example: Neisseria)
- Chains (**strepto-**) (example: Streptococci)
- Clusters (**staphylo-**) (example: Staphylococci)

The characteristics of bacteria have great clinical significance in the identification of the cause of disease in humans. The shape, group arrangement, and staining qualities of bacteria are important factors in their identification.

For example, round microorganisms grouped in chains are called streptococci. A very important member of this family is the *Streptococcus hemolyticus*, Figure 9–6. It causes septic sore throat and rheumatic fever.

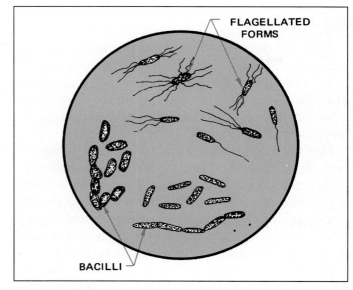

FIGURE 9–4.   Kinds of bacilli

Round organisms found in a cluster are called *staphylococci*. An example of this family is *Staphylococcus aureus*, Figure 9–7. Staphylococci cause many infections such as:

- Surgical wound infections
- Abscesses
- Boils
- Toxic shock

Round organisms found in pairs are called diplococci. A diplococcus, the *Neisseria gonorrheae*, Figure 9–8, causes gonorrhea.

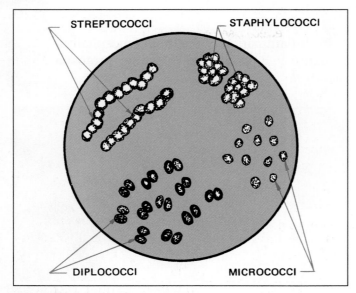

FIGURE 9–3.   Kinds of cocci

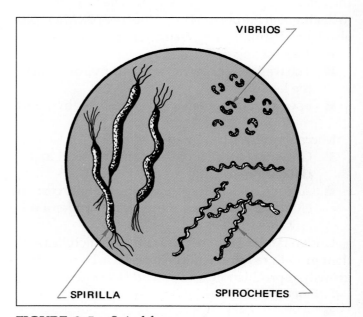

FIGURE 9–5.   Spiral forms

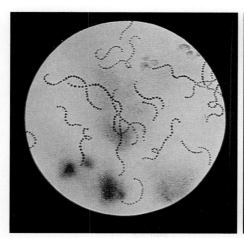

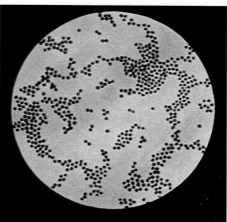

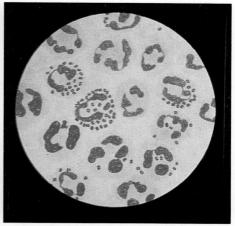

FIGURE 9–6. *Streptococcus hemolyticus* (*Courtesy of the Centers for Disease Control, Atlanta, GA*)

FIGURE 9–7. *Staphylococcus aureus* (*Courtesy of the Centers for Disease Control, Atlanta, GA*)

FIGURE 9–8. *Neisseria gonorrheae* (*Courtesy of the Centers for Disease Control, Atlanta, GA*)

Fungi (Fungus)

A **fungus** is classified as any of a major group (fungi) of saprophytic organisms that lack chlorophyll and include molds. (**Saprophytic** organisms live on dead organic matter.)

The two groups of fungi most commonly associated with infection in humans are:

- **Yeast**—any single-celled budding form of a fungus. Yeast can infect areas of the body such as:
  — Mouth/vagina *Candida albicans* (Fig. 9–9)
  — Skin   *Tinea capitis* (ringworm)
  — Feet   *Tinea pedis* (athlete's foot)
- **Mold**—saprophytic fungi that can cause mold or moldiness. A common mold that can cause infection in the lungs of humans is:
  — Lung   *Aspergillus*

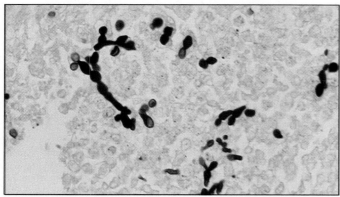

FIGURE 9–9. *Candida albicans* in human heart tissue (*Courtesy of the Centers for Disease Control, Atlanta, GA*)

Yeasts and molds are known as opportunistic parasites. Under normal conditions, the organisms are harmless. However, when the human immune system is impaired and unable to protect the body, these organisms can invade the body and cause severe infections. For example, a patient with AIDS is very susceptible to fungal infections because the immune system is not working properly.

Viruses

A **virus** is the smallest microbe in the world. It depends completely on the invaded host cell for reproduction (**replication**). The basic infectious material is the nucleic acid core (RNA or DNA). This material alone can usually penetrate (enter) susceptible cells and start infection. A special electron microscope is needed to see viruses in human tissue or body fluids. Viruses can be grown in the laboratory using special live animal tissue cultures. Several days or weeks are required for growth.

Viruses are classified according to:

- Type of nucleic acid core (DNA or RNA)
- Size
- Clinical properties
- Biologic and physical properties
- Mode of transmission

Viruses that cause disease in people are generally spread by people. The four primary modes of transmission of viral organisms from human to human are:

- Blood
- Respiratory secretions
- Enteric **excreta** (from the intestinal tract)
- Secretions from the reproductive tract

Common viral infections in humans include:

- Hepatitis, Figure 9–10
- Herpes, Figure 9–11
- Acquired immunodeficiency syndrome (AIDS)
- Influenza, Figure 9–12
- Common cold
- Measles

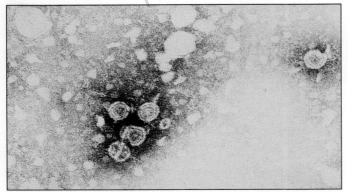

FIGURE 9–10. Electron micrograph of hepatitis B virus *(Courtesy of the Centers for Disease Control, Atlanta, GA)*

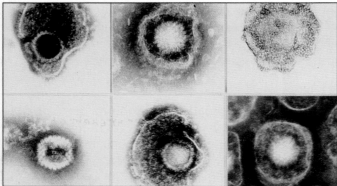

FIGURE 9–11. Electron micrographs of the various types of herpes simplex virus *(Courtesy of the Centers for Disease Control, Atlanta, GA)*

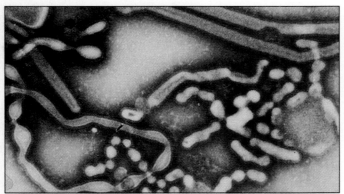

FIGURE 9–12. Electron micrograph of the influenza A virus, early passage *(Courtesy of the Centers for Disease Control, Atlanta, GA)*

Aerobic Organisms

Most microorganisms require oxygen to live. These **aerobic** microorganisms live best where there is plenty of oxygen available. Surfaces such as the skin are ideal for these microbes. A good example of an aerobic microorganism is the aerobic *staphylococcus* family. The organisms in this family:

- Are round in shape
- Are grouped in clusters
- Look white or yellowish when growing
- Require oxygen to live
- Are responsible for many hospital-acquired infections in patients

Hospital-acquired or **nosocomial** infection is an infection that develops after hospitalization. This type of infection was not incubating before the patient was admitted to the hospital. Nosocomial infections can be very serious and even life-threatening. In addition, a hospital-acquired infection can greatly increase the expense and length of hospital stay.

Two common and serious nosocomial infections are caused by bacteria: methicillin resistant *Staphylococcus aureus* (MRSA) and *Pseudomonas aeruginosa*. Both of these organisms have become resistant to the action of antibiotics. This makes infections caused by these organisms difficult to control.

Anaerobic Organisms

Anaerobic organisms live and multiply in the absence of oxygen. Many microbes in this group are important in breaking down waste products in the human digestive tract. Others may cause disease. An example of a disease-causing anaerobic organism is the anaerobic bacillus *Clostridium tetani*, Figure 9–13. This organism causes tetanus.

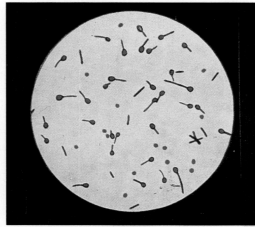

FIGURE 9–13. *Clostridium tetani* *(Courtesy of the Centers for Disease Control, Atlanta, GA)*

- The tetanus bacillus forms spores (inactive form of the bacteria) that can remain viable for years in soil and in animal feces.
- The bacilli are found in the soil where there is little free oxygen.
- The bacilli gain entrance into the body most frequently through a deep puncture wound. As the edges of such a wound close over, the oxygen is closed out and the bacilli grow.
- The organisms grow best when the kind of nourishment they need is present. Dead tissue is ideal food for this organism. There is always some tissue in a wound that has been destroyed by the injury.
- Growing in a wound, the tetanus bacilli cause the disease tetanus or lockjaw.

Because this organism is found in the soil, special care must be given to dirty wounds. They will frequently be washed out with hydrogen peroxide. When it is exposed to the air, hydrogen peroxide releases oxygen. The presence of the oxygen discourages the growth of the tetanus bacillus. Recall that this organism doesn't grow well in oxygen. A **hyperbaric chamber**, Figure 9–14, is used to deliver oxygen under pressure to the tissues of a patient with an anaerobic infection. Refer to Figure 9–15 for definitions of terms used in the previous discussion of microbes.

Infectious Disease Process

The process involved in the development of infectious disease in humans is referred to as the **chain of infection**, Figure 9–16. There are six components of this process:

1. Causative agent.
2. Reservoir of the agent

■ **Aerobic**—requires oxygen to live.
■ **Anaerobic**—grows best when oxygen is absent.
■ **Spore**—an inactive, resistant form that some bacteria can take when environmental conditions are unsuitable. Spore forms can become active again when conditions improve.
■ **Capsule**—a thickened wall around some organisms that protects them.
■ **Flagella**—whip-like appendages that allow some organisms to move freely through the body fluids.
■ **Saprophytes**—organisms that live on dead organic matter. An example is the *Clostridium tetani* (the tetanus bacillus).
■ **Parasites**—organisms that live on living organic matter. An example is *Entamoeba coli*

FIGURE 9–15.   Definitions of terms

3. Portal of exit of the agent from the reservoir
4. Mode of transmission of the agent
5. Portal of entry into the susceptible host
6. Susceptible host

The Causative Agent

The **causative agent** is the microorganism that can produce the disease process in humans. The most common biological agents of infectious disease are:

- Bacteria
- Viruses
- Fungi
- Protozoa

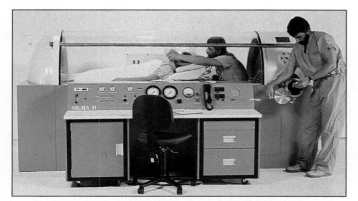

FIGURE 9–14.   Anaerobic organisms do not grow well in such high concentrations of oxygen as are found in the hyperbaric chamber *(Courtesy of Perry Baromedical Services)*

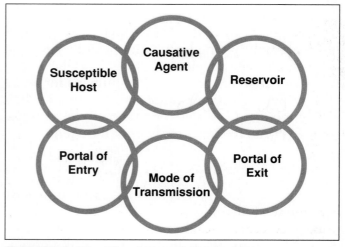

FIGURE 9–16.   The chain of infection

Reservoir of the Agent

The reservoir is where the causative agent can survive. It may or may not multiply in the reservoir. The four most common reservoirs are:

1. Humans—active cases and carriers
2. Animals
3. Environment
4. Fomites—objects that become contaminated with infectious material that contains the microbe. Fomites are anything that comes in direct contact with the excretions or secretions of an infected person. This includes:

   - Bedpans and urinals
   - Linens
   - Instruments
   - Containers with specimens for laboratory analysis

In the health care setting, the reservoirs include the:

- Patient
- Health care worker
- Environment
- Equipment

Human Reservoirs

The two major classifications of human reservoirs are cases and carriers.

- Cases—people with acute illness including obvious signs and symptoms. An example is a person with chicken pox.
- Carriers—those who have and transmit the disease organisms but do not have symptoms and do not display the evidence of the disease. Chronic (sustained or intermittent) carriers can spread the disease without being recognized because the illness is not apparent. Another type of carrier is one in whom the organisms are multiplying (incubating) before signs and symptoms develop.

Specific diseases can persist in humans for an indefinite period of time. Salmonella, hepatitis B, AIDS, and typhoid are examples of unknown carrier transmissions from the host reservoir of the agent.

Portals of Entry or Exit

Portals of Entry. Organisms enter the body through the following **portals of entry**:

- Breaks in the skin or mucous membranes— Many organisms that are part of the normal flora, such as staphylococci, enter through breaks in the skin.
- Respiratory tract—Organisms causing the common cold and many childhood communicable diseases such as mumps and measles may enter this way.
- Genitourinary tract—Organisms that cause syphilis, AIDS, gonorrhea and other sexually transmitted diseases enter this way.
- Gastrointestinal tract—Salmonellosis, typhoid fever, and hepatitis A are examples of diseases caused by organisms that enter the digestive tract.
- Circulatory system—Malaria, yellow fever, and meningitis are diseases that can enter the body this way through the bite of insects.
- Transplacental (mother to fetus) (AIDS and hepatitis B).

Portals of Exit. Infectious organisms leave the reservoir of the host through body secretions (**portals of exit**) including:

- Excretions of the respiratory tract (sputum) or genital tract (semen or vaginal excretions)
- Draining wounds
- Urine
- Feces
- Blood
- Saliva
- Tears

In infected persons, these products must be considered or capable of transmission of the disease agent.

Transmission of Disease

The mode of transmission of the potential disease agent is the way in which the agent is transferred from the reservoir of the host to a new, potentially susceptible host, Figure 9–17. The mode of transmission of these agents can vary depending on where they are found.

The major modes of transmission of disease are contact, common vehicle, airborne, and vectorborne.

- Contact. Direct contact is person-to-person spread, Figure 9–18. The actual physical contact is between patient and source. The presence of microbes on the source means that the source is **contaminated**. The most common source of transmission is the contaminated hands of the health care provider. For example, the fecal-oral spread of *Shigella* is an example of direct-contact spread.

MICROBES ARE SPREAD BY:

CONTACT

■ Direct contact of health care provider with patient:
   — Touching   — Toileting (urine and feces)
   — Bathing   — Secretions from patient
   — Rubbing

■ Indirect contact of health care provider with objects used by patients:
   — Clothing
   — Bed linens
   — Personal belongings
   — Personal care equipment
   — Instruments used in treatments
   — Specimen containers for laboratory analysis
   — Dressings
   — Diagnostic equipment
   — Health care equipment

■ Droplet spread within approximately three feet (no personal contact):
   — Coughing   — Talking
   — Sneezing

COMMON VEHICLE
   — Water   — Drugs   — Urine
   — Food   — Blood

AIRBORNE (DROPLET SPREAD)
■ Microbes carried by moisture or dust particles in air, which are inhaled

VECTORBORNE
■ Intermediate hosts such as insects and animals

FIGURE 9–17. Summary of the modes of transmission of microbes

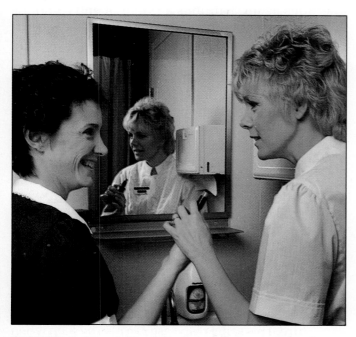

FIGURE 9–18. A lipstick shared between friends can spread microbes.

Indirect contact occurs when a patient or health care worker's hands come into direct contact with a contaminated intermediate object (fomite) and then spread the microbes to self, patients, or other health care workers. Handling equipment that comes in contact with a patient's body secretions during a diagnostic procedure is an example of how an intermediate object is involved in the transmission of pathogens.

Droplet spread occurs by person-to-person transmission at a distance of approximately three feet or less. There is no physical contact. The infected person and a susceptible host need only be within a short distance of each other for droplet spread to occur. Talking, sneezing, or coughing causes droplet spread of an infectious agent from person to person. The majority of common viral infections such as measles, influenza, and the common cold are transmitted in this manner.

■ Common vehicle. Microorganisms can live and/or multiply in a vehicle and cause an infectious process in a number of patients. This mode of transmission is called a common vehicle. An example of this type of transmission is *Salmonella* in food.

■ Airborne. Microbes are sometimes cast into the air and then inhaled by a susceptible host. The common cold, influenza, and tuberculosis are diseases transmitted in this way.

■ Vectorborne. This form of transmission requires an intermediate host such as a mosquito that can harbor the infectious agent. The mosquito that harbors the malaria parasite transmits the agent to humans but is not affected itself by the disease process. As another example, Lyme disease is caused by a spirochete. The organism is transmitted by tick bites. Intermediate hosts such as mosquitos, ticks, fleas, and flies are known as vectors and can spread various infectious diseases.

To illustrate the events in the chain of infection, let us assume that a patient has active tuberculosis. The tubercle bacillus (agent of infection) is found in the respiratory tract (reservoir) of the patient (host). The portal of exit from the host is the respiratory tract. When the patient coughs, airborne droplets (mode of transmission) carry the infectious agent to the respiratory tract (portal of entry) of the new, potentially susceptible host.

Host

The person who harbors infectious organisms is called a host. This person does not have enough resistance to the infectious agent. An infection develops in the host when infectious organisms:

- Penetrate the body
- Begin to multiply
- Cause damage to the host

Risk Factors. Specific characteristics of the host are known to influence the susceptibility to and severity of the resulting infectious disease. These characteristics are known as risk factors. They include:

- Age
- Heredity
- Sex
- Nutritional status
- Underlying diseases
- Immunization/vaccination
- Lifestyle
- Occupation
- Stress

In the beginning of this unit, you learned that microbes are everywhere. You may wonder why we are not ill all of the time because of the microorganisms we are exposed to. There are two major reasons:

1. Many microbes living in the body are not harmful. Some are even helpful in maintaining health.
2. Several factors influence the development of disease. They are the:
   - General health of the individual
   - Condition of the immune system
   - Numbers and strength of the organisms
   - Presence or absence of favorable conditions for growth

Susceptible hosts (likely to get infections) are old or young persons and those who are poorly nourished or in generally poor health. Large numbers of organisms or even a few of those that are very strong (aggressive) can cause a serious illness. Emotional stress and fatigue also play a role in the progress of an infectious disease.

Body Defenses. The body has some natural defenses to protect it from infectious agents. The most important natural, external defense the body has against the invasion of any pathogen is the skin. The intact skin acts as a mechanical barrier. Other defenses include:

- The respiratory, digestive, and reproductive tracts are lined with a special tissue called the mucous membrane. These membranes produce natural fluids called mucus. Secretions can kill or inhibit microbial invasion. The mucus is sticky. It traps foreign materials before they can cause damage.
- Cilia (fine microscopic hairs) lining the respiratory tract propel the mucus and the trapped infective agents out of the body.
- Coughing and sneezing remove foreign materials from the respiratory tract.
- Hydrochloric acid is produced in the stomach. It is a very strong chemical. It is harmful to most microbes.
- Eyes are protected by tears. Tears have special bacteria-killing chemicals (bacteriocides). Tears provide a flushing action. This action removes most microbes that enter the eyes.

The body also has a number of internal defenses against infectious agents, including:

- Fever
- Inflammation
- Special cells in the blood called phagocytes, which defend the body against invading microbes
- Immune response—the body develops protective proteins, which combat foreign microbes.

How Pathogens Affect the Body

The potential for infection depends upon a number of factors (listed previously). Two major factors are the susceptibility of the host and the amount of the infectious agent that finds a portal of entry into the host. Even then an infection does not always occur unless all the elements of the chain of infection are operating.

Microbes act in different ways to produce disease in the human body. Some pathogens:

- Attack and destroy the cells they invade. For example, the microscopic protozoan that causes malaria invades the red blood cells and begins to grow. The red blood cells eventually split. The person experiences chills, followed by fever.
- Produce poisons called toxins. Toxins harm the body. For example, the tetanus organism produces toxins that travel to and damage the nervous system.
- Cause sensitivity responses called allergies. For example, the person may have a runny nose and watery eyes but no rise in temperature. This same response can also be seen when pollens or dust irritate the respiratory membranes.

Disease Prevention

Asepsis

Asepsis is defined as the absence of disease-producing microorganisms. Generally, it is divided into two descriptive forms: medical asepsis and surgical asepsis.

Medical Asepsis

Medical asepsis refers to medical practices that reduce the numbers of microorganisms or interrupt transmission from one person to another person or from person to place or object. These practices are often referred to as clean technique.

It is not possible to eliminate all microorganisms in the human body or in the air. However, microbes can be reduced by the primary health practices of medical asepsis:

- ■ Handwashing
- ■ Using nonsterile gloves when in contact with body fluids
- ■ Cleaning and/or disinfecting equipment

Handwashing. Handwashing is the single most important health procedure any individual can

PROCEDURE 1	OBRA	SIDE 1		

HANDWASHING

1. Make sure the following equipment is available at a sink:
   - ■ Soap dispenser
   - ■ Waste container
   - ■ Paper towels
2. Turn the faucet on with a dry paper towel held between the hand and the faucet, Figure 9–19. Adjust water temperature until it is warm. Discard paper towel.
3. Wet hands. The fingertips must point downward at all times.
   CAUTION: Do not allow water to run up forearms. Keep hands pointed down at all times so water runs off fingertips.
4. Press hand soap dispenser or step on foot pedal, collecting soap in one hand.

5. Lather well, keeping hands pointed downward, Figure 9–20.
6. Rub the hands together in a circular motion, interlacing fingers, Figure 9–21. Continue for 10–15 seconds. Rub the fingernails against the palm of the opposite hand to force soap under nails for cleaning. OPTIONAL: Clean the fingernails with the blunt edge of an orange stick, Figure 9–22, or hand brush, Figure 9–23.
7. Rinse the hands with running water, fingertips down, Figure 9–24. Dry hands thoroughly.
8. Turn off the faucet with another clean, dry paper towel held between the hand and the faucet.
9. Drop the paper towel in the waste container.

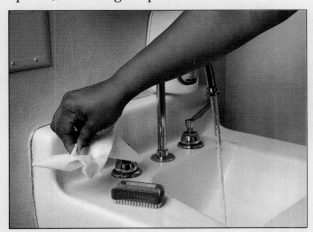

FIGURE 9–19. A dry, clean paper towel should be used to turn the faucet on or off.

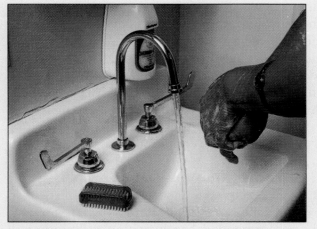

FIGURE 9–20. Point fingertips down while washing the hands.

continues

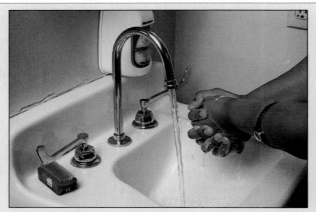

FIGURE 9–21. Interlace the fingers to clean between them.

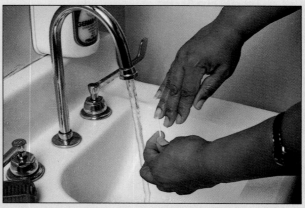

FIGURE 9–22. Use the blunt edge of an orange stick to clean under the fingernails.

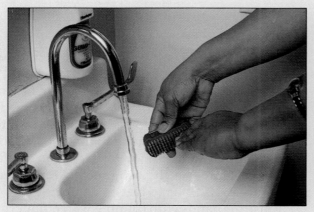

FIGURE 9–23. Another way to clean under the fingernails is to use a hand brush.

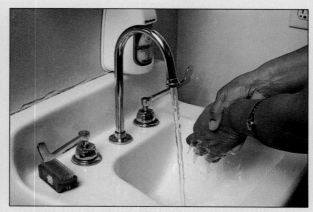

FIGURE 9–24. Rinse hands thoroughly with the fingertips down.

perform to prevent the spread of germs. Handwashing is a vigorous, short, rubbing together of all the surfaces of soap-lathered hands. It is followed by rinsing under a stream of running warm water.

The most important aspect of handwashing is the friction created by rubbing the hands together. This friction mechanically removes microbes from the hands. Routine handwashing with soap, running warm water, and friction by *all* medical personnel:

- Is the most significant control measure for the prevention of a nosocomial infection.
- Prevents cross-contamination between patients and between patients, the equipment, and health care providers.
- Is the single most important control measure to break the chain of infection.

The recommended handwashing technique will depend on the purpose of the handwashing. Hands can usually be washed effectively in 10–15 seconds. More time will be needed, however, if hands are visibly soiled.

CAUTION

Do not lean against the sink or allow your uniform to touch the sink. The sink is always considered to be contaminated (microbes are present). It is essential that each person use the same handwashing technique.

Handwashing should be performed before and after:

- Direct patient care
- Handling food
- Touching a wound
- Going to the bathroom

Warm water makes good lather. It is also less damaging to the skin than hot water.

In health care facilities, soap will be found in a dispenser. Bar soap is easily contaminated because microbes can grow in a wet soap dish.

Federal regulations require blood and body-fluid precautions be used for all patients. This means that health care providers must use barrier precautions to prevent exposure to infectious agents in the blood or other body fluids of patients. Barriers include disposable gloves and, as necessary, masks, protective eyewear, and gowns. This technique is known as **universal precautions** (see Unit 10, page 167).

Cleaning and Disinfecting. Keeping the patient's room and equipment clean contributes to maintaining a medically aseptic environment.

Concurrent cleaning goes on every day. It includes:
- Damp dusting of the unit
- Checking and, if necessary, cleaning the equipment on the bedside stand

Terminal cleaning is carried out after the patient is discharged. This is a thorough cleaning of the entire unit. This cleaning is performed by the housekeeping department. Terminal cleaning includes:
- Stripping the bed of linen and disposing of the soiled linen in the laundry, according to facility policy
- Washing and drying the mattress, pillow, and frame

PROCEDURE 2 | **OBRA** SIDE 1

REMOVING CONTAMINATED DISPOSABLE GLOVES

1. Slip gloved fingers of the dominant hand under the cuff of the opposite hand, touching the glove only, Figure 9–25. NOTE: If the glove does not have a cuff, grasp the outer part of glove at wrist with opposite gloved hand.
2. Pull glove down to the fingers, exposing the thumb, Figure 9–26.
3. Slip the uncovered thumb into the opposite glove at the wrist.
4. Allow the glove-covered fingers of the hand to touch only the outer portion of the soiled glove.

5. Pull the glove down over the dominant hand almost to the fingertips and slip the glove on to the other hand.
6. With the dominant hand touching only the inside of the other glove, continue pulling the glove over the dominant hand until only the clean surface is outermost.
7. Dispose of the soiled gloves according to facility policy.
8. Wash and dry hands thoroughly.

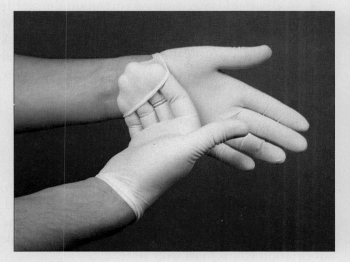

FIGURE 9–25.

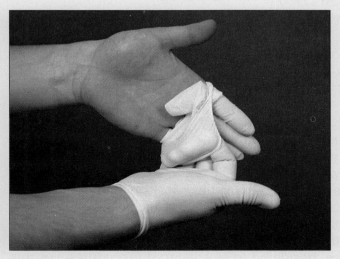

FIGURE 9–26.

- Cleaning the bedside cabinet and over-bed stand
- Cleaning and/or replacing bedside equipment
- Making a closed bed

The nursing assistant may be responsible for stripping and remaking the bed.

In the following units, precautions about the ways in which medical asepsis is promoted are given for all patient care procedures. Figure 9–27 summarizes the actions the nursing assistant must carry out and those that must be avoided in caring for patients.

Surgical Asepsis

Surgical asepsis refers to techniques that make and keep objects and clinical settings as free from microorganisms as possible. This is also known as sterile technique.

Surgical asepsis is:

- Carried out in the operating room using physical barriers and extraordinary control measures to maintain a sterile field. Physical barriers include sterile:
  — Gloves   — Gowns
  — Masks   — Drapes
  An infection control measure is the sterilization of objects by the use of chemicals and heat.
- Associated with procedures with high risk for infection. Examples are:
  — Insertion of catheters
  — Surgical wound dressing changes
  — Administration of injectable medications
- Associated with populations at high risk for infection. Examples are:
  — Burn patients
  — Transplant patients
  — Newborns (neonates)
  — Patients whose immune systems are depressed (such as cancer patients on chemotherapy and AIDS patients)

Nursing Assistant Responsibilities. There will be times when you will be asked to assist with a procedure that requires sterile technique. You must be aware of the special skills required to perform the correct technique in the clinical setting.

Sterile technique is used when handling sterile instruments, changing dressings, or carrying out other sterile procedures. Many of these procedures are considered to be advanced procedures. For this reason, they are covered in Unit 43. These procedures are:

- Putting on sterile gloves
- Opening a sterile package
- Transferring sterile items by forceps

The procedures are carried out only after adequate practice and supervision. They are done only in accordance with specific hospital policy regarding who is allowed to perform the procedures. A short discussion of the principles involved in these procedures is included here.

- The sterile field is the main area where sterile equipment and materials needed to perform a sterile procedure are placed during the procedure. This could be a table covered with a sterile drape.
- The designated sterile field should be kept sterile during the entire procedure.
- When you are assisting, never reach across or pass over the sterile field with unsterile items.
- Always keep your hands in front of you and above the waist to prevent accidental contamination with the unsterile areas.
- Before the sterile procedure, an antiseptic agent is used to prepare the patient's skin. The removal of hair might also be indicated.
- Barrier technique is required to maintain a sterile field during sterile procedures. Sterile gloves, masks, gowns, and drapes are used to decrease the transmission of microorganisms from personnel to patient.
- Special surgical suites or treatment rooms are used to maintain environmental and infection control measures.
- A dry field is necessary to maintain the sterile field. A sterile field that becomes wet is no longer a sterile field. Microbes can break through a wet barrier. Moisture-proof barrier drapes and gowns should be used when possible to maintain a dry sterile field.

Cleaning, Disinfecting, and Sterilizing Patient Care Equipment—Disposable Items

All patient-care disposable items should be handled with care since they might have come into contact with blood or body fluids containing blood. Disposing of these items properly protects you and the patient. It also keeps the environment safe. This information is found in Unit 10.

Although many facilities are using as much dispos-

DO

- Clean up dishes immediately after use.
- Damp-dust daily and be conscientious about concurrent cleaning.
- Provide a bag for the disposal of used tissues.
- Turn the face to one side so that the assistant and the patient are not breathing directly on each other.
- Cover the nose and mouth when coughing or sneezing.
- Protect the skin on the hands by using warm water, thorough drying, and applying lotion if needed.
- Treat breaks in the skin immediately, washing thoroughly, cleaning with an antiseptic and covering. Report any breaks in the skin to the nurse.
- Disinfect equipment, such as a stethoscope, that is used by more than one staff member or patient before and after each use.
- Gather or fold linen inward with the dirtiest area toward the center.
- Empty waste baskets frequently.

DO NOT

- Shake bed linens since any microbes present could be released into the air.
- Let dirty linens touch your uniform.
- Eat or share food from the patient's tray.
- Borrow personal care items from another patient or coworker.
- Permit the contents of urinals or bedpans to splash when being emptied.
- Report on duty if you are infectious.
- Permit linen to touch the floor, which must always be considered dirty.
- Do not carry clean linen against uniform.

FIGURE 9–27. Do's and Don'ts of infection control

---

able equipment as possible, there will always be reusable equipment. Reusable equipment must be disinfected and/or sterilized.

Disinfection

Cleaning is usually done by using water with or without detergents to remove soil physically. **Disinfection** is done to remove soil and reduce as many microorganisms as possible.

Disinfection occurs with the use of chemical germicides that kill pathogens.

- Carefully wash, rinse, and dry the article.
- Place the article in disinfectant. All parts should come into contact with the disinfectant.
- Soak item per the manufacturer's recommendation and for the time specified.
- Remove item, rinse well, and dry.
- Disinfect equipment used in cleaning.

Sterilization

The **sterilization** process destroys *all* microbes. This process can be accomplished by using heat in various forms:

- Many objects may be sterilized using steam under pressure. An example of this is sterilization by **autoclave**. This process is similar to the action of a pressure cooker.
- Some articles cannot be processed by steam because they are heat-sensitive. These articles require a special type of gas autoclave.

Special tape is used to secure the coverings on articles to be autoclaved. The tape changes color during the process, thus showing that sterilization has been achieved, Figure 9–28.

Opening a Sterile Package

Sterile equipment such as gloves, dressings, instruments, and procedure trays are double wrapped in cloth or special paper and sealed.

There are several guidelines to keep in mind:

- Most packages will have a seal that changes color to indicate that the sterilizing process has been completed.
- If the color code has not changed or a seal does not look intact, do not consider the article sterile. *If you have any questions, do not take a chance.* Dispose of the article according to facility policy.
- Touch only the outside of the package. Remember, only sterile surfaces may contact sterile surfaces.
- Commercially prepared products will be sealed. If the package is in poor condition, do not consider the article to be sterile. Discard the item if you are in doubt about its sterility.
- Transfer forceps are instruments used to pick up sterile equipment. They are processed by sterilization. They are to be used like sterile fingers. If you are trained to use the instrument, you must keep the entire instrument sterile. The forceps are lifted by the handle, being careful not to touch anything not sterile.

Opening Sterile Gloves

Gloves are sterilized in double-layered packages of paper or cloth.

■ The gloves are arranged in the package so that when it is opened, they are on the proper side for gloving. The palms will be up with the thumbs pointing to the outer edge. The wrist will be cuffed and folded over.

■ The inside of the glove comes in contact with the skin. Once it has been touched, it is considered contaminated.

■ When putting on gloves, the most important principle to remember is that glove surfaces must only touch glove surfaces, and skin surfaces must only touch skin surfaces.

The procedure for opening and putting on sterile gloves is found in Unit 43.

Immunization

An important way to protect yourself from pathogens is by maintaining your own general health. Sufficient rest, adequate nutrition, and stress management are ways you can contribute to your general resistance to disease.

Immunization is another excellent way to protect yourself. Immunization by vaccine allows your body to produce protective antibodies (proteins) to specific infectious organisms in a controlled way without becoming seriously ill. When you do contact the pathogens, the antibodies already formed in your body prevent you from becoming sick.

Immunizing vaccines do not exist for all infectious diseases. However, there are vaccines available for some serious infections. All health care providers are advised to take advantage of the protection these vaccines offer. Some diseases for which immunizing vaccines are available include:

■ Hepatitis B
■ Measles (Rubeola)
■ Mumps
■ German measles (Rubella)
■ Poliomyelitis
■ Tetanus
■ Influenza
■ Diphtheria
■ Whooping cough

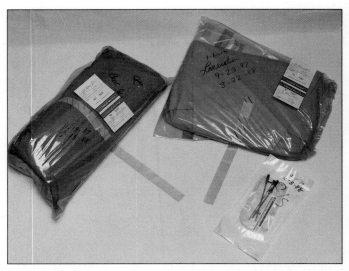

FIGURE 9–28. The packages have been sterilized with steam or gas. The strips below each package show how they look before sterilization. The strips shown on the packages have changed color because they have been sterilized.

You may have already received many of these vaccines as a child from your physician or health department.

Hepatitis B vaccine is effective against a serious form of liver infection. The virus (HBV) that causes hepatitis B can be passed in body fluids from an infected person to others. Health care providers may contact these body fluids as they give care.

Hepatitis B is more common than the AIDS virus. Currently, there is no vaccine for AIDS. Therefore, it is important that all health care providers be protected by receiving the hepatitis B vaccine.

The federal government requires all health care facilities to provide hepatitis B vaccination free of charge for their employees who come in contact with blood and body fluids of patients after they are educated about risks of occupational exposure. Currently there is no vaccine for HIV infection. Therefore, universal precautions must be followed carefully.

SUMMARY

Pathogens are microscopic organisms that cause disease. Pathogens differ from one another in the way they:

■ Look.
■ Cause disease.
■ Grow.

Pathogens:

■ Enter and leave the body by special routes known as portals of entry and exit.

■ Transmit disease by direct and indirect means. The spread of disease can be controlled by:

■ Handwashing
■ Proper medical and surgical asepsis
■ Practicing good sterile technique

Handwashing is the single most important procedure to break the chain of infection.

Immunization by vaccine to form antibodies against certain infectious diseases is an important form of protection.

UNIT REVIEW

A. Matching. Match Column I with Column II.

	Column I		Column II
f	1. microbes that require oxygen to grow	a.	staphylococci
k	2. spiral-shaped bacterium	b.	protozoan
i	3. organism that causes ringworm	c.	flagella
d	4. bacteria that grow in pairs	d.	diplococci
h	5. organism that causes AIDS	e.	spore
m	6. corkscrew-shaped bacterium	f.	aerobic
c	7. whip-like appendages that allow some microbes to move freely in body fluids	g.	streptococci
l	8. thickened wall around some microbes	h.	virus
a	9. bacteria that grow as clusters	i.	fungus
e	10. resistant form of some bacteria	j.	anaerobic
		k.	spirillum
		l.	capsule
		m.	spirochete

B. True/False. Answer the following true or false by circling T or F.

T **F** 11. Malaria is caused by a bacterium.

T **F** 12. Saprophytes exist on live organic matter.

T **F** 13. Normal body flora is the same in each part of the body.

T F 14. Sexually transmitted diseases use the genitourinary tract as the portal of entry.

T F 15. The feces is a common portal of exit for some infectious organisms.

T F 16. The general health of an individual is an important factor in determining if infectious disease will occur.

T F 17. Unbroken skin is a mechanical defense against infection.

T **F** 18. Bacteriocidal chemicals encourage the growth of microbes.

T F 19. The person who harbors an infectious organism is called a host.

T F 20. The presence of some microbes in the body causes an allergic response.

T **F** 21. Handwashing should be done in cold water.

T **F** 22. Always hold fingertips up when rinsing hands during handwashing.

T F 23. Proper handwashing is the single most important technique to prevent the spread of germs.

T F 24. Handling sterile equipment is a routine procedure for the nursing assistant.

T F 25. When disinfecting an instrument, every part of the instrument must come into contact with the disinfectant solution for a specific amount of time.

T F 26. An immunizing vaccine causes the body to produce antibodies that protect the person against certain infectious diseases.

T F 27. A nosocomial infection is hospital acquired.

T F 28. MRSA infections are easy to control. 154

T F 29. Bedpans and urinals can act as fomites.

T F 30. The respiratory tract is a common portal of exit for infectious organisms.

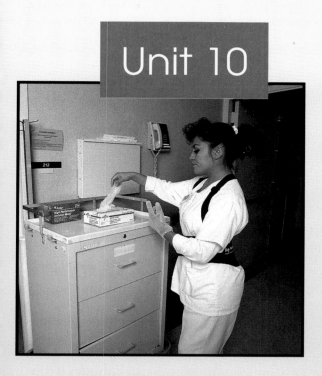

Universal Precautions and Isolation Techniques

As a result of this unit, you will be able to:

- Spell and define terms.
- Demonstrate universal precautions.
- Prepare an isolation unit.
- Demonstrate basic isolation techniques.
- Identify seven major isolation categories.

Learn the meaning and the correct spelling of the following words and phrases:

barrier
biohazard
blood-borne
   pathogens
category-specific
   isolation
   precautions
communicable
disease-specific
   isolation
   precautions
disposable
double-bagging
exposure incident
hepatitis B virus (HBV)

human immuno-
   deficiency virus
   (HIV)
isolation technique
isolation unit
occupational exposure
Occupational Safety
   and Health Act
   (OSHA)
personal protective
   equipment
potentially infectious
   materials
sharps
universal precautions

Unit 9 showed that microbes and host factors are very difficult to control. Therefore, efforts at breaking the chain of infection are usually directed at the mode of transmission. All patients are considered potentially infectious. Therefore, universal precautions are carried out with all patients. The following discussion of universal precautions and isolation techniques is based on this concept.

Universal Precautions

Health care providers at all levels are very much aware of the infection control problems related to the acquired immunodeficiency syndrome (AIDS) virus (HIV), hepatitis B virus (HBV), and other blood-borne pathogens. These diseases are caused by blood-borne pathogens. These are pathogenic microorganisms that are present in human blood and can cause disease in humans.

For several years, The Centers for Disease Control and Prevention (CDC) in Atlanta, Georgia (part of the Department of Health and Human Services) has published recommendations for preventing transmission of blood-borne diseases. However, these recommendations had no legal foundation and employers did not have to follow them.

In 1990, the Occupational Safety and Health Act (OSHA) was amended to include regulations that must be followed by all health care facilities. These regulations are laws that can be enforced by the federal government through the Department of Labor. The following list describes some of the items

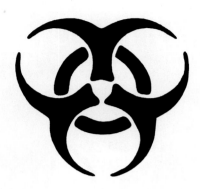

FIGURE 10–1. Containers for contaminated items and other potentially infectious wastes are identified with this label.

included in this legislation. All health care facility employers must:

- Determine which employees have occupational exposure.
  — This means reasonably anticipated skin, eye, mucous membrane, or parenteral contact with blood of other potentially infectious materials that may result from the performance of an employee's duties.

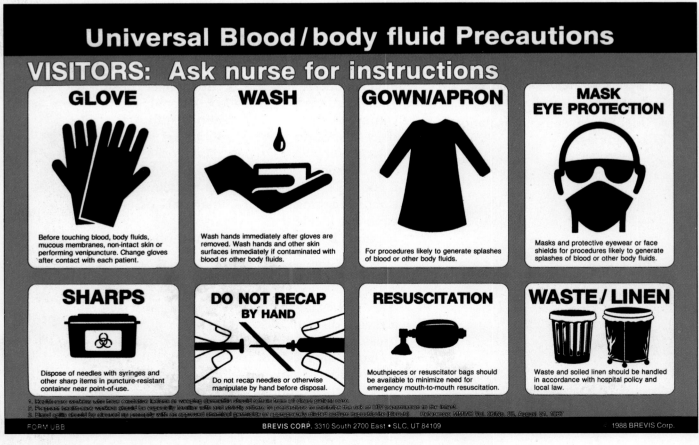

FIGURE 10–2A. Universal blood/body fluid precautions *(Courtesy of BREVIS Corporation)*

— Other potentially infectious materials include semen, vaginal secretions, fluids from other body cavities, and any body fluid that is visibly contaminated with blood. Many facilities consider urine and stool to be potentially infectious even if there is no visible blood.

■ Provide hepatitis B vaccine free of charge to all employees with occupational exposure.

■ Provide **personal protective equipment (PPE)** for all employees with occupational exposure.

— This equipment includes waterproof gowns, masks, gloves, goggles, and any other equipment needed to protect the employee.

■ Provide adequate handwashing facilities and supplies.

■ Provide training in regard to these rules to all employees with occupational exposure, on hiring and annually.

■ Provide evaluation and follow-up if an employee has an **exposure incident**

— An exposure incident means a specific eye, mouth, other mucous membrane, non-intact skin, or parenteral contact with blood or other potentially infectious material that results from the performance of the employee's duties. An accidental stick with a contaminated needle is an example of an exposure incident.

■ Provide appropriate containers for contaminated sharps and other potentially infectious wastes that are color coded (orange or orange-red) and labeled (Figure 10–1).

■ Provide an exposure control plan for staff to follow and post this information prominently.

These regulations must be carried out by health care providers in all settings of the health care delivery system. Health care facilities must require health care workers with occupational exposure to follow the regulations. Care providers whose activities involve contact with blood or other body fluids containing blood from patients are known to be at risk of acquiring HIV or other blood-borne illnesses, such as hepatitis B. There is no evidence that HIV is spread by casual contact, nor is it easily transmitted. Emphasis is placed on the health care provider's strict observance of these regulations to minimize the risk of exposure.

Universal precautions consist of procedures that incorporate these rules, Figure 10–2A:

■ Wash hands before and after contact with patients. Hands should always be washed after the use of gloves. If hands come in contact with blood and/or body fluids containing blood, wash them immediately with soap and water. (The procedure for handwashing is described in Unit 9.)

■ Wear gloves when contact with blood, body fluids, dressings, tissues, or surfaces contaminated with blood is likely.

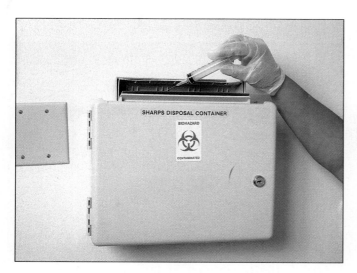

FIGURE 10–2B. All sharps should be disposed of in a special container.

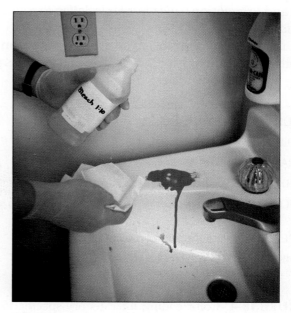

FIGURE 10–3. Clean all blood spills immediately using a 1:10 dilution of bleach.

- Wear a waterproof gown if blood splattering might occur.
- Wear masks and protective goggles if aerosolization (particles dispensed in a fine mist) and splattering of blood are likely to occur, such as in certain dental, surgical, and medical procedures.
- Place mouth-to-mouth resuscitation devices in convenient locations to minimize the need to give direct mouth-to-mouth resuscitation.
- Handle sharp objects, such as needles or blades (sharps), very carefully to prevent accidental needle cuts or punctures. Needles should never be bent, broken, or recapped by hand. Discard in appropriate sharps containers immediately after use, Figure 10–2B. Report incidents with sharps (exposure incident) immediately.
- Clean up blood spills promptly with a disinfectant solution such as 1:10 dilution of bleach, Figure 10–3.
- Consider laboratory specimens and specimen containers to be potentially infectious materials.

Directions for these procedures are included in isolation procedures.

Isolation Systems

The universal precautions do not eliminate the need for other isolation precautions. Isolation precautions are outlined in the Centers for Disease Control and Prevention *Guidelines for Isolation Precautions in Hospitals* (1983).

Diseases may be transferred from one person to another either directly or indirectly. Such diseases are

BLUE	Respiratory isolation
YELLOW	Strict isolation
ORANGE	Contact isolation
RED	Blood/body fluid precautions
BROWN	Enteric precautions (The term *enteric* relates to the intestines.)
GREEN	Drainage/secretion precautions
PINK	AFB isolation (Acid fast bacillus isolation for pulmonary tuberculosis), optional

FIGURE 10–4. Color coding for category-specific isolation

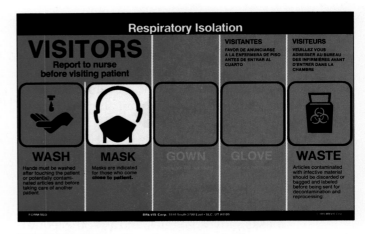

FIGURE 10–5. Respiratory isolation
(Courtesy of BREVIS Corporation)

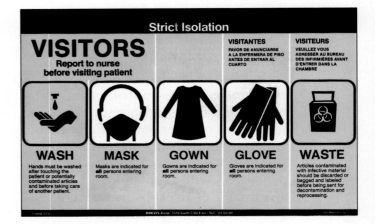

FIGURE 10–6. Strict isolation
(Courtesy of BREVIS Corporation)

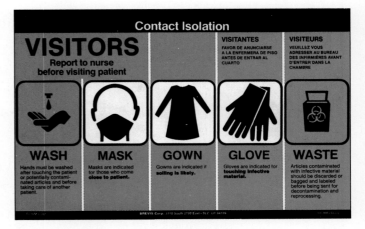

FIGURE 10–7. Contact isolation
(Courtesy of BREVIS Corporation)

salmonella

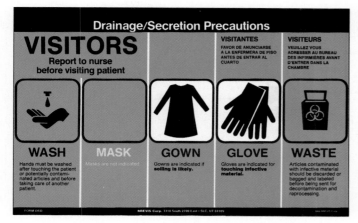

FIGURE 10–8. Enteric precautions
(Courtesy of BREVIS Corporation)

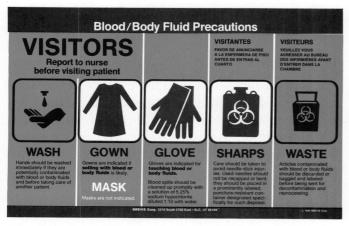

FIGURE 10–9. Drainage/secretion precautions
(Courtesy of BREVIS Corporation)

FIGURE 10–10. Blood and body fluids precautions.
(Courtesy of BREVIS Corporation)

called communicable diseases. Some diseases are transmitted more easily than others. Specific precautions must be taken to prevent their spread.

Communicable diseases may be spread:

■ Through upper respiratory secretions. An example of these are droplets from the nose and mouth.

■ By direct or indirect contact with feces.

■ Through draining wounds or infective materials such as blood on needles.

Each mode of transmission requires special precautions to interrupt the movement of microbes from the infected person to others.

The Centers for Disease Control has established isolation guidelines for diseases that are communicable and spread in specific ways. The CDC recommends that an isolation system be selected that will protect the patient and the employee from acquiring a communicable disease. This selection is determined by the facility.

The major isolation systems recommended are:

■ System A—Category-specific isolation precautions

■ System B—Disease-specific isolation precautions

Category-specific Isolation Precautions

The category-specific isolation precautions system groups diseases that require similar isolation precautions. This system includes seven isolation categories. Each category has a different set of precautions. The categories are color coded for easy identification, Figure 10–4. The system uses preprinted, color-coded instruction cards. A card is placed on the door or in the unit for each category of isolation. These cards are shown in Figures 10–5 to 10–10. An isolation category ending in the word *isolation* requires that the patient be in a private room. The categories ending in the word *precautions* require only that the patient be in a cubicle (unit).

Disease-specific Isolation Precautions

The disease-specific isolation precautions system considers each disease individually. The recommended precautions, such as private room, mask, gown, and gloves, are only those needed to interrupt transmission for the specific disease. An instruction card, Figure 10–11, is filled out, and adhesive symbols for the precautions needed are applied to the card. Usually the disease-specific requirements are posted next to the universal precautions on the door of the room as an added reminder. The card is placed on the door of the isolation unit. Remember that the use of universal precautions

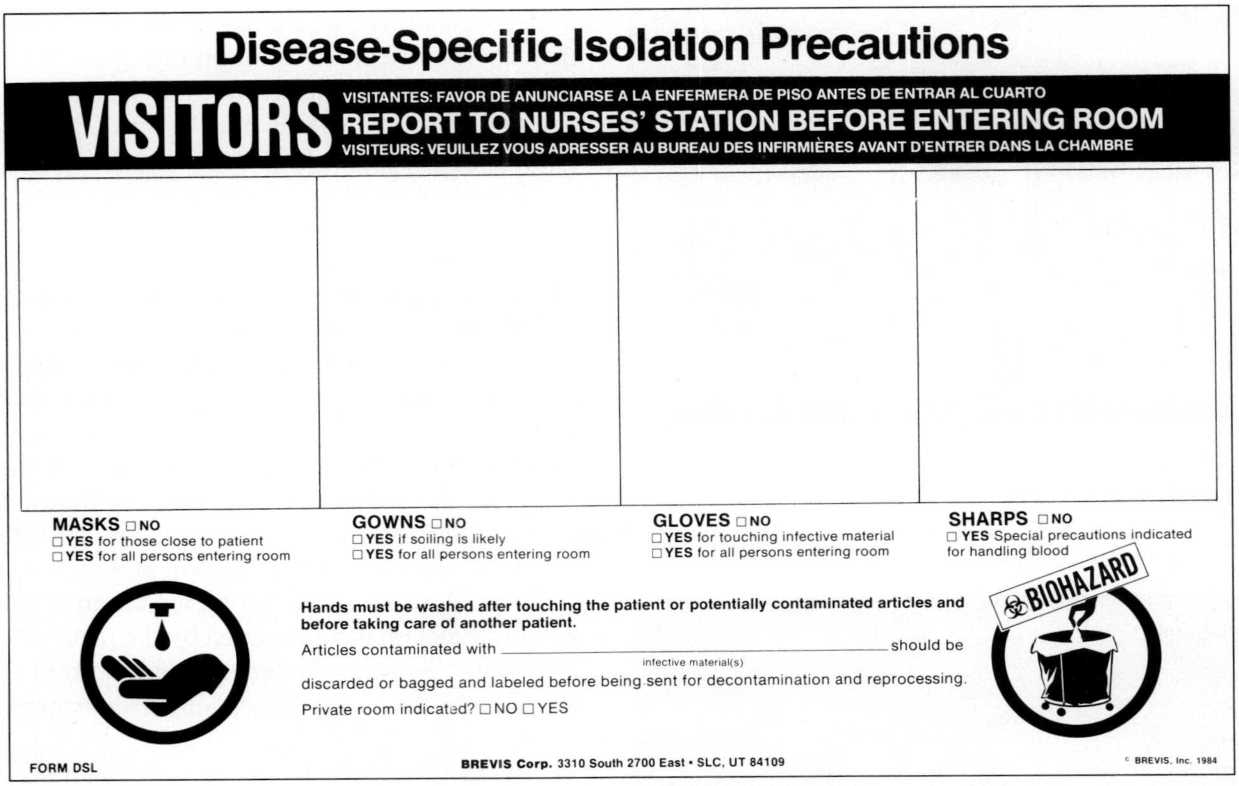

Disease-Specific Isolation Precautions

VISITORS VISITANTES: FAVOR DE ANUNCIARSE A LA ENFERMERA DE PISO ANTES DE ENTRAR AL CUARTO
REPORT TO NURSES' STATION BEFORE ENTERING ROOM
VISITEURS: VEUILLEZ VOUS ADRESSER AU BUREAU DES INFIRMIÈRES AVANT D'ENTRER DANS LA CHAMBRE

MASKS ☐ NO
☐ **YES** for those close to patient
☐ **YES** for all persons entering room

GOWNS ☐ NO
☐ **YES** if soiling is likely
☐ **YES** for all persons entering room

GLOVES ☐ NO
☐ **YES** for touching infective material
☐ **YES** for all persons entering room

SHARPS ☐ NO
☐ **YES** Special precautions indicated for handling blood

BIOHAZARD

Hands must be washed after touching the patient or potentially contaminated articles and before taking care of another patient.

Articles contaminated with _____ should be
                          infective material(s)
discarded or bagged and labeled before being sent for decontamination and reprocessing.

Private room indicated? ☐ NO ☐ YES

FORM DSL   **BREVIS Corp.** 3310 South 2700 East • SLC, UT 84109   © BREVIS, Inc. 1984

FIGURE 10–11. Disease-specific alert. This may be posted outside the patient's unit. It is recorded in the nursing care plan. *(Courtesy of BREVIS Corporation)*

does not mean that category- or disease-specific isolation precautions are no longer used. If a patient has infectious diarrhea, then the patient is placed on enteric precautions. A patient with pulmonary tuberculosis is put in respiratory isolation or AFB isolation.

Isolation Technique

There are three key points to be remembered at all times for isolation technique.

1. Isolation technique is the name given to the method of caring for patients with easily transmitted diseases.
2. It is essential that every person take responsibility and use the proper isolation technique to prevent the spread of the disease to others.
3. All items that come into contact with the patient's excretions, secretions, blood, or body fluids containing the known or suspected microbe are considered contaminated. This potentially infective material must be treated in a special way.

Isolation Unit

The isolation unit may be an area or a private room. A room with handwashing facilities and an adjoining room with bathing and toilet facilities is best. A private room is indicated for patients who:

- Are highly infectious.
- Have poor personal hygiene.
- Require special air control procedures within the room.

Handwashing

Handwashing is basic to the practice of the isolation technique. Handwashing is the single most important means of preventing the spread of infection for all isolation precautions. Health care providers wash their hands as described in Unit 9, even when gloves are used.

Cover Gown

A gown made of moisture-resistant material should be used when soiling with secretions or

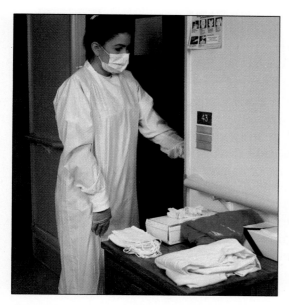

FIGURE 10–12. A clean cover gown is put on before entering the patient's room.

excretions is likely, Figure 10–12. The use of the gown prevents self-contamination. It also prevents contamination of the uniform with the infective material. When using a gown, it should be worn only once. Discard gowns in an appropriate place after use. Refer to Procedures 3 and 4.

Gloves

The use of disposable gloves (latex or vinyl) prevents the spread of infectious disease. Gloves should be worn for most health care procedures, depending on the diagnoses and condition of the patient. Gloves must be worn when carrying out procedures in which there may be contact with body fluids.

Face Mask

Masks are to be worn when exposure to droplet secretions may occur. For example, a suspected tu-

---

| PROCEDURE 3 | OBRA | SIDE 1 | | |

PUTTING ON A COVER GOWN

1. Remove your wristwatch and place on the clean side of an open paper towel.
2. Wash your hands.
3. Put on cover gown by slipping arms into sleeves, Figure 10–13A.
4. Slip fingers under inside neckband and grasp ties in the back, Figure 10–13B. Secure neckband with a simple bow, or fasten Velcro strips.

5. Reach behind and overlap the edges of the gown so that your uniform is completely covered. Secure waist ties with a simple bow, or fasten Velcro strips, Figure 10–13C.
6. NOTE: The watch will be carried with you into the isolation unit. It will remain on the paper towel so it can be referred to without being touched.

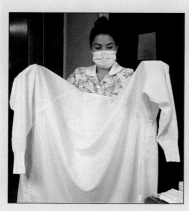

A. After tying on the mask, put on the gown outside the patient's room/unit.

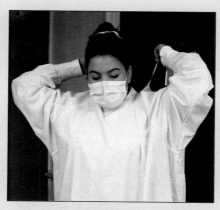

B. Slip fingers inside the neckband and tie gown.

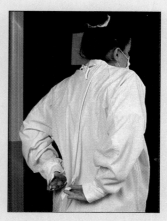

C. Reach behind, overlap the ends of the gown so the uniform is covered, and secure the waist ties.

FIGURE 10–13. Putting on the clean cover gown before entering the patient's room

PROCEDURE 4 | OBRA

REMOVING CONTAMINATED COVER GOWN, GLOVES, AND MASK

1. Remove gloves, turning them inside out. Dispose of gloves.
2. Undo waist ties of the gown.
3. Holding a clean paper towel, turn faucets on. Discard towel.
4. Wash your hands. Dry with paper towel.
5. Holding a dry paper towel, turn off faucets.
6. Undo mask (bottom ties first, then top ties). Holding by ties only, dispose of mask.
7. Undo the neck ties and loosen gown at shoulders.
8. Slip the fingers of the dominant hand inside the cuff of the other hand without touching the outside of the gown. Pull gown down over the other hand, Figure 10–14A.
9. With the gown-covered hand, pull the gown down over the dominant hand, Figure 10–14B.
10. Fold gown away from body with contaminated side inward, Figure 10–14C. Roll and dispose of in appropriate receptacle.
11. Wash hands using the technique described in steps 3–5.
12. Remove watch from clean side of paper towel. Holding clean side of paper towel, dispose of towel in wastepaper receptacle.

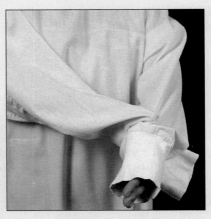

B. Using the gown-covered hand, pull the gown down over the dominant hand.

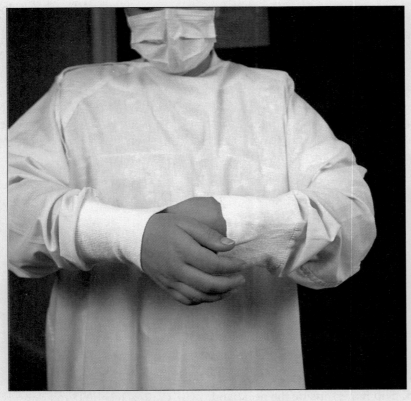

A. Slip fingers of the dominant hand inside the cuff of the other hand. Pull gown, as shown, over the other hand. Do not touch the outside of the gown with the dominant hand.

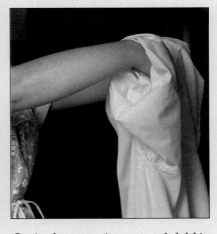

C. As the gown is removed, fold it away from the body with the contaminated side inward and then roll.

FIGURE 10–14. Removing the contaminated gown

| PROCEDURE 5 | OBRA | SIDE 1 |  | |

PUTTING ON AND TAKING OFF A DISPOSABLE PAPER FACE MASK

1. Wash your hands.
2. Adjust the mask over your nose and mouth. Be careful not to touch your face with your hands.
3. First tie top strings of the mask behind your head. Then tie bottom strings securely.
4. Replace mask if it becomes moist during procedure.
5. When ready to dispose of mask, wash your hands first.
6. Untie bottom strings first.
7. Untie top strings. Remove the mask by holding the top strings. Discard in appropriate infectious waste receptacle, located inside the patient's room.
8. Wash your hands.

berculosis patient who is coughing is releasing into the air moisture droplets containing the tuberculosis bacillus. When a mask is indicated, it is:

■ Used only once and discarded.
■ Discarded if it becomes moist.
■ Never left secured around the neck as it can contaminate the uniform and the environment.

A mask that covers both the nose and the mouth will give protection from the airborne spread of microbes. Refer to Procedure 5.

Equipment

Disposable (used once and discarded) patient-care equipment is used widely. It is ideal for patients on isolation precautions. Frequently used equipment remains in the patient's unit. Most articles will not require special handling unless they are contaminated (or likely to be contaminated) with infective material.

Special precautions are not necessary for dishes unless they are visibly contaminated with infective material. An example of this would be dishes that have blood, drainage, or secretions on them. Disposable dishes that have been contaminated with infective material can be handled as disposable patient-care equipment.

Containment of Articles

Contaminated articles leaving the patient's room must be handled so that pathogens will not be spread. It is important that contaminated equipment be bagged, labeled, and disposed of in accordance with the health care facility's policy for the disposal of infectious waste. Used articles are placed in an impenetrable bag (such as plastic) before they are removed from the room or unit of the patient. A single bag may be used if it is waterproof and sturdy enough to confine and contain the article without contaminating the outside of the bag.

Soiled linen is a source of pathogens and should be handled with care.

■ Handle linen as little as possible.
■ Fold dirtiest side inward.
■ Do not shake.
■ Bag before leaving the room.
■ Keep separate from general linen.
■ Transport soiled, wet linen in a leakproof bag.

Remember to perform these actions at the beginning and completion of each procedure, as appropriate. NOTE: Where there are open lesions, wet linen, or possible contact with patient body fluids or blood, disposable gloves are to be worn during the procedure. Put on gloves before contact with the patient or linen. Properly dispose of gloves after they are removed. **Always Apply Universal Precautions.**

■ BEGINNING PROCEDURE ACTIONS
— Wash your hands.
— Assemble equipment needed.
— Carry out precaution gowning and gloving.
— Go to the patient's room, knock, and pause before entering.
— Introduce yourself and identify the patient by checking the identification bracelet.
— Provide privacy.
— Explain what will happen and answer questions.

PROCEDURE 6   OBRA

COLLECTING A SPECIMEN IN THE ISOLATION UNIT

1. Bring a clean specimen container and cover into the unit. Place them on a clean paper towel.
2. Put on gloves. Place specimen into container without touching the container.
3. Cover specimen and label.
4. Remove gloves and wash your hands.
5. Using a clean paper towel, pick up specimen container and place it in a plastic transport bag.

PROCEDURE 7   OBRA

CARING FOR LINEN IN THE ISOLATION UNIT

1. Bring clean linen to the unit as needed.
2. Handle soiled linen as little as possible.
3. Place soiled linen in leakproof laundry bag in unit.
4. The bag should be labeled or identified by color code.
5. Secure the bag and route linen according to facility policy. Many facilities use a plastic-type outer bag that dissolves in the washer, freeing the linen.

PROCEDURE 8

TRANSPORTING THE PATIENT IN ISOLATION

1. Notify the department that the patient from isolation is being transported to their department. Identify the type of isolation technique required.
2. Cover transport vehicle with a clean sheet and wheel into the room.
3. Identify the patient and tell her what you plan to do and how she can assist you.
4. If required, put on appropriate barriers such as gown, mask, or gloves. Assist patient onto transport vehicle.
5. Mask the patient, if required.
6. Wrap the patient in a sheet, if required.
7. Remove your gown and other barriers as you leave the unit, following the proper technique.
8. Upon return from the other department, return the patient to the unit. Follow appropriate barrier technique as required and return patient to her bed.
9. Remove the sheet from transport vehicle and deposit in soiled linen hamper, or follow facility policy.
10. Wash your hands.

- — Allow patient to assist in procedure as much as possible.
- — Raise bed or table to comfortable working height.
■ PROCEDURE COMPLETION ACTIONS
  - — Position patient comfortably.
  - — Leave signal cord, telephone, and fresh water close at hand.
- — Return bed or table to lowest position.
- — Perform general safety check of patient and environment.
- — Carry out isolation technique.
- — Wash your hands.
- — Report completion of task.
- — Document action and your observations.

SUMMARY

When patients have communicable diseases that are easily transmitted to others, special techniques must be used. The patient is placed in isolation. Everyone coming into contact with the patient must practice appropriate isolation techniques. The emphasis is on the infective material that carries the specific microorganisms. The goal of the health care provider is to interrupt the chain of infection by preventing the transmission of the microbes. By working toward this goal, the health care provider protects the patient, the environment, and self.

UNIT REVIEW

A. True/False. Answer the following true or false by circling T or F.

T F 1. The Centers for Disease Control and Prevention has established isolation guidelines for diseases that are communicable.

T F 2. Color coding helps health care providers quickly identify the type of transmission to be controlled.

T F 3. Category-specific isolation precautions include ten isolation categories, each with a different set of precautions.

T F 4. The OSHA contains regulations to prevent transmission of blood-borne pathogens to health care providers.

T F 5. *Isolation technique* is the name given to the method of caring for patients with easily transmitted diseases.

T F 6. When a person has been placed on isolation precautions, only the nurse needs to be responsible for carrying out proper technique.

T F 7. The basic procedure to all isolation technique is proper bedpan care.

T F 8. When masks become moist, they must be discarded, since they are noneffective.

T F 9. Disposable patient care equipment is best when caring for a patient in isolation.

T F 10. A clean gown should be put on before entering the isolation unit.

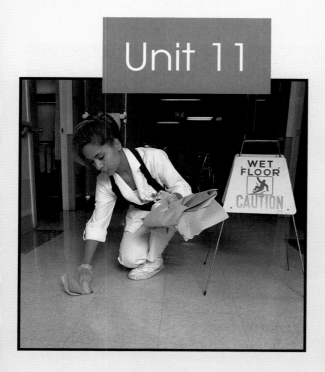

Environmental Control and Safety Measures

OBJECTIVES

As a result of this unit, you will be able to:

- Spell and define terms.
- Describe the patient's environment.
- Identify measures to provide for the safety and comfort of the patient.
- Describe safe transfer techniques to prevent falls when moving and transferring patients.
- List the purposes and guidelines for the use of postural supports/restraints.
- List the guidelines for fire safety.

VOCABULARY

Learn the meaning and the correct spelling of the following words and phrases:

ambulatory patient   semiprivate room
concurrent cleaning   side rails
private room   support
RACE   ward

The hospital bed is the patient's home while hospitalized, Figure 11–1A. The room becomes the patient's world. Yet the patient has little control over either the bed or the room. Cheerful and pleasant surroundings give the patient more of a sense of well-being. Consistent attention to safety factors help foster feelings of security in this foreign environment. *Both* aid in speeding recovery.

The nursing assistant helps keep the patient's unit safe and clean. All health care providers share in keeping the entire nursing unit safe and clean.

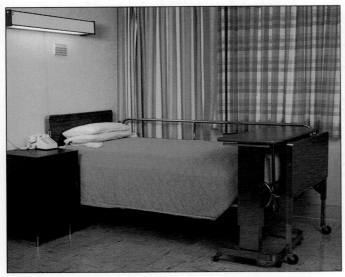

FIGURE 11–1A. The patient's unit becomes his home.

The Patient Environment

In a health care facility, the basic patient unit consists of a/an:

- Hospital bed with rails, Figures 11–1A and B
- Bedside table
- Chair
- Reading lamp
- Over-bed table
- Signal cord

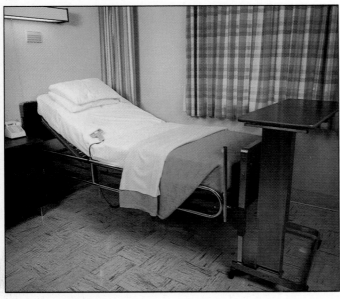

FIGURE 11–1B. Positions of hospital beds may be changed by controls, which are hand-held.

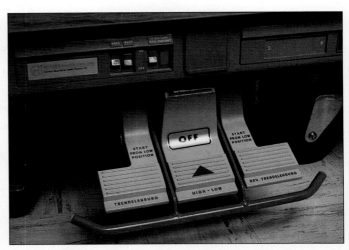

FIGURE 11–1C. Bed positions may also be operated by foot controls.

This equipment may be located in a single-, double-, or multiple-bed room. A **private room** contains only one bed. **Semiprivate rooms** contain two beds. **Wards** are multiple-bed rooms.

Each room is numbered. The beds are marked by letters or numbers. For example, Room 871 in a large medical center may be a four-unit ward. The beds are labeled A, B, C, D (or 1, 2, 3, 4). The patient in the fourth bed is in Unit 871–D or Unit 871–4.

The equipment from one unit should not be used by other patients. At home, the same unit elements will be present, but they will be modified. For example, there may not be an adjustable hospital bed or an over-bed table.

Hospital Beds

Hospital beds have mostly the same features, but there may be some differences. Hospital beds:

- Differ in the way in which they operate. Some are controlled electrically, Figures 11-1B and C. Others are operated by the turning of cranks or gatch handles.
- May be raised to the high horizontal position. At this position, there is less strain for those giving care. Beds must be left at the lowest horizontal position when leaving the room.
- Break in the middle so that the head may be raised.
- Break behind the knees to increase physical comfort for the bedridden patient.

Side rails are attached to the hospital-type bed. They protect the patient from falling. Side rails:

- Should be checked and attached securely before leaving the patient.

- Should only be down when beds are in the lowest horizontal position or if a release form has been signed by the patient.
- Are commonly raised at night since patients may become disoriented in dim light and unfamiliar surroundings.
- Should never be used for the attachment of tubes such as IV lines or catheters. Raising and lowering the side rails could put undue stress on such tubes.
- Are used whenever a patient is confused or disoriented.
- Should never be used for the attachment of restraints.
- May be viewed negatively by patients. Sometimes it may be necessary to reassure the patient that her condition is not becoming worse. The patient is told that the raising of side rails is hospital policy or is being done as a reminder of a new environment.

Temperature, Air Circulation, and Light

As you adjust and maintain the temperature, light, and ventilation, keep in mind the:

- Patient's condition.
- Patient's personal preference.
- Needs of the other patients in the room.
- Best temperature is about 70 degrees. A lower temperature may cause chilling and a higher one may make the patient uncomfortable.
- Movement of air and the temperature can be controlled by opening windows at the top and bottom if air conditioning is not being used.
- Patient can be shielded from drafts by screens or curtains.

In most hospitals and health facilities, rooms are automatically air conditioned. The thermostat is set from a central location or set individually in each patient's room.

Lighting comes from several sources. There will be times when less light will be desired. At other times, more light will be needed, Figure 11–2. Use as much light as needed to safely carry out your job. Be careful to shield other patients as much as possible.

Patients often find it difficult to sleep if lights are too bright. There should be only enough light at night to enable the staff to work safely.

- Rooms are equipped with lights above each bed. These illuminate a single patient bed.
- There may also be a ceiling light.

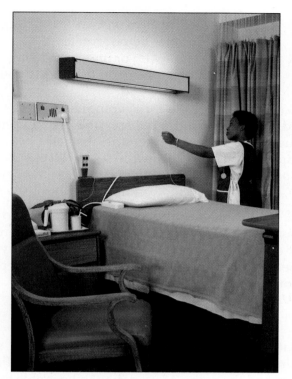

FIGURE 11–2. The best lighting is indirect lighting. The over-bed light can be adjusted to several lighting levels.

- Additional spotlights can be brought from the utility room when needed to provide extra light for delicate procedures.
- The best lighting is indirect since glare causes fatigue.
- Be sure to return extra lights as soon as you are finished because added clutter in a room is hazardous.
- Be sure to turn ceiling lights off when leaving the room.

Cleanliness, Noise Reduction, and Equipment

You are responsible for the cleanliness, quiet, and order of the patient units to which you are assigned. To contribute to the comfort of the patient:

- Report faulty equipment for repair.
- Speak quietly.
- Report wheels of equipment that need to be oiled to prevent squeaking.
- Avoid banging equipment and trays against other surfaces.

- Keep the area neat as you work. Check its overall appearance before you leave.
- Do not turn the TV on or up while giving care to patients unless the patient requests you do so.

You are responsible for keeping the patient supplied with fresh water, ice, disposable drinking cups, tissues, and straws. Make sure that all necessary equipment such as the wash basin, emesis basin, bedpan, urinal, soap, and towels are always available, clean, and in good condition, Figure 11–3.

Cleaning and care of basic equipment. The daily or **concurrent cleaning** of equipment is an important part of your job. It contributes to the safety of your patient. If damp dusting is needed and housekeeping is not available, see that it is done.

Safety Measures

Safety is the responsibility of everyone. A safe environment is essential for both the patient confined to bed and the **ambulatory patient** who is able to get up and walk around. Safety must be a part of everything you do. This concern covers not only the patient, but extends to the safety of the unit and the entire environment. Accidents involving patients and staff can be greatly reduced if simple measures are followed.

The signal cord must always function. It must be left within easy reach of the patient's hand. It is the patient's means of letting someone know of any needs.

The patient should be carefully instructed in the use of the signal cord. Allow the patient to show you how the signal cord is used so you can be sure that she understands. Inform the patient of the location of the emergency buttons located in each bathroom.

Equipment and Its Care

You can prevent accidents related to equipment by:
1. Reporting needed repairs promptly. Possible hazards include:
   a. Lost screws
   b. Frayed straps
   c. Loose wheels
   d. Broken control knobs
   e. Latches that do not hook
   f. Side rails that do not fasten correctly
   g. Faulty brakes on wheelchairs and stretchers
   h. Frayed electrical cords

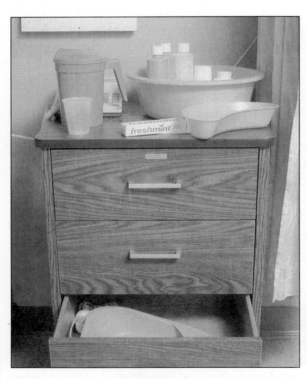

FIGURE 11–3. Standard equipment is included in each bedside stand.

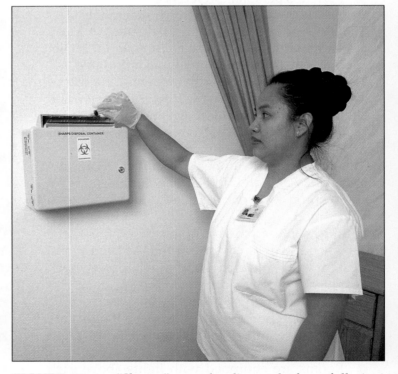

FIGURE 11–4. "Sharps" must be disposed of carefully in a safety container designed specifically for this use. Only authorized personnel may handle sharps such as syringes and IV needles.

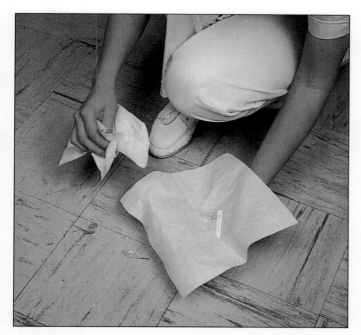

FIGURE 11–5. Small pieces of glass may be picked up carefully with a folded paper towel or tissues.

2. Disposing of equipment into proper containers. Facilities must dispose of "sharps," such as needles and blades, in special containers, Figure 11–4.
3. Never handle broken bits of glass with your hands. Larger pieces can be picked up with forceps. Small pieces can be picked up by moistening several thicknesses of paper towel and gently bringing the edges together so that your fingers do not touch the fragments, Figure 11–5.
4. Always know what you are handling and the proper method for its disposal.

Preventing Falls

Falls may occur for a variety of reasons. Patients may:

- Misjudge the distance from the bed to the floor.
- Feel weak or dizzy when trying to get up.
- Change position too rapidly and lose their balance when trying to rise from a chair. This is particularly common if the patient is older.
- Encounter hazards when walking.
- Be in unfamiliar surroundings.
- Take medications that make them less aware of surroundings.
- Be in a poorly lit area.

You must use great caution to avoid these mishaps.

- Always leave the bed in its lowest horizontal position when you have completed care.
- Leave side rails up and check for secure attachment, if applicable.
- Check and adjust protruding objects such as bed wheels or gatch handles.
- Clean and remove equipment when no longer needed.
- Do not permit blankets used by the patient sitting in a chair to touch the floor. Touching the floor contaminates the blanket. It can also cause tripping.
- Wipe up spills immediately.
- Encourage patients to use rails along corridor walls when walking.
- Observe ambulatory patients carefully for signs of weakness or unsteady gait.
- Make sure there is adequate lighting, especially during twilight and evening hours. Be sure that the patient has good foot support with nonskid soles.

Basic Guidelines for Moving or Transferring Patients

Transferring patients must be done carefully in order to avoid injury to you and the patient. Remember to employ good body mechanics and follow the exact procedures for each activity.

Specific procedures for carrying out transfer activities are covered in Unit 13. These are some general rules to keep in mind.

- Never use a footstool unless absolutely necessary. If it is necessary, keep it out of the traffic lane within the room. Place your foot firmly on top of it to keep it from slipping or hook your foot behind one leg of the stool when in use.
- When assisting the patient in any transfer, make sure the wheels of both the bed and the transfer vehicle, such as the stretcher or wheelchair, are locked, Figure 11–6.
- Brace chairs as patients rise or sit to prevent slipping. Hook one of your feet behind the front leg of the chair as your patient is being seated, Figure 11–7.
- Walk to the right in corridors. Stay to the right when moving patients in gurneys (stretchers or litters) and wheelchairs. Be especially careful at intersections, going up or down ramps, or when moving in narrow passageways.

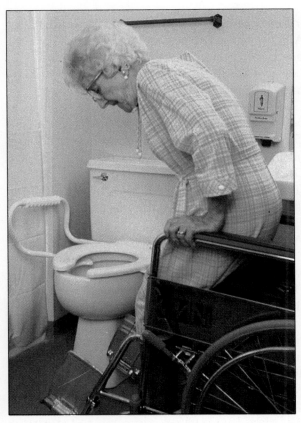

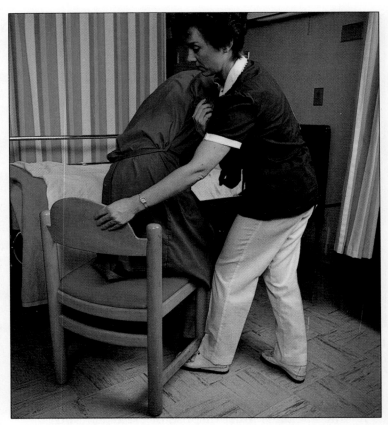

FIGURE 11–6. Locked wheelchair, grab bars, and safety rails on either side of the toilet improve the chance for a safe transfer.

FIGURE 11–7. When chairs do not have brakes, steady the chair by placing your foot behind a front leg.

- Always walk, never run, although you may feel pressured to move quickly at times.
- Never engage in horseplay. It is inappropriate and dangerous.
- Take care that a paralyzed patient's affected arm is placed in his lap. Do not allow it to hang over the spokes of the wheel where it may get caught. Paralyzed leg(s) should also be placed safely on the foot rests so as not to get caught under the chair when it is in motion. Remember to raise foot rests when patient is getting in or out of wheelchair, and to lock the brakes.
- In a home care environment, remove any scatter rugs which may cause the client to trip and fall. Place a nonslip mat in bathtub and shower.

Restraints/Safety Devices

It may be necessary sometimes to use devices (restraints) to ensure the patient's safety. These devices tend to restrict the patient's movement to some degree. Therefore, there are special guidelines for their use. These guidelines are discussed in Unit 3 and Unit 29. Positioning and safety devices position and support patients without restricting their movement, Figure 11–8.

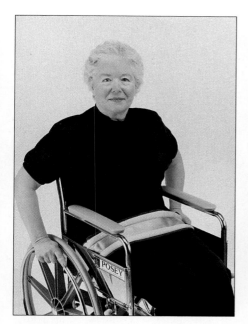
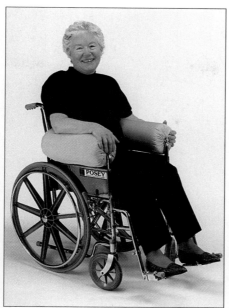
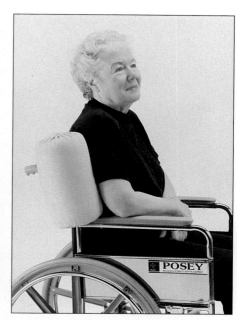

FIGURE 11–8. Supports help position patients and maintain body alignment without restricting movement. Patients are supported and protected without being restrained. *(Photos courtesy of J.T. Posey Co., Inc.)*

Fire Safety

It is a scientific fact that if three elements are present in the right proportions, Figure 11–9, there will be a fire. The three elements are heat, fuel, and oxygen.

It is the responsibility of every staff member to know and regularly practice the fire and evacuation plans for their facility.

- Role play the emergency procedures until you are completely secure. Remember that in any emergency the welfare and safety of the patients are most important.
- Learn the location of escape routes and the location and operation of all fire control equipment, Figure 11–10, such as:
  — Fire alarms
  — Extinguishers
  — Sprinklers
  — Fire doors
  — Fire escapes

- Know and practice fire drill procedures. These are conducted on a regular basis by each facility. Many patients could be injured during a fire because of the confusion and their inability to help themselves.
- Keep alert to all possible fire hazards. Report them immediately to the proper authorities.

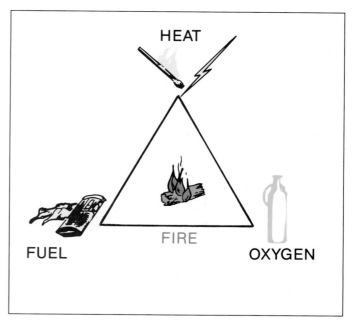

FIGURE 11–9. The fire triangle—elements needed for combustion (burning).

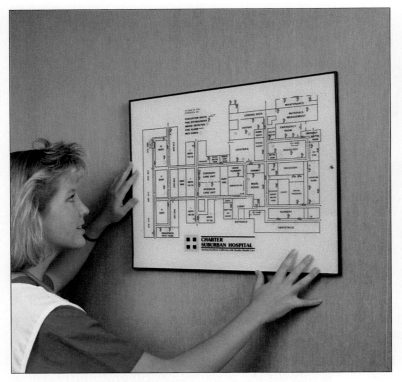 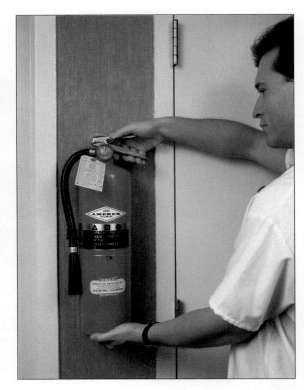

FIGURE 11–10. All personnel should know the escape plan in the event of a fire and should know where fire extinguishers are located.

Fire Hazards

Some possible fire hazards include:
- Frayed electrical wires
- Overloaded circuits
- Plugs that are not properly grounded
- Accumulated clutter such as papers and rags
- Improper protection during oxygen therapy
- Uncontrolled smoking; most health care facilities prohibit smoking throughout the facility
- Matches left where children or others may have unauthorized access to them
- Smoking in rooms where oxygen is in use

Fire Prevention

There is much you and every staff member can do to prevent the disaster of fire. In general:
- Check for frayed electrical wires.
- Do not overload circuits with too many electrical cords.
- Do not use a lightweight electrical cord with heavily powered equipment.
- Use three-prong grounded plugs.
- Do not allow clutter to accumulate in doorways or traffic lanes.
- Empty wastepaper cans in proper receptacles.
- Do not store oily rags or paint rags.
- Report any possible hazards right away.
- Report smoke and/or burning smells.
- Keep all fire exits clear of equipment and debris.
- Know and practice fire drill safety.
- Do not let visitors give cigarettes to patients.

Smoking

Smoking in bed should never be permitted unless the patient is supervised. Smoking should be strictly limited to specific areas, if permitted at all.

This applies to patients, visitors, and staff alike. Ashtrays should be large. The use of matches should be watched. Smoking materials are usually stored at the nurse's station. Patients who do not have smoking privileges should not have smoking materials. If you notice that a patient who is not allowed to smoke has smoking materials, collect the materials, and inform the nurse. Some smokers may need direct supervision in order to smoke.

Oxygen Precautions

The use of oxygen presents a specific hazard. When oxygen is in use:

- Never permit smoking, lighted matches, or open flames in the area.
- Do not use flammable liquids such as oils, alcohol, or nail polish.
- Do not use electrical equipment such as radios, hair dryers, electric razors, heating pads, or toys.
- Post a sign indicating that oxygen is in use.
- Use cotton blankets and gowns for the patient.
- Wear cotton uniforms and nonwool sweaters when providing care.
- Be certain there are no cigarettes and matches/lighters in the room.

In Case of Fire

You must be familiar with the fire policies and procedures for your facility. In case of fire, keep calm.

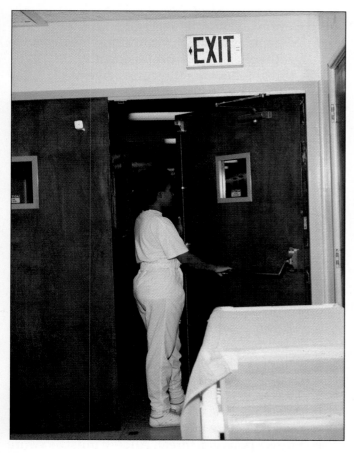

FIGURE 11–11. The nursing assistant is closing the fire door. When closed, fire doors retard the spread of a fire.

Be sure those in immediate danger are moved to safety. Then sound the alarm according to facility policy. Follow the evacuation plan as you have practiced. The patients may be confused and frightened. Therefore, the staff must be calm and in control. Remember:

- R = Remove patients. Move patients to safety. Patients who can walk can be escorted. In some cases, they may be called upon to assist others to escape routes. Patients may need to be moved in their beds out of the danger areas. If a person is unable to walk and the bed cannot be moved, bedsheets may be used as cradles and the patient pulled to safety.
- A = Alarm. Sound the alarm. Use the intercom, emergency signal bell, telephone, or fire alarm as directed by facility policy. Give the location and type of fire.
- C = Contain fire. Close windows and doors, Figure 11–11, to prevent drafts which cause the fire to spread more rapidly.
- E = Extinguish fire.
- Follow the fire emergency plan.
- Keep calm. Be prepared to follow directions when a person of authority takes charge.
- Shut off air conditioning and other electrical equipment.
- Shut off oxygen.
- Do not use elevators.

See Figure 11–12.

Use of a Fire Extinguisher

If you have been trained in the use of a fire extinguisher, it may be used on small fires, Figure 11–13.

- Fire extinguishers should be carried upright.
- Remove the safety pin.

R—Remove patient

A—Activate alarm

C—Contain fire

E—Extinguish fire

FIGURE 11–12. Remember the sequence of critical actions in case of a fire.

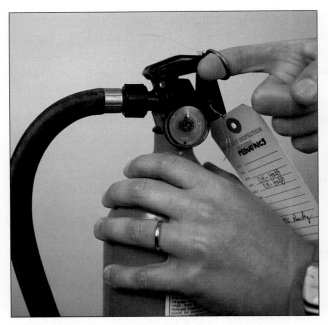

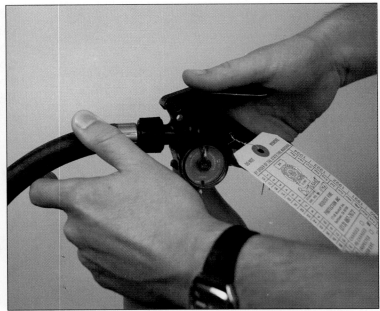

A. Remove pin.   B. Push top handle down.

FIGURE 11–13. Use of the fire extinguisher

■ Push the top handle down.
■ Direct the hose at the base of the fire.
Remember the letters PASS, Figure 11–14.
In all situations, get patients to safety, follow hospital policy, and keep calm.

Emergencies

Fire is only one of the emergency situations you may face. In general, remember:

■ In any emergency, keep calm.
■ Assess the situation.
■ Signal for help.

There may be other disasters for which your facility must be prepared. Tornadoes, hurricanes, floods, earthquakes, and bomb threats are examples of such disasters. Each facility has its own policies. Be sure you are familiar with them.

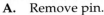

P— PULL the pin

A— AIM the nozzle at the base of the fire

S— SQUEEZE the handle

S— SWEEP back and forth along the base
      of the fire

FIGURE 11–14. Learn the meaning of the letters PASS so you will know how to operate a fire extinguisher.

■ Never leave the patient alone.
■ When help arrives, listen carefully to the nurse or other health care professional.
■ Closely follow the directions given.
■ Make safety rules and hazard prevention a growing part of your awareness.

As part of your training, you may receive instruction in basic first aid and cardiopulmonary resuscitation (CPR).

SUMMARY

The nursing staff is responsible for maintaining a safe, comfortable environment for the patient.

■ The bed and unit are the patient's home during his hospital stay.
■ All equipment must be readily available and kept in clean operating condition.
■ Safety is the business of everyone. Knowing the rules assures your full participation.
■ The cleanliness of the unit must be maintained on a daily basis. The unit must be completely cleaned before being used by a new patient.
■ Fire is a potential threat. All staff must be aware of those factors that contribute to a fire hazard and control them. Fire plans must be understood and followed in case of a fire.

UNIT REVIEW

A. Multiple Choice. Select the one best answer.

1. An ambulatory patient is
   a. confined to bed.
   b. sitting in a chair.
   c. walking around.
   d. receiving oxygen.

2. The patient's name is Phe Quan. She is in Room 116-D. From this information, you would understand that she is occupying a bed in a/an
   a. private room.
   b. rehabilitation department.
   c. semiprivate room.
   d. ward.

3. Side rails should be up and secure when
   a. the bed is higher than lowest horizontal height (unless when giving care).
   b. the patient is in bed for the night.
   c. leaving the patient after care unless there is a signed release.
   d. all of the above.

4. The best room temperature is approximately
   a. 45°F.
   b. 65°F.
   c. 70°F.
   d. 78°F.

5. Concurrent cleaning is performed
   a. twice daily.
   b. every day.
   c. weekly.
   d. when the patient is discharged.

6. You can help prevent falls by
   a. leaving the bed in the highest position when you have completed care.
   b. using a night light.
   c. keeping lighting low, especially at night.
   d. pushing equipment into the corner when no longer needed.

7. Which of the following represents a fire hazard?
   a. frayed electrical wire
   b. overloaded circuits
   c. uncontrolled smoking
   d. all of the above

8. Ashtrays should be emptied
   a. into a plastic container.
   b. into a metal container.
   c. into a paper sack.
   d. anywhere, since it really doesn't matter.

B. True/False. Answer the following true or false by circling T or F.

T F   9. The bed should be left in lowest horizontal position when the resident is sleeping.

T F 10. Confused patients should have side rails down so they will not feel confined.

T F 11. Attach restraints to the side rails for security.

T F 12. There should always be enough light to enable the staff to work safely.

T F 13. Noise and clutter are very disturbing to most people.

T F 14. Dry dusting is more effective than damp dusting.

T F 15. When doing terminal cleaning, anything left by the patient may be discarded.

T F 16. Washing the springs and frame of the bed is part of daily cleaning.

T F 17. Needed repairs should be reported immediately.

T F 18. The signal cord is the patient's way of letting the staff know that she is in need.

T F 19. A chair should be braced with your foot when assisting the patient to rise.

T F 20. Footstools are frequently used to help patients get in and out of bed.

T F 21. It is all right to play while at work as long as no one gets hurt.

T F 22. You are responsible for knowing and practicing fire drill procedures.

T F 23. In case of a fire, follow your own plan of action.

T F 24. Always carry a fire extinguisher in an upright position.

T F 25. It is wise to use an elevator during a fire emergency.

T F 26. In the event of any emergency, keep calm.

T F 27. Safety devices (restraints) may be needed for some patients.

T (F) 28. Smoking is permitted when oxygen is in use.

T (F) 29. A physician's order is not necessary before applying postural supports.

SELF-EVALUATION   Section 4

A. Define the following words:

1. protozoa _____

   _____

2. bacteria _____

   _____

3. contamination _____

   _____

4. fomites _____

   _____

5. autoclave _____

   _____

B. Match Column I with Column II on micro-organisms.

   Column I   Column II

____ 6. disease-causing   a. staphylococcus
        organisms
                                  b. pathogens
____ 7. arranged in pairs
                                  c. toxins
____ 8. arranged in
        chains   d. spores

____ 9. hard-to-destroy   e. streptococcus
        forms of microbes
                                  f. diplococcus
____ 10. poisons
                                  g. parasites
____ 11. grow on living
         organisms   h. vegetative

____ 12. arranged in
         clusters

C. Choose the phrase that best completes each of the following sentences by circling the proper letter.

13. Using proper handwashing technique, you should
    a. rinse with fingertips pointed up.
    b. use very hot water.
    c. not include the fingernails at this time.
    d. turn faucets on and off with a paper towel.

14. If the seal on a commercially prepared sterile package of gauze is broken, you will
    a. consider the package contaminated.
    b. use it anyway since the contents look clean.
    c. know the condition of the seal is not important.
    d. know that the seal has to be broken before use anyway.

15. When a patient is in isolation
    a. equipment can be moved in and out without special precautions.
    b. frequently used equipment remains in the patient unit.
    c. one person can move equipment safely in and out of the unit.
    d. contaminated equipment is labeled "clean."

16. Reverse isolation technique
    a. is used when the patient has a communicable disease.
    b. requires less extensive preparation than regular isolation.
    c. is used when patients have little resistance to disease.
    d. requires sterilization of all articles leaving the room.

17. When isolation technique is being used, a sign will be placed on the door which might read
    a. stop.
    b. keep clear.
    c. free area.
    d. barrier.

D. Complete the following statements correctly.

18. One very important way to control the spread of bacteria is by proper _____
    _____.

19. The special way of caring for patients with easily transferrable diseases is called _____
    _____.

20. Diseases spread through feces are called
    _____.

21. When leaving a patient, the bed should be in _____ position.

22. When patients are ambulating, there must be adequate lighting, especially during the _____ and _____ hours.

23. There must be a/an _____ before restraints may be applied.

24. Possible fire hazards include:
    a. _____
    b. _____
    c. _____
    d. _____
    e. _____

25. In any emergency situation, it is important that you keep _____
    _____.

E. Provide short answers to the following.

26. Write five procedures included in universal precautions.
    a. _____
    b. _____
    c. _____
    d. _____
    e. _____

27. List five factors to be considered when maintaining proper temperature, air circulation, and light.
    a. _____
    b. _____
    c. _____
    d. _____
    e. _____

28. Write out the guidelines for fire safety.
    a. _____
    b. _____
    c. _____
    d. _____
    e. _____
    f. _____

29. List the components of the patient's environment.
    a. _____
    b. _____
    c. _____
    d. _____
    e. _____
    f. _____

30. List four equipment repairs that, left undone, could be hazardous.
    a. _____
    b. _____
    c. _____
    d. _____

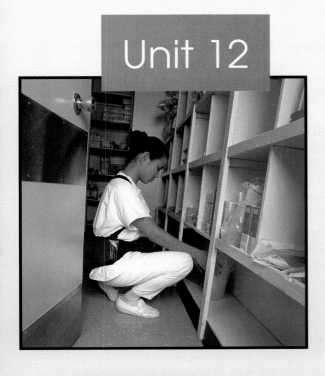

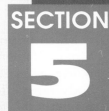

Unit 12

Principles of Body Mechanics

OBJECTIVES

As a result of this unit, you will be able to:

- Spell and define terms.
- Define body mechanics.
- List the basic rules for proper body mechanics.
- Describe the proper body alignment for the patient.
- List and describe the seven basic positions and the supportive measures to maintain body alignment.
- List the dangers of bedrest and immobility.

VOCABULARY

Learn the meaning and the correct spelling of the following words:

alignment
anorexia
body mechanics
constipation
contracture
dorsal recumbent
  position
fecal impaction
flexible
horizontal recumbent
  position

left lateral recumbent
  position
posture
prone position
right lateral recumbent
  position
semi-Fowler's position
Sims' position
supine position

Your body is like a well-organized machine. Each part is designed to do a special job. Your eyes see, your ears hear, and your muscles help you move. Some muscles help give your body shape and form. Others are attached to bones in such a way that it is possible for you to move or lift heavy objects. Muscle groups can do their best when used properly. Using the right muscles to do the job is called proper **body mechanics**

193

Body Mechanics for the Nursing Assistant

Much of your work will require physical effort. Moving patients, carrying equipment, and pushing wheelchairs require muscle power. You use your body most effectively when you use your muscles properly.

Posture

Good body mechanics start with proper posture. Proper posture means that there is a balance between the muscle groups, and body parts are in good alignment (position). Correct posture is the same in all positions—standing, sitting, and lying.

Good posture allows the body to function at its best in all activities. Correct posture makes lifting, pulling, and pushing easier.

Your spine is like a flexible (bendable) rod with a crossbar near the top and another near the bottom. Strong muscles attach the arms and legs to the back.

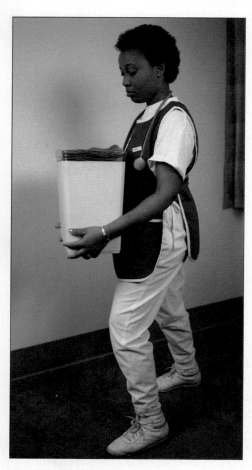

FIGURE 12–1. Keeping the feet separated provides a good base of support.

The muscles of the spine are small. They were not meant to lift heavy loads. Their main job is to bend the back in different directions and to hold the back steady, like an anchor, while the muscles of the legs and shoulders do the heavy work. To avoid straining your back muscles, bend from the hips and knees when you are moving an object. When you are carrying an object, hold it close to you.

Good standing posture begins by having the:

■ Feet flat on the floor, separated about 12 inches
■ Arms at the sides
■ Back straight
■ Abdominal muscles tightened
■ Knees very slightly flexed

Using Your Body Effectively

There are 10 basic rules to remember that will help your muscles work for you.

1. Keep your back straight.
2. Keep your feet separated to provide a good base of support, Figure 12–1.
3. Bend from the hips and knees to get close to the object. Do not bend from the waist, Figure 12–2.
4. Use the weight of your body to help to push or pull the object.
5. Use the strongest muscles to do the job.
6. Avoid twisting your body as you work and bend for long periods of time. Pivot the whole body.
7. Hold heavy objects close to your body.
8. Push or pull on an object rather than lifting it.
9. Always ask for help if you feel the patient or object is too heavy to move by yourself, Figure 12–3.
10. Synchronize movements. Prepare patient and other staff member by informing them when ready, or count to three and all move together on the word "go."

Be willing to help others. Do not take chances. Various mechanical devices are available to help in moving the helpless or heavy patient, Figure 12–4. When you are using one of the mechanical lifts, make sure that the support slings are positioned smoothly under the patient. Check to be sure that all parts of the equipment are safe and in working order.

Health care workers in many facilities have begun wearing body supports while they are working. These supports are designed to promote the use of good body mechanics, Figure 12–5. They are available in all sizes. It is important to wear the right size

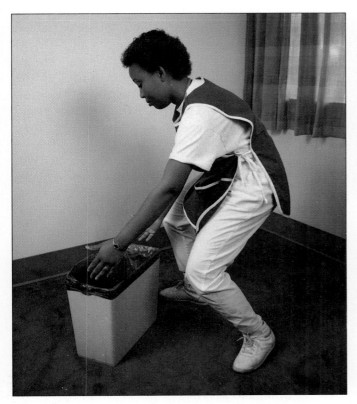

FIGURE 12–2. The correct way to maintain balance when picking up an object is to bend from the hips and knees.

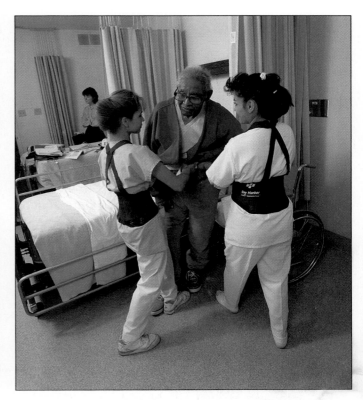

FIGURE 12–3. Get help whenever possible.

so maximum benefit is obtained. The support should fit snugly when the wearer is lifting or performing other strenuous tasks. It can be loosened at other times. However, the support should be worn throughout the shift so that it is in place when needed. The use of body supports has decreased the rate of work-related injuries in health care facilities.

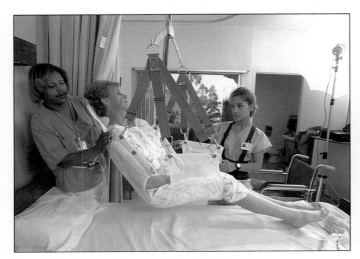

FIGURE 12–4. Use a mechanical device to move heavy or helpless patients.

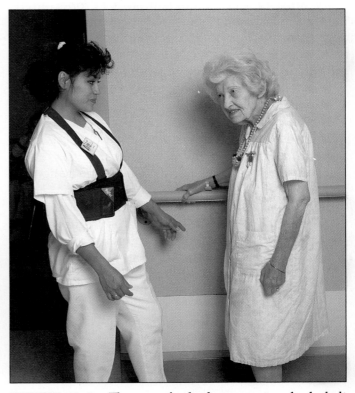

FIGURE 12–5. The use of a body support or body belt reduces the risk of work-related injury for nursing assistants.

Body Mechanics for the Patient

Body mechanics for the patient who is ambulatory are very similar to those for the health care team. While the patient is probably doing no lifting, whether heavy or not, good posture habits should not be neglected.

Good posture for the patient means that standing, walking, and changing positions will be done in a steady and safe manner.

Bed patients sometimes find it hard to stay in a position because they tend to slide toward the foot of the bed when the head of the bed is elevated.

Those patients who are incapacitated will not be able to change their position. Nor will they be able to help you change their position. Bed patients will need extra help to gain and maintain proper alignment.

Remember, whenever possible:

■ Get help.
■ Use turning or lifting sheets.
■ Use mechanical devices.
■ Change the patient's position frequently, at least every two hours.

Body Alignment and Positioning

Proper alignment (positioning) of the patient's body must be done conscientiously. Proper alignment means keeping a person in a position where the body can function at its best. Natural body curves need to be supported in their natural positions with pillows and rolled towels. Proper positioning:

■ Helps the patient feel more comfortable
■ Relieves strain
■ Helps the body function more efficiently
■ Prevents deformities and complications such as contractures and pressure sores

There are seven basic positions for the patient in bed.

1. **Dorsal recumbent, horizontal recumbent**, or back-lying (Figure 12–6A). This position is also known as the **supine position.**
   a. The bed is in the horizontal position.
   b. The patient is on the back.
   c. A pillow is placed under the patient's head for comfort.
   d. The arms are extended and supported by small pillows.
   e. A rolled towel may support the small of the back.
   f. A small pillow or rolled towel is placed along side the patient's thighs and tucked under to prevent external hip rotation.
   g. A padded footboard may be added to the bed to keep the feet in the proper position and to prevent foot drop or the patient may wear special shoes. A folded pillow may also be used.
   h. A folded pad or foam supports between calf and ankles reduces pressure on the heels, Figure 12–6B.

2. **Right lateral recumbent position** (Figure 12–6C). The patient is turned on the right side. The spine should be straight.
   a. Pillows may be used under the head, between the legs, and at the back.
   b. The right arm is flexed and brought under the pillow.
   c. The left arm is flexed and supported with a pillow.
   d. The left leg is slightly flexed. It is supported by a pillow to keep the proper relationship of legs to pelvis.

3. **Prone position** (face-lying) (Figure 12–6D). The patient is positioned on the abdomen. The spine is straight. The legs are extended. The arms are flexed and brought up to either side of the head. The patient's face is turned to the side.
   a. A small pillow is placed under the abdomen. This is especially important for female patients. It reduces pressure against the breasts. An alternate method is to roll a towel and place it under the shoulders to reduce pressure.
   b. Another pillow is placed under the lower legs. This prevents pressure on the toes and keeps the feet in proper position.
   c. The patient may also be moved to the foot of the bed so that the feet extend over the mattress. This is an alternate method of reducing pressure on the toes. It allows the foot to assume a normal standing position.

4. **Left lateral recumbent position.** The patient is positioned on the left side. The spine should be straight.
   a. A pillow may be used under the head at the back.

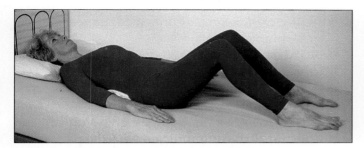

FIGURE 12–6A. Dorsal recumbent position

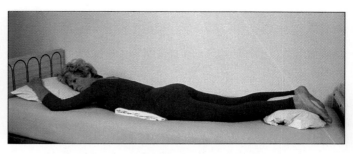

FIGURE 12–6D. Prone position (face-lying)

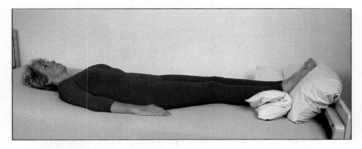

FIGURE 12–6B. Horizontal recumbent position

dorsal = supine } the same

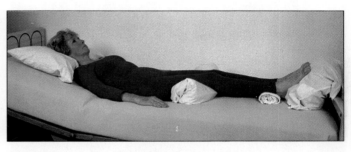

FIGURE 12–6E. Semi-Fowler's position

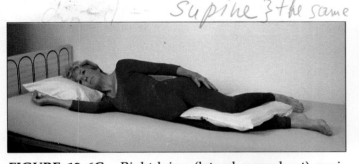

FIGURE 12–6C. Right-lying (lateral recumbent) position

left-lying

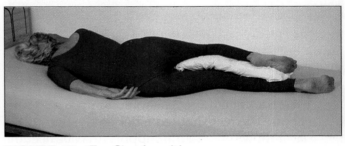

FIGURE 12–6F. Sims' position

the same   always left.

b. The right leg is flexed. It is supported by a pillow. This maintains the proper relationship of legs to pelvis.
c. A pillow in front of the patient extends up under the flexed right arm and shoulder.
d. The left arm is flexed and brought up beneath the head pillow.
5. **Semi-Fowler's position** (Figure 12–6E). The patient is positioned on the back. The head of the bed is elevated as follows.
   ■ semi-Fowler's—head elevated 30°
   ■ Fowler's—head elevated 45°-60°
   ■ high Fowler's—head elevated 90°
   a. One, two, or three pillows are used to support the head and shoulders.
   b. The knees may be slightly flexed and supported with a pillow.

c. A pillow may be placed under each arm for support.
d. A padded footboard or folded pillow keeps the feet in position.
6. **Sims' position** (Figure 12–6F). The patient is positioned on the left side with the left leg extended and the right leg flexed.
   a. The left arm is positioned behind the back and extended.
   b. The right arm is flexed and brought forward on the bed. It is supported by a pillow.
   c. A small pillow is placed under the head. This position is often used for rectal examinations and treatment, and enemas.
7. **Sitting position.** Patients should be positioned in a comfortable, well-constructed chair, so that the head and spine are erect, Figure 12–7.

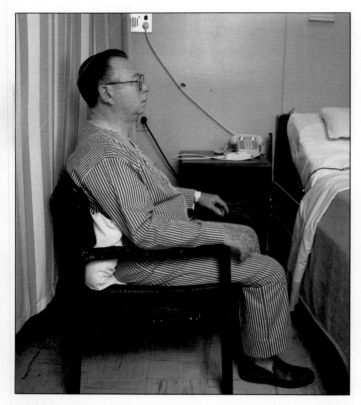

FIGURE 12–7. The correct sitting position does not permit the back of the patient's legs to rest against the chair. A small pillow supports the back.

The back and buttocks should be up against the chair. The feet should be flat on the floor.
a. Pillows or postural supports may be needed to maintain the position.
b. A small towel may be folded and placed at the small of the back to add comfort and support. A small pillow may also be used.
c. Do not permit the back of the patient's knees to rest against the chair.

Dangers of Bedrest and Immobility

- Lack of activity results in anorexia (loss of appetite), constipation (difficulty of bowel movement), and the severest form of constipation, fecal impaction
- Without frequent changes in position, the urinary system is less effective. Renal stones may form.
- When bones do not bear weight, calcium is lost from the bones. This makes them more easily broken.
- Contractures (deformities due to muscle shortening through lack of use) develop, Figure 12–8, and muscles atrophy.

- Lung expansion is diminished, increasing the risk of pneumonia.
- Circulation is impaired, increasing the risk of thrombophlebitis.
- There is greater likelihood of pressure sores developing, Figure 12–9.
- Frequent position changes give you an opportunity to communicate with the patient.

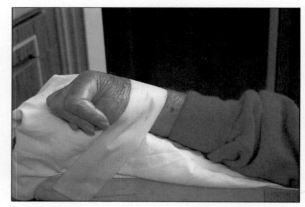

FIGURE 12–8. Immobility leads to deformities called contractures.

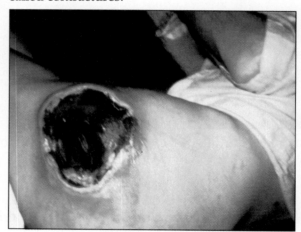

FIGURE 12–9. Deep (crater) lesion, also known as a decubitus ulcer *(Photo courtesy of Emory University Hospital, Atlanta, GA)*

SUMMARY

- Nursing tasks are easier when proper body mechanics are followed.
- Using large muscles to do the heavy work reduces fatigue and strain. It can also prevent serious injury.
- Care must be taken to keep the patient in good alignment and provide support at all times in all positions.

- Frequent change of position helps prevent deformities and decubiti. It also aids general body functions and contributes to comfort.
- Frequent position changes are essential to prevent:
  — Musculoskeletal deformities and bone loss of calcium from bones
  — Poor skin nutrition and the development of pressure sores
  — Respiratory complications such as pneumonia
  — Decreased circulation that could lead to thrombophlebitis and renal calculi
  — Loss of opportunities for social exchange between patient and staff

UNIT REVIEW

A. Matching. Match Column I with Column II.

	Column I		Column II
e	1. walking around	a.	bendable
h	2. semi-sitting position	b.	alignment
c	3. abnormal shortening of muscles	c.	contracture
		d.	decubitus ulcer
g	4. the way in which the body is aligned		
j	5. device to assist in moving patients	e.	ambulatory
a	6. flexible	f.	prone
i	7. backbone	g.	posture
b	8. position	h.	Fowler's
f	9. lying face down	i.	spine
d	10. bedsore	j.	mechanical lift

B. True/False. Answer the following true or false by circling T or F.

T F 11. Good standing posture is with the feet separated.

T **F** 12. The muscles of the spine are some of the strongest in the body.

T F 13. To avoid straining your back muscles, you should bend from the hips and knees when lifting an object.

T F 14. When you carry an object, you should hold it close to you.

T **F** 15. When working, it is alright to quickly twist your back as long as you don't remain in that position.

T F 16. The position of bed patients should be changed at least every two hours.

T F 17. Bath blankets can be used to decrease moisture accumulation when positioning patients.

T F 18. The large muscle groups should be used to do the heaviest jobs.

T **F** 19. When placing a woman in the prone position, it is especially important to place a bath blanket under the knees to prevent excessive pressure on the breasts.

T F 20. The left Sims' position is often used for rectal treatments, examinations, and enemas.

C. Completion.

21. Describe what good posture means.
22. State the characteristics of a good standing posture.
    a. feet flat _____
    b. feet separated _____
    c. back _____
    d. abdominal muscles _____
    e. knees _____
23. List four reasons why position should be frequently changed.
    a. _____
    b. _____
    c. _____
    d. _____

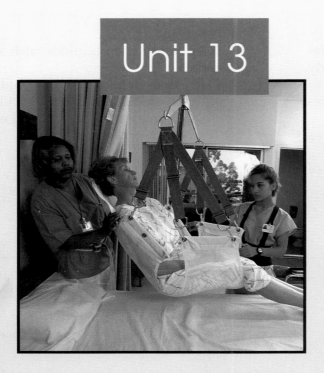

Moving, Lifting, and Transporting Patients

OBJECTIVES

As a result of this unit, you will be able to:

- Spell and define terms.
- List the elements that are common to all procedures.
- Describe and demonstrate the proper procedure for turning a patient.
- Describe and demonstrate the correct procedure for helping a patient sit up or move up in bed.
- Describe and demonstrate the correct procedure for helping a patient into a chair or wheelchair.
- Describe and demonstrate the proper procedure for lifting a patient using a mechanical device.
- Describe and demonstrate the correct procedure for transferring a patient from a bed to stretcher.
- Describe and demonstrate the proper procedure for log rolling the patient.
- Describe and demonstrate the proper procedure for ambulating a patient using a gait belt.
- Describe and demonstrate the proper procedure for helping a falling patient.
- Describe and demonstrate the proper procedure for transporting a patient by wheelchair or stretcher.

VOCABULARY

Learn the meaning and the correct spelling of the following words:

drawsheet	pivot
gait	procedure
gait belt	transfer belt
mechanical lift	turning sheet

Introduction to Procedures

Caring for patients safely means you must faithfully and carefully carry out specific routines. The routine manner of carrying out a task is called a procedure.

As you progress in your studies, you will learn the procedures for many nursing assistant tasks. You have already been introduced to the procedure for washing your hands. The procedures that follow give you step-by-step directions for carrying out tasks that involve patients.

Certain things must be done before you carry out patient care procedures. These actions are called preprocedure, or beginning procedure actions, Figure 13–1. At the completion of each patient care procedure, there are also a series of procedure completion actions to be followed, Figure 13–2.

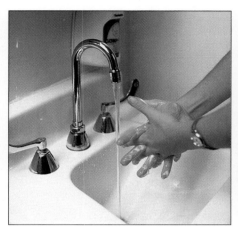

A. Wash your hands.

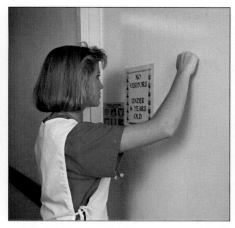

B. If the door is closed or the privacy curtains are drawn, knock or speak before entering.

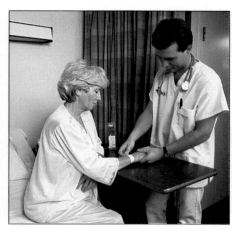

C. Identify the patient.

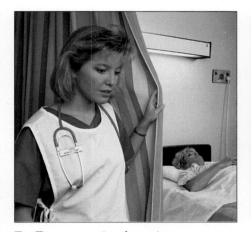

D. Draw curtains for privacy.

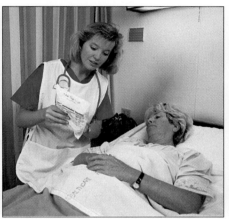

E. Explain to the patient what you are going to do.

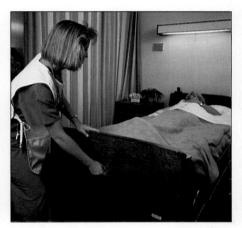

F. Raise the bed to a comfortable working height.

FIGURE 13–1. Before starting any patient care procedure, certain basic steps must be done.

Beginning Procedure Actions

Steps to be followed at the beginning of each procedure include the following:
- Wash hands thoroughly, Figure 13–1A.
- Assemble needed equipment.
- Go to patient's room, knock and pause before entering, Figure 13–1B.
- Introduce yourself and identify patient by checking the identification bracelet, Figure 13–1C.
- Ask visitors to leave the room and inform them where they may wait.
- Provide privacy, Figure 13–1D.
- Explain what will happen and answer questions, Figure 13–1E.
- Allow patient to assist as much as possible.
- Raise bed to comfortable working height, Figure 13–1F.

Procedure Completion Actions

Steps to be followed when the procedure is completed include the following:
- Position patient comfortably.
- Return bed to lowest horizontal position.

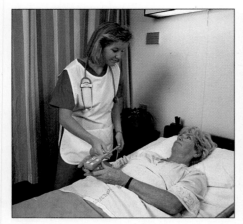

A. Lower the bed and place signal cord where patient can reach it.

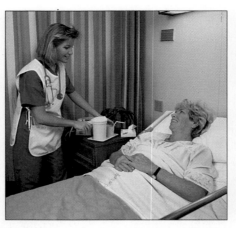

B. Make sure water is conveniently placed within the patient's reach.

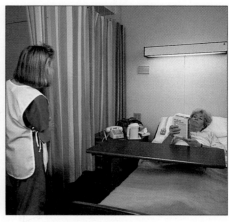

C. Open curtains.

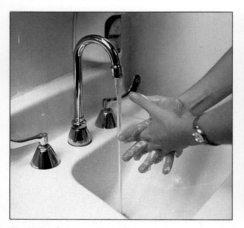

D. Wash your hands.

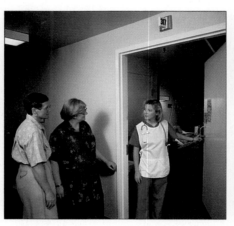

E. Let visitors know when they may reenter the patient's room.

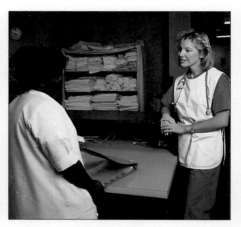

F. Report and document your actions and the patient's response.

FIGURE 13–2.   After completing any patient care procedure, certain basic steps must be done.

- Leave signal cord, Figure 13–2A, telephone, and fresh water where patient can reach them, Figure 13–2B.
- Perform a general safety check of patient and environment.
- Open curtains, Figure 13–2C.
- Care for equipment following facility policy.
- Wash hands, Figure 13–2D.
- Let visitors know when they may reenter, Figure 13–2E.
- Report completion of task, Figure 13–2F.
- Document action and your observations.

NOTE: Where there are open lesions, wet linen, or possible contact with patient body fluids or blood, disposable gloves are to be worn during the procedure. Put on gloves before contact with the patient or linen. Properly dispose of gloves after they are removed.

So much handwashing may seem to be unnecessary because of the short length of time that you are with the patient. Just remember that your hands can transmit germs. Patients already weakened by disease have a much lower resistance to germs.

Because the beginning procedure and procedure completion actions are the same for each patient care procedure, they will not be restated as individual steps with each procedure. Rather, a general reference will be made to these steps at the beginning and end of each procedure. You must, however, learn and faithfully complete each of these steps for each patient care procedure you perform.

Moving and Lifting Patients

Lifting, moving, and transporting patients is a major responsibility of the nursing assistant. Proper body mechanics and observance of safety rules will protect both you and your patients from injury. *Always* ask the nurse whether help is needed to lift or move a patient before proceeding with your assignment. Never be afraid to ask for help. By exercising caution, you are also preventing potentially serious injuries.

At times, two people or more will be needed to safely move or transport the patient and her equipment. For example, when the patient is:

- Receiving portable oxygen.
- Receiving intravenous fluids. There are portable intravenous (IV) stands which can move with the patient.
- Very heavy.
- Unable to assist in any way.

A good principle to follow is to *always get help to move or lift a patient when the patient weighs more than you do, or has problems with balance or standing on both feet.*

A turning sheet or drawsheet (folded large sheet or half sheet) may be placed under the heavy or helpless patient to make moving easier. The sheet must extend from above the shoulders to below the hips to be effective.

The following procedures should be followed when you are lifting, moving, or transporting patients. As you practice these procedures, keep in mind the 10 basic rules of good body mechanics that were discussed in Unit 12.

PROCEDURE 9   OBRA    SIDE 2

TURNING THE PATIENT TOWARD YOU

1. Carry out each beginning procedure action.
2. Remember to wash your hands, identify the patient, and provide privacy.
3. Lower near side rail. Cross the patient's far leg over the leg that is nearest to you.
4. Cross the far arm over the patient's chest. Bend the near arm at the elbow, bringing the hand toward the head of the bed.
5. Place your hand nearest the head of the bed on the patient's far shoulder. Place your other hand on the patient's hips on the far side, Figure 13–3A. You should brace your thighs against the side of the bed.
6. Roll the patient toward you. Do it slowly, gently, and smoothly. Help the patient bring the upper leg toward you and bend comfortably.
7. Put up the side rail. Be sure it is secure.
8. Go to the opposite side of the bed.
9. Place your hands under the patient's shoulders and then the hips. Pull toward the center of the bed, Figure 13–3B. This helps the patient maintain the side-lying position.
10. Make sure the patient's body is properly aligned and safely positioned, Figure 13–3C.

11. A pillow may be placed behind the patient's back. Secure it by pushing the near side under the patient to form a roll.
12. If the patient is unable to move self, position the arms and legs. Support them with pillows between the shoulders and hands and knees and ankles to prevent friction and

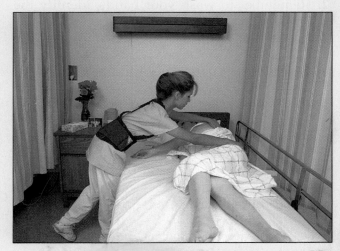

FIGURE 13–3A. Place your hands on the patient's far shoulder and hip.

continues

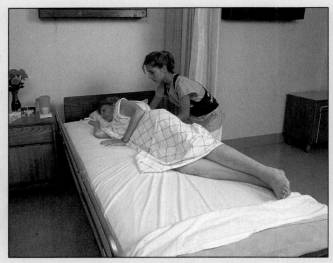

FIGURE 13–3B. Keeping your back straight, pull patient to center of bed.

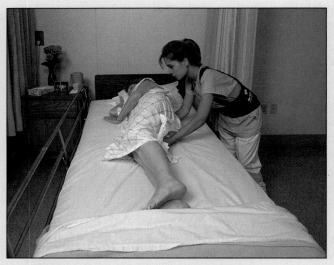

FIGURE 13–3C. Make sure patient is correctly positioned before adding pillows to maintain position and cushion pressure points.

contractures. If the patient has an indwelling catheter, make sure the tubing is not between the legs in order to prevent undue stress on it.

13. Carry out each procedure completion action.

Remember to wash your hands, report the completion of the task, and document the time, position changed (right lying—lateral), and patient reaction.

PROCEDURE 10 **OBRA**

SIDE
2

TURNING THE PATIENT AWAY FROM YOU

1. Carry out each beginning procedure action.
2. Remember to wash your hands, identify the patient, and provide privacy.
3. Lower near side rail. Be sure the side rail on the opposite side of the bed is up and secure.
4. Have patient bend knees, if able. Cross the arms on the chest, Figure 13–4A.
5. Place your arm nearest the head of the bed under the patient's head and shoulders. Place the other hand and forearm under the small of his back. Bend your body at the hips and knees. Keep your back straight. Pull the patient toward the edge of the bed.
6. Place your forearms under patient's hips and pull them toward you.
7. Move patient's ankles and knees toward you by placing one hand under the ankles and one under the knees.

8. Cross patient's nearer leg over the other leg at ankles, Figure 13–4B.

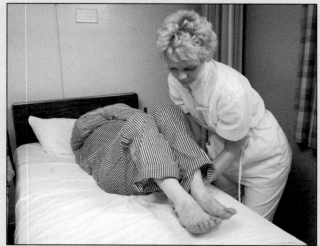

FIGURE 13–4A. Have patient cross arms and bend knees.

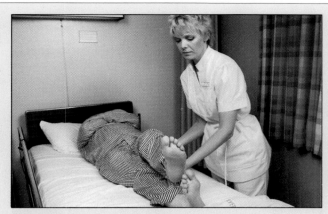

FIGURE 13–4B. Cross patient's near leg over far leg.

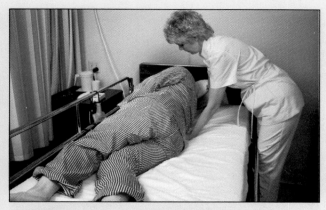

FIGURE 13–4C. Roll patient away from you.

9. Roll patient slowly and carefully away from you, Figure 13–4C, by placing one hand under the patient's shoulder and one hand under the hips.
10. Place your hands under the patient's head and shoulders. Draw them back toward the center of the bed.
11. Move patient's hips to the center of the bed as in step 5.
12. Place a pillow for support behind the patient's back.

13. Make sure that patient's body is in a good position. Support the upper leg with a pillow. Place the lower arm in a flexed position. Support the upper arm with a pillow.
14. Replace side rail on near side of the bed. Return bed to the lowest height.
15. Carry out each procedure completion action. Remember to wash your hands, report completion of task, and document the time, position changed (right or left lying—lateral), and patient reaction.

PROCEDURE 11   OBRA

ASSISTING THE PATIENT TO SIT UP IN BED

1. Carry out each beginning procedure action.
2. Remember to wash your hands, identify the patient, and provide privacy.
3. Lock the wheels of the bed. Be sure the bed is at a comfortable height. Lower near side rail.
4. Face the head of the bed. Keep one leg forward to give you a firm base of support, Figure 13–5A. Turn your head away from the patient's face.
5. Lock near arms (patient and assistant), Figure 13–5B.
6. Support the patient with the other arm by making a cradle for the head and shoulders, Figure 13–5C.
7. Bring the patient to a sitting position. Adjust the bed position. Provide pillows for support and comfort. Raise side rail.
8. Carry out each procedure completion action.

Remember to wash your hands, report completion of task, and document the time, action (assisted patient to sit up in bed), and patient's response.

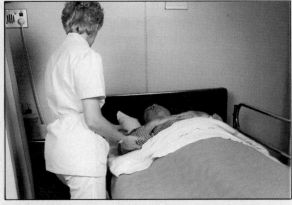

FIGURE 13–5A. Face head of bed and keep your outer leg forward.

continues

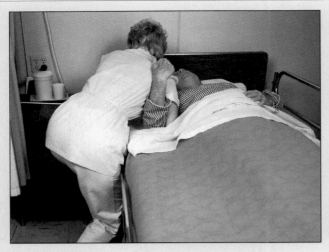

FIGURE 13–5B. Lock arms with patient.

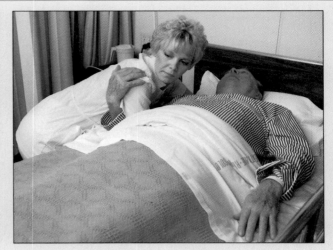

FIGURE 13–5C. Support patient's shoulders with your other arm by making a cradle.

PROCEDURE 12   OBRA

ASSISTING THE PATIENT TO MOVE TO THE HEAD OF THE BED

1. Carry out each beginning procedure action.
2. Remember to wash your hands, identify the patient, and provide privacy.
3. Lock wheels of bed. Raise bed to the high, horizontal position. Lower side rail on side nearest you.
4. Remove the pillow. Place it at the head of the bed, on its edge, for safety.
5. Face the head of the bed. Position your foot that is farthest away from the edge of the bed about 12 inches in front of the other foot.
6. Place your arm nearest the head of the bed under the patient's head and shoulders. Lock your other arm with patient's arm.
7. Instruct patient to bend knees, lift buttocks, and press in with heels as you lift shoulders. Move patient smoothly toward the head of the bed on a count of three, Figure 13–6. An alternate method is as follows:
   a. Place a pillow at the head of the bed on its edge.
   b. Have patient grasp head of bed or overhead trapeze with hands, if patient's condition permits.
   c. Slip your hands under the patient's back and buttocks.
   d. Have patient press in with heels and help the patient to raise hips and move to the head of the bed.
8. Replace pillow under the patient's head. Make patient comfortable.
9. Carry out each procedure completion action. Remember to wash your hands, report completion of task, and document the time, action (moved to head of bed), and patient's reaction.

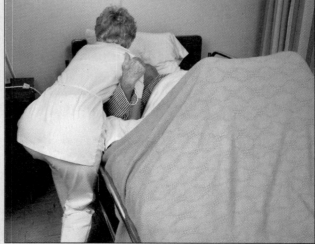

FIGURE 13–6. Instruct patient to press in with heels as you move patient to head of bed.

| PROCEDURE 13 | OBRA | SIDE 2 |  | |

MOVING A HELPLESS PATIENT TO THE HEAD OF THE BED

1. Carry out each beginning procedure action.
2. Remember to wash your hands, identify the patient, and provide privacy.
3. Ask a coworker to assist from the opposite side of the bed.
4. Lock wheels of bed. Raise bed to comfortable horizontal working height. Lower side rails.
5. Remove pillow. Place it at the head of the bed, on its edge, for safety.
6. Lift top bedding and expose drawsheet. Loosen both sides of the drawsheet.
7. Roll edges close to both sides of the patient's body, Figure 13–7.
8. Face the head of the bed. Grasp the drawsheet with the hand closest to the foot of the bed.
9. Position your feet 12 inches apart with the foot that is farthest from bed edge forward.
10. Place your free hand and arm under patient's neck and shoulders, cradling the head from both sides.
11. Bend your hips slightly.
12. Together, on a count of three, raise the patient's hips and back with the drawsheet, while supporting the head and shoulders. Move the patient smoothly toward the head of the bed.
13. Replace the pillow under the patient's head.

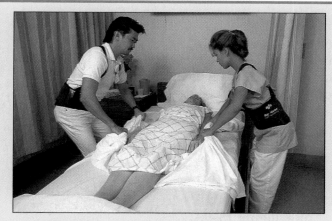

FIGURE 13–7. Roll both edges of the drawsheet close to the patient's sides.

14. Tighten and tuck in the drawsheet. Adjust top bedding.
15. Carry out each procedure completion action. Remember to wash your hands, report completion of task, and document the time, action (patient moved to head of bed), and patient's response.
   (All repositionings and turnings of patients should be recorded on the patient's chart.)
   NOTE: Do not leave the patient lying on his back for prolonged periods of time unless turning is contraindicated.

Refer to Figure 13–8 for guidelines for safe transfers.

- Know what type of transfer procedure you should use.
- Explain the procedure and tell the patient how to help.
- Place the bed in lowest position and lock the wheels.
- Place a transfer belt (gait belt) snugly around the patient's waist for standing transfers.
- Never place your hands or arms under the patient's shoulders. This practice can cause injury and pain.
- Never allow the patient's hands to be placed on your body. If the patient suddenly loses balance or is disoriented, the patient can inadvertently grab your neck. This can cause you to lose your balance and can cause severe injury to your neck.
- The patient should have on footwear with nonskid soles. Make sure these are on correctly before attempting to move the patient.
- Allow the patient to sit on the edge of the bed for 5 minutes before standing to avoid fainting or dizziness.
- Instruct the patient before standing to separate the knees for a wide base of support, to lean forward ("nose over toes"), and to move the feet back.
- When possible, transfer by leading with the patient's strongest side.

FIGURE 13–8. Guidelines for safe transfers.

PROCEDURE 14 | OBRA

USING A TRANSFER (GAIT) BELT

A transfer belt is 1-1/2 to 4 inches wide and 54 to 60 inches long. It is an assistive and safety device used to transfer patients from one surface to another. When it is used to ambulate patients, it is called a gait belt.

1. Explain the transfer or ambulation procedure to the patient.
2. Explain that the belt is a safety device and will be removed as soon as the transfer is completed.
3. Always apply the belt over the patient's clothing, Figure 13–9A.
4. Apply the belt around the patient's waist. Buckle the belt in front. Thread it through the teeth side first and place the belt through both openings to double lock, Figure 13–9B.
5. Use an underhand grasp when holding the belt to provide greater safety.
6. The belt should be snug enough to just get your fingers underneath, Figure 13–9C.
7. Check female residents to be sure the breasts are not under the belt.
8. Do not overuse the belt by pulling the patient up and down with too much force.

The transfer belt may not be appropriate for some patients. The nurse will provide you with this information.

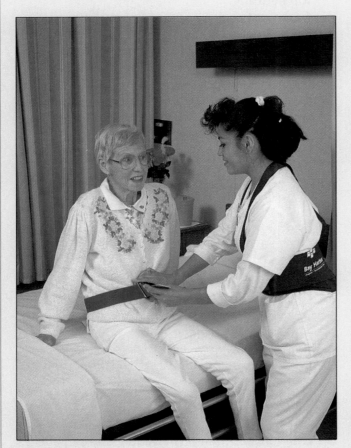

FIGURE 13–9A. Assist patient to a sitting position and place gait belt around the waist over clothing.

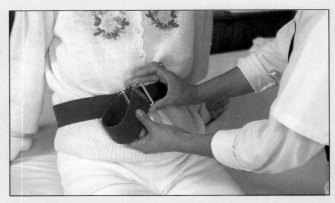

FIGURE 13–9B. Slip end of belt through toothed (serrated) portion of clasp and then through metal buckle.

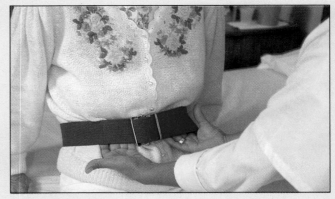

FIGURE 13–9C. Check for tightness and security.

ASSISTING THE PATIENT INTO A CHAIR OR WHEELCHAIR FROM BED

1. Carry out each beginning procedure action.
2. Remember to wash your hands, identify the patient, and provide privacy.
3. Obtain a wheelchair or chair (if not already at bedside).
4. Determine the patient's strongest side. Then place wheelchair so that it faces the foot of the bed on the same side. Lock the wheelchair, Figure 13–10A, and raise or remove the foot rests, Figure 13–10B.
5. Cover the chair or wheelchair with a cotton blanket.
   NOTE: Whenever possible, position the chair or wheelchair so that it is secure against a wall or solid furniture to ensure that it will not slide backward.
6. Lower the bed to the lowest horizontal position. Lock the bed and elevate the head.

These instructions are for getting out of the right side of the bed.

7. Instruct the patient to move toward the right side of the bed. (Stand against the right side of the bed.)
8. Have the patient roll over onto the right side, flexing the knees and bending the right arm so it can be used for propping. Bend the elbow of the top arm so this hand can be used to push off the bed, Figure 13–11A.
9. Instruct the patient to use the elbow of the right arm to raise the upper body and to push with the hand of the left arm to raise up to an upright position.
10. At the same time, instruct the patient to let the legs slide off the bed.
11. If assistance is needed, place one arm under the patient's shoulders (not the neck) and one arm over and around the knees, Figure 13–11B.
12. Bring the legs off the bed at the same time the shoulders are being raised off the bed.
13. Allow the patient to sit on the edge of the bed. Watch for signs of dizziness or fainting. Stand in front of the patient in case the patient loses balance.

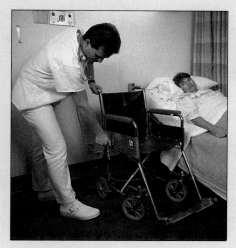

FIGURE 13–10A. Position wheelchair beside bed so it faces foot of bed on same side as patient's strongest side. Lock wheels.

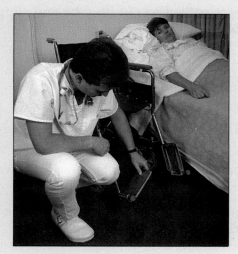

FIGURE 13–10B. Raise foot rests.

14. The patient should be sitting equally on both buttocks with the knees apart for a broad base of support, feet flat on the floor and arms at the sides.
15. Always protect a paralyzed arm and prevent it from dangling during the transfer. To avoid dangling, place the arm in a sling or place the

continues

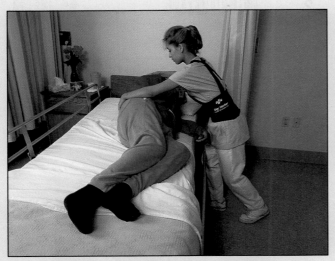

FIGURE 13–11A. Bend the elbow of the top arm so this hand can be used to push off the bed.

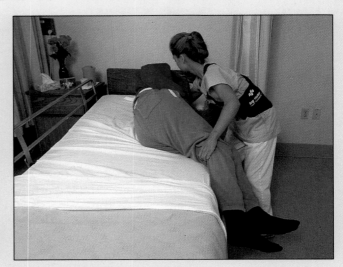

FIGURE 13–11B. Place one arm around the patient's shoulders (not the neck) and one arm over and around the knees.

hand in the patient's pocket. If neither of these are possible, carefully tuck the patient's fingers in the transfer belt until the patient is seated.
16. Assist patient to put on robe and slippers or shoes with nonskid soles.

17. Apply the transfer belt to the patient's waist if it is needed.
18. Proceed with a one or two person transfer as described below.

PROCEDURE 16   OBRA

TWO PERSON TRANSFER WITH TRANSFER BELT

Directions are given for transferring toward the patient's right side.

1. Complete pretransfer activities as described earlier.
2. The nursing assistants stand one on each side of the patient.
3. Each one places the hand closest to the patient through the belt with an underhand grasp in back of the patient. Coordination of movement is necessary.
4. The nursing assistant closest to the chair (on the patient's right side) stands in a position to step or pivot around in a smooth manner to allow the patient access to the chair. This person stands with the left leg further back than the right leg.

5. The other nursing assistant uses the left knee to brace the patient's weaker left leg. This person's right leg is further back than the left one.
6. Instruct the patient to bend forward (nose over toes) and to place the palms of the hands on the edge of the mattress in order to "push off."
7. The patient's knees should be spread apart. Have the patient put both feet back with the stronger foot slightly in back of the weaker foot.
8. The nursing assistants bend their knees, "squat," and assume a broad base of support.
9. On the count of three, the patient stands, Figure 13–12. Tell the patient to keep the head up. The nursing assistants help the patient pivot by slowly and smoothly pivoting their feet, legs,

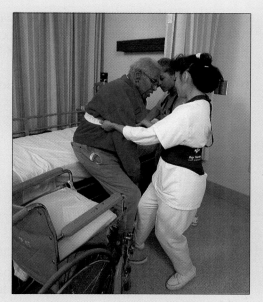

FIGURE 13–12. Both nursing assistants assist patient to rise. Note the underhand grasp on the transfer belt. The nursing assistants help the patient to pivot to the left to reach the wheelchair.

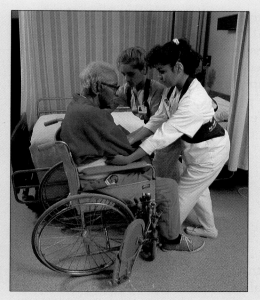

FIGURE 13–13. The nursing assistants continue to guide the patient until he is sitting safely in the wheelchair. The use of good body mechanics and the transfer belt assured a safe transfer for the patient and the nursing assistants.

and hips to their left. Allow the patient to stand for a moment and bear weight (if patient is allowed to do so.)

10. Have the patient place both hands (if possible) on the arms of the chair.
11. To sit, have the patient bend forward slightly,

bend the knees and lower into the chair, Figure 13–13. At the same time the patient reaches for the arms of the chair with both hands. Be sure that the patient's back is next to the back of the wheelchair and he is in good body alignment.

12. Remove the transfer belt.

PROCEDURE 17   OBRA

ONE PERSON TRANSFER WITH TRANSFER BELT

This method is used for the person who can bear weight in one or both legs and has good trunk stability and adequate balance. Remember to provide only the help that is necessary. Instructions are given for moving toward the patient's right side.

1. Carry out each beginning procedure action.
2. Follow instructions for bringing patient to sitting position on the side of the bed.
3. Secure transfer belt around the patient's waist.
4. The patient's hands should be grasping the edge of the bed. Bend your knees and assume

a broad base of support. If the patient has a weak leg, use your leg and foot to brace the weak foot and knee. Place your hands in the transfer belt with an underhand grasp.

5. Instruct the patient to bend forward and spread the knees apart. Both feet should be back with the stronger foot slightly in back of the weaker foot.
6. Ask the patient to push off the bed on the count of three and to stand up as you provide the necessary assistance.

continues

7. Allow the patient to remain standing for a time to stabilize position. Maintain your hands on the transfer belt and continue to brace the weak leg if necessary.
8. To complete the transfer, instruct the patient to step or pivot around to stand in front of the chair. Tell the patient to sit when the edge of the chair is touching the back of the legs.
9. To sit, have the patient bend forward slightly, bend the knees and lower into the chair. At the same time the patient reaches for the arms of the chair with both hands.
10. When the patient is safely positioned in the chair, remove the transfer belt.

PROCEDURE 18 OBRA

INDEPENDENT TRANSFER, STANDBY ASSIST

This method is appropriate for the patient who has good balance and strength and can understand instructions. Put a transfer belt on the patient the first time this is attempted.

1. Follow the instructions for coming to a sitting position on the side of the bed. For an independent transfer, the patient should be able to do this without help.
2. Now have the patient place the strongest foot slightly in back of the other foot. The patient's knees should be spread slightly apart.
3. Instruct the patient to place the palms of the hands at the edge of the bed and to lean slightly forward.
4. Tell the patient to press hands into the bed to push off at the same time the legs straighten to assume a standing position.
5. Once standing, have the patient reach for the far arm of the chair and then step or pivot to stand in front of the chair. Instruct the patient to sit when the edge of the seat is felt against the back of the legs.

PROCEDURE 19 OBRA

SIDE 2

ASSISTING THE PATIENT INTO BED FROM A CHAIR OR WHEELCHAIR

1. Carry out each beginning procedure action.
2. Remember to wash your hands, identify the patient, and provide privacy.
3. Check to see that the bed is in the lowest horizontal position and that the wheels are locked. Raise the head of the bed, fanfold the bedding to the foot, and raise the opposite side rail.
4. Determine the patient's strongest side. Then place chair or wheelchair so that it faces the foot of the bed on the same side. Lock the wheels of the wheelchair and lift the footrests.
5. Have the patient place feet flat on the floor.
6. Remove the bath blanket. Fold it and return it to the bedside stand.
7. Place transfer belt around patient's waist.
8. The nursing assistants stand one on each side of the patient.
9. Each one places the hand closest to the patient through the belt with an underhand grasp in back of the patient.
10. The nursing assistant closest to the bed (on the patient's right side) stands in a position to step or pivot around in a smooth manner to allow the patient access to the bed. This person stands with the left leg further back than the right leg.
11. The other nursing assistant uses the left knee to brace the patient's weaker left leg. This person's right leg is further back than the left one.
12. Instruct the patient to bend forward (nose over toes) and to place the palms of the hands on the

arms of the wheelchair in order to "push off."

13. The patient's knees should be spread apart. Have the patient put both feet back with the stronger foot slightly in back of the weaker foot.

14. The nursing assistants bend their knees, "squat," and assume a broad base of support.

15. On the count of three, the patient stands. Tell the patient to keep the head up. The nursing assistants help the patient pivot by slowly and smoothly pivoting their feet, legs, and hips to their left. Allow the patient to stand for a moment and bear weight (if patient is allowed to do so.)

16. Have the patient place both hands (if possible)

on the edge of the mattress.

17. To sit, have the patient bend forward slightly, bend the knees and lower onto the mattress.

18. Remove the transfer belt.

19. Remove the patient's robe and slippers.

20. Move the wheelchair out of the way.

21. Assist the patient to lie down in bed.

22. Position patient as necessary.

23. Draw the top bedding over the patient.

24. Carry out each procedure completion action. Remember to wash your hands, report completion of task, and document the time, action (assisting patient from wheelchair or chair to bed), and patient's reaction.

PROCEDURE 20 | **OBRA**

SIDE **2**

ONE PERSON TRANSFER FROM WHEELCHAIR TO BED

1. Follow steps 1 through 7 in Procedure 19.

2. The patient's hands should be grasping the arms of the wheelchair. Bend your knees and assume a broad base of support.

3. If the patient has a weak leg, use your leg and foot to brace the weak foot and knee. Place your hands in the transfer belt with an underhand grasp.

4. Instruct the patient to bend forward and spread the knees apart. Both feet should be back with the stronger foot slightly in back of the weaker foot.

5. Ask the patient to push off the chair on the count of three and to stand up as you provide the necessary assistance, Figure 13–14.

6. Allow the patient to remain standing for a time to stabilize position. Maintain your hands on the transfer belt and continue to brace the weak leg if necessary.

7. To complete the transfer, instruct the patient to step or pivot around to stand in front of the bed. Tell the patient to sit when the edge of the mattress is touching the back of the legs. To sit, have the patient bend forward slightly, bend the knees and lower himself onto the mattress.

8. When the patient is safely sitting, remove the transfer belt.

9. Remove the patient's robe and slippers.

10. Move the wheelchair out of the way.

11. Assist the patient to lie down in bed.

12. Position patient as necessary.

13. Draw the top bedding over the patient.

14. Carry out each procedure completion action. Remember to wash your hands, report completion of task, and document the time, action (assisting patient from wheelchair or chair to bed), and patient's reaction.

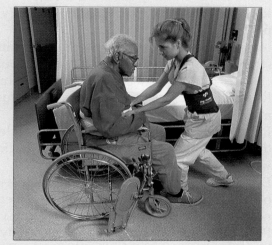

FIGURE 13–14. Keep your back straight and your base of support broad as you get ready to assist the patient to rise from the wheelchair.

PROCEDURE 21 | OBRA

ASSISTING THE INDEPENDENT PATIENT FROM WHEELCHAIR TO BED

1. Follow steps 1 through 7 in Procedure 19.
2. Have the patient place the strongest foot slightly in back of the other foot. The patient's knees should be spread slightly apart.
3. Instruct the patient to place the palms of the hands on the arms of the chair and to lean slightly forward.
4. Tell the patient to push off the chair seat at the same time the legs straighten to assume a standing position.
5. Once standing, have the patient step or pivot to stand in front of the bed. Instruct the patient to sit when the edge of the bed is felt against the back of the legs.
6. Remove the patient's robe and slippers.
7. Move the wheelchair out of the way.
8. Assist the patient to lie down in bed.
9. Position patient as necessary.
10. Draw the top bedding over the patient.
11. Carry out each procedure completion action. Remember to wash your hands, report completion of task, and document the time, action (assisting patient from wheelchair or chair to bed), and patient's reaction.

A mechanical lift is an electrically or hydraulically operated device that assists health care providers in moving heavy or helpless patients into and out of beds, tubs, and so on. A removable sling is placed under the patient's body for support. The sling is reattached to the lift and hydraulic action (or an electric motor) raises the lift to move the patient. All safety precautions relating to the use of the mechanical lift must be followed.

PROCEDURE 22 | OBRA

SIDE 4

LIFTING A PATIENT USING A MECHANICAL LIFT

1. Carry out each beginning procedure action.
2. Ask another nursing assistant to help.
3. Remember to wash your hands, identify the patient, and provide privacy.
   NOTE: Check the release mechanism, slings, straps, and chains for frayed areas or poorly closing clasps. Do not use defective equipment. Report need of repair and obtain safe equipment before taking to bedside.
4. Place a wheelchair or chair at right angles to the foot of the bed, facing the head. Lock the wheelchair.
5. Elevate the bed to a comfortable working height. Lock the wheels of the bed. Lower the nearest side rail. Roll the patient toward you.
6. Position slings beneath the patient's body behind the shoulder, thighs, and buttocks, Figure 13–15A. Be sure the sling is smooth.
7. Roll the patient back onto the sling and position properly under shoulders and hips, Figures 13–15B and 13–15C.
8. Position the lift frame over the bed with base legs in maximum open position and lock, Figure 13–15D.
9. Attach suspension straps to the sling, Figure 13–15E. Check fasteners for security.
10. Attach suspension straps to the frame. Position the patient's arms inside the straps and chains with hooks facing outward.
11. Secure restraint straps, if needed.
12. Talking to the patient, slowly lift the patient free of the bed, Figure 13–15F.
13. Guide the lift away from the bed.
14. Position the patient close to the chair or wheelchair. Make sure that the wheels of the wheelchair are locked.
15. The second nursing assistant holds the sling and helps lower the patient slowly into the

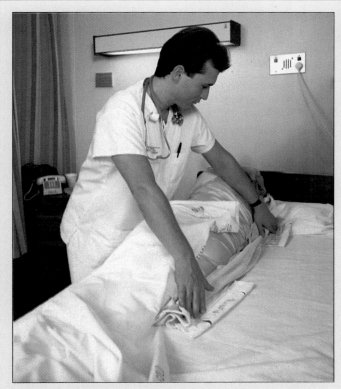

FIGURE 13–15A. Roll patient toward you and place sling smoothly under patient's body.

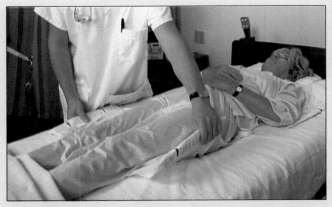

FIGURE 13–15B. Make sure top of sling is positioned under shoulders so it extends above them.

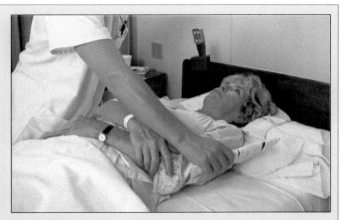

FIGURE 13–15C. Position sling smoothly under hips.

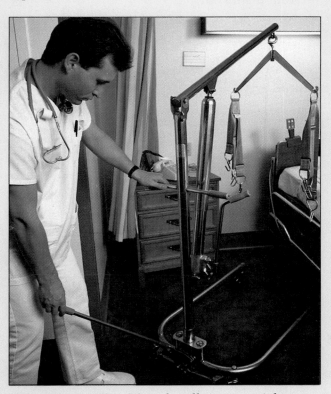

FIGURE 13–15D. Move handle to your right to release lock pin. Then bring handle toward you in a complete half circle. Lock legs in full open position, then slide legs under bed.

chair or wheelchair. Pay particular attention to the position of the patient's feet and hands.

16. Unhook the suspension straps and remove lift.

17. If the patient is to remain up for a period of time in the chair, make sure she is comfortable and secured in the chair before leaving.

18. Carry out each procedure completion action. Remember to wash your hands, report completion of task, and document the time, action (patient transferred from bed to chair using a mechanical lift), and patient's response.

continues

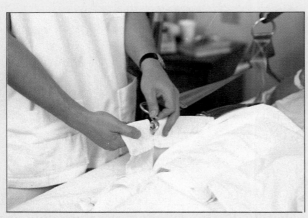

FIGURE 13–15E. Hook straps of lift to sling from inside out.

FIGURE 13–15F. Lift patient free of bed. (Second nursing assistant is out of camera range.)

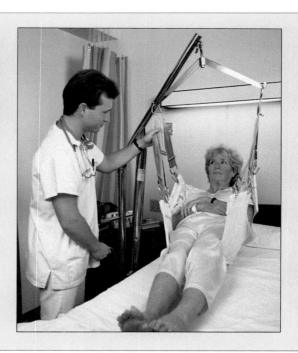

PROCEDURE 23

TRANSFERRING A CONSCIOUS PATIENT FROM A BED TO STRETCHER

1. Carry out each beginning procedure action.
2. Remember to wash your hands, identify the patient, and provide privacy.
3. Elevate the bed to the level of the stretcher.
4. Move the stretcher (litter) against and parallel to the bed. Lock both the stretcher and bed, Figure 13–16. Double check to be sure both are secure.
5. Cover the patient with a bath blanket. Fanfold the bedding to the foot of the bed.
6. With one person beside the stretcher and the other person on the opposite side of the bed, assist the patient to move onto the stretcher, Figure 13–17. If only one person is available, raise the opposite side rail and stand beside the stretcher to brace.
7. Secure the stretcher restraint and raise the side rails of the stretcher.
8. Transport the patient to the desired destination.
9. Carry out each procedure completion action. Remember to wash your hands, report completion of task, and document the time, action (transferred patient to stretcher), and patient's reaction.

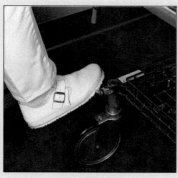

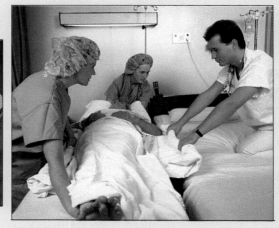

(A)   **(B)**

FIGURE 13–16. Make sure wheels of both stretcher **(A)** and bed **(B)** are locked.

FIGURE 13–17. The staff helps transfer patient from bed to stretcher.

PROCEDURE 24

TRANSFERRING A CONSCIOUS PATIENT FROM A STRETCHER TO BED

1. Carry out each beginning procedure action and secure help.
2. Remember to wash your hands, identify the patient, and provide privacy.
3. Lock the wheels of the bed. Raise the bed to a horizontal position equal to the height of the stretcher. Fanfold the bedding to the foot of the bed.
4. Push the stretcher against the bed and lock the wheels.
5. Position one assistant next to the stretcher and another assistant against the opposite side of the bed.
6. Loosen the stretcher restraints and blanket covering patient.
7. If the patient is able to move, hold the covering loosely and assist the patient to slide from the stretcher to the bed, Figure 13–18.
8. If a turning or drawsheet is used, roll the sheet to the edges of the patient's body. Place one arm under the patient's shoulders while grasping the turning sheet with the other.
9. At an agreed upon signal, lift the turning sheet and slide the patient onto the bed.
10. Move the stretcher out of the way.
11. Assist the patient to a comfortable position in the center of the bed.
12. Pull the top bedding up over the patient. Withdraw the bath blanket from underneath the patient.
13. Return the bed to the lowest horizontal position. Adjust the side rails in the up position.
14. Carry out each procedure completion action. Remember to wash your hands, report completion of task, and document the time, action (transfer of patient from stretcher to bed), and patient's response.

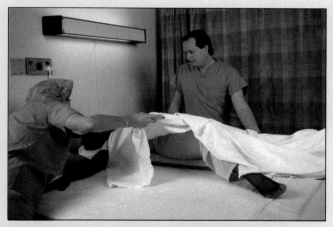

FIGURE 13–18. The conscious patient can assist in transferring into bed.

PROCEDURE 25

TRANSFERRING AN UNCONSCIOUS PATIENT OR A PATIENT UNABLE TO ASSIST FROM STRETCHER TO BED

1. Carry out each beginning procedure action.
2. Remember to wash your hands, identify the patient, and provide privacy.
3. Lock the wheels of the bed. Raise the bed to a horizontal position equal to the height of the stretcher. Lower the side rail. Fanfold the bedding to the foot of the bed.
4. Position one nursing assistant against the opposite side of the bed and one nursing assistant at the foot of the stretcher. You will be the third person and will stand on the opposite side of the stretcher, Figure 13–19A.
5. Position the stretcher against the bed. Lock the wheels and lower the side rails of the stretcher.
6. Loosen the stretcher restraints and bath blanket covering the patient.
7. Roll the turning sheet close to the patient's body.
8. The assistant on the opposite side of the bed uses both hands to grasp the turning sheet. Lift

continues

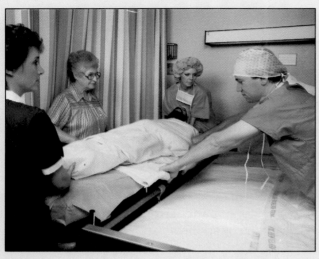

FIGURE 13–19A. Position a nursing assistant at head and foot of patient.

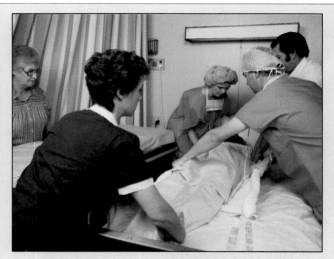

FIGURE 13–19C. Move stretcher away while supporting patient.

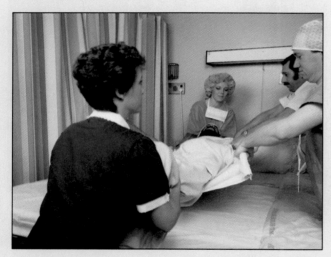

FIGURE 13–19B. At the count of three, all nursing assistants raise lifting sheet and move patient onto bed.

and draw the patient onto the bed, Figure 13–19B. It may be necessary for this assistant to kneel on the bed to reach.

9. The assistant at the foot of the bed lifts the patient's feet and legs.

10. The assistant opposite the stretcher places one arm for support under the patient's head and shoulders. With the other hand, the assistant grasps the turning sheet to guide the patient. All assistants must coordinate their activities and move together as a signal is given.

11. Move the stretcher out of the way.

12. Using the turning sheet, position the patient in bed, Figure 13–19C.

13. Pull the top bedding up over the patient. Remove the blanket from underneath the patient.

14. Carry out each procedure completion action. Remember to wash your hands, report completion of task, and document the time, action (transfer of patient to bed from stretcher), and patient's response.

PROCEDURE 26

TRANSFERRING AN UNCONSCIOUS PATIENT FROM A BED TO STRETCHER

1. Carry out each beginning procedure action.
2. Remember to wash your hands, identify the patient, and provide privacy.
3. Secure the help of three other nursing assistants.

4. Lock the wheels of the bed. Raise the bed to a horizontal position equal to the height of the stretcher. Lower the side rails. Place the stretcher parallel to and against the bed. Lock the wheels.

5. Position:
   - One assistant against the opposite side of the bed.
   - One at the foot of the bed, facing the head of the bed.
   - Third assistant against the stretcher.
   - Fourth person at the head of the stretcher facing the foot.
6. Lower the side rails. Position the stretcher close to the bed. Lock the stretcher wheels.
7. Loosen the turning sheet and roll it against the patient.
8. At a prespecified signal, all assistants act together as follows:
   - Assistant at the foot of the bed lifts the patient's feet and legs.
   - Assistant against the side of the bed lifts and guides the patient's body with the turning sheet.
   - Assistant against the stretcher grasps the turning sheet with both hands, raises and draws patient onto stretcher.
   - Assistant at the head of the stretcher cradles the patient's head and neck with hands under shoulders, arms together.
9. Center the patient on the stretcher. Cover the patient with a bath blanket.
10. Secure the stretcher restraint. Raise the side rails of the stretcher.
11. Transport the patient as directed.
12. Carry out each procedure completion action. Remember to wash your hands, report completion of task, and document the time, action (transfer of patient from bed to stretcher), and patient's response.

PROCEDURE 27	OBRA

SIDE
2

LOG ROLLING THE PATIENT

NOTE: This procedure is performed when the patient's spinal column must be kept straight, such as following spinal surgery or spinal cord or vertebral column injury.

1. Carry out each beginning procedure action.
2. Remember to wash your hands, identify the patient, and provide privacy.
3. Secure help from another nursing assistant.
4. Elevate the bed to waist-high horizontal position. Lock the wheels.
5. Lower the side rail on the side opposite to which the patient will be turned. Both assistants should be on the same side of the bed.
6. One assistant places hands under the patient's head and shoulders. The second person places hands under the patient's hips and legs. Then move the patient as a unit toward you.
7. Place a pillow lengthwise between the patient's legs. Fold the patient's arm over chest.
8. Raise the side rail. Check for security.
9. Go to the opposite side of the bed and lower the side rail.
10. Turning the patient to side may be done by:
    a. Using a turning sheet which has been previously placed under the patient.
       - Reach over the patient, grasping and rolling the turning sheet toward the patient, Figure 13–20A.
       - One nursing assistant should be positioned beside the patient to keep the patient's shoulders and hips straight.
       - Second assistant should be positioned to keep the patient's thighs and lower legs straight.
    b. If a turning sheet is not in position, the first assistant should position hands on the patient's far shoulder and hips.
       - Second assistant positions hands on the patient's far thigh and lower leg.
11. At a specified signal, the patient is drawn toward both assistants in a single movement, keeping the patient's spine, head, and legs in a straight position, Figure 13–20B.

continues

12. Place additional pillows behind the patient to maintain position. A small pillow or folded bath blanket may be permitted under the patient's head and neck. Leave a pillow between the patient's legs. Position small pillows or folded towels to support the patient's arms.
13. Carry out each procedure completion action.

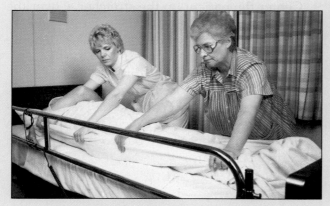

FIGURE 13–20A. Roll turning sheet against patient.

Remember to wash your hands, report completion of task, and document the time, action (log rolling patient to side—right or left), and patient's response.

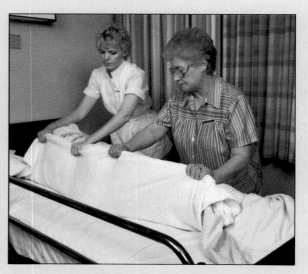

FIGURE 13–20B. Pulling together, turn patient to side in one smooth movement.

Transporting Patients

You may be assigned to transport patients from their unit to some other hospital department. For example, patients may need to have tests done or receive treatments which cannot be performed in their rooms. On occasion, the entire bed will be used for transport but, more often than not, transportation will be by wheelchair or stretcher.

If the patient being transported has an IV or drainage, additional precautions should be taken.
- Keep the IV bag above the infusion site.
- Keep a drainage bag below the drainage site.
- Keep tubes free of kinking or twisting.
- Keep tubes free of stress at all times.

PROCEDURE 28   OBRA

ASSISTING PATIENT TO GET OUT OF BED AND AMBULATE

1. Carry out each beginning procedure action.
2. Remember to wash your hands, identify the patient, and provide privacy.
3. Have slippers and robe or other clothing ready.
4. Place a chair at right angles beside the bed, facing the head of the bed.
5. Lower the side rail nearest you.
6. Drape the patient with a bath blanket. Fanfold the top covers to the foot of the bed.
7. Gradually elevate the head of the bed.
8. Allow the patient to sit on the edge of the bed for a few minutes. Note the patient's color, pulse, and response, Figure 13–21.
9. Help the patient to dress or put on robe.
10. Put on the patient's shoes or slippers.
11. Instruct the patient to swing his legs over the side of the bed.

NOTE: If the patient becomes dizzy, lay him back down, secure the side rails, and report to the nurse.

12. Lower the bed to the lowest position.
13. Help the patient to stand with your arm behind the patient's back for a few minutes.
    NOTE: If the patient becomes weak or tired, pivot to the right and seat the patient in a chair or return to bed. Recheck the patient's pulse.
14. Transfer your arm behind the patient's waist and turn so you face in the same direction. Let the patient grasp your hand.
15. Follow, walking behind and to one side, until you are sure the patient is stable. Start off on the same foot as the patient and keep in step.
16. Observe the patient frequently for signs of fatigue or light-headedness.
17. Return the patient to bed following ambulation by reversing the procedure.
18. Carry out each procedure completion action. Remember to wash your hands, report completion of task, and document the time, action (assisted patient out of bed and ambulated) and amount of time, and patient's response.

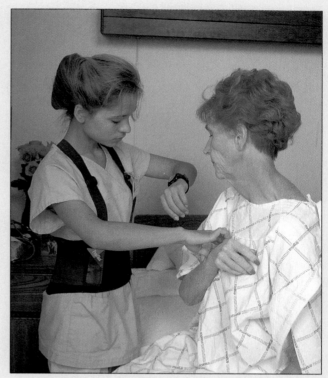

FIGURE 13–21. Note patient's pulse, color, and response.

PROCEDURE 29 | OBRA

ASSISTING PATIENT WHO IS OUT OF BED TO AMBULATE

1. Carry out each beginning procedure action.
2. Remember to wash your hands, identify the patient, and provide privacy.
3. Assist the patient to stand slowly. Keep one hand under the patient's bent arm for support. Check the patient's pulse.
4. If a gait belt is to be used, apply the belt. See Procedure 14.
5. Walk behind and to one side of the patient during ambulation, Figure 13–22. Start with the same foot as the patient and keep in step. Maintain a firm hold on the gait belt.
6. Encourage the patient to use hand rails.
7. Watch for signs of fatigue. Check the patient's pulse. If the patient becomes fatigued, help the patient to sit.

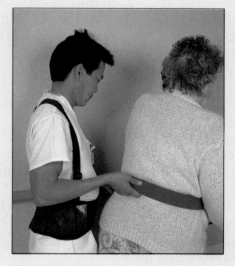

FIGURE 13–22. Be sure you have a firm underhand grasp on the gait (transfer) belt.

continues

8. Talk to the patient during the procedure. Be on guard for anything in the way that might cause the patient to fall.
9. Return to the patient's room. Assist the patient back to the bed or chair. Remove the gait belt, if it was used.

10. Carry out each procedure completion action. Remember to wash your hands, report completion of task, and document the time, action (assisted with ambulation of patient for— amount of time), and patient's response.

NOTE: Some patients will use crutches when they ambulate. The physical therapist or nurse will measure the patient for the crutches and will instruct the patient on which gait to use. The word gait refers to how the patient walks with the crutches. If any of the patients use crutches, check the following to make sure the crutches are safe to use:

■ The screws that hold the crutches together are tight and secure

■ The rubber tips on the bottoms of the crutches are in good condition
■ The handgrips are secure and properly placed
■ The pads on the top of the crutches are in good condition.

Report any problems with the crutches to the nurse.

PROCEDURE 30 | **OBRA**   SIDE **2**

CARE OF THE FALLING PATIENT

1. Keep your back straight as you assist a falling patient, Figure 13–23. If the patient is wearing a gait belt, keep a firm hold on the belt.
2. Ease the patient to the floor. Be sure to protect head.
3. Stay with the patient.
4. Call for help.
5. Do not move the patient until patient has been examined.
6. Assist in returning the patient to bed.
7. Place the signal cord close at hand.
8. Leave the patient comfortable and the unit tidy.
9. Wash your hands. Report the incident to your supervisor.
10. Document your witness of the fall in an incident report. Include:
    a. Date and time
    b. Objective account of the incident
    c. Patient's reaction

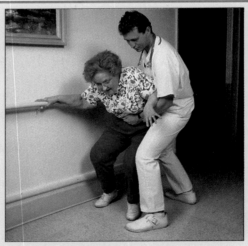

FIGURE 13–23. Note nursing assistant's wide base of support. The patient is eased to the floor. Remember to protect patient's head.

PROCEDURE 31 | OBRA

TRANSPORTING A PATIENT BY WHEELCHAIR

1. Carry out each beginning procedure action.
2. Remember to wash your hands, identify the patient, and provide privacy.
3. Determine the patient's strongest side. Position the wheelchair beside the bed on the patient's strongest side. The wheelchair should face the head of the bed.
4. Lock the wheelchair wheels and raise the footrests.
5. Place a bath blanket opened on the wheelchair to cover the patient once seated.
6. Follow the procedure for assisting a patient into a wheelchair.
7. Once seated, cover the patient with the bath blanket. Be sure it does not drag on the floor.
8. Position the patient's feet on the footrests. Secure the patient's feet with restraint straps.
9. Unlock the wheels of the chair.
10. Guide the chair from behind, Figure 13–24, carrying out the following precautions:
    a. Stay to the right of corridors.
    b. Be careful when approaching intersecting hallways.
    c. Back down slanted ramps.
    d. Back into and out of elevators and doorways, turning your head to ensure clearance, Figure 13–25.
    e. Once in the elevator, turn the wheelchair so the patient's back is to the door.
11. Check to see if the patient's chart is to accompany the patient.
12. Transport the patient to the assigned area. *Do not leave the patient alone.* Wait until another health care provider assumes responsibility for the patient's care.
13. Unless instructed to wait, return to the unit.
14. Carry out each procedure completion action. Remember to wash your hands, report completion of task, and document the time, action (transporting of patient by wheelchair), and patient's response.

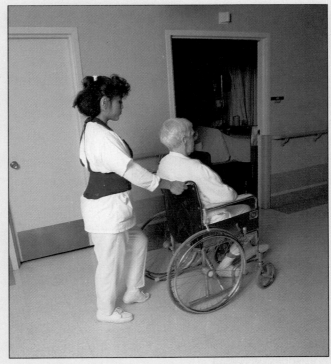

FIGURE 13–24. Guide the wheelchair from behind.

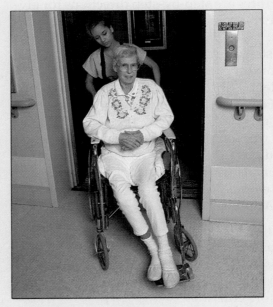

FIGURE 13–25. Always back into doorways and elevators when transporting a patient by wheelchair.

PROCEDURE 32

TRANSPORTING A PATIENT BY STRETCHER

1. Carry out each beginning procedure action.
2. Remember to wash your hands, identify the patient, and provide privacy.
3. Lock the wheels of the bed. Raise the bed to a horizontal height at the same level as the stretcher. Lower the side rails on one side.
4. Cover the patient with a bath blanket. Fanfold the bedding to the foot of the bed.
5. Position the stretcher against the bed. Lock the wheels.
6. Assist the patient to move onto the stretcher while keeping the patient covered with the bath blanket. To move the helpless patient, see Procedure 26.
7. Secure the strap over the patient's legs. Raise both side rails.
8. Check to see if the patient's chart is to accompany the patient.
9. Assume a position at the patient's head and push the stretcher.
   a. Stay to the right of corridors.
   b. Back down slanted ramps and through doorways.
   c. Be careful when approaching intersections.
   d. Back into elevators.
10. Transport the patient to the assigned area. *Do not leave the patient alone.* Wait until another health care provider assumes responsibility for the patient's care.
11. Unless instructed to wait, return to the unit.
12. Carry out each procedure completion action. Remember to wash your hands, report completion of task, and document the time, action (transporting of patient by stretcher), and patient's response.

SUMMARY

- Procedures are step-by-step directions for giving patient care. They must be followed faithfully.
- Some steps are common to all procedures. The beginning procedure actions and procedure completion actions include the following.
  NOTE: Where there are open lesions, wet linen, or possible contact with patient body fluids or blood, disposable gloves are to be worn during the procedure. Put on gloves before contact with the patient or linen. Properly dispose of gloves after they are removed. **Always Apply Universal Precautions.**

Beginning Procedure Actions
- Wash your hands.
- Assemble all of the necessary equipment.
- Go to the patient's room, knock, and pause before entering.
- Introduce yourself and identify the patient by checking the identification bracelet.
- Ask visitors to leave and inform them where they can wait.
- Provide privacy.
- Explain what will happen and answer any questions.
- Allow patient to assist as much as possible.
- Raise the bed to a comfortable working height.

Procedure Completion Actions
- Position the patient comfortably.
- Return the bed to the lowest position.
- Leave the signal cord, telephone, and fresh water close at hand.
- Perform a general safety check of the patient and environment.
- Open curtains.
- Care for equipment following facility policy.
- Wash your hands.
- Let visitors know they may reenter.
- Report completion of task.
- Document action and your observations.

- Special procedures in this unit relate to moving, lifting, and transporting patients in a safe, appropriate manner using proper body mechanics.

UNIT REVIEW

A. Matching. Match the following by matching Column I with Column II.

Column I

_____ 1. making a record of an action

_____ 2. liftsheet

_____ 3. turning a patient in a straight, single movement

_____ 4. turn

_____ 5. device used to assist in moving patients

_____ 6. step-by-step directions for performing nursing assistant tasks

Column II

a. document

b. mechanical lift

c. log rolling

d. procedure

e. drawsheet

f. pivot

B. True/False. Answer the following true or false by circling T or F.

T F 7. Before attempting to move a patient, determine if help is needed.

T F 8. Each documentation should include the date and time.

T F 9. When turning a patient toward you, cross the patient's near leg over the leg that is farthest from you.

T F 10. You must wash your hands before and after completing every nursing assistant task.

T F 11. After patient care, the bed should be left in the highest horizontal position.

T F 12. Before using a mechanical lift, always check the slings and straps for frayed areas.

T F 13. Privacy should be provided before carrying out care.

T F 14. You should always explain what you plan to do even if the patient seems not to hear.

T F 15. One person can safely transfer an unconscious patient from a stretcher to the bed.

T F 16. Turning sheets make moving heavy patients an easier task.

T F 17. When transferring a patient from a bed to a stretcher, raise the bed to the same horizontal height as the stretcher.

T F 18. When transporting a patient in a wheelchair, always walk on the left of the corridor.

T F 19. Always back in as you push a patient on a stretcher into an elevator.

T F 20. You should back down a ramp when transporting a patient in a wheelchair.

T F 21. The unconscious patient should be secured with support restraints during transport.

T F 22. During transfer, always keep the drainage bag above the drainage site.

T F 23. Test the snugness of the gait belt between the belt and the patient.

C. Completion. Complete the following statements in the space provided.

24. Nine actions to be taken at the beginning of each patient care procedure are:

a. _____
b. _____
c. _____
d. _____
e. _____
f. _____
g. _____
h. _____
i. _____

25. Ten actions to be taken to complete each patient care procedure are:

a. _____
b. _____
c. _____
d. _____
e. _____
f. _____
g. _____
h. _____
i. _____
j. _____

SELF-EVALUATION Section 5

A. **Choose the phrase that best completes each of the following sentences by circling the proper letter.**

1. Proper body mechanics include
   a. keeping knees and hips straight as you bend.
   b. keeping your back flexed.
   c. twisting your body as you work.
   d. using the strongest muscles to do the job.
2. When turning a patient in bed, remember to
   a. unlock the bed.
   b. roll the patient toward you.
   c. place your hand under the patient's near shoulder.
   d. All of the above.
3. In assisting the patient to sit up in bed, remember to
   a. keep your feet close together.
   b. keep your face close to the patient's face.
   c. lock arms with the patient.
   d. lock hands with the patient.
4. In assisting a patient to move to the head of the bed, you should
   a. unlock the bed wheels.
   b. add a pillow under the patient's head.
   c. face the head of the bed.
   d. place the foot farthest away from the bed edge behind the other foot.
5. If you are alone and assisting a patient to move to the head of the bed
   a. lower the bed.
   b. raise the head of the bed.
   c. have the patient grasp the head of the bed.
   d. ask the patient to keep his knees straight.
6. When moving a helpless patient to the head of the bed
   a. ask a coworker to assist.
   b. lower bed to lowest possible horizontal position.
   c. tighten lower bedding.
   d. position feet close together.
7. When assisting a patient into a wheelchair
   a. place chair at end of bed.
   b. lower foot pedals.
   c. lock bed and chair wheels.
   d. raise bed.

8. When lifting a patient using a mechanical lift
   a. check the slings and straps for safety.
   b. place the chair so that it faces the bed.
   c. unlock the wheels.
   d. position lift frame over bed with base legs close together.
9. To transfer a conscious patient alone from bed to stretcher
   a. unlock bed wheels.
   b. place stretcher parallel against bed.
   c. stand beside bed.
   d. lower both side rails.
10. When transporting a patient by wheelchair
    a. keep footrests up.
    b. guide chair from the side.
    c. do not allow bath blanket to drag.
    d. keep wheels of chair locked.
11. When transporting any patient
    a. keep to the left of corridors.
    b. be careful approaching intersections.
    c. head down slanted ramps.
    d. move forward into elevators.
12. When transporting using a gurney
    a. leave side rails down.
    b. secure straps.
    c. keep wheels locked.
    d. keep to the left of corridors.
13. Good standing posture includes
    a. feet close together.
    b. arms out straight.
    c. feet separated.
    d. abdominal muscles relaxed.
14. One basic rule of good body mechanics is
    a. keep feet close together.
    b. bend from hips and knees.
    c. twist your body as you work.
    d. keep your back relaxed.
15. Another basic rule of good body mechanics is
    a. use the weight of your body to help move objects.
    b. stand an arm's length away from the object being moved.
    c. keep your feet close together.
    d. bend from your waist.

16. When a patient has an IV in place and must be moved, remember
    a. avoid stress on tubes.
    b. tubes are flexible and can be twisted.
    c. it is all right to allow the tube to drop below the infusion site.
    d. None of the above.
17. If the patient being moved has a drainage tube in place
    a. slight stress creates no problem.
    b. do not allow the drainage container to drop below the drainage site.
    c. never allow the drainage container to be raised above the drainage site.
    d. All of the above.
18. Staying in one position for long periods leads to
    a. improved circulation.
    b. skin breakdown.
    c. more flexible joints.
    d. greater comfort.
19. When carrying an object
    a. hold it with extended arms.
    b. use your back muscles.
    c. hold it close to the body.
    d. keep knees straight and tensed.
20. Proper alignment can be maintained with
    a. turning sheets.
    b. drawsheets.
    c. pillows and foam pads.
    d. cradles.
21. When using a turning sheet
    a. roll it closely to patient's side.
    b. move one side at a time.
    c. it should extend just under the shoulders.
    d. it should extend just under the hips.

B. Match Column I with Column II.

Column I	Column II
_____ 22. pivot	a. bendable
_____ 23. alignment	b. position
_____ 24. decubitus ulcer	c. twisting motion
_____ 25. flexible	d. bedsore
	e. rigid
	f. muscle relaxation

C. Provide short answers to the following.

26. List the ten rules to help your muscles work efficiently.
    a. _____
    b. _____
    c. _____
    d. _____
    e. _____
    f. _____
    g. _____
    h. _____
    i. _____
    j. _____
27. List five dangers of immobility.
    a. _____
    b. _____
    c. _____
    d. _____
    e. _____

D. Complete the following statements correctly.

28. A gait belt is also called a _____.
29. To be sure the gait belt is not too tight ____
    _____.
30. As you assist the patient to ambulate, grasp the belt with an _____ grasp or by the special loops.

Body Temperature

OBJECTIVES

As a result of this unit, you will be able to:

- Spell and define terms.
- Name and identify the three types of clinical thermometers and tell their uses.
- Read a thermometer.
- Demonstrate the procedure for using each type of clinical thermometer.
- Convert thermometer readings between Fahrenheit and Celsius.
- Identify the range of normal values.
- Describe the nursing assistant actions for hypothermia and hyperthermia.

VOCABULARY

Learn the meaning and the correct spelling of the following words:

aural thermometer	fever
axillary temperature	flagged
body core	groin temperature
body shell	hyperthermia
Celsius scale	hypothermia
clinical thermometers	metabolism
diurnal	probe
electronic thermometer	pyrexia
Fahrenheit scale	vital signs

Measurement of body temperature is a common nursing assistant task. Body temperature is one of the vital (living) signs. The patient's other vital signs include the pulse, respiration, and blood pressure. Although they are not part of the vital signs, the height and weight of the patient are other values commonly measured.

Specific equipment is used to determine or measure these values. They must be accurately measured because they tell us a great deal about the patient's condition. Do not tell the patient the results. This is not your responsibility. Tell the patient you will ask the nurse to discuss the results with him. Although they are usually determined as a combined procedure, each vital sign will be discussed in a separate unit. Measuring height and weight are discussed in Unit 17.

Many facilities use electronic equipment that automatically registers the four vital signs simultaneously.

Temperature Values

Temperature values may be expressed in either of two scales. They are the:

- **Fahrenheit scale**, which is indicated by an *F*.
- **Celsius scale**, which is indicated by a *C*.

A small ° after either capital letter indicates degrees or levels of temperature.

A formula can be used to convert temperature readings from Celsius to Fahrenheit and from Fahrenheit to Celsius. See Figure 14–1 for some important equivalents. Figure 14–2 compares the markings of the Fahrenheit and Celsius thermometers.

Definition of Body Temperature

Temperature is the measurement of body heat. It is the balance between heat produced and heat lost.

Body temperature is:

- Fairly constant. There is a daily (**diurnal**) variation of 1–3°F. Body temperature is lowest in the morning. It is higher in the afternoon and evening.
- The body temperature is lower the closer to the body surface it is measured. The temperature

	Celsius (C)	Fahrenheit (F)
Freezing	0°	32°
Body Temperature	37°	98.6°
Pasteurization	63°	145°
Boiling	100°	212°
Sterilizing (Autoclave)	121°	250°

Conversion Formulas

F › C $C = \frac{5}{9}(F - 32)$

C › F $F = \frac{9}{5}C + 32$

For example:	To convert a Celsius temperature of 100 to Fahrenheit, follow the procedure: $100 \times \frac{9}{5} = \frac{900}{5} = 180 + 32 = 212°F$
For example:	To convert a Fahrenheit temperature of 212 to Celsius, follow the procedure: $\frac{5}{9} = (212 - 32) = \frac{5}{9} \times 180 = 100°C$

FIGURE 14–1. Formulas for converting Fahrenheit and Celsius temperature readings

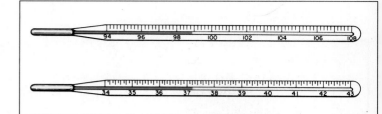

FIGURE 14–2. Fahrenheit and Celsius thermometers

	Oral	Axillary	Rectal
Average Temperature	98.6°F	97.6°F	99.6°F
Range	97.6–99.6°F (36.5–37.5°C)	96.6–98.6°F (36–37°C)	98.6–100.6°F (37–38.1°C)

FIGURE 14–3. Temperature variations in the same person

Age	Temperature
3 months	99.4°F
6 months	99.5°F
1 year	99.7°F
3 years	99.0°F
5 years	98.6°F
9 years	98.0°F

FIGURE 14–4. Average temperatures in infants and children. Temperature control in infants and children is less stable.

at the center of the body (**body core**) is much higher than the temperature at the surface of the body.

- Different in the same person when determined from different body areas, Figure 14–3. It is important to know the "normal" temperature for an individual since the normal may vary from person to person.
- Less stable in children. Figure 14–4 shows average temperatures in infants and children.
- Affected by
  - illness
  - external temperature/environment
  - medication
  - age
  - infection
  - time of day
  - exercise
  - emotions
  - pregnancy
  - menstrual cycle
  - crying
  - hydration
- Excessive body temperature puts stress on vital body organs.

Temperature Control

Activities to control and regulate body temperature are managed by special cells in the brain.

- Heat is produced by chemical reactions (**metabolism**) in the body core and muscular contractions. For this reason, rectal temperature is highest.
- Blood carries the heat to the skin (**body shell**). The heat is lost from the skin to the outside.
- Heat loss is largely controlled by regulating the amount of blood reaching the skin and through perspiration.
- Average oral temperature range is 96.8°F (36°C)–100.4°F (38°C). Average temperature is 98.6°F (37°C).

Measuring Body Temperature

There are four body areas in which temperature is usually measured. They are:

- mouth (oral)—most common
- ear (aural)—takes the least amount of time
- rectal—most accurate of commonly used sites (mouth, rectal, axillary); rectal temperature registers 1°F higher than oral
- axillary or groin—least accurate. (This method is used only when the patient's condition does not permit the use of oral, aural, or rectal sites.)

An axillary or groin temperature registers 1°F (or 0.6°C) lower than oral temperature.

The patient's condition determines which is the best site for measuring the temperature. The most common site used is the mouth. It is not, however, always the best or safest site to use. In some situations, it would be wiser to use the rectal site.

For example, if the patient is a child or irrational, a glass thermometer in the mouth could result in injury. Patients with respiratory problems, mouth breathers, or those who are very weak or unconscious may not be able to keep the oral thermometer in their mouths for a long enough period of time to ensure an accurate recording. In these situations, the best choice is the aural site because the care provider holds the aural thermometer in the ear. The reading registers within seconds so the aural thermometer is a good choice for restless patients as well. If the aural thermometer is not available, the rectal site might be used. Use a rectal thermometer inserted in the anus for the proper time. Be sure to hold the rectal thermometer in place to avoid possible injury.

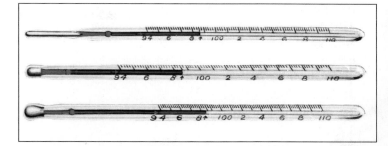

FIGURE 14–5. Clinical thermometers: from top to bottom—oral, security, rectal.

Clinical Thermometers

The Glass Clinical Thermometer

A patient's temperature is determined by using a clinical thermometer. There are several types of clinical thermometers in use. The glass **clinical thermometer** is a slender glass tube containing mercury, which expands when exposed to heat. Three types of glass clinical thermometers are in general use, Figure 14–5. They are the oral, security, and rectal thermometers. They differ mainly in the size and shape of the bulb. The bulb is the end that is inserted into the patient. When only the security or stubby type is in use, the rectal thermometers are marked with a red dot at the end of the stem.

Electronic Thermometer

The **electronic thermometer**, Figure 14–6, is used in many hospitals. One unit can serve many patients by simply changing the disposable sheath which fits over the probe.

- The electronic thermometer is battery-operated. It registers the temperature on the viewing screen in a few seconds.
- The portion called the **probe** is inserted into the patient.
- The probes are colored red for rectal use and blue for oral use.
- The probe is covered by a plastic sheath before use. The plastic sheath stays on during use. It is discarded after use.

Disposable Oral Thermometers

Plastic or paper thermometers are used in some facilities. They are used once and discarded. They have dots on them. The dots are treated to change color from brown to blue, according to the patient's temperature.

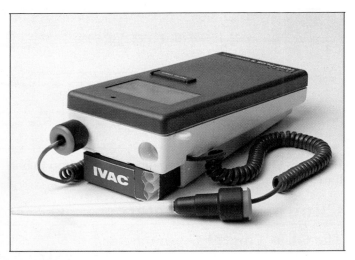

FIGURE 14–6. An electronic thermometer. The temperature is registered in large, easy-to-read numerals. The disposable protective sheath is placed over the probe tip. The probe is then inserted in the patient's mouth in the usual manner. *(Photo courtesy of IVAC Corporation, San Diego, CA)*

Refer to Figure 14–7 to review the beginning procedure actions and the procedure completion actions.

The aural (ear) thermometer is a relatively new way of determining body temperature, Figure 14–8A. The instrument measures the temperature from blood vessels in the tympanic membrane in the ear, Figure 14–8B. This provides a reading close to the core body temperature. The instrument has a built-in converter that provides the equivalent temperature in rectal or oral values (in both the Fahrenheit or Celsius system). The type of temperature reading (mode) is selected by the user. The disposable speculum is inserted into the ear canal, gently sealing the canal. The instrument is activated, usually by pressing a button, and within a few seconds registers the temperature of the blood flowing through the vessels in the eardrum.

Reading the Glass Thermometer

The glass thermometer is a long, cylindrical, calibrated tube that contains a column of mercury.

- Starting with 94°F (34°C), each long line indicates a 1-degree elevation in temperature.
- Only every other degree is marked with a number.
- In between each long line are four shorter lines.
- Each shorter line equals two-tenths (2/10 or 0.2) of 1 degree.

Mercury (the solid color line shown in Figure 14–9) in the bulb of the thermometer rises in the hollow center of the stem as heat is registered. To read the thermometer:

- Hold it at eye level.
- Find the solid column of mercury.
- Look along the sharper edge between the numbers and lines.

BEGINNING PROCEDURE ACTIONS	PROCEDURE COMPLETION ACTIONS
■ Wash your hands. ■ Assemble equipment needed. ■ Go to the patient's room, knock, and pause before entering. ■ Introduce yourself and identify the patient by checking the identification bracelet. ■ Ask visitors to leave and inform them where they can wait. ■ Provide privacy. ■ Explain what will happen and answer questions. ■ Allow patient to assist in procedure as much as possible. ■ Raise bed to comfortable working height.	■ Position patient comfortably. ■ Leave signal cord, telephone, and fresh water close at hand. ■ Return bed to lowest position. ■ Perform general safety check of patient and environment. ■ Wash your hands. ■ Report completion of task. ■ Let visitors know when they may reenter. ■ Document action and your observations.

NOTE: Where there are open lesions, wet linen, or possible contact with patient body fluids or blood, disposable gloves are worn during the procedure. Put on gloves before contact with the patient or linen. Properly dispose of gloves after they are removed. ALWAYS APPLY UNIVERSAL PRECAUTIONS.

FIGURE 14–7. Review of beginning procedure actions and procedure completion actions

■ Read at the point at which the mercury ends.
■ If it falls between two lines, read it to the closest line.

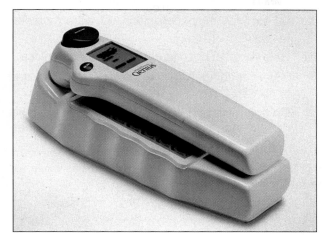

FIGURE 14–8A. Cordless, hand-held aural thermometer. The window on the handset indicates the digital temperature reading. *(Photo courtesy of Intelligent Medical Systems, Carlsbad, CA)*

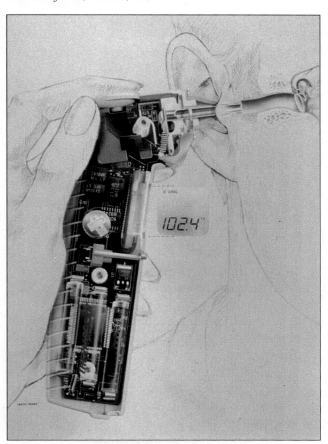

FIGURE 14–8B. The aural thermometer measures the temperature of the tympanic membrane in the ear. *(Courtesy of THERMOSCAN®, San Diego, CA)*

Some glass thermometers come individually prepackaged for patient use. The patient receives it as part of the Admission Package.

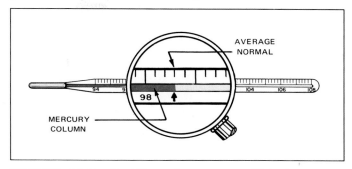

FIGURE 14–9. Reading a thermometer. This thermometer reads 98.6°F. Most Fahrenheit thermometers have an arrow indicating 98.6°.

Oral Temperature
Do not use if the patient is:
■ Uncooperative
■ Restless
■ Unconscious
■ Chilled
■ Confused
■ Coughing
■ Infant or child
■ Unable to breathe through the nose
■ Has had oral surgery
■ Irrational
■ Very weak
■ Receiving oxygen (except nasal prongs)
■ On seizure precautions
NOTE: An oral temperature reading could be false on denture wearers.
NOTE: To measure an oral temperature accurately, wait 15 minutes after patients have been smoking, eating, or drinking hot or cold liquids.

Rectal Temperature
Do not use if the patient has:
■ Diarrhea
■ Fecal impaction
■ Combative behavior
■ Rectal bleeding
■ Hemorrhoids
■ Had rectal surgery or rectal or colonic disease
NOTE: Always hold a rectal thermometer with probe in place the entire time.

Figure 14–10 lists general safety precautions to follow when using thermometers.

NOTE: Refer to Figure 14–7 to review the beginning procedure actions and procedure completion actions.

■	Check glass thermometers for chips.
■	Shake mercury down before use. Shake away from the patient or hard objects.
■	Do not leave the patient alone with a thermometer in place.
■	Hold rectal and axillary thermometers in place.
■	Before reading, wipe the thermometer from end to tip with an alcohol wipe or cotton ball.
■	Do not touch bulb end that has been in patient's mouth (oral thermometer) or anus (rectal thermometer).

FIGURE 14–10. General safety precautions when using thermometers.

SIDE 3

PROCEDURE 33 | OBRA

MEASURING AN ORAL TEMPERATURE (GLASS THERMOMETER)

1. Carry out each beginning procedure action.
2. Remember to wash your hands, identify the patient, and provide privacy.
3. Assemble the following equipment on a tray:
   - Container with clean thermometers
   - Container for used thermometers
   - Container for soiled tissues
   - Container with tissues
   - Pad and pencil
   - Watch with second hand
   - Gloves, if indicated
4. Have patient rest in a comfortable position in bed or chair.
5. Remove thermometer from container by holding stem end. Rinse thermometer with cold water and wipe with tissue from stem to mercury bulb end if thermometer has been in disinfectant. Check to be sure the thermometer is intact. Read the mercury column. It should register below 96°F. If necessary, shake down. (To shake down, Figure 14–11A, move away from table or other hard objects. Grasp the stem tightly between your thumb and fingers. Shake down with downward motion.) If used in your facility, place in disposable plastic cover sheath.
6. Ask patient if he or she has had hot or cold liquids to drink or smoked within the last 15 minutes. Wait 15 minutes before taking oral temperature if the answer is "yes."
7. Insert bulb end of thermometer under patient's tongue, toward side of mouth, Figure 14–11B. Tell patient to hold thermometer gently with lips closed for 3 minutes.
8. Remove thermometer, holding by stem. Wipe from stem end toward bulb end, Figure 14–11C.
9. Discard tissue in proper container.
10. Read thermometer and record on pad, Figure 14–11D.
11. Place thermometer in container for used thermometers. If thermometer is to be reused for this patient:
    - Wash it in cold water and soap twice with two separate cotton balls, wiping from stem to bulb.
    - Rinse and dry it.
    - Return it to the individual disinfectant-filled holder.

12. Carry out each procedure completion action. Remember to wash your hands, report completion of task, and document on patient's chart the date, time, temperature reading, and patient's reaction.

13. Report any unusual variations to the nurse at once.

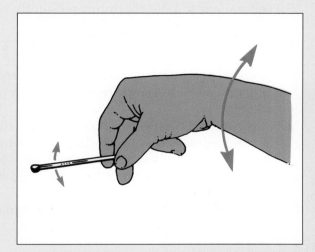

FIGURE 14–11A. Shake mercury down in column by holding the thermometer by the stem and snapping the wrist. Check the reading. Repeat until the reading is below 96°F.

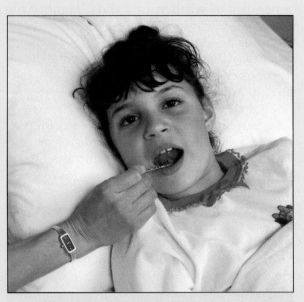

FIGURE 14–11B. The bulb end of the thermometer is inserted under the tongue, left 3 minutes, then removed.

FIGURE 14–11C. Wipe thermometer after removing it from patient's mouth. Always wipe from stem to bulb. Do not touch bulb.

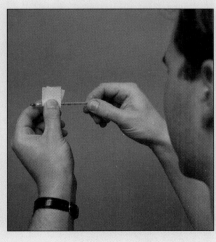

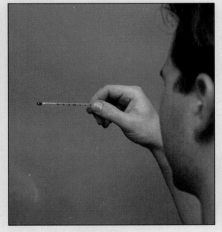

FIGURE 14–11D. Hold thermometer at eye level. Locate the column of mercury and read to the next closest line.

PROCEDURE 34   OBRA

MEASURING TEMPERATURE USING A SHEATH-COVERED THERMOMETER

1. Carry out each beginning procedure action.
2. Remember to wash your hands, identify the patient, and provide privacy.
3. Assemble needed equipment:
   - Clinical thermometer with protective sheath (unopened package), Figure 14–12A.
   - Pad and pencil
   - Gloves, if indicated
4. Have patient rest in a comfortable position.
5. Ask patient if he or she has had hot or cold liquids to drink or smoked within the last 15 minutes. Wait 15 minutes before taking oral temperature if the answer is "yes."
6. Open thermometer package by pulling apart at one end.
7. Carefully grasp thermometer and protective sheath covering it and pull from package, Figures 14–12B and C.
8. Keeping protective sheath over thermometer, Figure 14–12D, insert bulb end of thermometer under patient's tongue, toward side of mouth.
9. Tell patient to hold thermometer gently with lips closed for 3 minutes.
10. Remove thermometer and record reading on pad.
11. Discard sheath. Thermometer can be stored in patient's bedside stand for reuse with a new sheath.
12. Carry out each procedure completion action. Remember to wash your hands, report completion of task, and document on patient's chart the date, time, temperature reading, and patient's reaction.
13. Report any unusual variations to the nurse at once.

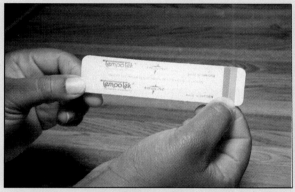

FIGURE 14–12A. Sheath-covered clinical thermometer.

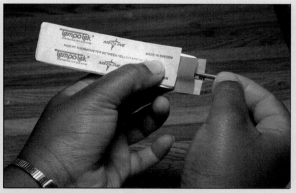

FIGURE 14–12B. Grasp thermometer and sheath and remove from outside cover.

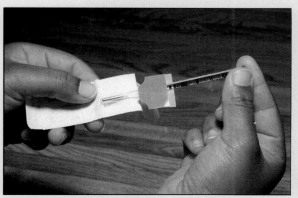

FIGURE 14–12C. Thermometer, sheath, and outer covering.

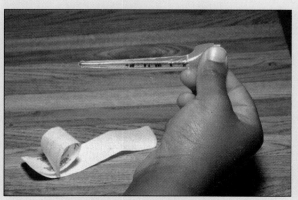

FIGURE 14–12D. The sheath-covered thermometer is inserted into patient's mouth. After temperature is recorded, the sheath is discarded. This technique makes disinfection unnecessary.

PROCEDURE 35

MEASURING AN ORAL TEMPERATURE (PLASTIC THERMOMETER)

NOTE: Latest findings indicate that temperature readings taken with this type of thermometer may not be entirely accurate.

1. Carry out each beginning procedure action.
2. Remember to wash your hands, identify the patient, and provide privacy.
3. Obtain an unused packaged plastic thermometer, and gloves, if indicated.
4. Ask patient if he or she has had hot or cold liquids to drink or smoked within the last 15 minutes. Wait 15 minutes before taking oral temperature if the answer is "yes."
5. Open package by grasping separated end (indicated by the words *open here*).
6. Expose end of thermometer to be handled.
7. Remove thermometer from package. Do not touch end to go in patient's mouth.
8. Place tip in patient's mouth under tongue in the usual manner.
9. Leave thermometer in place one minute.
10. Remove thermometer and read at once.
11. Carry out each procedure completion action. Remember to wash your hands, report completion of task, and document date, time, temperature reading, and patient's reaction.

PROCEDURE 36 | OBRA

SIDE 3

MEASURING AN ORAL TEMPERATURE (ELECTRONIC THERMOMETER)

1. Carry out each beginning procedure action.
2. Remember to wash your hands, identify the patient, and provide privacy.
3. Obtain electronic thermometer, disposable sheaths, and gloves, if indicated.
4. Ask patient if he or she has had hot or cold liquids to drink or smoked within the last 15 minutes. Wait 15 minutes before taking oral temperature if the answer is "yes."
5. Cover probe (blue) with protective sheath.
6. Insert covered probe under patient's tongue toward side of mouth.
7. Hold probe in position. Ask patient to close mouth and breathe through nose.
8. When buzzer signals temperature has been determined, take reading and record on pad.
9. Discard sheath in wastepaper basket. Do not touch sheath.
10. Return probe to proper position and entire unit to charging.
11. Carry out each procedure completion action. Remember to wash your hands, report completion of task, and document date, time, temperature reading, and patient's reaction.

PROCEDURE 37 | OBRA

SIDE 3

MEASURING A RECTAL TEMPERATURE (GLASS THERMOMETER)

1. Carry out each beginning procedure action.
2. Remember to wash your hands, identify the patient, and provide privacy.
3. Assemble equipment on a tray:
   - Container with clean rectal thermometer
   - Container for used thermometers
   - Container for soiled tissues
   - Lubricant
   - Container with tissues
   - Pad and pencil
   - Watch with second hand
   - Disposable gloves (universal precautions)
4. Put up opposite side rail. Lower backrest of bed. Ask patient to turn to left side, if possible. Assist patient, if necessary.
5. Place small amount of lubricant on tissue.

continues

6. Put gloves on. Remove thermometer from container by holding stem end. Read mercury column. Be sure it registers below 96°F. Check condition of thermometer.
7. Apply small amount of lubricant to bulb with tissue.
8. Fold the top bedclothes back to expose anal area.
9. Refer to Figure 14–13. Separate buttocks with one hand. Insert the thermometer gently into rectum 1-1/2 inches. Hold in place. Adjust bedclothes as soon as thermometer is inserted.
10. Thermometer should remain inserted 3–5 minutes. (Follow facility policy.) Hold thermometer in place for full time.
11. Remove thermometer, holding by stem. Wipe from stem toward bulb end.
12. Discard tissue in proper container.
13. Read thermometer. Record reading on pad.
14. Wipe lubricant from patient. Discard tissue.
15. Remove gloves and handle per hospital policy. Place thermometer in container for used thermometers. If thermometer is to be reused for this patient:

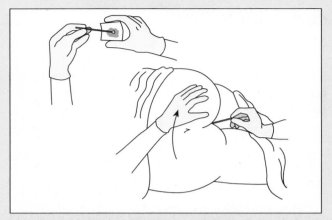

FIGURE 14–13. The rectal thermometer is lubricated and then inserted 1-1/2 inches into the rectum.

a. Wash it in cold water and soap.
b. Rinse and dry it.
c. Return it to the individual disinfectant-filled holder.
16. Lower opposite side rail.
17. Carry out each procedure completion action. Remember to wash your hands, report completion of task, and document date, time, temperature reading (R), and patient's reaction.

PROCEDURE 38   **OBRA**

SIDE
3

MEASURING A RECTAL TEMPERATURE (ELECTRONIC THERMOMETER)

1. Carry out each beginning procedure action.
2. Remember to wash your hands, identify the patient, and provide privacy.
3. Assemble equipment on a tray:
   - Electronic thermometer
   - Red sheaths
   - Gloves
4. Lower backrest of bed. Ask patient to turn on his side. Assist patient, if necessary.
5. Put on gloves. Place a small amount of lubricant on the tip of the sheath.
6. Fold the top bedclothes back to expose anal area.
7. Separate buttocks with one hand. Insert

sheath-covered probe about one and one-half inches into rectum. Hold in place. Replace bedclothes as soon as thermometer is inserted.
8. Read temperature when registered on digital display. Note reading on pad.
9. Remove probe and discard sheath. Wipe lubricant from patient. Discard tissue.
10. Remove gloves and dispose of according to facility policy.
11. Carry out each procedure completion action. Remember to wash your hands, report completion of task, and document the date, time, temperature reading (R), and patient's reaction.

PROCEDURE 39 · OBRA

MEASURING AN AXILLARY OR GROIN TEMPERATURE (GLASS THERMOMETER)

1. Carry out each beginning procedure action.
2. Remember to wash your hands, identify the patient, and provide privacy.
3. Assemble equipment on a tray:
   - Container with clean oral thermometers
   - Container for used thermometers
   - Container for soiled tissues
   - Container with tissues
   - Pad and pencil
   - Watch with a second hand
   - Gloves
4. Wipe the area dry and place the thermometer. Put on gloves if groin area is used for temperature measurement.
   a. The patient's arm is held close to his body if axillary site is used, Figure 14–14.
   b. Thermometer must be in the fold against the body if groin site is used.
   c. Leave the thermometer in place 10 minutes.
   d. Remove, wipe, and read thermometer. Note reading on pad.
   e. Clean and replace as with oral thermometer if it is to be reused.
5. If the groin area was used, remove gloves and discard according to facility policy.

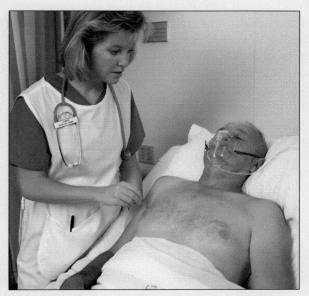

FIGURE 14–14. When the thermometer is placed in the axilla, it must be held in place.

6. Carry out each procedure completion action. Remember to wash your hands, report completion of task, and document date, time, temperature reading (AX or GR), and patient's reaction.

PROCEDURE 40 · OBRA

MEASURING AN AXILLARY TEMPERATURE (ELECTRONIC THERMOMETER)

1. Carry out each beginning procedure action.
2. Remember to wash your hands, identify the patient, and provide privacy.
3. Equipment needed: same as for oral temperature measurement using an electronic thermometer.
4. Wipe axillary area dry and place covered probe in place. Keep patient's arm close to the body. Hold probe in place until temperature records on digital display and buzzer signals.
5. Remove thermometer probe. Dispose of sheath.
6. Carry out each procedure completion action. Remember to wash your hands, report completion of task, and document date, time, temperature reading (AX), and patient's reaction.

Cleaning Glass Thermometers

Glass thermometers are reusable. They, therefore, need to be cleaned and disinfected between use. If each patient has an individual thermometer kept in solution at the bedside, you must clean and disinfect it after each use. If a general supply of thermometers is used to determine routine temperature, they too must be disinfected before reuse, Figure 14–15.

Each used thermometer must be carefully washed with soapy, cold, running water to remove saliva or other body secretions. It must be rinsed to remove the soap and then carefully dried before disinfecting.

Remember that glass breaks very easily so use care in washing and drying the thermometer. Check each one for chips before putting it into disinfectant and before placing the thermometer in the patient.

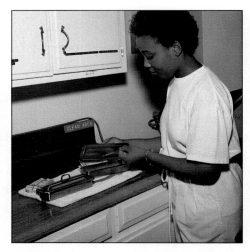

FIGURE 14–15. Remove clean thermometer from container and measure the patient's temperature.

PROCEDURE 41	SIDE 3		

CLEANING GLASS THERMOMETERS

1. Wash your hands and assemble the following equipment:
   - Tray
   - Towel
   - Label
   - Washcloth
   - Soiled thermometers in container of soapy water
   - Container for clean thermometers
   - Liquid soap
   - Container of cotton balls
   - Disinfectant, according to facility policy
   - Disposable gloves, according to facility policy
2. Take tray of equipment to utility room.
3. Place towel on sink side.
4. Wash and dry container and cover for clean thermometers. Place on towel with cover top up.
5. Place gauze in bottom of container.
6. Clean sink with cleanser. Then place washcloth in bottom of sink and fill sink 1/3 full with cool water. This is in case you drop a thermometer. It is less likely to break. Put on gloves.
7. Slowly turn on cold water faucet.
8. Moisten a sponge/cotton ball and apply soap.
9. Pick up one thermometer at a time, holding by the stem. Proceed as follows:
   a. Using a circular motion, cleanse the thermometer from stem to bulb.
   b. Discard cotton ball.
   c. Carefully rinse each thermometer.
   d. Using a circular motion and a dry cotton ball for each, dry each thermometer.
   e. Check thermometers for chips and shake down to 96°F (21°C) or below before placing in clean container, Figure 14–16A.
   f. Fill container 1/2 full with disinfectant, Figure 14–16B.
   g. Empty water from dirty container.
10. Shut off faucet. Squeeze out washcloth and put into laundry. Shut basin drain and add hot water and soap.
11. Wash, rinse, and dry dirty thermometer container.
12. Remove gloves and discard according to facility policy.

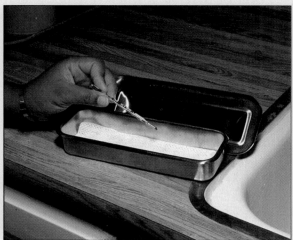

FIGURE 14–16A. Place in a clean container that has folded gauze on the bottom to prevent breakage of thermometers.

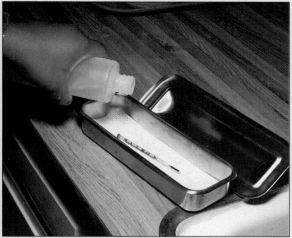

FIGURE 14–16B. Add disinfectant solution, being sure to cover entire thermometer.

13. Add disinfectant, if necessary, so that each thermometer is completely covered by it.
14. Place cover on container. Place label with date, time, and your initials on container. Remember that disinfectants take time to be effective.
15. Place washcloth and towel in laundry. Dispose of used sponges in trash.
16. Leave area neat and tidy.
17. After disinfecting:
    a. Remove label. Remove thermometers.
    b. Empty disinfectant.
    c. Wash and dry container.
    d. Place 4 × 4 folded sponge on the bottom of the container.
18. Rinse and dry thermometers.
19. Place dry, clean thermometers on sponge in container and cover, Figure 14–16C.
20. Store per facility policy in clean area.
21. Wash your hands and report completion of task to the nurse.

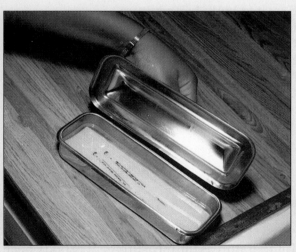

FIGURE 14–16C. Allow thermometers to soak the required time. Then remove and rinse well before storing in a clean, dry container.

Special Situations

Hypothermia

Hypothermia is a drop in core body temperature below 95°F (35°C) rectally. This can occur:
- When people are exposed to cold without adequate protection.
- In the elderly, when a person is exposed to external temperatures as warm as 60°F.
- Deliberately induced before surgery to slow body metabolism.

Indications of hypothermia to report include:
- Drop in body temperature
- Poor coordination and confusion
- Slurred speech
- Decreased respiratory and heart rates

Nursing Assistant Actions

- Report observations to the supervisor.
- Check the environmental temperature and adjust it.
- Provide external warmth with a sweater or blanket.
- Reduce drafts with screens or curtains.
- If permitted, give something warm to drink.
- Check vital signs.

Hyperthermia

Hyperthermia is an elevation of core body temperature to 104°F (40°C) rectally or higher. This can occur:

- When a person is exposed to high external temperature.
- In serious injuries such as burns.
- When there is damage to the temperature control center in the brain.
- With infections.

Indications of hyperthermia to report include:

- Elevated body temperature
- Hot, flushed skin
- Faintness
- Headache
- Nausea
- Convulsions

Fever or pyrexia is when core body temperature rises to at least 101°F (rectally). Fever is often associated with infections, injury, surgery, and serious trauma. Indications of fever are the same as those for general hyperthermia.

NOTE: In children, temperatures tend to rise higher than in adults. This puts children at greater risk for seizures.

Nursing Assistant Actions

- Report observations to the supervisor.
- Check environmental temperature and adjust it.
- Reduce external warmth. Cover the patient only with a gown or sheet.
- If permitted, give cooling drink.
- Carry out cooling procedures as ordered. For example, give cooling baths or enemas.
- Check vital signs frequently.

Documentation

In many facilities, temperatures are recorded on a temperature clipboard. They are then transferred to the individual patient charts. Changes in readings may be flagged (specially noted) by placing a circle around the reading or a star beside it. Make sure to report any changes from previous temperature readings directly to the nurse. Your accurate observations, reporting, and documentation contribute to the nurses' evaluation and assessment of the patient.

SUMMARY

- Temperature is the measurement of body heat. It varies in different areas in the same person.
  — Average oral temperature is 98.6°F.
  — Average rectal temperature is 99.6°F.
  — Average axillary temperature is 97.6°F.
- Measurements of temperature may be made using the Fahrenheit (F) or Celsius (C) scale.
- Three kinds of clinical thermometers are commonly used to measure the body temperature. They are the:
  — Oral
  — Security
  — Rectal
- There are different colored thermometer tips for rectal and oral use.

- In addition to glass thermometers, there are other types of thermometers in use. They are the:
  — Battery-operated electronic thermometer. It has different colored tips for rectal and oral use.
  — Plastic thermometer. It has dots which change color according to the body temperature.
  — Aural thermometer. A probe placed in the external auditory canal measures body temperature at the tympanic membrane.
- The procedure for measuring body temperature should be carefully followed, including beginning procedure and procedure completion activities.

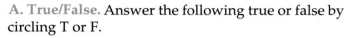

UNIT REVIEW

A. True/False. Answer the following true or false by circling T or F.

T F 1. When charting an axillary temperature, always print an *AX* after the reading.

T F 2. Readings taken with a plastic thermometer may not be entirely accurate.

T F 3. Temperature is the measurement of body heat.

T F 4. The most common method of measuring the temperature of a cooperative adult is by mouth.

T F 5. To measure a rectal temperature, the patient had best be positioned on her back.

T F 6. 96.8°F is an average oral temperature.

T F 7. Only temperature variations of more than 5°F need to be reported to the nurse.

T F 8. Clinical thermometers can be identified by the shapes of their bulbs.

T F 9. The probe of an electronic thermometer is covered with a red sheath for rectal use.

T F 10. The axillary temperature of a patient will register approximately one degree higher than his oral temperature.

T F 11. The aural temperature reading is the most accurate.

T F 12. A freezing temperature registered in Celsius readings would be 32°.

T F 13. It would be unsafe to use glass oral thermometers with children.

T F 14. If safely placed, rectal thermometers need not be held.

T F 15. Wait five minutes after the patient has taken hot liquids to measure an oral temperature.

T F 16. When washing used glass thermometers, always wash them in hot, soapy water.

T F 17. Always wipe the axillary area before placing a thermometer.

T F 18. When using an electronic thermometer, you should not allow your fingers to touch the probe sheath.

T F 19. All rectal thermometers should be lubricated before insertion.

T F 20. The oral thermometer should remain in place one minute.

T F 21. The mercury column in a glass oral thermometer should register below 96°F at the beginning of the procedure.

T F 22. There may be times when a temperature may have to be measured in the groin area.

T F 23. Each long line on the stem of a clinical thermometer indicates an increase of two degrees of temperature.

T F 24. Each short line on the stem of the clinical thermometer indicates a 0.2-degree increase in temperature.

T F 25. Measuring the temperature in the groin area gives the most accurate indication of body temperature.

Pulse and Respiration

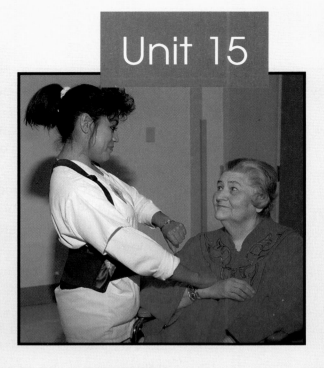

As a result of this unit, you will be able to:

- Spell and define terms.
- Define pulse.
- Explain the importance of monitoring a pulse rate.
- Locate the pulse sites.
- Identify the range of normal pulse and respiratory rates.
- Measure the pulse at different locations.
- List the characteristics of the pulse and respiration.
- Describe and demonstrate the use of the stethoscope.
- Measure the respiratory rate.

Learn the meaning and the correct spelling of the following words and phrases:

accelerated	pulse deficit
apical pulse	radial pulse
apnea	rales
bradycardia	rate
Cheyne-Stokes	respiration
respirations	rhythm
cyanosis	stertorous
dyspnea	symmetry
expiration	tachycardia
inspiration	tachypnea
pulse	volume

The pulse and respiration of the patient are usually counted during the same procedure. Because breathing is partly under voluntary control, a person is able to stop or alter breathing temporarily for a short period. For example, when a patient realizes that her breathing is being watched and counted, she alters her breathing pattern without meaning to do so. To avoid this, the respirations are counted immediately following the pulse count without telling the patient. The patient's hand is kept in the same position, and your fingers remain upon the pulse so that you seem to still be taking the pulse.

The Pulse

The **pulse** is:

■ The pressure of the blood felt against the wall of an artery as the heart alternately contracts (beats) and relaxes (rests).

■ More easily felt in arteries that come fairly close to the skin and can be gently pressed against a bone.

■ The same in all arteries throughout the body.

■ An indication of how the cardiovascular system is able to meet the body's needs.

■ The **radial pulse** is the most commonly mea-sured pulse. It is measured at the radial artery in the wrist.

Figure 15–1 shows areas of the body where other large blood vessels come close enough to the surface to be sites for counting the pulse. Conscious patients can be checked at the radial artery. Unconscious patients should be checked at the carotid artery or apically (over the heart).

Pulse measurement includes determining the:

1. Rate or speed
   a. **Bradycardia**—an unusually slow pulse
   b. **Tachycardia**—an unusually fast pulse
2. Character
   a. **Rhythm**—regularity
   b. **Volume** or fullness

Report:

■ Pulse rates over 100 beats per minute (bpm) (tachycardia)

■ Pulse rates under 60 bpm (bradycardia)

■ Irregularities in character (rhythm and volume)

Pulse rates can be affected by:

■ Illness   ■ Sex
■ Emotions   ■ Position
■ Age   ■ Physical training
■ Exercise   ■ Lowered temperature
■ Elevated   ■ Drugs
  temperature

Figure 15–2 shows average pulse rates.

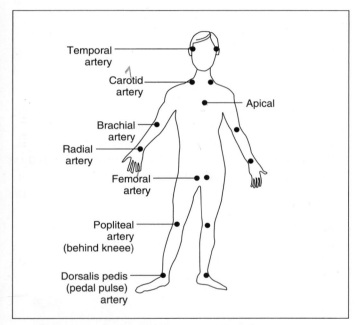

FIGURE 15–1. Pulse sites in the body *(From Simmers, Diver-sified Health Occupations, 1988, Delmar Publishers Inc.)*

Adult men	60–70	beats per minute
Adult women	65–80	beats per minute
Children over 7 years	75–100	beats per minute
Preschoolers	80–110	beats per minute
Infants	120–160	beats per minute

FIGURE 15–2. Average pulse rates

PROCEDURE 42   OBRA

SIDE **3**

COUNTING THE RADIAL PULSE RATE

1. Carry out each beginning procedure action.
2. Remember to wash your hands, identify the patient, and provide privacy.
3. Place patient in a comfortable position. The palm of the hand should be down and the arm should rest on a flat surface.

4. Locate the pulse on the thumb side of the wrist with the tips of your first three fingers, Fig-ure 15–3. Do not use your thumb since it con-tains a pulse which may be confused with the patient's pulse.

continues

5. When the pulse is felt, exert slight pressure. Use second hand of watch and count for one minute. It is the practice in some hospitals to count for one-half minute and multiply by two and to record the rate for one minute. A one-minute count is preferred and must be done if the pulse is irregular.

6. Carry out procedure completion actions. Remember to wash your hands, report completion of task, and document date, time, pulse rate and character, and patient's reaction.

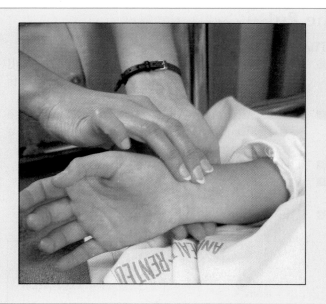

FIGURE 15–3. Locate the pulse on the thumb side of the wrist with the tips of your fingers.

The Apical Pulse

An **apical pulse** is counted by placing the stethoscope on the chest over the apex (tip) of the heart and listening for the heart sounds that indicate closing of the valves. These sounds occur as the heart pumps the blood into the arteries. The sounds should occur at the same rate as the pulse that is felt as an expansion of the radial artery, Figure 15–4. The apex of the heart is found:

- On the left side of the front of the chest
- Between the fifth and sixth ribs
- Just below the left nipple
- In women, under the left breast

Listen carefully for two sounds. (Lub dub) The louder sound (Lub) corresponds to the contraction of the ventricles pushing the blood forward through the arteries, and the closing of the valves to prevent the back-flow of blood. This is the sound to be counted. The softer sound (dub) corresponds to the relaxation of the ventricles as they fill with blood before the next contraction and the closing of the semilunar valves to prevent back-flow from the arteries.

Sometimes the contraction of the heart is so weak, it fails to send sufficient blood to the arteries to expand them. When this happens, no pulse is felt. In this case, the number of loud sounds do not correspond with the number of pulses felt in the radial artery.

The difference between the apical pulse (the loud sounds heard over the heart) and the radial pulse (the expansion felt over the radial pulse) is called a **pulse deficit**. Apical pulse rates are checked:

- Whenever a pulse deficit exists or is suspected.
- Before the registered nurse administers drugs that profoundly alter the heart rate or rhythm.
- In children whose rapid rates might be difficult to count at the radial artery.
- For one full minute.
- On any child 12 months of age or younger.
- Whenever you are uncertain of the accuracy of the radial pulse or it is irregular.

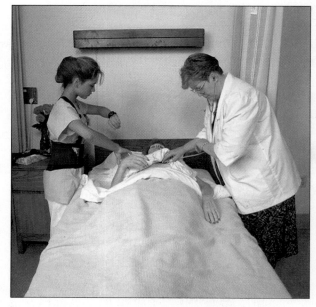

FIGURE 15–4. The nurse takes the apical pulse while the nursing assistant takes the radial pulse.

PROCEDURE 43

COUNTING THE APICAL PULSE

1. Carry out each beginning procedure action.
2. Remember to wash your hands, identify the patient, and provide privacy.
3. Clean stethoscope earpieces and bell with disinfectant.
4. Place stethoscope earpieces in your ears.
5. Place the stethoscope diaphragm or bell over the apex of the patient's heart. If it is cold, warm diaphragm with hands before placing it on patient's chest.
6. Listen carefully for the heartbeat.
7. Count the louder sounding beats for one minute.
8. Check radial pulse for one minute. The best way to obtain these numbers is to have the nurse count the apical pulse while you take the radial pulse, Figure 15–4.
9. Note results on a pad for comparison.
10. Clean earpieces and bell of stethoscope with disinfectant.
11. Carry out each procedure completion action. Remember to wash your hands, report completion of task, and document date, time, pulse values as in example, character (e.g., weak and irregular), and patient's reaction.

Example: Apical pulse   = 108
Radial pulse   =   82
Pulse deficit   =   26 (108 – 82 = 26)

Respiration

The main function of respiration is to supply the cells in the body with oxygen and to rid the body of excess carbon dioxide. When respirations are inefficient, there is less oxygen in the blood available for body needs. In addition, carbon dioxide is released less efficiently. The skin takes on a bluish color and the condition is known as cyanosis

There are two parts to each respiration: one inspiration (inhalation) followed by one expiration (exhalation). Special terms describe different breathing patterns:

- Tachypnea—rapid, shallow breathing
- Dyspnea—difficult or labored breathing
- Shallow—breaths that partially fill the lungs
- Apnea—a period of no respirations
- Cheyne-Stokes respirations—a period of dyspnea followed by periods of apnea
- Stertorous—Snoring-like respirations
- Rales (gurgles)—moist respirations. At times, fluid (mucus) will collect in the air passages. This causes a bubbling type of respiration. Rales are common in the dying patient.

Respirations should be checked for:

- Rate—number of respirations per minute
- Rhythm—regularity
- Symmetry—ability of the chest to expand equally due to air entry into each lung
- Volume—depth of respiration
- Character—terms used to describe the character of respirations include:

- Regular
- Irregular
- Shallow
- Deep
- Labored (difficult)

The rate of respiration is determined by counting the rise or fall of the chest for one minute with a watch equipped with a second hand.

- The average rate for adults is 16 to 20 per minute.
- If the rate is more than 25 per minute, it is said to be accelerated. Accelerated respiration should be reported.
- If the rate is less than 12 per minute, it is too slow. It should be reported.

Remember that, if possible, respirations should be counted without the patient's awareness since the rate and volume may be changed if the patient knows they are being counted. You might count respirations before or after counting the radial pulse. Continue pressing on the pulse area while counting.

The factors affecting respiratory rates are listed in Figure 15–5.

PROCEDURE 44 — OBRA

COUNTING RESPIRATIONS

1. When the pulse rate has been counted, you may leave your fingers on the radial pulse and start counting the number of times the chest rises and falls during one minute.

2. Note depth and regularity of respirations.
3. Record the time, rate, depth, and regularity of respirations.

■ Illness	■ Age
■ Emotions	■ Exercise
■ Elevated temperature	■ Position
■ Sex	■ Drugs

FIGURE 15–5. Factors affecting respiratory rates

Temperature, pulse, and respiration (TPR) values are recorded in a notebook and then transferred to the patient's chart, Figure 15–6.

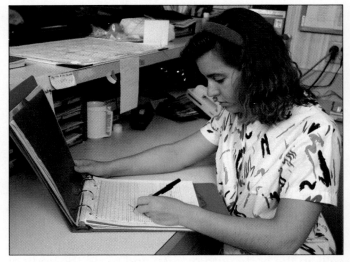

FIGURE 15–6. TPR readings are recorded on the patient's record.

SUMMARY

- Pulse and respiratory rates and character are determined as part of the vital signs.
- The values are usually determined in a single procedure.
- Differences in apical and radial pulse rates are known as pulse deficits.

- Accurate values for respirations are best made when the patient is unaware that the procedure is being carried out.
- Unusual findings should be reported to the nurse.

UNIT REVIEW

A. True/False. Answer the following true or false by circling T or F.

T F 1. A pulse deficit develops when there is a difference between the apical and radial pulses.

T F 2. The pulse is the pressure of blood against the arterial wall.

T F 3. Cheyne-Stokes respirations are deep and regular.

T F 4. Pulses differ when counted at different pulse sites.

T F 5. The pulse rate of an infant is between 110–130 bpm.

T F 6. An apical pulse should be counted in children.

T F 7. The most often used pulse site is the carotid artery.

T F 8. The respiratory system rids the body of excess carbon dioxide.

T F 9. Mucus in the air passages causes rales.

T F 10. A pulse is best counted using the thumb placed over the artery.

B. Matching. Match Column I with Column II.

Column I	Column II
_h_ 11. Snoring types of respiration	a. accelerated
_d_ 12. Bluish discoloration to the skin	b. apnea
_g_ 13. Regularity	c. bradycardia
____ 14. Periods of no respiration	d. cyanosis
_e_ 15. Difficult breathing	e. dyspnea
_i_ 16. Rapid respirations	f. rate
_a_ 17. Increased or speeded up	g. rhythm
_k_ 18. Expiration	h. stertorous
_f_ 19. Speed	i. tachypnea
_c_ 20. Slow pulse	j. inspiration
	k. exhalation

Cause

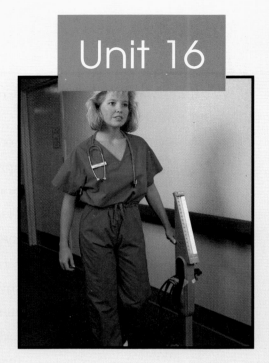

Unit 16

Blood Pressure

OBJECTIVES

As a result of this unit, you will be able to:

- Spell and define terms.

- Describe the factors that influence blood pressure.

- Identify the range of normal blood pressure values.

- Identify the causes of inaccurate blood pressure readings.

- Demonstrate the use of the stethoscope.

- Demonstrate the use of the sphygmomanometer.

- Measure and record patients' blood pressure.

- Select the proper sized blood pressure cuff.

- List precautions associated with use of the sphygmomanometer.

VOCABULARY

Learn the meaning and the correct spelling of the following words and phrases:

aneroid gauge
ausculatory gap
blood pressure
brachial artery
depressant
diastolic pressure
elasticity
fasting
hypertension

hypotension
palpated systolic
  pressure
pulse pressure
sphygmomanometer
stethoscope
stimulant
systolic pressure

Blood pressure is the fourth vital sign. It is the measure of the force of the blood against the walls of the arteries. Figure 16–1 shows an instrument that measures all vital signs. Blood pressure depends upon the:

- Volume (amount of blood in the circulatory system).

- Force of the heartbeat.

- Condition of the arteries. Arteries that have lost their elasticity (stretch) give more resistance. The pressure is greater in these arteries.

- Distance from the heart. Blood pressure in the legs is lower than in the arms.

Blood pressure is elevated by:

- Sex of the patient (males slightly higher than females before menopause)

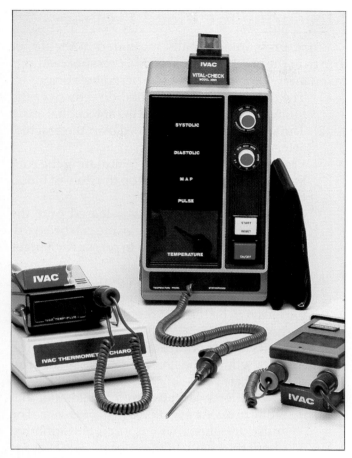

FIGURE 16–1. All vital signs may be checked with a single instrument. *(Photo courtesy of IVAC Corporation, San Diego, CA)*

- Exercise
- Eating
- **Stimulants** (substances that speed up body functions)
- Emotional stress such as anger, fear, and sexual activity
- Disease conditions such as arteriosclerosis (hardening of the arteries)
- Hereditary factors
- Pain
- Obesity
- Age
- Condition of blood vessels

Blood pressure is lowered by:
- **Fasting** (not eating)
- Rest
- **Depressants** (drugs that slow down body functions)
- Weight loss
- Emotions (such as grief)

■ Age	■ Heredity
■ Sleep	■ Sex
■ Weight	■ Viscosity of blood
■ Emotion	■ Condition of blood vessels

FIGURE 16–2. Factors influencing blood pressure readings

- Abnormal conditions such as hemorrhage (loss of blood) or shock

The factors affecting blood pressure are summarized in Figure 16–2.

Equipment

The **sphygmomanometer** (blood pressure apparatus) consists of:
- A cuff (different sizes are available) that fits around the patient's arm. There is a rubber bladder inside the cuff. A pressure control button is attached to the cuff. It is important to use the proper size cuff when measuring blood pressure. Cuffs that are too wide or too narrow will give inaccurate readings, Figure 16–3. The width of the cuff should measure approximately two-thirds the diameter of the patient's arm.
- Two tubes. One tube is connected to the pressure control bulb and to the bladder inside the cuff. The other tube is connected to the pressure gauge.

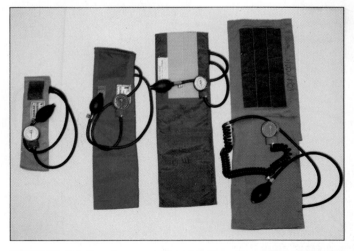

FIGURE 16–3. Improperly sized cuffs will give false readings.

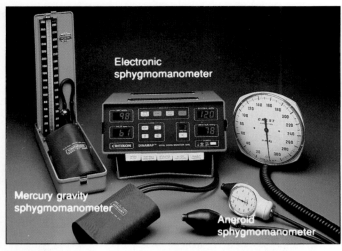

FIGURE 16–4. Types of sphygmomanometers *(Photos courtesy of Critikon, Inc.)*

■ A pressure gauge, which may be a round aneroid gauge dial or a column of mercury, Figure 16–4. Both are marked with numbers.

The stethoscope, Figure 16–5, magnifies sounds. It consists of:

■ A bell or diaphragm.
■ Tubing that carries sounds to listener.
■ Earpieces that direct the sounds into the listener's ears. The earpieces and diaphragm must be cleaned with antiseptic before and after each use to prevent transmission of disease.

Electronic sphygmomanometers with attached cuffs are used in some facilities. These units do not require a stethoscope but automatically register the readings on a digital display. Check with your nurse for specific operating instructions.

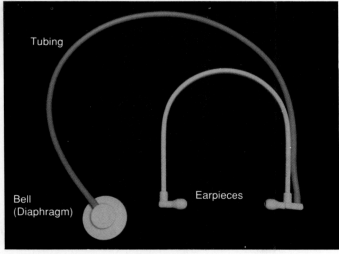

FIGURE 16–5. The stethoscope

Measuring the Blood Pressure

Blood pressure is usually measured in the upper arm over the brachial artery. Blood pressure readings taken anywhere else must be ordered by doctor.

1. The cuff is smoothly applied directly over the brachial artery (2 cm above the antecubital area).
2. The stethoscope bell is placed over the brachial artery.
3. Pressure is then increased by inflating the rubber bladder in the cuff to stop the flow of blood through the artery.
   a. The pressure is slowly released and the sounds of heart valves closing can be heard. The sounds correspond to pressure changes in the blood.
4. The blood pressure is measured:
   a. At its highest point as the systolic pressure. This will be the first regular sound you will hear.
   b. At its lowest point as the diastolic pressure. This will be the change or last sound you will hear.
   c. The difference between systolic and diastolic pressure is called pulse pressure. The pulse pressure gives important information about the health of the arteries. The average pulse pressure in a healthy adult is about 40 mm Hg (range 30–50 mm Hg). There are, however, factors in health and disease that can bring about an alteration in the pulse pressure. An increase in blood volume or heart rate or a decrease in the ability of the arteries to expand may result in an increased pulse pressure.
5. Blood pressure readings are recorded as an improper fraction; e.g., systolic/diastolic or 130/92.
6. Blood pressure values:
   a. Average resting adult brachial artery pressure is between 90–140 millimeters of mercury (mm Hg) systolic and between 60–90 millimeters of mercury (mm Hg) diastolic.
   b. Hypertension (high blood pressure) is when values are greater than 140 mm Hg systolic and 90 mm Hg diastolic.
   c. Hypotension (low blood pressure) is when values are less than 100 mm Hg systolic and 60 mm Hg diastolic.

Inaccurate Blood Pressure Readings

Causes of inaccurate blood pressure readings include:

- Use of a wrong size cuff
- An improperly wrapped cuff
- Incorrect positioning of arm
- Not using the same arm for all readings
- Not having the gauge at eye level
- Deflating the cuff too slowly
- Mistaking an auscultatory gap (sound fadeout for 10–15 mm Hg which then begins again) as the diastolic pressure

CAUTION

Do not attempt to measure blood pressure using an arm that is the site of an intravenous infusion, paralyzed, injured, the site of an A-V shunt, or if edema is present.

How to Read the Gauge

The gauges are marked with a series of lines. The large lines are at increments of 10 mm (millimeters) of mercury (Hg) pressure. The shorter lines are at 2-mm intervals. For example, the first small line above 80

mm is 82 mm. The first small line below 80 mm is 78 mm, Figure 16–6.

To properly read the mercury gauge:

- It should be at eye level.
- It should not be tilted.
- The reading should be taken at the top of the column of mercury. It should not be taken at the "hump" in the middle of the mercury when you hear the first sound.

To properly read the aneroid gauge, observe the gauge at eye level. Do not read it at an angle.

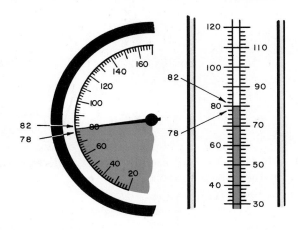

FIGURE 16–6. The aneroid gauge (*left*) and the mercury gravity gauge (*right*). Take reading at the closest line.

PROCEDURE 45 | OBRA

TAKING BLOOD PRESSURE

SIDE 3

1. Carry out each beginning procedure action.
2. Remember to wash your hands, identify the patient, and provide privacy.
3. Assemble the equipment needed:
   — Sphygmomanometer
   — Stethoscope (Clean earpieces and bell with antiseptic solution, Figure 16–7.)
4. Place the patient's arm palm-upward, supported on bed or table. Place pillow lengthwise under the arm if patient is seated in a chair without a table.
5. Roll sleeve of gown up about 5 inches above elbow. Be sure it is not tight on the arm.
6. Apply cuff smoothly and evenly 1–1 1/2 inches above the elbow. The center of the rubber bladder should be directly over the brachial artery. If the cuff is marked with an arrow, place cuff

so that the arrow points over the brachial artery.

7. Tuck ends of cuff under a fold. Hook to secure or use Velcro™ closure. Be sure cuff is secure but not too tight. Check by slipping two fingers between cuff and patient's arm.
8. Locate the radial artery and palpate it as you:
   a. Close valve attached to hand pump (air bulb) by turning it clockwise.
   b. Quickly inflate cuff until the gauge registers 50 mm Hg.
   c. Continue to inflate cuff in 10 mm Hg increments until radial pulse cannot be felt. This pressure indicates the palpated systolic pressure. Note the pressure.
   d. Quickly deflate cuff by turning the closed valve counterclockwise.

continues

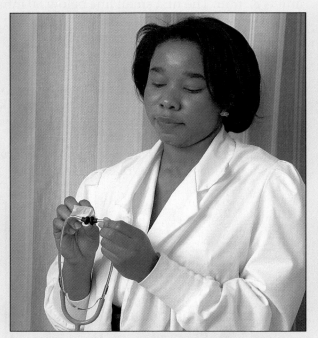

FIGURE 16–7. Carefully clean earpieces of the stethoscope before use.

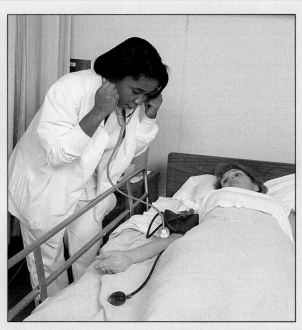

FIGURE 16–8. Place earpieces of the stethoscope comfortably in your ears.

9. Ask the patient to raise the arm and flex fingers.
10. Locate the brachial artery with the fingers. The brachial artery is located on the inside of the arm (medial aspect) just inside the elbow.
11. Place earpieces in ears, Figure 16–8. Place bell of stethoscope directly over the artery, Figure 16–9.
12. Close valve and reinflate cuff quickly until gauge registers 20 mm above palpated systolic pressure.
13. Listen carefully as you open valve of bulb by turning counterclockwise.
14. Let air escape slowly (between 1–3 mm per second) until first heart sound is heard, Figure 16–10. Note reading on gauge as the systolic pressure.
15. Continue to release the air pressure slowly until there is an abrupt change of the sound from very loud to a soft muffled sound. The reading at which this change is heard is the diastolic pressure. In some facilities, the last sound heard is taken as the diastolic pressure.
16. Rapidly deflate cuff and remove, expel air from the cuff, and replace apparatus. Clean

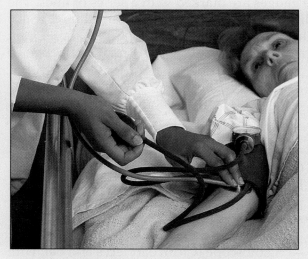

FIGURE 16–9. Place stethoscope diaphragm or bell right over the brachial artery.

earpieces and bell of stethoscope with antiseptic solution.
NOTE: If repeat procedure is necessary, wait at least one minute.
   a. Ask patient to raise arm and flex fingers.
   b. Repeat procedure.

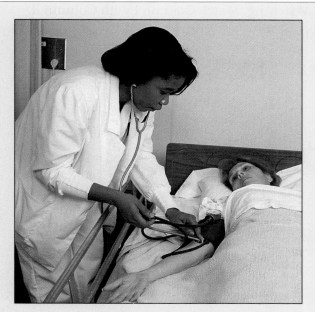

FIGURE 16–10. Release the valve and listen to the first and change sounds. Read gauge carefully.

17. Carry out each procedure completion action. Remember to wash your hands, report completion of task, and document date, time, systolic and diastolic reading as an improper fraction, patient's reaction, and site of reading if other than the brachial artery, Figure 16–11.

> Report if:
> ■ Unable to hear reading
> ■ Blood pressure is higher than in previous reading
> ■ Blood pressure is lower than in previous reading
> ■ Site of reading is other than brachial artery

FIGURE 16–11. Blood pressure reportables

SUMMARY

Blood pressure is the fourth vital sign. It must be determined and recorded accurately by watching the gauge and listening with the stethoscope.
■ Note and record the first regular sound as the systolic pressure.
■ Note and record the change sound or last sound as the diastolic pressure, as determined by facility policy.

■ Recheck unusual readings after one minute.
■ Report unusual blood pressures to the nurse.
■ Document the blood pressure as an improper fraction with the systolic reading above the diastolic reading.

UNIT REVIEW

A. True/False. Answer the following true or false by circling T or F.

(T) F 1. The volume of blood in the circulatory system helps determine the blood pressure.

T (F) 2. Exercise decreases blood pressure.

(T) F 3. To accurately measure a blood pressure, you will need both a sphygmomanometer and a stethoscope.

T (F) 4. Blood pressures taken over arteries closer to the heart will be lower than those taken over arteries farther from the heart.

T (F) 5. A blood pressure below 100/70 would signal hypotension.

T F 6. The large lines on the blood pressure gauge are in increments of 20 mm of Hg pressure.

T (F) 7. Depressant drugs elevate the blood pressure.

(T) F 8. Using a blood pressure cuff of the wrong size will give an inaccurate reading.

T F 9. When measuring a blood pressure, the gauge should always be at eye level.

T F 10. Stethoscope earpieces should be cleaned both before and after use.

B. Matching. Match Column I with Column II.

Column I

_g_ 11. high blood pressure

____ 12. lowest blood pressure reading

_h_ 13. stretch

_a_ 14. most common artery used to determine blood pressure

_e_ 15. blood pressure apparatus

Column II

a. brachial

b. diastolic

c. stethoscope

d. femoral

e. sphygmo-manometer

f. hypotension

g. hypertension

h. elasticity

i. systolic

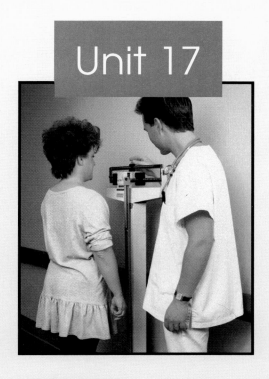

Unit 17

Measuring Height and Weight

As a result of this unit, you will be able to:

■ Spell and define terms.

■ Measure and record the patient's height and weight using an upright scale.

■ Demonstrate the proper use of an over-bed scale.

■ Demonstrate the technique of measuring a patient who must remain in bed.

■ Convert pounds to kilograms and kilograms to pounds.

■ Convert inches to centimeters and centimeters to inches.

VOCABULARY

Learn the meaning and the correct spelling of the following words:

balance bar
baseline
calibrated
centimeter (cm)

increments
kilogram (kg)
pounds (lb)

Changes in weight are a frequent indicator of the patient's condition:

■ `A baseline (original) measurement of height and weight is usually obtained on admission.

■ Weights are frequently measured when patients are given drugs (diuretics) to increase their urine output.

■ Measurements of weight and height must be accurately made and recorded according to facility policy because medications may be ordered according to the patient's size.

■ Height measurements may be recorded in feet (') and inches (") or in centimeters (cm)

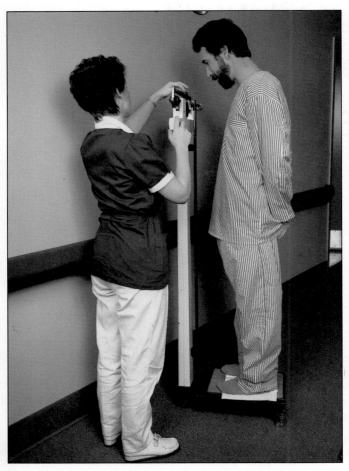

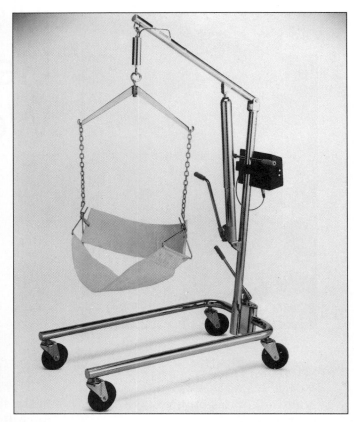

FIGURE 17–1B.   The scale with the mechanical lift is used when patients are not ambulatory. *(Photo courtesy of Health o meter®)*

FIGURE 17–1A.   The upright scale is used for ambulatory patients.

- Weight measurements may be recorded as **pounds (lb)** or **kilograms (kg)**
- The upright scale is used for ambulatory patients, Figure 17–1A.
- In-bed scales are also available for weighing patients who must remain in bed, Figure 17–1B.
- Chair scales are available for weighing patients in wheelchairs, Figure 17–1C.

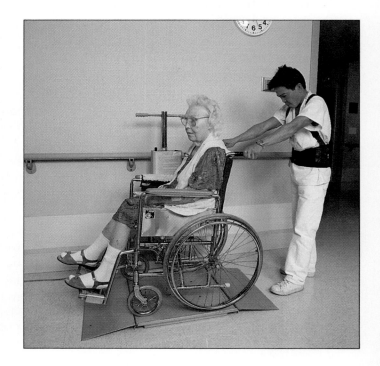

FIGURE 17–1C.   The wheelchair scale can weigh the patient who is in a wheelchair.

WEIGHING AND MEASURING THE PATIENT USING AN UPRIGHT SCALE

1. Carry out each beginning procedure action.
2. Remember to wash your hands, identify the patient, and provide privacy.
3. Check previous weight as documented. Then escort the patient to the scales.
4. Place a paper towel on the platform of the scale.
5. Be sure the weights are to the extreme left and the balance bar (bar with weight markings hangs free.
   - The lower bar (large indicator) is calibrated (marked) in increments (amounts) of 50 pounds.
   - The upper bar (small indicator) is calibrated in increments of single pounds.
   - The even-numbered pounds are marked with numbers.
   - The long line between even numbers indicates the odd-numbered pounds.
   - Each small line indicates one quarter of a pound.

6. Assist the patient to remove his shoes and help him step up onto the scale platform. The balance bar will rise to the top of the bar guide. The patient should not hold the bar or other parts of the scale.
7. Move the large weight to the closest estimated patient weight.
8. Move the small weight to the right until the balance bar hangs free half-way between the upper and lower bar guides.
9. Add the two figures and record the total as the patient's weight in pounds or kilograms, according to hospital policy. For example, the weight shown in Figure 17–2 is determined as follows:

Large indicator	150 pounds
Small indicator	4 pounds
Total	154 pounds

   or 154 ÷ 2.2 = 70 kilograms. Refer to Figure 17–3 for kilogram/pound conversions.
10. While the patient continues standing on the platform, facing away from the balance bar, raise the height bar until it is level with the top of the patient's head, Figure 17–4A.

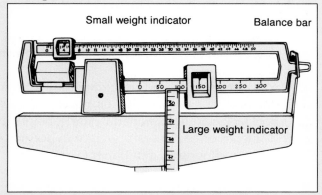

FIGURE 17–2. The weight shown on the lower bar is added to the weight shown on the upper bar.

Kilogram/Pound Conversions

1 kilogram is equal to 2.2 pounds.
- To convert from kilograms to pounds, multiply the number of kilograms by 2.2.
  Example: 70 kg × 2.2 = 154 lb
- To convert from pounds to kilograms, divide the number of pounds by 2.2.
  Example: 154 lb ÷ 2.2 = 70 kg

FIGURE 17–3. Some facilities record weights in kilograms. Others record weights in pounds.

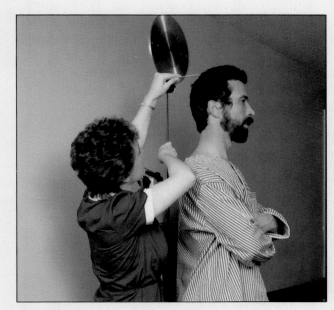

FIGURE 17–4A. Height may be measured right after the weight is measured.

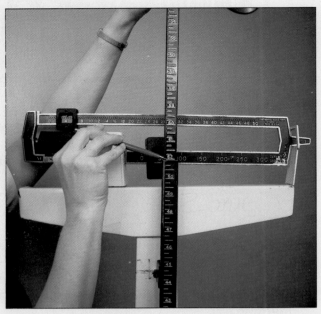

FIGURE 17–4B. The patient's height is read at the movable point of the ruler.

1 foot is equal to 12 inches.
- ■ To convert from feet to inches, multiply the number of feet by 12.
  Example: 6 feet × 12 = 72 inches
- ■ To convert from inches to feet, divide the number of inches by 12.
  Example: 72 inches ÷ 12 = 6 feet

1 inch equals 2.5 centimeters
- ■ To convert from inches to centimeters, multiply inches by 2.5
  Example: 6 inches × 2.5 = 15 centimeters
- ■ To convert from centimeters to inches, divide centimeters by 2.5.
  Example: 15 centimeters ÷ 2.5 = 6 inches

MULTIPLES OF 12	
12 × 1 = 12	12 × 7 = 84
12 × 2 = 24	12 × 8 = 96
12 × 3 = 36	12 × 9 = 108
12 × 4 = 48	12 × 10 = 120
12 × 5 = 60	12 × 11 = 132
12 × 6 = 72	12 × 12 = 144

FIGURE 17–5. Some facilities measure height in feet and inches. Other facilities measure height in centimeters.

11. The reading is made at the movable point of the ruler, Figure 17–4B.
12. Note the number of inches indicated. Record this information according to facility policy in inches ("), feet (') and inches ("), or centimeters (cm). Remember, there are 12 inches to 1 foot, and 2.5 centimeters equal 1 inch. For example, the height shown in Figure 17–4B is 62 inches. This may be recorded as 62 inches; 5 feet 2 inches (62 ÷ 12 = 5 feet 2 inches); or as 155 centimeters (62 inches × 2.5). Record on your note pad. Refer to Figure 17–5 for conversions from feet to inches and inches to feet and from inches to centimeters and centimeters to inches.
13. Assist the patient to put on his shoes and return to the room.
14. Carry out each procedure completion action. Remember to wash your hands, report completion of task, and document date, time, height in feet/inches or centimeters, weight in pounds/ounces or kilograms, and patient's reaction.

PROCEDURE 47   **OBRA**   SIDE **4**

MEASURING AND WEIGHING THE PATIENT IN BED

1. Carry out each beginning procedure action.
2. Remember to wash your hands, identify the patient, and provide privacy.
3. Obtain assistance from coworker.
4. Assemble equipment needed:
   - ■ Over-bed scale
   - ■ Tape measure
   - ■ Pencil
5. Check scale sling and straps for frayed areas or poorly closing straps.
6. Lower side rail on your side. Make sure side rail on other side is up.
7. Fanfold top linen to foot of bed.
8. Position patient flat on his back with arms and legs straight and body in good alignment.

9. Make a small pencil mark at the top of the patient's head on the sheet.
10. Make a second pencil mark even with the feet.
11. Using the tape measure, measure the distance between the two marks.
12. Note this on a pad as the patient's height in feet and inches.
13. Remove the scale sling from suspension straps and position half under the patient.
    a. Turn the patient away from you.
    b. Place the sling folded lengthwise under the patient.
    c. Return patient to recumbent position and place sling so that the patient rests securely within it.
    d. Attach sling to suspension straps. Check to be sure attachments are secure.
14. Position lift frame over bed with base legs in maximum open position and lock.
15. Elevate head of bed and bring patient to sitting position.
16. Attach suspension straps to frame. Position patient's arms inside straps.
17. Slowly raise sling so patient's body is free from bed. Be reassuring.
18. Guide the lift away from the bed so that no part of the patient touches the bed.
19. Adjust weights to balance scale.
20. Take and note reading.
21. Reposition sling over center of bed.
22. Release knob slowly, lowering patient to bed.
23. Remove sling by reversing the process in Step 12.
24. Assist patient into a comfortable position.
25. Move over-bed scale out of the way.
26. Replace top bed linen over patient. Raise side rail and lower bed to lowest horizontal height.
27. Carry out each procedure completion action. Remember to wash your hands, report completion of task, and document time, weight (lb/oz or kg) determined using over-bed scale, height (ft/in., in., or cm) measurement taken in bed, and patient's reaction.

PROCEDURE 48 | OBRA

WEIGHING A PATIENT ON THE WHEELCHAIR SCALE

1. Carry out each beginning procedure action.
2. Remember to wash your hands, identify the patient, and provide privacy.
3. Unless wheelchair was previously weighed:
    a. Take wheelchair to wheelchair scale.
    b. Position ramps on either side of scale platform.
    c. Be sure scale registers 00 or that weights are to the extreme left and balance bar hangs free.
    d. Push wheelchair onto platform. Remove hands and weigh. Note weight.
4. Take wheelchair to patient and assist patient into it.
5. Return to scale with patient in wheelchair.
6. Position patient in wheelchair facing ramp.
7. Roll patient in wheelchair up ramp and onto platform. Lock wheels of wheelchair.
8. Weigh patient in wheelchair and note reading.
9. Unlock wheels and roll patient and wheelchair down ramp. Lock wheelchair wheels.
10. Return ramps to closed position.
11. Unlock wheelchair wheels and return patient to room.
12. Record patient's weight as combined wheelchair and patient weight minus wheelchair weight.
13. Carry out each procedure completion action. Remember to wash your hands, report completion of task, and document date, time, patient weight, and patient reactions.

SUMMARY

Measurement of the patient's height and weight is usually taken on admission. Additional weight measurements are made during the patient's stay. The original weight is used as the basis for comparison with later weight measurements.

- Medications are often given according to the patient's weight.
- Weight changes may reflect the patient's condition and progress.

Measurements of height are made in:

- Feet (')
- Inches (")
- Centimeters (cm)

Measurements of weight are made in:

- Pounds (lb)
- Kilograms (kg)

Different techniques and equipment are used to make height and weight determinations depending on the patient's condition.

UNIT REVIEW

A. True/False. Answer the following true or false by circling T or F.

T (F) 1. A man who weighs 154 pounds also weighs 78 kilograms.

T (F) 2. One inch is equal to 2 centimeters.

T (F) 3. The lower bar on the scale indicates pounds in increments of 25. *50*

(T) F 4. Always check the over-bed scale for needed repairs before use.

(T) F 5. To obtain a proper reading, the scale balance bar must hang freely.

(T) F 6. One foot is equal to 12 inches.

(T) F 7. The most common scale used to weigh ambulatory patients in care facilities is the upright scale.

T (F) 8. A patient who cannot get out of bed cannot be measured.

(T) F 9. When using an overbed scale, the patient's body must be free of the bed.

T (F) 10. To measure a patient confined to bed, first help her assume the left Sims' position.

SELF-EVALUATION Section 6

A. Choose the phrase that best completes each of the following sentences by circling the proper letter.

1. To read a thermometer properly, you should
   a. hold it straight up and down.
   b. hold it by the bulb.
   c. hold it at eye level.
   d. turn it rapidly.

2. When a patient has just finished a cool drink, it is best to
   a. wait 15 minutes to take the temperature.
   b. take the temperature right away since the mouth will be moist.
   c. omit the temperature until next time temperatures are regularly taken.
   d. take the temperature by the axillary method.

3. In order to take the patient's pulse accurately, you will need
   a. pencil and pad.
   b. watch with a second hand.
   c. oral thermometer.
   d. lubricant.

4. When you take a rectal temperature, remember to
   a. hold the thermometer in place.
   b. lubricate the tip.
   c. use a rectal thermometer.
   d. All of the above.

5. When patients have individual thermometer holders by the bedside, remember to
   a. replace the thermometer directly into the solution.
   b. wash the thermometer before putting it back into the solution.
   c. lubricate the thermometer before inserting it into the patient's mouth.
   d. None of the above.

6. To take an axillary temperature accurately, the thermometer must be in place
   a. 2 minutes.
   b. 20 minutes.
   c. 3 minutes.
   d. 10 minutes.

7. The respirations are best counted
   a. without letting the patient know.
   b. while the patient is eating.
   c. while the patient is talking.
   d. after telling the patient what you plan to do.

8. The most common place to take the pulse is at the
   a. temple.
   b. bend in the elbow.
   c. wrist.
   d. knee.

9. The pulse of an adult male patient is 72 beats per minute. You quickly realize this rate is
   a. too fast and must be reported.
   b. too slow and must be reported.
   c. about average for an adult.
   d. about average for a young child.

10. The function of respiration is
    a. to circulate blood.
    b. to bring oxygen into the body.
    c. to rid the body of carbon dioxide.
    d. Both b and c.

11. When taking blood pressure, it is important that the
    a. mercury column or dial be at eye level.
    b. armband is smooth and tight.
    c. stethoscope is placed over the radial artery.
    d. mercury column or dial be tilted.

**B. Read and record the temperatures on each ther-
mometer and insert the value on the proper line.**

12. _____

14. _____

13. _____   *98.6*

15. _____

C. Complete the following statements.

16. To indicate on a graphic chart that the temperature has been taken other than orally,
you should _____
_____.

17. The following equipment is needed to determine vital signs: _____
_____.

18. Four sites, other than the wrist, where the
pulse may be taken are _____
_____.

19. The three types of clinical thermometers in
general use are _____
_____.

20. Height may be recorded in feet and inches or
_____.

21. Weight may be recorded in pounds or _____
_____
_____.

D. Match Column I with Column II.

Column I	Column II
_____ 22. moist, bubbling respirations	a. bradycardia
_____ 23. abnormally slow pulse rate	b. systolic
_____ 24. highest blood pressure reading	c. diastolic
_____ 25. difficult respirations	d. tachycardia
	e. dyspnea
	f. apnea
	g. gurgles

**E. Identify four times when the nursing assistant
should report a blood pressure reading:**

26. _____

27. _____

28. _____

29. _____

Admission, Transfer, and Discharge

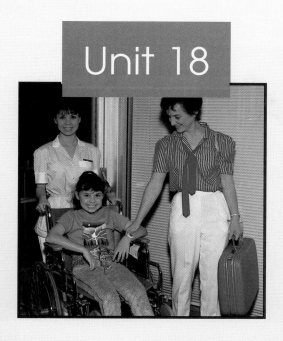

OBJECTIVES

As a result of this unit, you will be able to:

- Spell and define terms.
- List the ways the nursing assistant can help in the processes of admission, transfer, and discharge.
- Demonstrate the procedure for admitting a patient to the hospital unit.
- Demonstrate the procedure for transferring a patient.
- Demonstrate the procedure for discharging a patient.

VOCABULARY

Learn the meaning and the correct spelling of the following words:

admission   discharge
baseline assessment   transfer

The nurse is responsible for overseeing and carrying out hospital procedures and physician's orders regarding all admissions, transfers, and discharges. You will usually help the nurse by carrying out the routine procedures associated with these activities.

A nursing assistant, a volunteer, or someone from the admissions office will accompany the patient to the unit. Someone must always escort the patient from the unit during transfer or discharge.

You can do much to make these activities easier for the patient, family, and the other staff members by:

- Having equipment and materials prepared for the activity.
- Being very observant during each activity.
- Documenting observations carefully and accurately. These make a valuable contribution to the nurse's initial baseline assessment of the patient's condition. Refer to Unit 7 to recall the importance of accurate observations.
- Reporting observations directly to the nurse.

265

■ Giving attention to the details of each procedure.

■ Being aware of the emotional stress these activities cause patients and their families.

■ Being courteous to everyone, Figure 18–1.

Admission

When a person enters a health care facility for treatment of an illness or injury, the necessity for the admission process is usually a cause of concern to the patient, family, and friends. The first impression created is very important. Since you will be one of the first staff members to see the patient, it is important that you be courteous, confident and efficient.

When a patient is ready for admission, ask if:

■ The patient requires a gurney or wheelchair to reach the unit.

■ Any special equipment such as oxygen or a fracture bed is needed.

■ There are any special instructions such as withholding fluids or foods.

Introduce yourself and observe the patient carefully. Listen for complaints as you escort and assist the patient to the room and to bed. Initial observations are very important. They become the basis of comparison for future observations.

If it is necessary to ask visitors to leave, this must be done in a kindly manner since they are most anxious to remain and see the patient settled and comfortable.

■ Show them where they may wait.

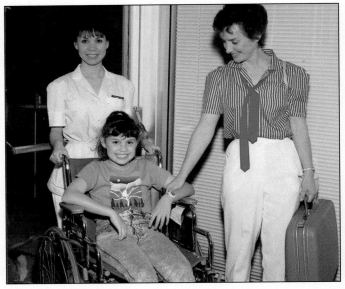

FIGURE 18–1. Be courteous to the family accompanying the patient. Remember, they are anxious and concerned.

■ Let them know about how long they will have to wait.

■ Tell them where they can get refreshments.

■ Answer questions they may have about where to find a chapel and telephones, and visiting hours.

■ After you have completed your part of the admission procedure, locate visitors and let them know they may return to the patient's room.

Figure 18–2 is a review of procedure beginning and procedure completion activities.

BEGINNING PROCEDURE ACTIONS	PROCEDURE COMPLETION ACTIONS
■ Wash your hands.	■ Position patient comfortably.
■ Assemble equipment needed.	■ Leave signal cord, telephone, and fresh water close at hand.
■ Go to the patient's room, knock, and pause before entering.	■ Return bed to lowest position.
■ Introduce yourself and identify the patient by checking the identification bracelet.	■ Perform general safety check of patient and environment.
■ Ask visitors to leave and inform them where they can wait.	■ Care for equipment according to facility policy.
■ Provide privacy.	■ Wash your hands.
■ Explain what will happen and answer questions.	■ Report completion of task.
■ Allow patient to assist in procedure as much as possible.	■ Let visitors know when they may reenter.
■ Raise bed to comfortable working height.	■ Document action and your observations.

NOTE: Where there are open lesions, wet linen, or possible contact with patient body fluids or blood, disposable gloves are worn during the procedure. Put on gloves before contact with the patient or linen. Properly dispose of gloves after they are removed. ALWAYS APPLY UNIVERSAL PRECAUTIONS.

FIGURE 18–2. Beginning procedure actions and procedure completion actions

PROCEDURE 49

ADMITTING THE PATIENT

1. Wash hands and assemble the following equipment:
   - ■ Equipment for urine specimen collection
   - ■ Equipment for taking temperature
   - ■ Pad and pencil
   - ■ Patient's chart or worksheet
   - ■ Stethoscope
   - ■ Admission kit, Figure 18–3
   - ■ Scale
   - ■ Blood pressure cuff and manometer
   - ■ Watch with second hand
   - ■ Disposable gloves (if urine specimen is required)
2. Prepare the unit for the patient by:
   a. Making sure that all necessary equipment and furniture are in their proper places and in good working order.
   b. Checking the unit for adequate lighting.
   c. Making a toepleat (Unit 19).
   d. Opening the bed, Figure 18–4.

■ Water pitcher	■ Towel
■ Glass	■ Basin
■ Liquid soap	■ Lotion
■ Wash cloth	■ Mouth wash

FIGURE 18–3. Contents of the admission kit

3. Identify the patient both by asking the name and checking the identification bracelet.
   a. Introduce yourself.
   b. Take the patient and family to the unit.
   c. Do not appear to rush the patient.
   d. Be courteous and helpful to the patient and family.
4. Ask the patient to be seated.
   a. Ask the family to go to the lounge or lobby while the patient is being admitted.
   b. Introduce the patient to the other patients in the room, unless it is a private room.
   c. As permitted, explain what will happen in the next hour.
5. Screen the unit to provide privacy, Figure 18–5.
6. Help the patient to undress and put on a hospital gown or night clothes from home. Care for clothing according to facility policy.

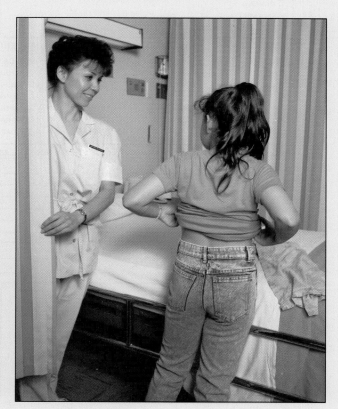

FIGURE 18–5. Provide privacy as the patient undresses.

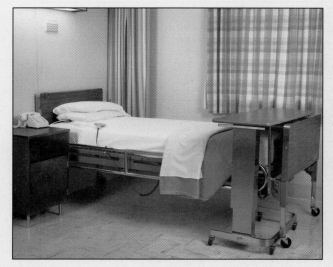

FIGURE 18–4. An open bed lets patients know that they are expected and welcome.

continues

PATIENT PREFERS TO BE ADDRESSED AS:

Extended care facility

FROM: □ E.R.   □ E.C.F.   □ HOME   □ M.D.'S OFFICE

COMMUNICATES IN ENGLISH: □ WELL   □ MINIMAL   □ NOT AT ALL   □ OTHER LANGUAGE (SPECIFY)____

□ INTERPRETER (NAME PERSON) _____   □ NONE

MODE OF TRANSPORTATION:
□ AMBULATORY   □ OTHER   **SMOKER:** Y □ N □
□ WHEELCHAIR ____
□ STRETCHER ____

HOME TELEPHONE NO. (   ) ____
WORK TELEPHONE NO. (   ) ____

ORIENTATION TO ENVIRONMENT:
□ ARMBAND CHECKED   □ CALL LIGHT
□ BED CONTROL   □ PHONE
□ TV CONTROL   □ SIDE RAIL POLICY
□ BATH ROOM   □ VISITATION POLICY
□ PERSONAL PROPERTY POLICY   □ SMOKING POLICY

PERSONAL BELONGINGS: (CHECK AND DESCRIBE)
□ CLOTHING ____
□ JEWELRY ____
□ MONEY ____
□ WALKER ____
□ WHEELCHAIR ____
□ CANE ____
□ OTHER ____

DENTURES: □ UPPER □ PARTIAL □ LOWER □ NONE
CONTACT LENSES: □ HARD □ SOFT □ LT □ RT
GLASSES: □ Y □ N   **HEARING AID:** □ Y □ N
PROSTHESIS: □ Y □ N
(DESCRIBE) ____

DISPOSITION OF VALUABLES:
□ PATIENT
□ HOME   GIVEN TO: ____
         RELATIONSHIP: ____
□ PLACED
  IN SAFE ____
        (CLAIM NO.)

IN CASE OF EMERGENCY NOTIFY: _Relatives_
NAME: ____
RELATIONSHIP: ____
HOME TELEPHONE NO. (   ) ____
WORK TELEPHONE NO. (   ) ____

VITAL SIGNS
TEMP: ____ □ ORAL □ RECTAL □ AXILLARY
PULSE: ____ □ RADIAL □ APICAL   RESPIRATORY RATE ____
B/P: ____ □ RT □ LT □ STANDING □ SITTING □ LYING
HEIGHT: ____ WEIGHT: ____ □ BEDSIDE □ STANDING

ALLERGIES:
MEDICATIONS: □ NONE KNOWN   FOOD: □ NONE KNOWN
□ PENICILLIN □ TAPE   (SHELLFISH, EGGS, MILK, ETC.)
□ SULFA □ OTHER (LIST)
□ IODINE
□ ASPIRIN
□ MORPHINE
□ DEMEROL

MEDICATIONS: (PRESCRIPTIVE/NON PRESCRIPTIVE)   DOSE/FREQUENCY   LAST DOSE (DATE/TIME)
1. _q.d. every day_
2.
3.
4.
5.
6.

DISPOSITION OF MEDICATIONS:
□ NONE BROUGHT TO HOSPITAL
□ SENT HOME ____ WITH ____
□ TO PHARMACY: (LIST)

ADMITTING DIAGNOSIS: ____
NURSE'S SIGNATURE ____ RN/LVN   DATE ____ TIME ____

CHARTER SUBURBAN HOSPITAL
16453 SOUTH COLORADO AVENUE
PARAMOUNT, CALIFORNIA 90723

NURSING ADMISSION ASSESSMENT PAGE 1 of 6

FIGURE 18–6. Careful completion of the admission form supports the nursing baseline assessment. _(Form courtesy of Charter Suburban Hospital, Paramount, CA)_

7. Check the patient's vital signs, weight, and height.
8. Help the patient get into bed. Adjust side rails as needed.
9. If the patient is wearing any jewelry or has valuables:
   a. Make a list of them and ask the patient to sign it. This protects the facility and the patient.
   b. Ask the relatives also to sign the list and take the valuables home, or
   c. After checking and signing, give them to the nurse to put in the hospital safe.
10. Tell the patient if a urine specimen is necessary.
    a. Put on gloves and assist the patient as necessary.
    b. Allow patient to use the bathroom, if ambulatory, or offer the bedpan or urinal.
11. Pour the patient's specimen from the bedpan into the specimen bottle. Put on the cap. Remove gloves and dispose of according to facility policy. Be sure to label the specimen correctly (Unit 24).
12. An admission form is usually completed at this time, Figure 18–6. Vital information includes:
    - Observations
    - Vital signs (TPR, BP, height, weight)
    - Known allergies
    - Medications being taken
    - Food preferences and dislikes
13. If admission is to a long-term care facility, name labels must be added to belongings.
14. Orient the patient to the unit by explaining:
    - Visiting hours
    - How to use the phone and/or television
    - How to use the call light system for assistance
    - Standard hospital regulations
    - TV rental procedures, if available
    - Any questions about facility routines
    - When meals and refreshments are provided, as necessary
15. Carry out each procedure completion action. Remember to wash your hands, report completion of task, and document time, admitted to unit (room number), values of vital signs, height and weight, method of transport, and patient's reaction.

Transfer

It may be necessary for the patient to be moved to another unit, Figure 18–7. Preparations for the transfer will be handled by the nurse, but you may be asked to assist.

The transfer may be the patient's own preference or because a change in the patient's condition requires a different type of care. The patient may or may not fully understand the reasons for the transfer. Be positive and supportive in your attitude. Recognize that the patient may be feeling very anxious. It would be helpful to know what the patient has been told about the reasons for the transfer.

All details must be taken care of according to facility policy. Following facility policy ensures that there is no interruption of health care services. Some facilities have transportation services for transferring patients.

After the new unit has been notified and prepared for the move, you will:
- Tell the patient what you are doing.
- Gather all the patient's belongings together. Explain to the patient what you are doing.

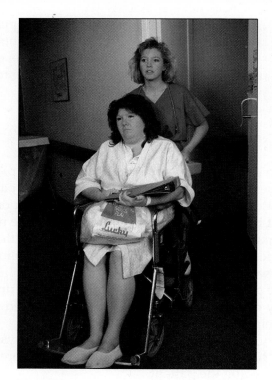

FIGURE 18–7. Transfers should be carried out in a calm and efficient manner.

■ Secure the medicines, charts, and other personal data from the nurse.
■ Assist in the physical transfer.
■ Give the records and medication directly to the nurse on the new unit. **CAUTION: Never leave the patient, the records, or medications unattended.**
■ Make sure the patient is comfortable in her new environment before returning to your own unit.

PROCEDURE 50 | OBRA

TRANSFERRING THE PATIENT

1. Determine the unit to which the patient will be transferred. Check to see that it is ready.
2. Learn from the nurse in charge the method of transfer. Get the necessary vehicle (wheelchair, stretcher, or patient's own bed).
3. Check to see if any equipment is to be transferred with the patient.
4. Carry out each beginning procedure action.
5. Remember to wash your hands, identify the patient, and provide privacy.
6. Explain to the patient what you are doing.
7. Gather all patient's belongings together.
   a. Place disposables in paper bag to transport with you.
   b. Check against clothes list.
8. Assist patient to put on robe and slippers, if permitted. Assist patient into wheelchair or stretcher, as directed. The entire bed is often used. Make sure side rails are up during transport.
9. Obtain from the nurse:
   ■ Patient's chart
   ■ Nursing care plan
   ■ Medications
   ■ Paper bag
10. Transport patient and belongings to new unit. Use all precautions related to safe transport.
11. Give any transferred medications, nursing care plan, and chart to nurse in charge.
12. Introduce patient to staff. Proceed to patient's room.
13. Assist staff in helping patient into bed. Assist in putting away patient's belongings and helping patient to become settled.
14. Before leaving the unit, carry out each procedure completion action. Remember to wash your hands, report completion of task, and document time, transfer to (unit) (facility) per (wheelchair), and patient's reaction.

Discharge

The **discharge** or authorized release of a patient requires the written order of the physician. If a patient indicates an intention of leaving without an order, report it to your supervisor immediately. The nurse will make the necessary arrangements. Health care facilities have special policies that must be followed in these cases.

The patient should be spared any fatigue or unnecessary delay when being routinely discharged. You can help if you:
■ Check with the nurse to see that the physician has written an order for discharge before preparing the patient.
■ Gather all the patient's belongings and assist in packing, if necessary. Patients who are well enough prefer to assemble their own things. You will need to do this activity completely for other patients.
■ Carefully check the closet and bedside table. Disposable equipment is often sent home with the patient. If this is the policy in your facility, be sure that the equipment is clean.
■ Check with the nurse for any medications or other treatment-related equipment that should be sent home with the patient.
■ Verify that the patient has received discharge instructions from the nurse, physician, or discharge coordinator.
■ Never allow a patient to leave the health care facility unassisted. The patient is the staff's responsibility until he has left the building.

PROCEDURE 51

DISCHARGING THE PATIENT

1. Check to be sure the physician has ordered the patient discharged. If the discharge has not been written, check with the supervisor before proceeding, Figure 18–8.
2. Carry out each beginning procedure action.
3. Remember to wash your hands, identify the patient, and provide privacy.
4. Help the patient to dress, if necessary.

5. Collect the patient's personal belongings. Help the patient check them against the admission list.
   a. Pack, if necessary.
   b. Check valuables against list according to facility policy.
   c. Make sure that all of the patient's belongings have been removed from the closet and bedside stand.

LEAVING THE HOSPITAL AGAINST ADVICE   Date/Time _____

Patient _____   Age _____

This is to certify that _____ a patient in   Charter Suburban Hospital, is leaving the hospital against the advice of the attending physician(s) and hospital authorities. I am aware of the dangers involved by leaving at this time and I accept all responsibility for any results caused by this premature departure. Therefore, I release the hospital and the attending physician(s) from all liability for any ill effects which may result from this action

Patient _____   Other person responsible - Relationship _____

Witness _____

RELEASE OF SIDE RAILS   Date/Time _____

Patient _____   Age _____

Having been informed that protective side rails should be placed on my bed and raised for my personal protection against injury, I instruct the hospital and its employees NOT to place or raise protective side rails on my bed. I accept all risks of injury resulting from this action and release the hospital, its employees and my physician(s) from any and all liability for any injury or damage which may arise from the lack of such protection

Patient _____   Other person responsible - Relationship _____

Witness _____

PERMIT FOR USING ELECTRICAL APPLIANCES   Date/Time _____

Patient _____   Age _____

I hereby agree that in using _____ and/or similar appliances in my room while a patient in Charter Suburban Hospital, I do so at my own risk and hereby absolve the hospital from any and all responsibility for burns, injuries or property damage which may result to, from or because of the appliance.

Patient _____   Other Person responsible - Relationship _____

Witness _____

CHARTER SUBURBAN HOSPITAL

16453 South Colorado Avenue
Paramount, California 90723

CONSENT FORMS

FIGURE 18–8. Patients who leave against their physician's advice must sign a form before discharge. (*Form courtesy of Charter Suburban Hospital, Paramount, CA*)

    d. Check to see if medications or other equipment are to go home with the patient.

    e. Verify that the patient has received discharge instructions from the nurse, physician, or discharge coordinator.

6. Tell the patient or a member of the family how to collect valuables from the facility safe, if valuables were put there.

7. Help patient into wheelchair.

8. Take patient to the discharge entrance of the facility.

    a. Help patient to transfer safely into the vehicle.

    b. Be gracious as you say goodbye.

9. Return wheelchair.

10. Return to patient unit.

    a. Strip bed. Dispose of linen according to facility policy.

    b. Clean and replace equipment used in care of patient, according to facility policy.

11. Wash your hands.

12. Record discharge in accordance with facility policy. Include:
- Time
- Method of transport
- Patient's reaction
- Signature

13. Report completion of task to nurse.

SUMMARY

The nursing assistant has specific responsibilities related to the admission, transfer, and discharge of the patient. These responsibilities include:

- Providing emotional support to both patient and family.
- Assisting in the safe physical transport of the patient.
- Carrying out the specific procedures relating to admission, transfer, and discharge.
- Preparing and disassembling the patient unit before and after use.
- Reporting and documenting observations.

UNIT REVIEW

A. True/False. Answer the following true or false by circling T or F.

T F 1. When transferring a patient, it is alright to leave the patient unattended and return immediately to your own unit.

T F 2. Use all precautions related to safe transport when admitting or discharging a patient.

T F 3. You do not need to waste time introducing a new patient to others since facility stays are very short anyway.

T F 4. It is alright to allow patients to simply leave a health care facility.

T F 5. After discharge, the patient's unit is stripped, cleaned, and restocked.

T F 6. The patient's unit should be prepared as soon as you are notified that there will be an admission.

T F 7. During a transfer, the patient's medications remain on the original unit.

T F 8. Measuring the patient's height and weight is part of the admission procedure.

T F 9. The discharge order is written by the physician.

T F 10. Careful observation of the patient should take place during the admission procedure.

B. Multiple Choice. Select the one best answer to each of the following sentences by circling the proper letter.

11. The assistant can do much to help facilitate the admission procedure by
   a. preparing equipment after the patient arrives on the unit.
   b. letting the nurse make all the observations.
   c. giving attention to the details of the procedure.
   d. recognizing that admission to the facility causes more anxiety to the staff than to the patient.

12. When dealing with the newly admitted patient's family, you should
   a. treat them with courtesy and consideration.
   b. send them home.
   c. let the nurse deal with them.
   d. allow them to stay at the patient's bedside at all times.

13. Part of the admission procedure includes
   a. securing a stool specimen.
   b. obtaining a sputum specimen.
   c. working in a hurried manner so the patient knows you are efficient.
   d. measuring vital signs.

14. Valuables that accompany the patient to her unit should be
   a. taken away.
   b. listed and signed for.
   c. left in the bedside stand.
   d. tucked under the pillow for safety.

15. When a patient is transferred, you should include his
   a. personal belongings
   b. chart.
   c. medications.
   d. all of the above.

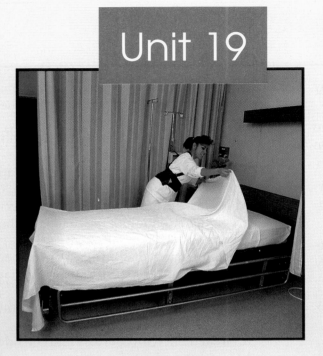

Unit 19

Bedmaking

VOCABULARY

Learn the meaning and the correct spelling of the following words and phrases:

box (square) corner
Circ O lectric® bed
closed bed
electric bed
gatch bed

mitered corner
open bed
Stryker frame
toepleats

The room, to say nothing of the bed, is the patient's home while hospitalized. A well-made bed offers both comfort and safety. It is an extremely important contribution to the well-being of the patient.

Operation and Uses of Beds in Health Care Facilities

The types of beds and the methods used in their operation may vary in different health care facilities, but the basic principles of bedmaking are the same. The two most common beds are the:

- Gatch bed—a stationary bed about 26 inches high. Modern facilities are equipped with beds that can be raised to the desired height for bedside nursing or lowered to 13 inches to accommodate the out-of-bed patient. The position of the head and knee areas of the

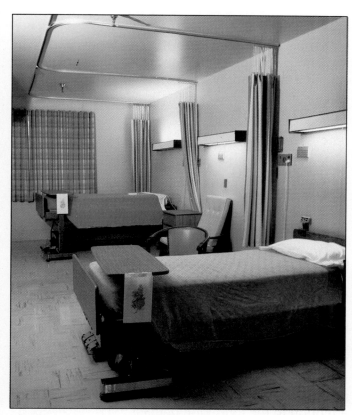

FIGURE 19–1. A typical hospital bed that can be adjusted for height and position. Note that the bed by the window has been raised.

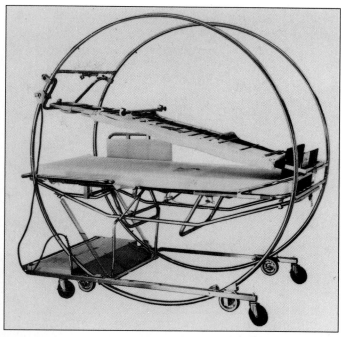

FIGURE 19–2. The Circ O lectric® Circle bed (*Photo courtesy of Stryker Corporation*)

bed can be adjusted for comfort. This operation may be done manually by turning the cranks.

- **Electric bed**—a bed similar to the gatch in that it can be raised or lowered and the knee and head can be adjusted. It is operated electrically, Figure 19–1. You will be using this bed most often in a large facility.

- **Circ O lectric® bed**—a special bed frame placed within a circular frame, Figure 19–2. The circular frame can be rotated. The patient is secured on the inner frame before moving the bed. The entire inner frame is rotated forward. This allows for position change without any stress on the patient. This bed is operated electrically. After rotating, the patient is on the abdomen.

- **Stryker frame or spinal bed**—a turning frame that serves the same purpose as the Circ O lectric® but is operated manually. Once the patient is secured by placement of the upper frame, a crank is used to turn the entire frame and patient. After turning, the patient is on the abdomen. The patient lies on the frame until turned once more, Figure 19–3.

Patients with severe burns or spinal injuries are examples of patients who are often placed on special

beds like the Circ O lectric® or Stryker frame for their safety. These beds allow patients to be repositioned with minimal handling of their bodies.

This procedure is frightening for many patients. Reassure the patient that he is secure and that turning will proceed without incident. In most facilities a licensed nurse must be present during turning.

Another type of bed is available for the treatment of patients with multiple or advanced pressure ulcers, flaps, grafts, burns and intractable pain. The Clinitron® bed, Figure 19–4, is a special unit that supports the patient's body evenly. It is filled with a sand-like material. Warm, dry air circulates through the material to maintain an even temperature and support the body evenly.

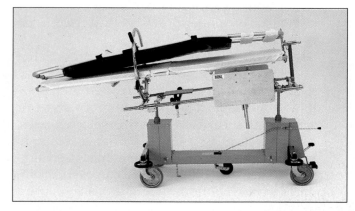

FIGURE 19–3. The turning frame or spinal bed (*Photo courtesy of Stryker Corporation*)

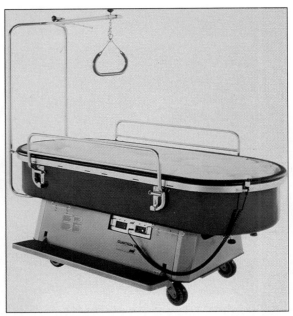

FIGURE 19–4. CLINITRON® Air Fluidized Therapy Unit Model CII *(Courtesy of Support Systems International, Inc., Charleston, SC)*

Correct operation of any bed or equipment is important to the safety of the patient. Always seek help and instruction from the nurse or another health care professional when using any specialized beds. Never try to operate any bed or equipment with a patient in it without first practicing and gaining security and skill in the operations.

Bedmaking

The Closed Bed

Bed linen is always changed when soiled. It is routinely changed:

- daily in the acute care facility.
- two or three times a week in long-term care facilities.

Residents in long-term care may prefer to use their own pillows, blankets, and spreads.

The **closed bed** is made following the discharge of the patient and after the unit is cleaned (terminal cleaning). It remains closed until a new patient is to be admitted. Details are important. The same procedure is followed when making an unoccupied bed but the bed is opened as a final step when a patient is to occupy is shortly. The closed bed will be properly made and comfortable for the patient if you give attention to the following details:

PROCEDURE 52 | **OBRA**

SIDE 4

MAKING A CLOSED BED

1. Wash your hands and assemble the following equipment:
   - 2 pillowcases
   - Pillow
   - Spread
   - Blankets, as needed
   - 2 large sheets (90" × 108")
   - Cotton drawsheet or half sheet*
   - Plastic or rubber drawsheet* (if used in facility)
   - Mattress pad and cover, if mattress is not plastic treated

   *NOTE: Mattresses that are treated with plastic do not require a moisture-proof sheet or cotton half sheet (drawsheet). In selected cases, the half sheet is used as a lifter to assist in moving the patient. It is sometimes used simply to keep the bottom sheet clean. Some facilities use fitted bottom sheets. If this is so, use a fitted sheet in place of one of the large sheets.

2. Elevate the bed to a comfortable working height in the horizontal position. Lock bed wheels so the bed will not roll. Place chair at the side of the bed.

3. Arrange linen on chair in order in which it is to be used.

4. Position mattress at the head of the bed by grasping mattress handles (or the edge of the mattress, if no handles are present).

5. If used, place mattress cover on mattress. Adjust it smoothly for corners. You will work entirely from one side of the bed until that side is completed. Then go to the other side of the bed. This conserves time and energy.

6. Place mattress pad even with the top of the mattress and unfold.

7. Place on the bed and unfold the bottom sheet, right side up, wide hem at the top. The small hem should be brought to the foot of the mattress, Figure 19–5. Center fold should be at the center of the bed. If a fitted bottom sheet is

used, fit it smoothly around one corner, Figures 19–6A and B.

8. Tuck 12 to 18 inches of sheet smoothly over the top of the mattress, Figures 19–7A to 7C.

9. Make a mitered corner, Figures 19–8A to 8F. The square corner, preferred by some facilities, is made in a similar way to the mitered corner.

10. Tuck in the sheet on one side, keeping the sheet straight. Work from the head to the foot of the bed. If using a fitted sheet, adjust it over the head and bottom ends of mattress.

11. If used, place the plastic drawsheet and half sheet with upper edge about 14 inches from head of mattress and tuck under one side. Be sure that the half sheet covers the plastic sheet. It should cover the area above the patient's shoulders and below the hips.

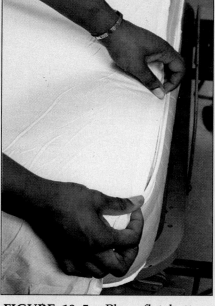

FIGURE 19–5. Place flat bottom sheet even with end of mattress at foot of bed.

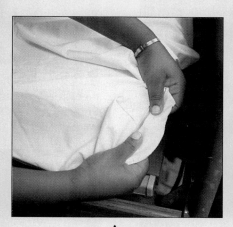

A.

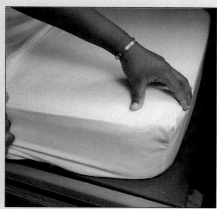

B.

FIGURE 19–6. If a fitted bottom sheet is used, fit it properly and smoothly around one corner.

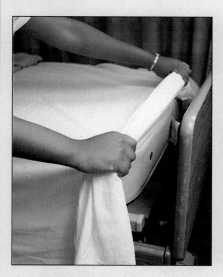

FIGURE 19–7A. Gather about 12 to 18 inches of top sheet at bottom of bed.

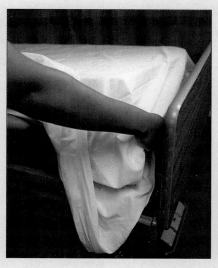

FIGURE 19–7B. Face foot of bed and lift mattress with near hand.

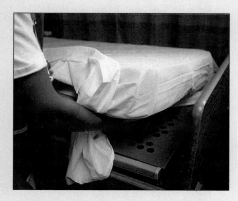

FIGURE 19–7C. Bring sheet with opposite hand smoothly over end of mattress.

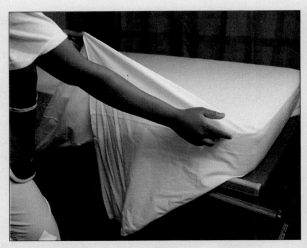

FIGURE 19–8A. To make a mitered corner, pick up sheet hanging at side of bed, about 12 inches from bed, forming a triangle.

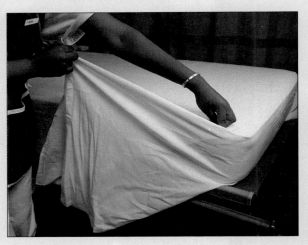

FIGURE 19–8B. Place your finger on bed to form sharp corner.

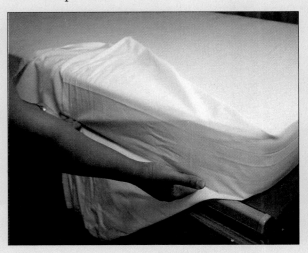

FIGURE 19–8C. Using two hands, tuck sheet well under the mattress.

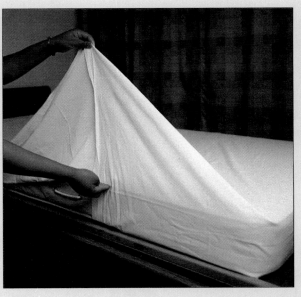

FIGURE 19–8D. Using fingers as a guide, allow sheet to drop straight down. Run fingers along edge of mattress to end, forming the mitered triangular corner.

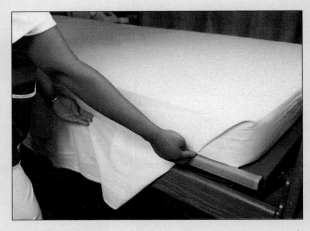

FIGURE 19–8E. Finish tucking in corner and smooth.

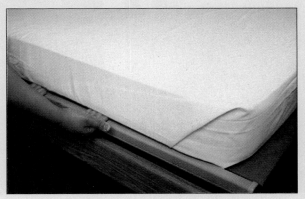

FIGURE 19–8F. The finished mitered corner should look like this.

12. Place the top sheet, wrong side up, hem even with the upper edge of the mattress, and center fold in the center of the bed.

13. Spread the blanket over the top sheet and foot of mattress. Keep blanket centered.

14. Tuck top sheet and blanket under mattress at the foot of the bed as far as the center only. Make a **box (square) corner**, Figures 19–9A to 9C.

15. Place spread with top hem even with head of mattress. Unfold to foot of bed.

16. Tuck spread under mattress at the foot of bed and make mitered corner. Sometimes the spread may be placed directly on top of the sheet. Rather than tucking the sheet, blanket, and/or spread under the end of the mattress separately and forming separate corners, all of the covers may be tucked under at the same time and one corner formed, Figures 19–10A to 10E.

17. Go to other side of the bed. Fanfold the top covers to the center of the bed in order to work with lower sheets and pad.

18. Tuck bottom sheet under head of mattress and make mitered corner. Working from top to bottom, smooth out all wrinkles and tighten these sheets as much as possible to provide comfort. (Adjust fitted bottom sheet smoothly and securely around mattress corners.)

19. Grasp protective drawsheet, if used, and cotton drawsheet in the center. Tuck these sheets under the mattress.

20. Tuck in top sheet and blanket at foot of bed and make mitered corner.

21. Fold top sheet back over blanket, making an 8–inch cuff.

22. Tuck in spread at foot of bed and make a mitered corner. Bring top of spread to head of mattress.

23. Insert pillow into pillowcase in the following way.
    a. Place hands in the clean case, freeing the corners.
    b. Grasp the center of the end seam with hand outside the case and turn case back over hand.
    c. Grasp the pillow through the case at the center of one end. Pull case over pillow with free hand.
    d. Adjust the corners of the pillow to fit in the corners of the case.

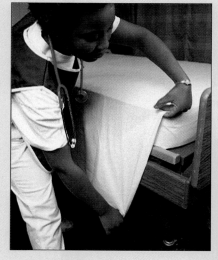

FIGURE 19–9A. Make the square (box) corner following the steps shown in Figures 19–8A to 19–8E. Then, holding corner with left hand, grasp bottom of sheet and pull it straight down until fold is even with edge of mattress. Tuck as in Figure 19–8E.

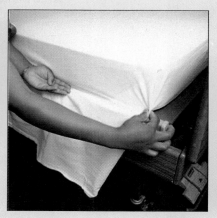

FIGURE 19–9B. Holding the square corner in place, tuck remaining sheet under mattress.

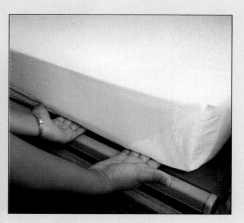

FIGURE 19–9C. Finished square corner should look like this.

24. Place pillow at head of bed with open end away from the door.
25. Lower bed to lowest horizontal position.
26. Arrange room as follows:
    a. Replace bedside table parallel to bed. Place chair in assigned location.
    b. Place over-bed table over the foot of the bed opposite the chair.
    c. Place signal cord or call panel within easy reach of the patient.
    d. Leave side rails down.
    e. Check for possible hazards such as crank handles out of place.

27. Leave unit neat and tidy.
28. Wash your hands.
29. Report completion of task to the supervisor.

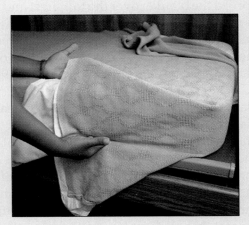

FIGURE 19–10C. Continue as in the procedure for a mitered corner.

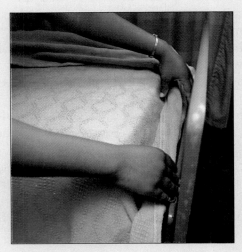

FIGURE 19–10A. Gather top sheet and spread together and smooth evenly over end of mattress.

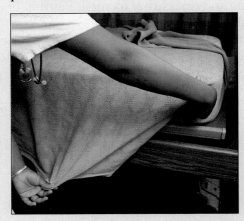

FIGURE 19–10D. Slide finger to the end to make a smooth edge.

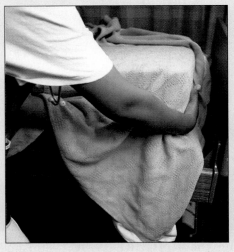

FIGURE 19–10B. Tuck sheet and spread under mattress together.

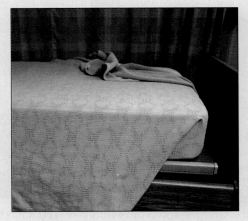

FIGURE 19–10E. The completed top bedding. The procedure is repeated on the opposite side.

- The bottom sheet must be free of wrinkles and carefully tucked in at the corners.
- The top covers must be neatly adjusted and firmly tucked under the mattress at the foot of the bed.
- The spread is evenly and properly placed.

The Unoccupied Bed

Beds are often made while patients are up in a shower or chair. Follow the procedure for making a closed bed but then fanfold the top bedding half way down. This "opens" the bed and makes it easier for the person to get into it.

The Open Bed

The **open bed** is like a sign saying "welcome" to the new patient, Figure 19–11. It indicates that the arrival of the patient has been made known to the assistant. It also shows that the unit has been prepared. In long-term care beds are not opened unless the resident is going to bed soon.

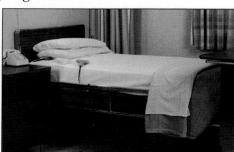

FIGURE 19–11. The closed bed is opened by drawing the bedding to foot and fanfolding.

PROCEDURE 53 | OBRA

OPENING THE CLOSED BED

1. Wash your hands.
2. Check assignment for bed location.
3. Raise bed to comfortable working height in the horizontal position. Move over-bed table to one side.
4. Lock bed wheels.
5. Loosen top bedding. Make **toepleats** at foot of bed, Figures 19–12A to 19–12C. **NOTE:** The toepleat provides extra room for the patient's feet to lessen the pressure of the covers.
6. Facing head of bed, grasp top sheet and spread and fanfold to foot of bed.
7. Return bed to lowest horizontal position. Place over-bed table over foot of bed.
8. Place call bell under pillow or within easy reach.
9. Leave unit neat and tidy.
10. Wash your hands.
11. Report completion of task to the nurse.

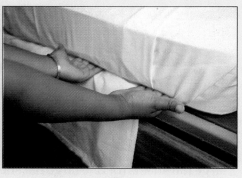

B.

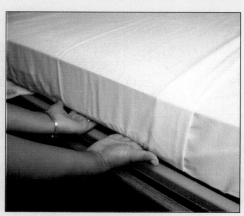

FIGURE 19–12. Making a toepleat. Before tucking in corner, make a 3-inch fold toward foot of bed (A) and then tuck in the sheet (B). (C) shows completed toepleat.

A.

C. Completed toepleat.

BEGINNING PROCEDURE ACTIONS	PROCEDURE COMPLETION ACTIONS
■ Wash your hands. ■ Assemble equipment. ■ Go to the patient's room, knock, and pause before entering. ■ Introduce yourself and identify the patient by checking the identification bracelet. ■ Ask visitors to leave and inform them where they can wait. ■ Provide privacy. ■ Explain what will happen and answer questions. ■ Raise bed to comfortable working height.	■ Position patient comfortably. ■ Leave signal cord, telephone, and fresh water close at hand. ■ Return bed to lowest position. ■ Perform general safety check of patient and environment. ■ Care for equipment according to facility policy. ■ Wash your hands. ■ Report completion of task. ■ Let visitors know when they may reenter the patient's room. ■ Document action and your observations.

NOTE: Where there are open lesions, wet linen, or possible contact with patient body fluids or blood, disposable gloves are worn during the procedure. Put on gloves before contact with the patient or linen. Properly dispose of gloves after they are removed. ALWAYS APPLY UNIVERSAL PRECAUTIONS.

FIGURE 19–13.   Beginning procedure actions and procedure completion actions.

The Occupied Bed

Unless the patient is permitted out of bed by physician's order, the bed is made with the patient in it. The patient frequently enjoys this refreshing procedure if the nursing assistant is skillful. Making the bed usually follows the bed bath, while the patient is covered with a bath blanket. It may, however, be done any time it would add to the comfort of the patient.

Remember to perform the actions shown in Figure 19–13 at the beginning and completion of each procedure, as appropriate.

PROCEDURE 54	OBRA	SIDE 4		

MAKING AN OCCUPIED BED

1. Carry out each beginning procedure action.
2. Remember to wash your hands, identify the patient, and provide privacy.
3. Assemble the equipment needed:
   - ■ Cotton drawsheet or turning sheet for selected patients
   - ■ 2 large flat sheets (or one large flat sheet and one fitted bottom sheet)
   - ■ 2 pillowcases
   - ■ Laundry hamper
   - ■ Disposable gloves (if linens are soiled with blood or body fluids)
4. Place bedside chair at the foot of the bed.
5. Arrange clean linen on chair in the order in which it is to be used.
6. Bed should be flat with wheels locked unless otherwise indicated. Raise to working horizontal height. Lower side rail on your side of bed.
7. If bed linens are soiled with blood or other body fluids, put on disposable gloves.

8. Loosen the bedclothes on your side by lifting the edge of the mattress with one hand and drawing bedclothes out with the other. Never shake the linen. This spreads germs.
9. Put side rail up and go to opposite side of bed.
10. Adjust mattress to head of bed, Figure 19–14. Get help, if possible.
11. Remove top covers except for top sheet, one at a time. Fold to bottom. Pick up in center. Place over the back of chair.
12. Place the clean sheet or bath blanket over top sheet. Have the patient hold the top edge of the clean sheet if he is able. If the patient is unable to help, tuck the sheet beneath the patient's shoulder.
13. Slide the soiled sheet out, from top to bottom. Put it in hamper.
14. Ask the patient to move to the side of the bed toward you. Assist if necessary. Move one pillow with the patient and remove the other

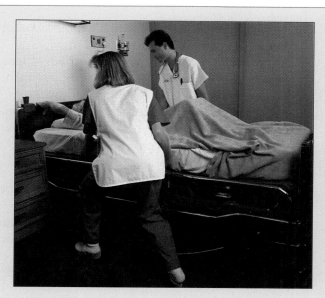

FIGURE 19–14. The patient grasps head of bed and pushes in with heels while two nursing assistants pull mattress to head of the bed.

pillow. Pull up the side rail. (Alternatively, you may ask the patient to turn toward the opposite side of the bed, holding onto the raised side rail. You would then fanfold the sheet, as in Step #15, but there would be no need to go to the other side of the bed.)

15. Go to the other side of the bed. Fanfold the soiled cotton drawsheet, if used, and bottom sheet close to the patient, Figures 19–15A and B.

16. Straighten mattress pad. If bottom sheet is to be changed, place a clean sheet on the bed so that the narrow hem comes to the edge of the mattress at the foot. The seamed side of the hem is toward the bed. The lengthwise center fold of the sheet is at the center of the bed. Fanfold opposite side of sheet close to patient.

17. Tuck top of sheet under the head of the mattress.

18. Make mitered corner.

19. Tuck side of sheet under mattress, working toward the foot of the bed.

20. Position fresh turning sheet. If drawsheet is used, position and tuck it under the mattress.

21. Ask or assist patient to roll toward you, over the fanfolded linen. Move the pillow with the patient.

22. Raise side rails. Test for security.

23. Go to the other side of the bed. Lower side rail. Remove the soiled linen by rolling the edges inward. *Keep soiled linen away from your uniform.* Place soiled linen in hamper.

24. Pull the clean bottom sheet into place. Tuck it under the mattress at the head of the bed. Make a mitered corner.

25. Pull gently to eliminate wrinkles. Then tuck the side of the sheet under the mattress, working from top to bottom.

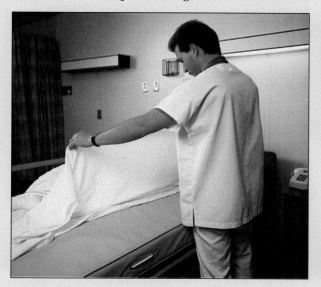

FIGURE 19–15A. Fanfold soiled bottom sheet to center of bed as close to patient as possible.

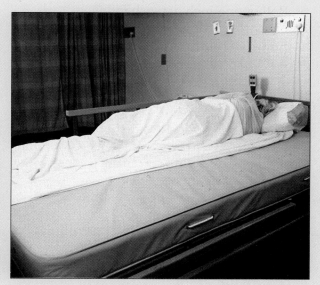

FIGURE 19–15B. Note that the bottom linen is flat and patient is positioned to far side of bed.

continues

26. Pull the drawsheet smoothly into place. Tuck firmly under the mattress.
27. Place the top sheet over the patient. Remove the bath blanket.
28. Complete the bed as an unoccupied bed, making toepleats in top sheet and blanket. Another way to reduce pressure is to grasp the top bedding over the toes and pull straight up.

Some patients prefer not to have the blanket and top sheet or spread tucked in.
29. Assist the patient to turn on his back. Place clean pillowcase on pillow not being used. Replace pillow. Change other pillowcase.
30. Carry out each procedure completion action, remembering to wash hands, report completion of task, and note patient's reaction.

The Surgical Bed

The surgical bed provides a safe, warm environment to receive the postsurgical patient. It must be made in such a way that movement from gurney to bed is made with maximum safety and with a mini-mum of effort. For this reason, the bed should be left open and at stretcher height.

All equipment needed to monitor vital signs and to supervise recovery should be in place and ready for use. You should also keep alert for the patient's return so you can help in the safe transfer from stretcher to bed.

PROCEDURE 55

MAKING THE SURGICAL BED

1. Wash your hands.
2. Check assignment for unit location.
3. Assemble the following equipment:
   - Articles for basic bed
   - One extra drawsheet
   - Bath blanket for warmth
   - One protective (rubber or plastic) draw-sheet (if used in facility)
   - Roll of one-inch gauze bandage
   - Equipment for monitoring vital signs
   - Emesis basin (from bedside stand)
   - Box of tissues
4. Lock bed. Strip and discard used linen.
5. Make bottom foundation bed as instructed earlier in this unit. (Steps 1–11 in *Making a Closed Bed*. Repeat on opposite side of bed.)
6. Place protective drawsheet over head of mattress sheet. Cover with cotton drawsheet. Miter corners and tuck in on sides.
7. Place top sheet, blanket, and spread in usual manner. Do not tuck in.
8. Fold linen back at foot of bed even with edge of mattress.
9. Fanfold upper covers and top sheet to far side of bed, Figure 19–16.
10. Tie waterproof pillow to head of bed with gauze bandaging or place according to facility policy.

11. Position bed so there is adequate room to position stretcher next to it. Leave bed locked and at same height as stretcher.
12. Check unit for obvious hazards.
13. Leave the room neat and tidy.
14. Wash your hands.
15. Report completion of task to nurse.

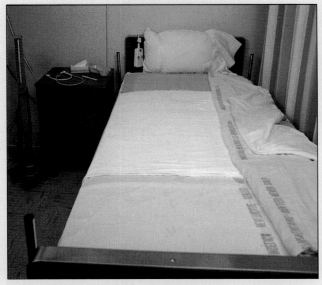

FIGURE 19–16. The bed is prepared for a patient returning from surgery by fanfolding cover to far side of bed and placing bed at stretcher height.

Modern surgical techniques have shortened the time many patients stay in an acute care facility after surgery. Patients are often admitted on the morning of surgery to special units, have the surgery performed, return to these same units immediately after surgery, and are discharged the same day to recuperate at home. These units are called short-term or day care units. To prepare a postsurgical bed in one of these units:

- Tighten the bottom linen.
- Fanfold top linen to the side or foot of bed.
- Raise bed to gurney height and lock wheels.
- Place equipment to check vital signs, emesis basin, and tissues by recovery bed.

SUMMARY

Proper bedmaking is an important part of your work.

- A skillfully made bed provides comfort and safety for the patient.
- Beds may be built to meet specific patient needs and conditions. Each type of bed will be made differently.
- Types of beds include:
  — Circ O lectric® bed
  — Stryker frame
  — Clinitron®
  — Electric
  — Gatch
- Bedmaking methods include
  — Closed beds
  — Occupied beds
  — Unoccupied beds
  — Surgical beds

- Drawsheets or turning sheets may be used, depending on individual situations.
- Some facilities are using fitted bottom sheets. The procedure may be changed to accommodate this difference.
- See precautions listed in Figure 19–17.

- Wear gloves if linen is wet or soiled with blood or body fluids.
- Do not shake linen.
- Avoid touching uniform with soiled linen.
- Fold linen in from the outside edges.
- Check for obvious hazards such as the position of the bed cranks (on nonelectric beds).
- Put soiled linen in proper receptacle.

FIGURE 19–17. Remember these precautions when making beds.

UNIT REVIEW

A. True/False. Answer the following true or false by circling T or F.

T F 1. The patient is most comfortable in a closed bed.

(T) F 2. The Stryker frame is used to turn patients easily.

(T) F 3. You should not attempt to operate a bed until you have been thoroughly supervised.

(T) F 4. The closed bed is made following the completion of terminal cleaning.

T (F) 5. Bottom bed linen can be loosely tucked as long as there are no wrinkles when you have finished.

T F 6. A mitered corner is tucked in, forming a triangle.

(T) F 7. Shaking linen as you change the bed spreads germs.

(T) F 8. The open bed is like a sign saying "Welcome."

T F 9. Before making an occupied bed, adjust the mattress to the head of the bed.

(T) F 10. The side rail opposite you must be up as you make an occupied bed.

B. Multiple choice. Select the one best answer to each of the following statements or questions by circling the proper letter.

11. Toepleats are made
    a. to improve the appearance of the bed.
    b. in unoccupied beds.
    c. as folds in the bottom sheet.
    d. to reduce pressure on the toes.

12. When making an unoccupied bed, make the
    a. entire bottom first.
    b. far side of the bottom and top first.
    c. near side of the entire bed first.
    d. far side of the bottom first.

13. Before making an unoccupied bed
    a. elevate to comfortable working height.
    b. keep the bed at lowest horizontal height.
    c. raise the head portion.
    d. raise bed to highest horizontal height.

14. Before making any bed always
    a. raise side rails.
    b. lower bed to lowest horizontal height.
    c. lock the bed wheels.
    d. raise the bed to its highest horizontal height.

15. Sheets should be smoothly tucked in over the head of the mattress
    a. 5"–7".
    b. 12"–18".
    c. 20"–24".
    d. any amount as long as the job is quickly done.

16. If a drawsheet or lift sheet is used, it should be placed so that it covers the area under the patient's
    a. head and shoulders.
    b. heels and lower legs.
    c. buttocks only.
    d. shoulders and buttocks.

17. When placing the case on the pillow
    a. tuck it under your chin.
    b. lay the pillow on the bed.
    c. pull the case over while grasping the pillow with the opposite hand.
    d. lay the pillow on the bedside stand.

18. When opening a closed bed
    a. fanfold top bedding to the foot.
    b. loosen all top bedding.
    c. leave the bed at its highest horizontal height.
    d. raise the head of the bed.

19. The top bedding in a surgical bed is
    a. untucked and draped.
    b. tucked in on two sides.
    c. untucked and fanfolded.
    d. made with toepleats.

20. A common element to all bedmaking is
    a. toepleats.
    b. leaving the unit neat and tidy.
    c. leaving the bed at its highest horizontal height.
    d. using the same linen and equipment

Patient Bathing

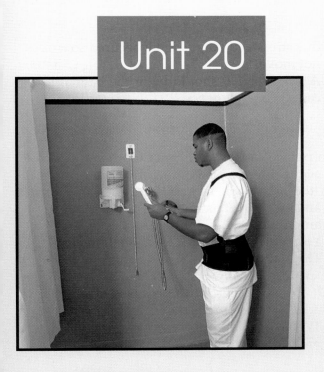

OBJECTIVES

As a result of this unit, you will be able to:

- Spell and define terms.
- Describe the safety precautions for patient bathing.
- List the purposes for bathing patients.
- Assist the patient with a tub bath or shower.
- Give a bed bath.
- Give a partial bath.
- Bathe patient in tub with whirlpool feature.
- Give female perineal care.
- Give male perineal care.
- Give routine hand and fingernail care.
- Give routine foot and toenail care.
- Give a bed shampoo.

VOCABULARY

Learn the meaning and the correct spelling of the following words:

axillae   perineal care
cuticle   perineum
genitalia   pubic

A daily bath is as important for the patient as it is for you. Following the bath, the patient feels relaxed, clean, and refreshed. A bath with warm water and mild soap:

- Removes dirt and perspiration
- Increases circulation
- Provides the patient with mild exercise
- Provides an opportunity for close observation

You as the care giver are able to see first-hand how the patient's condition is improving, declining, or changing in any way. Your observations are valuable aids to accurate nursing assessments.

With the physician's permission, the patient may be allowed to take regular tub baths or showers. Other patients will be bathed in bed. Care of the hair, teeth, and nails usually follows the bath procedure but may be carried out as independent procedures. Range of motion exercises frequently follow bathing.

A partial bath assures cleaning of the hands, face, back, axillae, buttocks, and genitals. It is very refreshing. Many patients will be able to help with the bath process. Whenever possible, encourage them to do so.

Patient Bathing

Some patients will be bathed in bed. Others, with permission, may be allowed to take regular tub baths or showers.

There are safety precautions, Figures 20–1A and B, which you must take to guard the patient against injury during the bathing procedure.

- The room should be comfortably warm and free from drafts to guard the patient against chilling.
- Cotton bath blankets can be used to cover the patient during a bed bath. They may also be used for added warmth following the tub bath or shower.
- The temperature of the water, whether shower, tub, or bed bath, should be maintained at about 105°F. Use a bath thermometer to check the temperature of the water.
- Nonskid strips can be placed in the tub and floor of the shower to prevent slipping.
- Handrails can be secured to the walls to help prevent falls as the patient transfers in and out of the tub.
- The patient should be assisted in all transfer activity related to the bath.
- Placing a chair in the shower can prevent un-

due stress and fatigue if it is secured so it does not move.
- A safety signal should be in the bath area in case of an emergency.

Safety Measures

If a patient falls or feels faint, do not leave him alone. Signal for help, using the emergency call button in the bathroom. In addition, since the warm water and exertion of bathing may tire the patient or make him feel faint, be sure that:

- You remain with the patient at all times.
- The bathroom door remains unlocked.

The patient receiving special treatments can be bathed. These patients, however, need special care. They include, for example, the patient who is receiving an IV, has drainage tubes, or is receiving oxygen.

Be careful as you bathe and move the patient that you:

- Do not put stress on the tubes.
- Never lower the IV container below the level of the infusion site.
- Never raise the drainage tube above the drainage site.

Review Figure 20–2 to be sure you perform all of the beginning procedure actions and procedure completion actions.

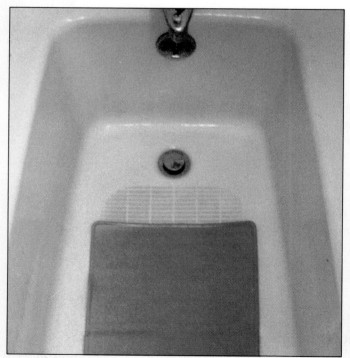

FIGURE 20–1A. Nonskid rubber strips or a rubber pad placed in the bottom of the tub help prevent slipping.

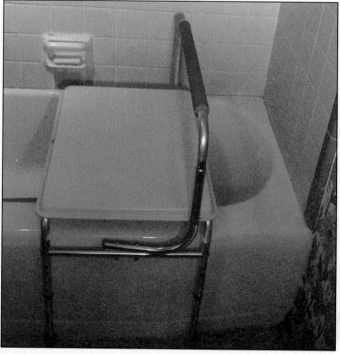

FIGURE 20–1B. Grab bars and shower seats provide solid support.

BEGINNING PROCEDURE ACTIONS	PROCEDURE COMPLETION ACTIONS
■ Wash your hands. ■ Assemble equipment. ■ Go to the patient's room, knock, and pause before entering. ■ Introduce yourself and identify the patient by checking the identification bracelet. ■ Ask visitors to leave and inform them where they can wait. ■ Provide privacy ■ Explain what will happen. Answer questions. ■ Raise bed to comfortable working height.	■ Position patient comfortably. ■ Leave signal cord, telephone, and fresh water close at hand. ■ Return bed to lowest position. ■ Perform general safety check of patient and environment. ■ Care for equipment according to facility policy. ■ Wash your hands. ■ Report completion of task. ■ Let visitors know when they may reenter. ■ Document action and your observations.

NOTE: Where there are open lesions, wet linen, or possible contact with patient body fluids or blood, disposable gloves are worn during the procedure. Put on gloves before contact with the patient or linen. Properly dispose of gloves after they are removed. ALWAYS APPLY UNIVERSAL PRECAUTIONS.

FIGURE 20–2. Beginning procedure actions and procedure completion actions

PROCEDURE 56 **OBRA**

SIDE **5**

ASSISTING WITH THE TUB BATH OR SHOWER

1. Carry out each beginning procedure action.
2. Remember to wash your hands, identify the patient, and provide privacy.
3. Assemble equipment needed:
   - ■ Disposable gloves
   - ■ Liquid soap
   - ■ Washcloth
   - ■ 2–3 bath towels
   - ■ Bath blanket
   - ■ Bath lotion
   - ■ Chair or stool beside shower or tub
   - ■ Bath or shower chair, as needed
   - ■ Patient's gown, robe, and slippers
   - ■ Bath mat
4. Take the supplies to the bathroom. Prepare bathroom for patient. Make sure tub is clean.
5. Fill tub half full with water at 105°F or adjust shower flow. Use a bath thermometer to check the water temperature, Figure 20–3A. If a bath thermometer is not available, test the water with your wrist. The water should feel comfortably warm.
6. Help the patient put on robe and slippers. Escort patient to bathroom.
7. Place towel in the bottom of the tub to prevent patient from slipping (if nonskid strips are not present in tub).

8. Help the patient to undress. Give the patient a towel to wrap around the waist.
9. Position shower chair in tub or shower, if needed, Figure 20–3B.
10. Assist the patient into the tub or shower.
11. Wash the patient's back.

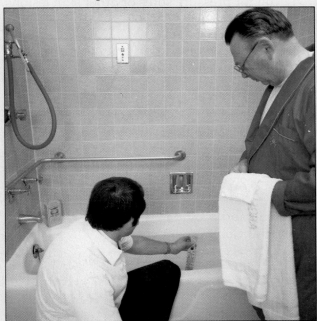

FIGURE 20–3A. Check temperature of water in bathtub before allowing patient to enter.

continues

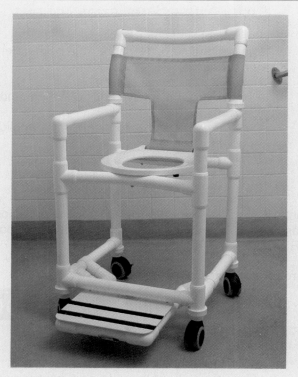

FIGURE 20–3B. The shower chair allows the patient to bathe in safety.

■ Observe the skin for signs of redness or breaks. See Unit 32 for information on caring for pressure sores or other skin lesions.

■ The patient may be left alone to wash the genitalia (external reproductive organs).
■ If the patient is not able to wash the genitalia, then you will also perform this part of the bath.
■ If the patient shows any signs of weakness:
  — Get help. Use the call button.
  — Remove the plug and let the water drain.
  — Turn off the shower.
  — Allow the patient to rest until feeling better before making any attempt to assist patient out of the tub or shower.
  — Keep the patient covered with a bath blanket to avoid chilling.
12. Hold the bath blanket around the patient who is stepping out of the tub. The patient may choose to remove wet towel under bath blanket.
13. Assist the patient to dry, dress, and return to the unit.
14. Return supplies to the patient's unit.
15. Clean the bathtub and disinfect. Wash your hands.
16. Carry out each procedure completion action. Remember to wash your hands, report completion of task, and document time, tub or shower bath, and patient reaction.

PROCEDURE 57 **OBRA**   SIDE **5**

GIVING A BED BATH

NOTE: Disposable gloves should be worn if the patient has draining wounds.
1. Carry out each beginning procedure action, Figures 20–4 and 20–5.
2. Remember to wash your hands, identify the patient, and provide privacy.
3. Assemble equipment needed:
   ■ Disposable gloves
   ■ Bed linen
   ■ Bath blanket
   ■ Laundry bag or hamper
   ■ Bath basin with water at 105°F
   ■ Bath thermometer
   ■ Soap and soap dish, or liquid soap
   ■ Washcloth
   ■ Face towel
   ■ Bath towel
   ■ Hospital gown/patient's night clothes
   ■ Lotion
   ■ Equipment for oral hygiene
   ■ Nail brush, emery board, and orangewood stick
   ■ Deodorant
   ■ Brush and comb
   ■ Bedpan and cover or urinal/paper towel or protector
4. Make sure windows and door are closed and fans are off to prevent chilling the patient.
5. Put clean towels and linen on chair in order of use, Figure 20–6. Place laundry hamper nearby.

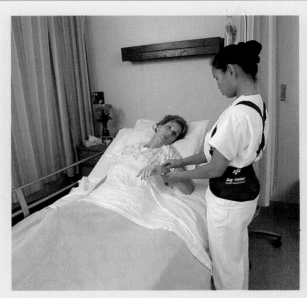

FIGURE 20–4. Identify the patient and explain what you plan to do and how the patient can help.

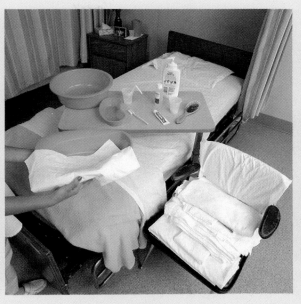

FIGURE 20–6. Assemble equipment and place on chair next to bed.

6. Offer bedpan or urinal, Figure 20–7. If patient wants to use the bedpan or urinal, put on gloves. Empty and clean bedpan or urinal before proceeding with bath. Remove gloves and discard according to facility policy. Wash your hands.
7. Lower the back of the bed and the side rails, if permitted.
8. Loosen top bedclothes. Remove and fold blanket and spread. Place bath blanket over top sheet, Figure 20–8, and remove by sliding it out from under the bath blanket.

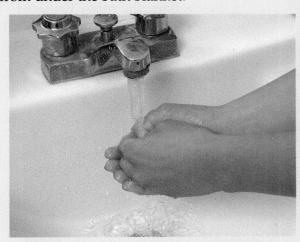

FIGURE 20–5. Wash your hands before assembling equipment.

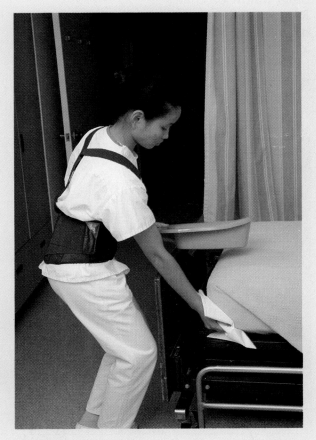

FIGURE 20–7. Offer the bedpan to patient before beginning procedure.

continues

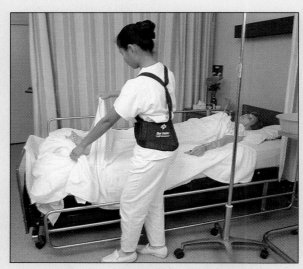

FIGURE 20–8.   Replace top bedding with a bath blanket.

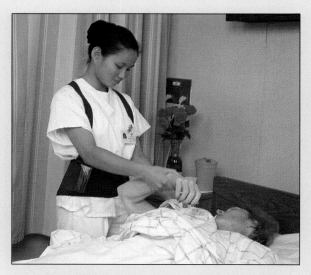

FIGURE 20–10A.   Remove gown from arm opposite infusion site.

9. Leave one pillow under patient's head. Place other pillow on chair.
10. Remove patient's night wear and place in laundry hamper (assuming no IV).
    a. Loosen gown from neck.
    b. Slip gown down arms.
    c. Make sure patient is covered by bath blanket, Figure 20–9.

d. If patient has an IV line in place:
    1. Slip gown away from body toward arm with IV line in place, Figure 20–10A.
    2. Gather gown at arm and slip downward over arm and line. Be careful not to disturb line.
    3. Gather material of gown in one hand so there is no pull or pressure on line, Figure 20–10B, and slowly draw gown over tip of fingers, Figure 20–10C.
    4. With free hand, lift IV free of standard and slip gown over bottle, Figure 20–10D. Be sure at no time to lower the bottle. Raise the gown. Replace IV container on standard.

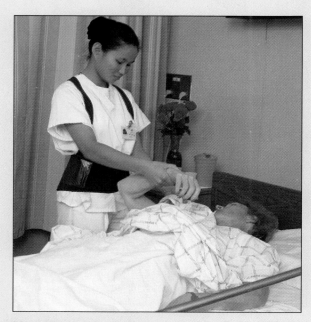

FIGURE 20–9.   Keeping patient covered with bath blanket, remove patient's gown.

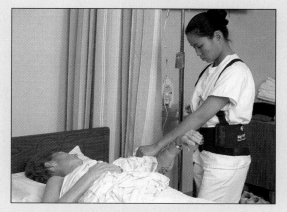

FIGURE 20–10B.   Gather up gown to form a tunnel while supporting infusion site.

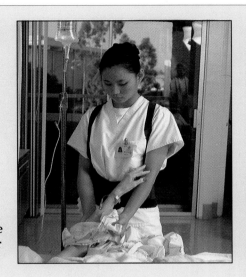

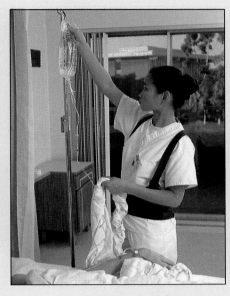

FIGURE 20–10C. Ease the gown over infusion site.

FIGURE 20–10D. Remove IV from stand and move gown up over the tubing. Pass IV container through sleeve. Rehang IV.

e. If the patient has a weak or paralyzed arm always undress the patient in this manner:
   1. Untie the gown and remove the back sides of the gown from underneath the patient.
   2. Remove the gown from the stronger arm first.
   3. Bring the gown across the patient's chest and slide the gown down over the weak arm.
   4. Gently lift the patient's weak arm to finish removing the gown over the patient's hand.
   5. Reverse the procedure to put a clean gown on the patient by putting the gown over the weaker arm first.

11. Fill bath basin two-thirds full with water at 105°F. Use a bath thermometer to be sure of the proper temperature.

12. Assist patient to move to the side of the bed nearest you.

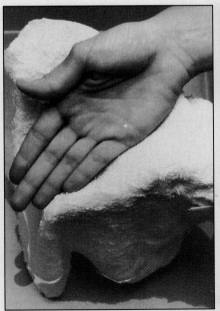
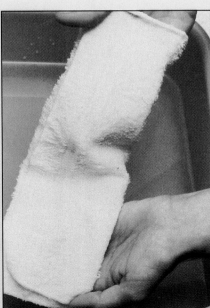
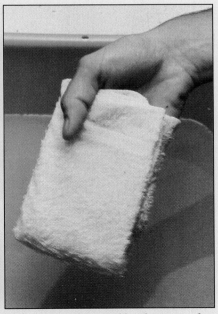

FIGURE 20–11. To make a bath mitt: Wrap the washcloth around one hand, bringing free end back over palm, and back up tucking in the end.

continues

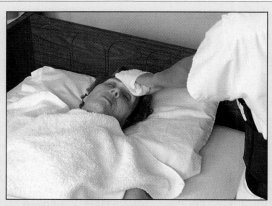

FIGURE 20–12. Wash face carefully. Always do eyes separately and do not use soap when washing eyes.

13. Foid face towel over upper edge of bath blanket to keep it dry. Put on gloves if needed.
14. Form a mitten by folding washcloth around hand, Figure 20–11.
    a. Wet washcloth.
    b. Wash eyes, using separate corners of cloth.
    c. Wipe from inside to outside corner.
    d. Do not use soap near eyes.
    e. Do not use soap on face unless patient requests it.
15. Rinse washcloth and apply soap if patient desires. Squeeze out excess water. Do not leave soap in water.

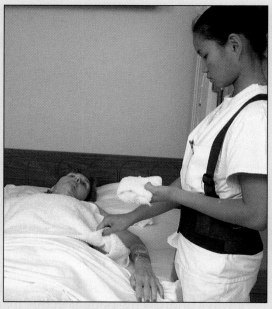

FIGURE 20–14. Cover chest with a towel and draw bath blanket down to waist.

16. Wash and rinse patient's face, Figure 20–12, ears, and neck well. Use towel to dry.
17. Expose patient's far arm. Protect bed with bath towel placed underneath arm, Figure 20–13.
    a. Wash, rinse, and dry arm and hand.
    b. Repeat for other arm.

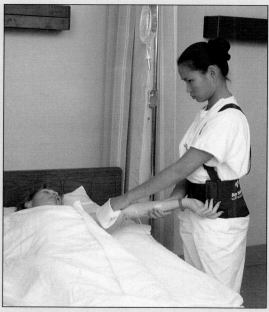

FIGURE 20–13. Place towel under near arm and support arm as you wash it.

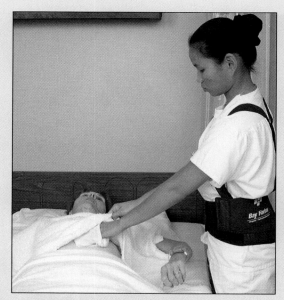

FIGURE 20–15. Lift towel with one hand and use other hand to wash underneath.

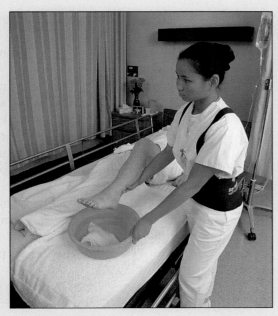

FIGURE 20–16. Support leg and place the foot in the basin.

c. Be sure **axillae** (armpits) are clean and dry.
d. Apply deodorant if patient requests it.

18. Care for hands and nails as necessary. Check with the nurse first to see if there are any special instructions.
    a. Place hands in basin of water. Wash each hand carefully. Rinse and dry. Push **cuticle** (base of fingernails) back gently with towel while wiping the fingers.
    b. Clean under nails with orangewood stick. Shape with emery board. Be careful not to file nails too close. Do not cut nails if patient is diabetic. Inform the nurse if attention is needed.

19. Put bath towel over patient's chest. Then fold blanket to waist, Figure 20–14. Under towel:
    a. Wash, rinse, and dry chest, Figure 20–15.
    b. Rinse and dry folds under breasts of female patient carefully to avoid irritating the skin.

20. Fold bath blanket down to **pubic** area (location of external genitalia). Wash, rinse, and dry abdomen. Fold bath blanket up to cover abdomen and chest. Slide towel out from under bath blanket.

21. Ask patient to flex knee, if possible. Fold bath blanket up to expose thigh, leg, and foot. Protect bed with bath towel.
    a. Put bath basin on towel.

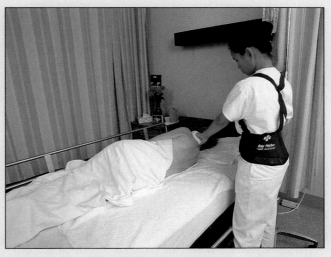

FIGURE 20–17. Change water and wash patient's back.

    b. Place patient's foot in basin, Figure 20–16.
    c. Wash and rinse leg and foot.
    d. When moving leg, support leg properly, Figure 20–16.

22. Lift leg and move basin to the other side of the bed. Dry leg and foot. Dry well between toes.

23. Repeat for other leg and foot. Take basin from bed before drying leg and foot.

24. Care for nails as necessary. Apply lotion to feet of patient with dry skin.
    ■ Do not attempt to cut thickened nails.
    ■ File nails straight across.
    ■ Do not round edges.
    ■ Do not push back the cuticle because it is easily injured and infected.

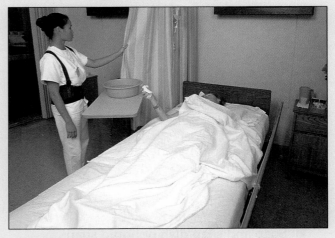

FIGURE 20–18. Leave wash water within easy reach so patient can do own perineal care, if condition permits.

continues

25. Change water and check for correct temperature with bath thermometer. It may be necessary to change water before this point in the patient's bath if it becomes cold or too soapy.
26. Help patient to turn on side away from you. Help him to move toward the center of the bed. Place bath towel lengthwise next to patient's back.
    ■ Wash, rinse, and dry neck, back, and buttocks, Figure 20–17.
    ■ Use long, firm strokes when washing back.
27. A back rub is usually given at this time (see Unit 21).
28. Help patient to turn on back.
29. Place a towel under the buttocks and upper legs. Change water in basin and check for correct temperature. Place washcloth, soap, basin, and bath towel within convenient reach of the patient, Figure 20–18. Have patient complete bath by washing genitalia. Assist the patient, if necessary. You must take the responsibility for the procedure if the patient has difficulty. Many times patients are reluctant to acknowledge the need for help. If assisting a patient, always put on disposable gloves.
    ■ For a female patient, wash from front to back, drying carefully.
    ■ For a male patient, be sure to carefully wash and dry penis, scrotum, and groin area.
30. Carry out range of motion exercises as ordered. (See Unit 35 for procedures.)
31. Cover pillow with towel. Comb or brush hair.

Oral hygiene is usually given at this time (see Unit 21).
32. Discard towels and washcloth in laundry hamper.
33. Provide clean gown. If the patient has an IV, check with the nurse before proceeding with steps a through f. Find out if the gown is to (1) go over the arm with the IV or (2) remain off the arm and be draped over the shoulder (as with multiple IVs or an infusion pump). If situation #1 is the case, then:
    a. Gather the sleeve on the IV side in one hand.
    b. Lift the bottle free of the standard, maintaining height.
    c. Slip the IV bottle through the sleeve from the inside and rehang.
    d. Guide the gown along the IV tubing to bed.
    e. Slip gown over hand. Do this very carefully so as not to disturb the infusion site.
    f. Position gown on infusion arm. Then insert opposite arm.
34. Clean and replace equipment according to facility policy.
35. Put clean washcloth and towels in bedside stand or hang according to facility policy.
36. Change the linen following occupied bed procedure. Replace and discard soiled linen in laundry hamper.
37. Carry out each procedure completion action. Remember to wash your hands, report completion of task, and document time, bed bath, and patient reaction.

PROCEDURE 58   OBRA

GIVING A PARTIAL BATH

1. Carry out each beginning procedure action.
2. Remember to wash your hands, identify the patient, and provide privacy.
3. Assemble equipment needed:
   ■ Disposable gloves
   ■ Bed linen
   ■ Bath blanket
   ■ Bath thermometer
   ■ Soap and soap dish or liquid soap
   ■ Washcloth
   ■ Face towel
   ■ Bath towel
   ■ Gown
   ■ Laundry bag or hamper
   ■ Bath basin—water at 105°F
   ■ Lotion
   ■ Equipment for oral hygiene
   ■ Nail brush, emery board, and orangewood stick
   ■ Brush, comb, and deodorant
   ■ Bedpan or urinal and cover
   ■ Paper towels or protector

4. Make sure windows and door are closed and fans are off to prevent chilling the patient.
5. Put towels and linen on chair in order of use. Place laundry hamper conveniently.
6. Offer bedpan or urinal (see Unit 21). Empty and clean before proceeding with bath. Wash your hands.
7. Elevate head rest, if permitted, to comfortable position.
8. Loosen top bedclothes. Remove and fold blanket and spread. Place bath blanket over top sheet. Remove top sheet by sliding it out from under the bath blanket.
9. Leave one pillow under patient's head. Place other pillow on chair.
10. Assist patient to remove gown. Place it in laundry hamper. Make sure patient is covered with bath blanket.
11. Place paper towels or bed protector on over-bed table.
12. Fill bath basin two-thirds full with water 105°F. Place basin on over-bed table.
13. Push over-bed table comfortably close to patient.
14. Place towels, washcloth, and soap on over-bed table within easy reach.
15. Tell patient to wash as much as she is able and that you will return to complete the bath.
16. Place call bell within easy reach. Ask patient to signal when ready.
17. Wash hands and leave unit.
18. Wash hands and return to unit when patient signals.
19. Change the bath water. Complete bathing those areas the patient couldn't reach. Make sure the face, hands, axillae, buttocks, back, and genitals are washed and dried. Put on disposable gloves to wash buttocks and genitalia.
20. Give a back rub with lotion.
21. Assist the patient in applying deodorant and a fresh gown.
22. Cover pillow with towel. Comb or brush hair. Assist with oral hygiene, if needed (see Unit 21).
23. Clean and replace equipment according to facility policy.
24. Put clean washcloth and towels in stand or hang according to facility policy.
25. Change the linen following occupied bed procedure. Replace and discard soiled linen in laundry hamper.
26. Carry out each procedure completion action. Remember to wash your hands, report completion of task, and document time, partial bath, and patient reaction.

Century Tub Bathing

The Century tub, Figure 20–19, is a special bathtub that provides the value of whirlpool activity with cleansing activity. (See Procedure 59)

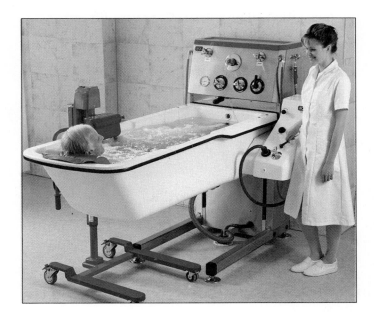

FIGURE 20–19. Arjo-Century's height-adjustable bathing system with hydromassage (whirlpool action) and lift hygiene chair (not shown) *(Courtesy of Arjo-Century, Inc.)*

PROCEDURE 59

BATHING A PATIENT IN A CENTURY TUB

1. Prepare bath before transporting patient to bath area.
   a. Wash your hands.
   b. Check to be sure that the tub is clean.
   c. Fill tub with water at 105°F to approximately 8 inches from the top.
   d. Check that room temperature is approximately 70°F.
   e. Add one capful of liquid soap, or as facility policy states.
   f. Have ready the following:
      — Lotion
      — Deodorant
      — 2 bath towels
      — 1 bath blanket
      — Patient's clothing
      — Disposable gloves
2. Wash your hands. Get Saf-Kary chair. Take chair to bedside.
3. Carry out each beginning procedure action.
4. Remember to wash your hands, identify the patient, and provide privacy.
5. Help patient to undress.
6. Position patient in Saf-Kary chair and secure straps. Cover patient with bath blanket.
7. Transport patient to tub room.
8. Replace bath blanket with two towels. Fold blanket for later use.
9. Position chair with back against lift arms.
10. Step on *up* pedal of lift to engage seat on Saf-Kary chair.
11. Check to see that both pins are engaged in lift arm slots.
12. Latch safety latches.
13. Raise seat to maximum height.
14. Rotate seat on lift arm 90 degrees so patient faces you.
15. Facing patient, slowly guide chair to tub edge so patient is parallel and over tub edge.
16. Lift patient's feet and guide them over tub edge toward lower well of tub.
17. Lower patient into tub by stepping gently on *down* pedal. Water should be chest high.
18. Press turbine button, activating whirlpool for 5 minutes.
19. Put on gloves.
20. Bathe face and upper body.
21. Step on *up* pedal, raising patient until feet are level with whirlpool outlet.
22. Dry upper body.
23. Raise lift to maximum height.
24. Pull chair and patient toward you, rotating seat as you lift feet from tub. Dry feet and legs.
25. Cover patient with bath blanket.
26. Raise safety latch on Saf-Kary chair.
27. Apply deodorant. Give lotion backrub. Remove gloves and discard according to facility policy.
28. Slowly lower lift and Saf-Kary chair until it is flat on the floor.
29. Return patient to unit.
30. Carry out each procedure completion action. Remember to wash your hands, report completion of task, and document time, bathed in Century tub, and patient reaction.
31. Return to tub room and clean tub according to facility policy.

Perineal Care

The perineum is the area between the legs. In females, it is the area between the vagina and the anus. In males, it is the area between the scrotum and the anus. Perineal care means to wash the area including the genitals and anus (see Procedures 60 and 61).

PROCEDURE 60 | OBRA

GIVING FEMALE PERINEAL CARE

1. Carry out each beginning procedure action.
2. Remember to wash your hands, identify the patient, and provide privacy.
3. Assemble equipment needed:
   - Bath blanket
   - Bedpan and cover
   - Liquid soap
   - Basin with warm water (105°F)
   - Bath thermometer
   - Disposable gloves
   - Bed protector
   - Washcloth and towel
4. Lower side rail on side where you will be working. Be sure opposite side rail is up and secure.
5. Remove bedspread and blanket. Fold and place on back of chair.
6. Patient is to be on back. Cover patient with bath blanket and fanfold sheet to foot of bed.
7. Ask patient to raise hips while you place bed protector underneath patient.
8. Offer bedpan to patient. If used, put on gloves.
   a. When the patient is finished, remove bedpan and cover.
   b. Put up side rail.
   c. Take bedpan to bathroom or utility room, empty and wash it, and return it to the proper storage place.
   d. Remove gloves and discard according to facility policy.
   e. Return to patient and lower side rail.
9. Position bath blanket so only the area between the legs is exposed.
10. Ask patient to separate her legs and flex knees.

NOTE: If patient is unable to spread legs and flex knees, the perineal area can be washed with the patient on the side with legs flexed. This position provides easy access to the perineal area.

11. Put on disposable gloves.
12. Wet washcloth, make mitt, and apply soap.

NOTE: Heavy soap application may be difficult to rinse off completely. Soap residue is irritating.

13. Use one gloved hand to stabilize and separate the vulva. With the other gloved hand, proceed as follows.
    a. Bring soaped washcloth in one downward stroke along the far side of outer labia to perineum.
    b. Rinse washcloth, remake mitt, and rinse area just cleaned.
    c. Repeat Steps a and b, washing and rinsing inner far labia.
    d. Repeat Steps a and b, washing and rinsing outer near labia.
    e. Repeat Steps a and b, washing and rinsing inner near labia.
    f. With gloved hands, separate labia. Clean and rinse inner part of vulva to perineum.
    g. Dry washed area with towel.
14. Turn patient away from you. Flex upper leg slightly if permitted.
15. Make a mitt, wet and apply soap lightly.
16. Expose anal area. Wash area, stroking from perineum to coccyx.
17. Rinse well in the same manner.
18. Dry carefully.
19. Return patient to back.
20. Remove and dispose of bed protector according to facility policy.
21. Cover patient with sheet.
22. Remove, fold, and store bath blanket according to facility policy.
23. Replace top covers, tuck under mattress, and make mitered corners.
24. Remove and dispose of gloves according to facility policy
25. Put up side rail.
26. If patient used bedpan, measure contents if patient is on I&O.
27. Empty bedpan, clean, and return to stand.
28. Empty water, clean equipment, and dispose of or store, according to facility policy.
29. Carry out each procedure completion action. Remember to wash your hands, report completion of task, and document time, perineal care completed, and patient's reaction.

PROCEDURE 61   OBRA

SIDE
5

GIVING MALE PERINEAL CARE

1. Carry out each beginning procedure action.
2. Remember to wash your hands, identify the patient, and provide privacy.
3. Assemble equipment needed:
   - Bath blanket
   - Urinal or bedpan and cover
   - Liquid soap
   - Basin with warm water (105°F)
   - Bath thermometer
   - Disposable gloves
   - Bed protector
   - Wash cloth and towel
4. Lower side rail on side where you will be working. Be sure opposite side rail is up and secure.
5. Remove bedspread and blanket. Fold and place on back of chair.
6. Patient is to be on back. Cover patient with bath blanket and fanfold sheet to foot of bed.
7. Ask patient to raise hips while you place bed protector underneath patient.
8. Offer urinal or bedpan to patient. Put on gloves.
   a. When the patient is finished, remove bedpan and cover.
   b. Put up side rail.
   c. Take bedpan to bathroom or utility room, empty and wash it, and return it to the proper storage place.
   d. Remove gloves and discard according to facility policy.
   e. Return to patient and lower side rail.
9. Position bath blanket so only the area between the legs is exposed.
10. Ask patient to separate his legs and flex knees.

NOTE: If patient is unable to spread legs and flex knees, the perineal area can be washed with the patient on the side with legs flexed. This position provides easy access to the perineal area.

11. Put on disposable gloves.
12. Wet washcloth, make mitt, and apply soap.

NOTE: Heavy soap application may be difficult to rinse off completely. Soap residue is irritating.

13. Grasp penis gently with one hand and wash. Begin at the meatus and wash in a circular motion toward the base of the penis.
14. If patient is not circumcised, draw foreskin back and be sure entire penis is washed.
15. Wash scrotum. Lift scrotum; wash perineum.
16. Rinse washcloth, remake mitt, and rinse area just washed.
17. Dry washed area with towel. Reposition foreskin if necessary.
18. Turn patient away from you. Flex upper leg slightly if permitted.
19. Make a mitt, wet and apply soap lightly.
20. Expose anal area. Wash area, stroking from perineum to coccyx.
21. Rinse well in the same manner.
22. Dry carefully.
23. Return patient to back.
24. Remove and dispose of bed protector according to facility policy.
25. Cover patient with sheet.
26. Remove, fold, and store bath blanket, according to facility policy.
27. Replace top covers, tuck under mattress, and make mitered corners.
28. Remove and dispose of gloves according to facility policy.
29. Put up side rail.
30. If patient used urinal or bedpan, measure contents if patient is on I & O.
31. Empty urinal or bedpan, clean, and return to bedside stand.
32. Empty water, clean equipment, and dispose of or store, according to facility policy.
33. Carry out each procedure completion action. Remember to wash your hands, report completion of task, and document time, perineal care completed, and patient's reaction. Be sure to note any redness, edema or abnormal discharge and report.

PROCEDURE 62 | OBRA

GIVING HAND AND FINGERNAIL CARE

NOTE: Check with nurse and nursing care plan to learn if this procedure is permitted for the patient or if it is to be modified because of the patient's condition.

1. Carry out each beginning procedure action.
2. Remember to wash your hands, identify the patient, and provide privacy.
3. Assemble equipment needed:
   - Basin
   - Soap
   - Bath towel
   - Lotion
   - Plastic protector
   - Nail clippers
   - Nail file
   - Orangewood stick
4. Elevate head of bed, if permitted. Adjust over-bed table in front of patient. If patient is allowed out of bed, help patient move to a chair. Position over-bed table waist high across lap.
5. Place plastic protector over the bedside table.
6. Fill basin with warm water approximately 105°F. Place basin on over-bed table.

7. Instruct patient to put hands in basin.
   - Soak for approximately 20 minutes.
   - Place towel over basin to help retain heat.
   - Add warm water, if necessary.
8. Wash patient's hands. Push cuticles back gently with washcloth.
9. Lift hands out of basin and dry with towel.
10. Use nail clippers to cut fingernails, if permitted by facility policy.
    - Cut nails straight across.
    - Do not cut below tips of fingers
    - Keep nail cuts on protector, to be discarded.
11. Shape and smooth fingernails with nail file.
12. Pour small amount of lotion in your palms and gently smooth on patient's hands.
13. Empty basin of water. Gather equipment. Clean and store according to facility policy.
14. Return over-bed table to foot of bed. If patient has been sitting up for the procedure, assist into bed.
15. Carry out each procedure completion action. Remember to wash your hands, report completion of task, and document time, hand and fingernail care, and patient reaction.

PROCEDURE 63 OBRA

GIVING FOOT AND TOENAIL CARE

NOTE: Check with nurse and nursing care plan to learn if this procedure is permitted for the patient or if it is to be modified because of the patient's condition. Older patients will be more comfortable during this procedure if you squat so they do not have to extend their legs.

1. Carry out each beginning procedure action.
2. Remember to wash your hands, identify the patient, and provide privacy.
3. Assemble equipment needed:
   - ■ Wash basin
   - ■ Soap
   - ■ Bath mat
   - ■ Lotion
   - ■ Disposable bed protector
   - ■ Bath towel/washcloth
   - ■ Orangewood stick
4. If permitted, assist patient out of bed and into chair.
5. Place bath mat on floor in front of patient.
6. Fill basin with warm water (105°F). Put basin on bath mat.
7. Remove slippers and allow patient to place feet in water, Figure 20–20A. Cover with bath towel to help retain heat, Figure 20–20B.

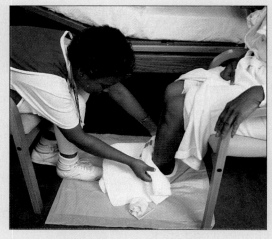

FIGURE 20–20B. Cover feet and basin with towel to hold in warmth.

8. Soak feet approximately 20 minutes.
   - ■ Add warm water as necessary.
   - ■ Lift feet from water while warm water is being added, Figure 20–20C.

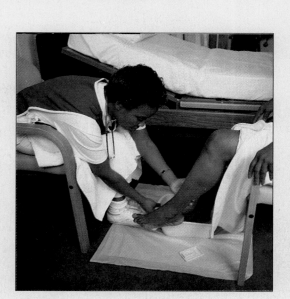

FIGURE 20–20A. Soak feet in warm water.

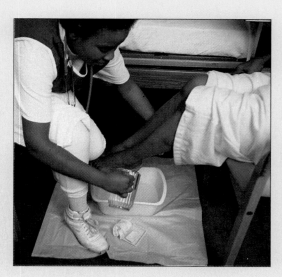

FIGURE 20–20C. Lift feet while warm water is being added.

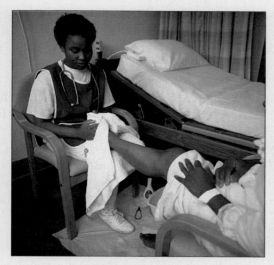

FIGURE 20–20D. Dry feet and inspect for any abnormalities.

9. At end of soak period:
   - ◼ Wash feet with soap.
   - ◼ Use washcloth to scrub roughened areas.
   - ◼ Rinse and dry, Figure 20–20D.
   - ◼ Note any abnormalities like corns or callouses.
10. Remove basin, covering feet with towel.
11. Use the orangewood stick gently to clean toenails, Figure 20–20E. If nails are long and need to be cut, report this fact to the nurse. *Do not* undertake this task yourself.
12. Dry feet.
13. Pour lotion into palms of hands. Hold hands together to warm lotion. Apply to patient's feet, Figure 20–20F. Do not apply lotion between the toes.
14. Assist patient with slippers and to return to bed unless ambulatory.
15. Carry out each procedure completion action. Remember to wash your hands, report completion of task, and document date, time, foot and toenail care, and patient reaction.

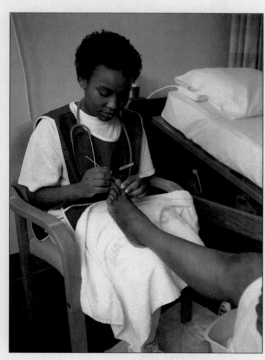

FIGURE 20–20E. Clean toenails carefully with an orangewood stick.

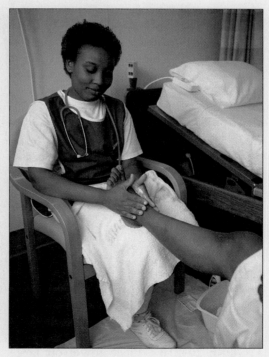

FIGURE 20–20F. Apply lotion to feet and smooth on.

PROCEDURE 64 | OBRA

GIVING A BED SHAMPOO

1. Carry out each beginning procedure action.
2. Remember to wash your hands, identify the patient, and provide privacy.
3. Assemble equipment needed:
   - Shampoo tray—plastic sheeting that has the top and two sides rolled forming a drain may be used if regular tray is not available, Figure 20–21A to 21C.
   - Shampoo
   - Washcloths
   - 3 bath towels
   - Bath blanket
   - Basin of water (105°F)
   - Safety pin
   - 2 bed protectors
   - Waterproof covering for pillow
   - Large bucket to collect used water
   - Hair dryer, if available (portable)
   - Hairbrush and comb
   - Small empty pitcher or cup
   - Larger pitcher of water (105°F)—use if additional water is needed
4. Place large, empty basin on floor under spout of shampoo tray.
5. Arrange on bedside stand within easy reach, Figure 20–22A:
   - Large pitcher of water (105°F)
   - Washcloth
   - 2 bath towels
   - Shampoo
   - Small pitcher of water (105°F)
6. Replace top bedding with bath blanket.
7. Ask patient to move to side of bed nearest you.
8. Replace pillowcase with waterproof covering.
9. Cover head of bed with bed protector. Be sure it goes well under the shoulders.
10. Loosen neck ties of gown.
11. Place towel under patient's head and shoulders. Brush hair free of tangles, working snarls out carefully.

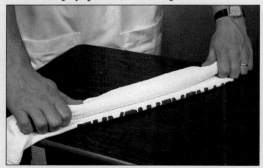

FIGURE 20–21A. If a shampoo tray is not available, roll a towel lengthwise.

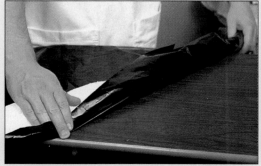

FIGURE 20–21B. Place towel on large piece of plastic and roll forming a trough at the top and on both sides.

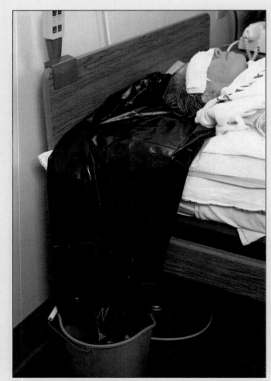

FIGURE 20–21C. Place end of plastic trough into a bucket. Position patient's head in trough. The trough allows water to drain into the collecting bucket.

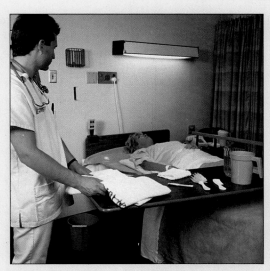

FIGURE 20–22A. Assemble equipment.

12. Bring towel down around patient's neck and shoulders and pin. Position pillow under shoulders so that head is tilted slightly backward.
13. Raise bed to high horizontal position.
14. Raise patient's head and position shampoo tray, Figure 20–22B, so that drain is over the edge of bed directly above basin.
15. Give patient washcloth to cover eyes, Figure 20–22C.
16. Recheck temperature of water in the basin.
17. Using the small pitcher, Figure 20–22D, pour a small amount of water over hair until thor-

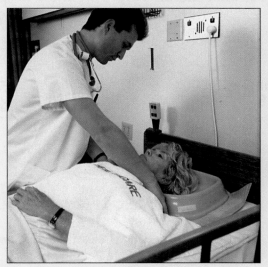

FIGURE 20–22B. Position with head on shampoo tray. Protect patient with a towel and bed with a protector.

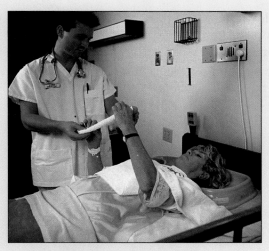

FIGURE 20–22C. Give patient folded washcloth to protect her eyes.

oughly wet. Use one hand to help direct the flow away from the face and ears.
18. Apply a small amount of shampoo, working up a lather, Figure 20–22E. Work from scalp to hair ends.
19. Massage scalp with tips of fingers. Do not use fingernails.
20. Rinse thoroughly, pouring from hairline to hair tips. Direct flow into drain. Use water from pitcher if needed, but be sure to check temperature of water before use.
21. Repeat procedure a second time.
22. Lift patient's head. Remove tray and bed protector. Adjust pillow and slip a dry bath towel underneath head.
23. Place tray on basin. Wrap hair in towel. Be sure to dry face, neck, and ears as needed.
24. Dry hair with towel. If available and not otherwise counterindicated, a portable hair dryer may be used to complete the drying process. Brushing the hair as you blow dry helps the hair to dry. Be sure to keep the dryer moving and not too close to the hair.
25. Comb hair appropriately. Remove protective pillow cover. Replace with cloth cover.
26. Lower height of bed to comfortable working position.
27. Replace bedding and remove bath blanket.
28. Help patient assume a comfortable position. Lower bed to lowest horizontal position. Leave call bell within reach.

continues

29. Allow patient to rest undisturbed. Length of procedure may tire patient.
30. Empty water from collection basin.

31. Carry out each procedure completion action. Remember to wash your hands, report completion of task, and document time, bed shampoo, and patient reaction.

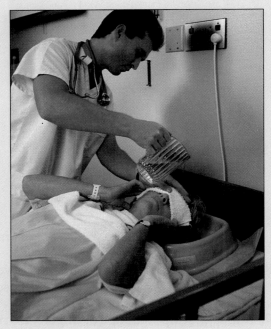

FIGURE 20–22D. Use warm water to wet hair.

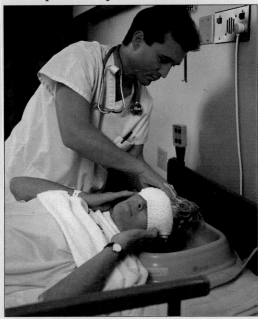

FIGURE 20–22E. Apply shampoo and work into a lather.

Dressing a Patient

Patients in hospitals generally wear hospital gowns because they are in bed most of the time. However, some patients may prefer to wear their own night-gowns or pajamas and will need assistance in dressing. You may also need to assist patients to dress when they are discharged from the hospital. It is usually easier to help people dress while they are still in bed.

PROCEDURE 65	OBRA

DRESSING AND UNDRESSING THE PATIENT

These directions are for helping a patient dress after a bath.

1. Carry out each beginning procedure action.
2. Remember to wash your hands, identify the patient, and provide privacy.
3. If possible, allow the patient to select the clothing.
4. Elevate head of bed to sitting position.
5. Cover patient with bath blanket and fanfold top bedclothes to foot of bed.
6. Bra: slip straps over patient's hands and move straps up arms and position on shoulders, hook bra.
7. Undershirt or any garment that slips over the head:
   a. Gather undershirt and slip over patient's head.
   b. Grasp patient's hand and guide it through

arm hole by reaching into the arm hole from outside.

   c. Repeat procedure with opposite arm.

   d. Assist resident to sit forward, adjusting undershirt so it is smooth and over upper body.

8. Alternate procedure for slipover garments: (garment must be sufficiently large and/or of stretchy fabric for this procedure)

   a. Start with garment lying face down on patient's lap with opening facing away from patient.

   b. Put both of the patient's hands into the garment from the bottom and into the sleeve holes.

   c. Pull the sleeves up the patient's arms as far as possible.

   d. Gather up the back of the garment with your hand and slip the garment over the patient's head.

   e. Smooth the garment down and position garment comfortably on patient's body.

9. Shirts or dresses that fasten in the front:

   a. Insert your hand through sleeve of garment and grasp hand of patient, drawing sleeve over your hand and patient's.

   b. Adjust sleeve at shoulder.

   c. Assist patient to sit forward. Arrange clothing across back.

   d. Gather sleeve on opposite side by slipping your hand in from the outside.

   e. Grasp patient's wrist and pull sleeve of garment over your hand and patient's hand. Draw upward and adjust at shoulder.

   f. Button, zip, or snap garment.

10. Underwear or slacks:

   a. Facing foot of bed, gather patient's underwear from waist to leg hole.

   b. Slip underwear over feet and draw up the legs as high as possible.

   c. Assist patient to raise buttocks and draw garment over buttocks and up around waist. (Have patient roll first to one side and then to the other to adjust clothing if this is easier).

   d. Fasten garment if necessary.

11. Socks:

   a. Roll socks and adjust over toes, draw up over foot. Adjust so socks lie flat and smooth.

12. Pantyhose:

   a. Gather pantyhose and adjust over toes and feet. Draw up over feet and legs as high as possible.

   b. Assist patient to raise hips and position pantyhose as directed above.

13. Shoes:

   a. Slip shoes on—use shoehorn if necessary.

14. Carry out each procedure completion action. Wash your hands, report completion of task.

SUMMARY

Bathing makes a patient feel refreshed and clean. Full or partial baths may be carried out in:

- Bed
- Showers
- Regular bathtubs
- Century tubs

Personal hygiene measures include care of the:

- Teeth
- Hair
- Nails

Range of motion exercises are frequently performed during the bath procedure, according to the patient's needs and orders. See Unit 35. The daily hygiene routine gives you a chance to make close observations of the patient.

UNIT REVIEW

A. True/False. Answer the following true or false by circling T or F.

(T) F   1. The nursing assistant should carefully observe the patient during the bath procedure.

(T) F   2. Patients are submerged in the water of a Century tub and the whirlpool action is turned on for 20 minutes.

T (F)   3. Perineal care is given with the patient positioned on a bedpan.

(T) F   4. Range of motion exercises are often performed after the bath procedure begins.

T F (5.) The bath can be omitted if the patient is receiving an IV.

(T) F   6. During the bed bath, only the part being bathed should be exposed.

(T) F   7. Patients should be encouraged to use handrails when getting in and out of the bathtub.

T (F)   8. Stress may be placed on drainage tubes as long as they are not disconnected.

T (F)   9. Since soap is used during the bathing procedure, the tub need not be cleaned between patient use.

(T) F 10. The bathing procedure can provide the patient with a mild form of exercise.

(T) F 11. Disposable gloves should be worn if the patient has draining wounds.

B. Matching. Match the words in Column II with the statements in Column I.

	Column I	Column II
_c_	12. External reproductive organs	a. axillae
_d_	13. Area at base of nails	b. midriff
_A_	14. Area under the arms	c. genitalia
		d. cuticle
_f_	15. Apparatus that provides whirlpool action	e. shampoo
		f. Century tub

C. Multiple Choice. Select the correct answer to each of the following statements by circling the proper letter.

16. The room temperature during the bath procedure should be about
    a. 62°F.
    b. 68°F.
    (c.) 70°F.
    d. 78°F.

17. Patients needing special care during the bath period are those who
    a. have drainage tubing.
    b. are receiving an IV.
    c. are receiving oxygen.
    (d.) All of the above.

18. Bath water temperature should be approximately
    (a.) 105°F.
    b. 90°F.
    c. 100°F.
    d. 115°F.

19. When giving foot care, the feet should be soaked approximately
    a. 1 hour.
    b. 1/2 hour.
    (c.) 20 minutes.
    d. 5 minutes.

20. The best way to warm lotion before applying it to the feet is to
    a. shake the lotion bottle.
    (b.) pour lotion into hands and hold hands together.
    c. wrap it in a bath towel.
    d. None of the above.

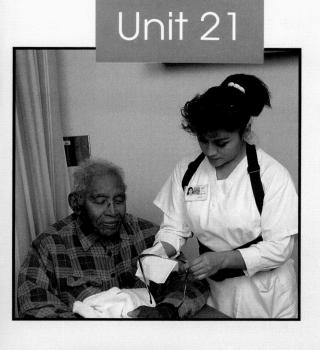

Unit 21

General Comfort Measures

OBJECTIVES

As a result of this unit, you will be able to:

- Spell and define terms.
- Identify patients who require frequent oral hygiene.
- List the purposes of oral hygiene.
- Assist the patient with oral hygiene, both routine and special.
- Explain nursing assistant responsibilities for a patient's dentures and eyeglasses.
- State the purpose of back rubs.
- Give a back rub.
- Describe safety precautions when shaving a patient.
- Describe the importance of hair care.
- Explain the use of comfort devices.
- Assist the patient with use of the bedpan, urinal, or commode.

VOCABULARY

Learn the meaning and the correct spelling of the following words:

bridging	footdrop
caries	halitosis
dentures	oral hygiene
feces	trochanter roll
footboard	

There is much that you can do for your patients that will add to their general comfort and feeling of well-being. This includes:

- Caring for oral hygiene
- Giving back rubs
- Brushing hair
- Shaving
- Using pillows and special equipment to maintain comfortable positions

Oral Hygiene

Oral hygiene is the care of the mouth and teeth.

- Routine oral hygiene should be performed at least three times a day.
- Patients should be encouraged to do as much as possible for themselves.
- Special oral hygiene is the cleansing of the mouth of the helpless patient using commercially prepared lemon and glycerine swabs and other preparations.

Patients requiring more frequent oral hygiene include those who are:

- Unconscious
- Vomiting
- Experiencing a high temperature
- Receiving certain medications
- Dehydrated
- Mouth breathers

- Receiving oxygen
- Dying

Proper cleansing of the teeth and mouth helps
- Prevent tooth decay (**caries**)
- Eliminate bad breath (**halitosis**)
- Contribute to the patient's comfort

Refer to Figure 21–1 for a recap of the beginning procedure actions and procedure completion actions you are to perform for each patient care procedure.

BEGINNING PROCEDURE ACTIONS	PROCEDURE COMPLETION ACTIONS
■ Wash your hands. ■ Assemble equipment. ■ Go to the patient's room, knock, and pause before entering. ■ Introduce yourself and identify the patient by checking the identification bracelet. ■ Ask visitors to leave and inform them where they can wait. ■ Provide privacy. ■ Explain what will happen. Answer questions. ■ Raise bed to comfortable working height.	■ Position patient comfortably. ■ Leave signal cord, telephone, and fresh water close at hand. ■ Return bed to lowest position. ■ Care for equipment according to facility policy. ■ Perform general safety check of patient and environment. ■ Wash your hands. ■ Report completion of task. ■ Let visitors know when they may reenter the patient's room. ■ Document action and your observations.

NOTE: Where there are open lesions, wet linen, or possible contact with patient body fluids or blood, disposable gloves are worn during the procedure. Put on gloves before contact with the patient or linen. Properly dispose of gloves after they are removed. ALWAYS APPLY UNIVERSAL PRECAUTIONS.

FIGURE 21–1. Beginning procedure actions and procedure completion actions

PROCEDURE 66 | OBRA   SIDE **6**

ASSISTING WITH ROUTINE ORAL HYGIENE

1. Carry out each beginning procedure action.
2. Remember to wash your hands, identify the patient, and provide privacy.
3. Assemble equipment needed:
   - Disposable gloves and face mask
   - Toothbrush
   - Toothpaste or powder
   - Mouthwash solution in cup
   - Emesis basin
   - Bath towel
   - Drinking tube
   - Tissues
   - Cup of fresh water
   - Paper bag
4. Raise back of bed so that the patient may sit up, if condition permits.
5. Place bath towel over patient's gown and bedcovers.
6. Pour water over toothbrush and put toothpaste on brush.
7. Put on disposable gloves and face mask.
8. Brush teeth as follows, Figure 21–2:
   a. Insert toothbrush into the mouth with bristles in a downward position.
   b. Turn toothbrush with bristles toward teeth.
   c. Brush all tooth surfaces with an up-and-down motion.
9. Give patient water in cup to rinse mouth. Use straw, if necessary. Turn the patient's head to one side with emesis basin near chin for return of fluid.

10. Repeat Steps 8 and 9 as necessary. Offer mouth-wash. Dilute mouthwash, if desired by patient.
11. Remove basin. Wipe patient's mouth and chin with tissue. Discard tissue in paper bag.
12. Remove towel.
13. Rinse toothbrush with water.
14. Remove and dispose of gloves according to facility policy.
15. Carry out each procedure completion action. Remember to wash your hands, report completion of task, and document date, time, mouth care/oral hygiene, and patient reaction.

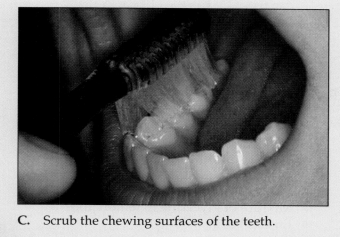

C. Scrub the chewing surfaces of the teeth.

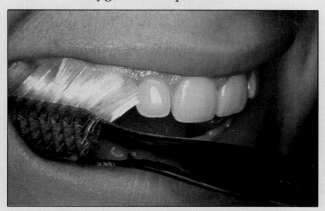

A. Place the head of your toothbrush beside the teeth, with the bristle tips at a 45-degree angle against the gumline. Move the brush back and forth in short (half-a-tooth-wide) strokes several times, using a gentle "scrubbing" motion. Brush the outer surfaces of each tooth, upper and lower, keeping the bristles angled against the gumline.

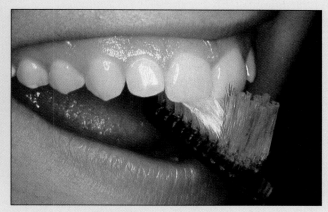

D. To clean the inside surfaces of the front teeth, tilt the brush vertically and make several gentle up-and-down strokes with the "toe" (the front part) of the brush.

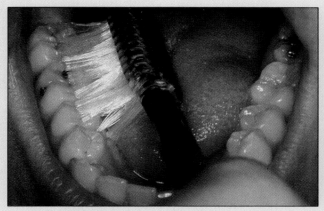

B. Use the same method on the inside surfaces of all the teeth, still using short back-and-forth strokes.

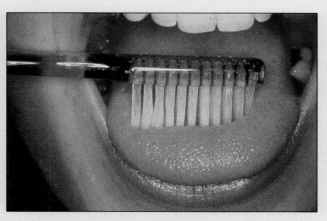

E. Brushing the patient's tongue will help freshen breath and clean the mouth by removing bacteria.

FIGURE 21–2. Brush the teeth as they grow and across the chewing surfaces. *(Toothbrushing photos and descriptions compliments of the American Dental Association)*

PROCEDURE 67 | **OBRA**   SIDE **6**

ASSISTING WITH SPECIAL ORAL HYGIENE

NOTE: Special oral hygiene is provided when the patient cannot participate actively in such care.

1. Carry out each beginning procedure action.
2. Remember to wash your hands, identify the patient, and provide privacy.
3. Assemble equipment needed:
   - Disposable gloves
   - Mouthwash or solution in cup or
   - Mixture of glycerine in lemon juice
   - Emesis basin
   - Bath towel
   - Paper bag
   - Applicators
   - Tissues
   - Tongue depressor
   - Lubricant for lips
4. Cover pillow with towel and turn patient's head to one side and slightly forward so any excess fluid will not run down throat. Place emesis basin under patient's chin.
5. Put on gloves.
6. Open mouth gently with tongue depressor.
7. Dip applicators into mouthwash solution or glycerine mixture. (In some cases, a physician may order hydrogen peroxide solution.)
8. Using moistened applicators, wipe gums, teeth, and inside of mouth, Figure 21–3.
9. Discard used applicators in paper bag.
10. Apply lubricant to lips.
11. Clean and replace equipment.

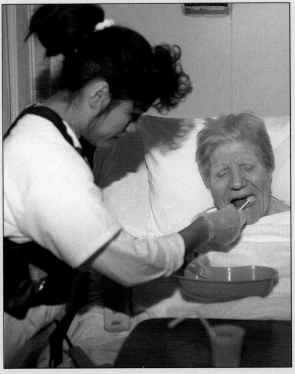

FIGURE 21–3. Using moistened applicators, wipe gums, teeth, and tongue.

12. Remove and dispose of gloves properly.
13. Carry out each procedure completion action. Remember to wash your hands, report completion of task, and document date, time, special mouth care/oral hygiene, and patient reaction.

PROCEDURE 68 | **OBRA**

ASSISTING PATIENT TO BRUSH TEETH

1. Carry out each beginning procedure action.
2. Remember to wash hands, identify patient, and provide privacy.
3. Assemble equipment needed:
   - Disposable gloves
   - Emesis basin
   - Toothbrush
   - Toothpaste
   - Glass of cool water
   - Mouthwash (if permitted)
   - Hand towel
   - Bed protector
4. Elevate the head of bed. Help patient into a comfortable position.
5. Lower side rails and position over-bed table across patient's lap.
6. Cover table with plastic protector.
7. Place emesis basin and glass of water on over-bed table.
8. Place towel across patient's chest.

9. Be prepared to help as patient brushes teeth, Figure 21–4.
10. After patient has brushed his teeth:
    a. Push over-bed table to the foot of the bed.
    b. Remove towel, fold, and place in table.
11. Carry out each procedure completion action. Remember to wash your hands, report completion of task, and document date, time, assisted with oral hygiene, and patient reaction.

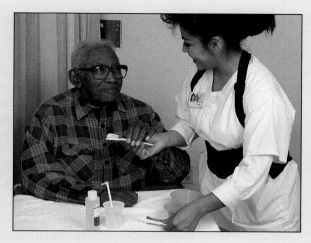

FIGURE 21–4. Assist the patient as needed.

Dentures and Eyeglasses

Dentures are artificial teeth that are removable. They must be cleaned. The patient may feel embarrassed about wearing dentures and even more so when seen after the dentures have been removed. Therefore, always provide privacy when dentures are to be removed and cleaned.

When a patient wears dentures, it is your responsibility to:
- Use extreme care when handling dentures.
- See that the dentures are kept clean.
- See that the dentures are not lost or broken.
- Store dentures safely when out of the patient's mouth.

— Keep dentures in bedside stand.
— Keep in container labeled with patient's name on the side.
— Plastic dentures must be kept dry.

Eyeglasses and contact lenses need special care and attention. They should:
- Be kept clean with special lens paper or soft, nonabrasive tissue.
- Be stored in their container in the bedside stand when not in use.
- Always be kept within easy reach of the patient.

Patients should be encouraged to wear dentures and glasses whenever possible.

PROCEDURE 69 | **OBRA**

SIDE **6**

CARING FOR DENTURES

1. Carry out each beginning procedure action.
2. Remember to wash your hands, identify the patient, and provide privacy.
3. Assemble equipment needed:
   - Disposable gloves
   - Tissues
   - Emesis basin
   - Toothbrush or denture brush
   - Toothpaste or powder
   - Gauze squares
   - Denture cup
4. Allow the patient to clean dentures if able to do so. If the patient cannot:
   a. Put on gloves.
   b. Give tissue to patient.
   c. Ask patient to remove dentures.
   d. Assist, if necessary.
5. If patient cannot remove dentures:
   a. Ask patient to open mouth.
   b. Firmly grasp lower dentures. Gently ease up and forward and remove from mouth.
   c. Firmly grasp upper dentures. Gently ease down and forward and remove from mouth.

continues

6. Place dentures in denture cup or emesis basin padded with gauze squares. Take to bathroom or utility room.
7. Place approximately 2–3 inches of cool water in the bottom of the emesis basin. Also place a washcloth or paper towel on the bottom of the container. Hold dentures over emesis basin as they are cleaned. This will protect the dentures in case they are dropped.
8. Put toothpaste or tooth powder on toothbrush. Hold each denture under a gentle stream of warm water and brush until all surfaces are clean.
9. Rinse dentures thoroughly under cold running water. Rinse denture cup.
10. Place fresh gauze squares in denture cup. Place dentures in cup and take them to bedside.
11. Assist patient to rinse mouth with mouthwash.
12. A soft toothbrush or applicator should be used to clean the mouth while dentures are out. Carefully observe and report the condition of the teeth, mouth, tongue, lips, and dentures.
13. Use tissue or gauze to hand the wet dentures to patient. The upper denture is inserted first. If necessary; the nursing assistant replaces the dentures.
14. Remove and dispose of gloves according to facility policy.
15. Carry out each procedure completion action. Remember to wash your hands, report completion of task, and document date, time, denture care, and patient reaction.

NOTE: Store dentures in a denture cup inside the bedside stand when not in use. Some patients prefer storing their dentures dry. Others prefer to store their dentures in a special solution.

Back Rubs

When properly given, back rubs can be:
- Stimulating to the patient's circulation.
- A major aid in preventing skin breakdown (decubiti).
- Soothing.
- Refreshing.

Keep your nails short to prevent injuring the patient. The back rub procedure provides a good opportunity for you to observe the condition of the patient's skin. Report all observations to the nurse. Look for:
- Reddened areas that do not blanch (whiten) when pressed
- Raw areas of skin
- Condition of skin over bony prominences

Unless contraindicated, the back rub is given:
- Routinely as part of the cleansing bed bath or partial bath.
- Following use of the bedpan.
- When changing the position of the helpless patient.
- At bedtime.
- When it could be a comfort to the patient.

Long, smooth strokes are relaxing. Short, circular strokes tend to be more stimulating.

The back rub is given with warmed lotion.

| PROCEDURE 70 | OBRA | SIDE 6 |  | |

GIVING A BACK RUB

1. Carry out each beginning procedure action.
2. Remember to wash your hands, identify the patient, and provide privacy.
3. Assemble equipment needed:
    - Disposable gloves (if resident has draining wounds)
    - Basin of water (105°F)
    - Bath towel
    - Soap or lotion
4. Put up far side rail. Raise bed to comfortable horizontal height.
5. Place lotion in basin of water to warm, Figure 21–5.
6. Turn the patient on his side with his back toward you.
7. Expose and wash the back and dry.

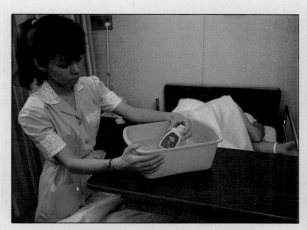

FIGURE 21–5. The lotion can be warmed in the basin of water.

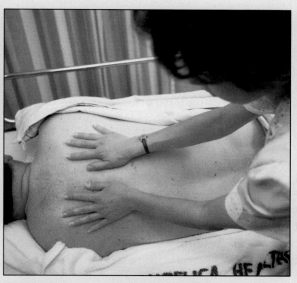

FIGURE 21–6. Use long, smooth strokes as you apply the lotion.

8. Pour a small amount of lotion into one hand.
   a. Hold between hands to warm.
   b. Apply to the skin.

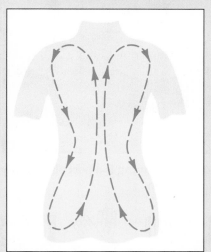

A. Soothing strokes

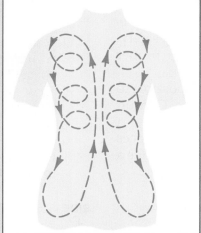

B. Circular movement

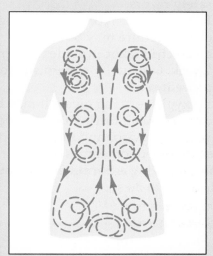

C. Passive movement

FIGURE 21–7. Strokes to be used during the back rub

   c. Rub with a gentle but firm stroke, Figure 21–6.
   d. Give special attention to all bony parts.
9. Begin at the base of the spine and with long, soothing strokes rub up the center, around the shoulders, and down the sides of the back and buttocks, Figure 21–7A. This procedure stimulates circulation over the bony places.
   a. Repeat this step four times, using the long, soothing upward stroke and a circular motion on the downstroke, Figure 21–7B.
   b. Repeat, but on the downward stroke, rub in a small circular motion with the palm of the hand,

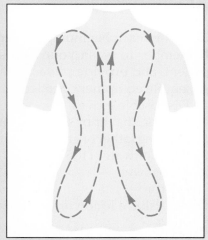

D. Soothing strokes

continues

Figure 21–7C. Be sure to include area over coccyx.
c. Repeat the long, soothing strokes to muscles for 3–5 minutes, Figure 21–7D.
d. Dry carefully.
e. If pressure areas are noted, be sure to report to the nurse. (See Unit 32 for information on care and treatment of pressure sores.)

10. Straighten and tighten drawsheet.
11. Change the patient's gown, if needed.
12. Carry out each procedure completion action. Remember to wash your hands, report completion of task, and document date, time, back rub/back care, and patient reaction.

Daily Shaving

Daily shaving is part of the routine self-care of most men. It should not be neglected in a care facility. When patients are unable to shave themselves and a barber is not available, it is your responsibility, Figure 21–8.

■ Use the patient's own shaving equipment if possible. Otherwise, use disposable, one-use safety razors.
■ If the patient is receiving anticoagulants, a special procedure may be required. For example, an electric razor provides the greatest safety. Check with your supervisor for the proper procedure.
■ If oxygen is being given, it may be possible to discontinue it during this procedure. Consult your supervisor and follow hospital policy.

Elderly women sometimes grow hair on their faces and chins. Shaving is permitted but you must have a specific order to do so.

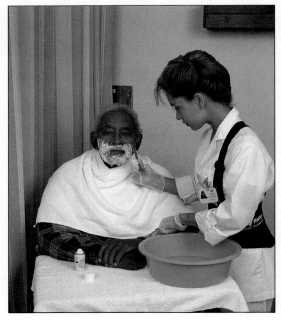

FIGURE 21–8. Shaving is a part of the daily routine of most men.

PROCEDURE 71 | **OBRA**

SHAVING A PATIENT

1. Carry out each beginning procedure action.
2. Remember to wash your hands, identify the patient, and provide privacy.
3. Assemble equipment needed:
   ■ Disposable gloves
   ■ Electric shaver or safety razor
   ■ Shaving lather or an electric preshave lotion
   ■ Basin of water (105°F)
   ■ Face towel
   ■ Mirror
   ■ Aftershave lotion or powder

4. Put up far side rail. Raise the head of the bed. Place equipment on over-bed table.
5. Put on disposable gloves.
6. Place face towel across patient's chest.
7. Moisten face and apply lather.
8. Starting in front of the ear:
   a. Hold skin taut.
   b. Bring razor down over cheek toward chin.
   c. Repeat until lather on cheek is removed and area has been shaved.
   d. Repeat on other cheek.

e. Remove hair from under nose and above upper lip by moving the razor in short, downward strokes from nose toward lip.

f. Shave chin carefully. Having the patient tense the area helps smooth out the tissue.

g. Ask patient to raise chin. Shave neck area on each side, bringing razor up toward chin.

h. Use firm, short strokes. Rinse razor often.

i. Be sure to shave under nose.

9. Lather neck area and stroke up toward the chin in a similar manner.

10. Wash face and neck. Dry thoroughly.

11. Apply aftershave lotion or powder, if desired.

12. If the skin is nicked:
   a. Apply pressure directly over the area.
   b. Report incident to nurse.

13. Remove disposable gloves and dispose according to facility policy.

14. Dispose of razor blade in sharps container or according to facility policy.

15. Carry out each procedure completion action. Remember to wash your hands, report completion of task, and document date, time, face shaved, and patient reaction.

NOTE: Women may need assistance in applying makeup.

Daily Hair Care

Daily care of the hair, for both male and female patients, is usually performed after the patient's bed bath. Brushing the hair:

- Stimulates circulation of the scalp.
- Refreshes the patient.
- Removes dust and lint.
- Helps to keep the hair shiny and attractive.

If additional care is needed, a fluid dry cleaner to shampoo the hair is available. It leaves the hair soft and manageable and the hair set intact. This procedure is so simple that it is often used instead of the regular shampoo for bed patients.

Sometimes, however, a shampoo may be advisable for the patient in bed. Approval for the procedure must be obtained from the doctor. Bed shampoos should be given every two weeks when the patient is bed bound for an extended period. The procedure for giving a bed shampoo is given in Unit 20.

The following procedure assumes that the patient is a female. Hair care for a male is very similar, however, so the procedure can easily be adapted.

PROCEDURE 72 | **OBRA**

GIVING DAILY CARE OF THE HAIR

1. Carry out each beginning procedure action.
2. Remember to wash your hands, identify the patient, and provide privacy.
3. Assemble equipment needed:
   - Towel
   - Comb and brush
4. Ask the patient to move to the side of the bed nearest you or to a chair, if permitted.
5. Cover the pillow with a towel.
6. Part or section hair and comb with one hand between scalp and end of hair.
7. Brush carefully and thoroughly.
8. Have patient turn so hair on the back of the head may be combed and brushed. If hair is snarled:
   - Work section by section.
   - Unsnarl the hair, beginning near the ends and working toward the scalp.
   - Gum may be removed with ice.
9. Complete brushing and arrange attractively. Braid long hair to prevent repeated snarling.
10. Carry out each procedure completion action. Remember to wash your hands, report completion of task, and document date, time, hair care, and patient reaction.

Comfort Devices

Bed Cradle

The bed cradle, Figure 21–9, prevents the weight of the bedclothes from falling on some part of the body. It can be used therapeutically or as a comfort device. It is used:

- Over fractured limbs.
- When there are burns.
- To prevent skin lesions.

Coverings that maintain some degree of warmth within the cradle may also be needed to keep the patient comfortable. Lights may be suspended from a cradle to provide extra external heat to promote

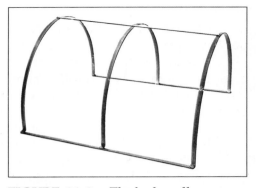

FIGURE 21–9. The bed cradle

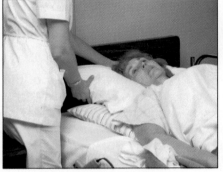

A. One pillow is placed crosswise under the patient's shoulders and the other under her head.

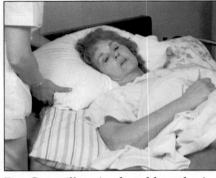

B. One pillow is placed lengthwise along each shoulder and the third supports the patient's head.

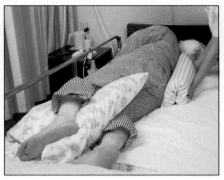

C. Pillows between the legs and the back increase comfort by maintaining the proper position.

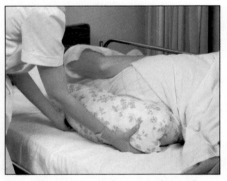

D. The patient is lying on his side, and a pillow is doubled over and placed lengthwise to support his back.

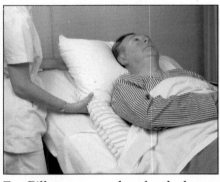

E. Pillows are used under the lower back and head for support.

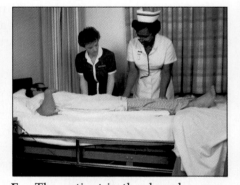

F. The patient in the dorsal recumbent position needs support with a rolled bath blanket or trochanter roll to prevent external hip rotation. The knees are slightly flexed and the heels are free from pressure.

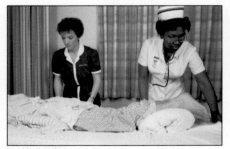

G. In the prone position, a small pillow under the abdomen reduces pressure on the thorax. The knees are slightly flexed to prevent pressure on the toes.

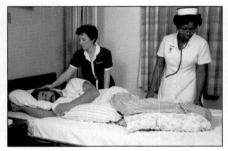

H. A pillow between the legs and in front of the abdomen supports the pelvis and shoulders in proper alignment.

FIGURE 21–10

healing. An order is required before a bed cradle and heat are used. Care must be taken with heat lamps to prevent burns.

The patient must not come close to the metal of the cradle or the light. Care must be taken to position the limb within the cradle. It may be necessary to pad the cradle edges.

Footboard or Footrest

The **footboard** or footrest is a device placed between the mattress and bed to keep the foot at right angles to the legs (natural standing position). A footboard is always padded in use. It is used to prevent **footdrop**. Footdrop may happen when the patient must remain in bed over a long period of time. In footdrop, the muscle in the calf of the leg tends to tighten, causing the toes to point downward. Even a brief period in bed is sufficient to cause a degree of footdrop that makes walking difficult when the patient does get out of bed.

If a footboard is not available, a pillow folded lengthwise may be placed against the foot of the bed and may serve the same purpose.

Pillows

Pillows can be used as comfort devices and to maintain alignment when properly arranged. Figures 21–10A through 21–10H show different arrangements. For directions on properly altering the patient's positions, refer again to Unit 13.

A **trochanter roll** or support can be made as follows:
1. Fold a bath blanket lengthwise in thirds.
2. Position patient in center of folded bath blanket. Blanket should extend from mid thigh to above the waist.

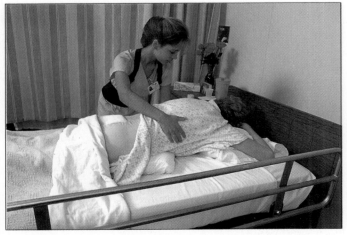

FIGURE 21–11. This patient is positioned on his abdomen and pillows are used to form a bridge, preventing pressure on his genitals.

Chart of Positions	
■ Semi-Fowler's	■ Left lateral recumbent
■ Dorsal recumbent	■ Right lateral recumbent
■ Prone	

FIGURE 21–12. Unless contraindicated, patients are routinely positioned in a sequential manner.

3. Roll each side of the blanket under and toward the patient until the blanket roll is firmly against the patient. Then tuck roll inward toward bed and patient to maintain patient's position.

Pillows are also used to relieve pressure. This technique is called **bridging**, Figure 21–11. See Figure 21–12 for a chart of positions.

Range of Motion Exercises

Range of motion (ROM) exercises are routinely performed during the morning care. They are also done at other times during the day, Figure 21–13. ROM exercises:
- ■ Prevent deformities.
- ■ Increase respiratory and circulatory activity.
- ■ Help maintain muscle tone.
- ■ Reduce the discomfort of stiffness.
- ■ Are presented in Unit 35.

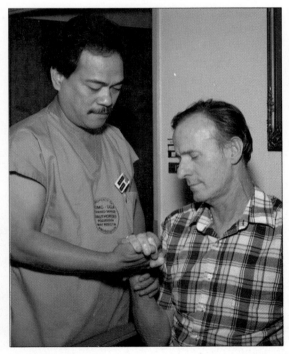

FIGURE 21–13. Range of motion exercises help prevent permanent deformities.

Elimination Needs

Regular, periodic elimination of body wastes is essential for maintaining health. Patients who are confined to bed must rely on you to help them with this physical task. You have learned about the structure and function of the urinary system and the bowel in Unit 4. You should also know that:

- The patient must regularly empty the bladder by urinating (voiding).
- A urinal (duct or bottle) is used by male patients when they need to urinate. A bedpan is used by female patients to void when they are confined to bed.
- A regular bowel movement (which is the discharge of solid waste from the body) is also important to a patient's health.
- The solid waste produced by the patient is called feces or stool.

- Both male and female patients use a bedpan for solid elimination when confined to bed.
- Many patients are somewhat sensitive about using a bedpan or urinal.
- Personal hygiene is exceedingly important in carrying out these procedures properly.
- Bedpans are very uncomfortable.

Four important factors must be kept in mind. You must:

1. Wear disposable gloves.
2. Wash your hands immediately before and after the procedure. This will help prevent the transmission of any disease to others and to yourself.
3. Provide privacy for the patient. Obtain the proper bedpan according to patient needs.
4. As soon as possible answer the light indicating the patient is finished.

PROCEDURE 73 | **OBRA**   SIDE **7**

GIVING AND RECEIVING THE BEDPAN

1. Carry out each beginning procedure action.
2. Remember to wash your hands, identify the patient, and provide privacy.
3. Assemble equipment needed:
   - Bedpan and cover
   - Basin of warm water
   - Washcloth
   - Disposable gloves
   - Paper towels/protector
   - Toilet tissue
   - Soap
   - Towel
4. If raised, lower the head of the bed.
5. Take the bedpan and tissue from the bedside stand.
   - Place protector on bedside chair. Place bedpan, Figure 21–14, on it.
   - Never place it on the side stand or over-bed table.
   - Put the remainder of the articles on the bedside table.
6. Place bedpan cover at the foot of the bed between the mattress and springs.
   - The bedpan may be warmed by running hot water into it and then emptying it.
   - In hot weather, talcum powder may be used on the bedpan to prevent the patient's skin from sticking to it.

- Plastic bed pans may be comfortable without warming.

NOTE: Never carry or allow a used bedpan to sit uncovered. If a bedpan cover is not available, cover the bedpan with a towel, pillowcase, or paper towels.

7. Put on disposable gloves.
8. Fold top bedcovers back at a right angle. Raise the patient's gown. If the patient is thin or has

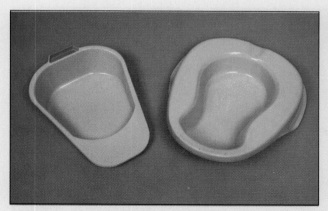

FIGURE 21–14. Orthopedic bedpan (left) and regular bedpan (right)

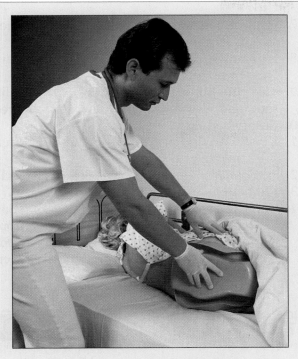

FIGURE 21–15. Roll patient away from yourself while supporting patient with one hand on patient's hip and arm. Place bedpan with the other hand. Then roll patient back onto bedpan.

a pressure sore, consult the nurse for the appropriate action. The nursing care plan may have specific instructions for such cases. For example, it may be necessary to pad the bedpan with a folded towel or take some other action.

9. Ask patient to flex knees and rest weight on heels, if able.
10. Help the patient to raise buttocks by:
    - Putting one hand under the small of the patient's back and lifting gently and slowly with one hand.
    - With the other hand, place the bedpan under the patient's hips.
    - If the patient is unable to raise the buttocks, two assistants may be needed to lift the patient.
    - The pan may also be placed by rolling the patient to one side, positioning the bedpan against the buttocks, and rolling the patient back on it, Figure 21–15. Check to be sure bedpan is positioned properly.

- Alternatively, if a trapeze is in place over the bed, place the bedpan under the patient as the patient lifts self using the trapeze, Figure 21–16.
- The patient's buttocks should rest on the rounded shelf of the bedpan.
- The narrow end should face foot of bed.

11. Replace top bedcovers. Raise the head of the bed to a comfortable height. Remove gloves and dispose of properly.
12. Make sure the signal cord is within easy reach of the patient. Leave the patient alone unless contraindicated in the nursing care plan.
13. Wash your hands. Watch for patient's signal.
14. Answer the patient's call signal immediately. Fill the basin with warm water and get soap, washcloth, and towel. Put on disposable gloves.
15. Remove bedpan from under patient.
    - Ask the patient to flex knees and rest weight on heels. Place one hand under the small of the back and lift gently to help raise the buttocks off bedpan. Take the bedpan with the other hand. Cover it and place it on the chair.

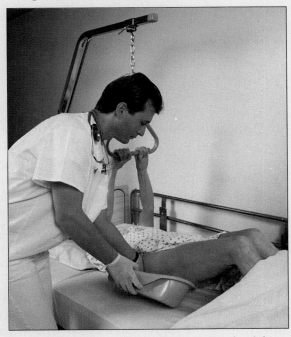

FIGURE 21–16. The patient assists by lifting with the trapeze as the nursing assistant places the bedpan under patient. Note that the nursing assistant supports the patient's back with hand.

continues

■ If the patient is unable to raise the buttocks, two assistants may be needed to lift. Otherwise, roll the patient off the pan to the side and remove the pan. Lift and move carefully. Hold the pan firmly with one hand.

■ Many patients have difficulty cleaning adequately after using the bedpan. You may need to clean and dry the patient yourself.

16. Assist the patient to a clean area of the bed, if necessary.

■ Discard tissue in bedpan unless specimen is to be collected.

■ Cover bedpan again and place protector on chair.

■ Cleanse patient with warm water and soap, if necessary.

17. Replace bedclothes, changing linen or protective pads as necessary.
18. Encourage the patient to wash hands and freshen up after the procedures.
19. Take the bedpan to the bathroom or utility room and observe contents. Measure, if required.
20. Empty bedpan.
21. Rinse with cold water and disinfectant. Rinse, dry, and cover bedpan.
22. Remove gloves and dispose of them properly.
23. Put bedpan inside patient's bedside table.
24. Carry out each procedure completion action. Remember to wash your hands, report completion of task, and document time, voided/defecated—amount/character, and patient reaction.

PROCEDURE 74 — OBRA

SIDE 7

GIVING AND RECEIVING THE URINAL

1. Carry out each beginning procedure action.
2. Remember to wash your hands, identify the patient, and provide privacy.
3. Assemble equipment needed:
   ■ Urinal, Figure 21–17
   ■ Basin of warm water
   ■ Soap
   ■ Washcloth
   ■ Towel
   ■ Disposable gloves
4. Put on gloves. Lift the top bedcovers and place the urinal under the covers so the patient may grasp the handle. If he cannot do this you must place the urinal in position and ensure the penis is placed in the opening.
5. Remove gloves and dispose of them properly. Make sure the signal cord is within easy reach of the patient. Leave the patient alone if possible, but watch for his signal.
6. Answer the patient's signal immediately. Never leave urinal in position for any length of time during the night. Fill a basin with warm water, and lay out the soap, washcloth, and towel, so patient can wash and dry hands.
7. Put on gloves. Ask the patient to hand the urinal to you. Cover it. Rearrange bedclothes if necessary.

8. Take the urinal to the bathroom or utility room and observe the contents. Measure, if required. Do not empty urinal if anything unusual (such as blood) is observed. Rather, save the contents of the urinal for your supervisor's inspection.
9. Empty the urinal. Rinse with cold water, and clean with warm soapy water. Rinse, dry, and cover urinal. Remove gloves and dispose of them properly.
10. Place urinal inside patient's bedside table. Clean and replace other articles.
11. Carry out each procedure completion action. Remember to wash your hands, report completion of task, and document time, voided—amount/character, and patient reaction.

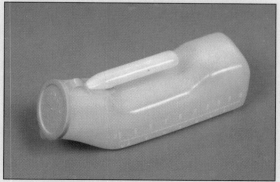

FIGURE 21–17. Male urinal

PROCEDURE 75 | OBRA

SIDE 7

ASSISTING WITH THE USE OF THE BEDSIDE COMMODE

1. Carry out each beginning procedure action.
2. Remember to wash your hands, identify the patient, and provide privacy.
3. Assemble equipment needed:
   - Portable commode
   - Toilet tissue
   - Basin of warm water
   - Washcloth and soap
   - Towel
   - Disposable gloves
4. Position commode beside bed, facing head. Lock wheels and remove cover. Be sure receptacle is in place under seat, Figure 21–18.
5. If bed and side rails are elevated, lower side rail nearest you and lower bed to lowest horizontal position. Lock bed wheels.
6. Assist patient to sitting position. Swing patient's legs over edge of bed.
7. Put slippers on patient. Assist patient to stand.
8. Have patient place hands on your shoulders. If needed, use a transfer belt.
9. Support patient with hands on either side of the chest. Remember to use proper body mechanics. Pivot patient to the right and lower to commode.
10. Leave call bell and tissue within reach.
11. When patient signals, return promptly. Draw warm water in basin. Bring basin to bedside along with soap, towel, and washcloth. Put on gloves.
12. Assist patient to stand.
13. Cleanse anus or perineum if patient is unable to help self.
14. Allow patient to wash and dry hands.
15. Assist patient to return to bed. Adjust bedding and pillows for comfort.

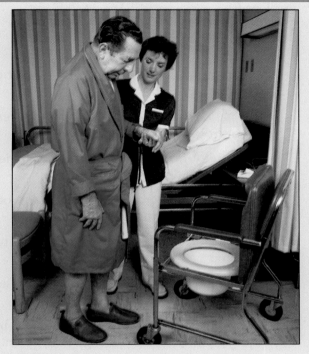

FIGURE 21–18. The bedside commode

16. Leave signal cord within easy reach.
17. Put cover on commode.
18. Remove receptacle. Cover with bedpan cover.
19. Take to bathroom. Note contents and measure if required.
20. Empty and clean per facility policy. Return to commode. Remove and dispose of gloves properly.
21. Put commode in proper place.
22. Carry out each procedure completion action. Remember to wash your hands, report completion of task, and document time, voided/defecated—amount/character, and patient reaction.

SUMMARY

There are several measures that you can take to add to the general comfort of the patient. These measures include:
- Caring for the patient's teeth and hair.
- Shaving the patient.
- Using specific devices such as footboards and bed cradles.
- Giving back rubs to soothe and stimulate.
- Meeting elimination needs promptly and providing privacy.

UNIT REVIEW

A. True/False. Answer the following true or false by circling T or F.

(T) F 1. Plastic dentures should be stored in an antiseptic solution.

(T) F 2. Back rubs are routinely given as part of the bath procedure.

(T) F 3. A padded footboard is used to prevent footdrop.

T (F) 4. Routine oral hygiene should be carried out once daily.

(T) F 5. Proper oral hygiene helps prevent tooth decay.

T (F) 6. When not in the patient's mouth, dentures should be left on the bedside stand.

(T) F 7. Glycerine and honey swabs are often used for special oral care.

(T) F 8. The assistant's long fingernails could injure a patient when care is being given.

(T) F 9. Disposable gloves should be used by a nursing assistant giving oral care.

T (F) 10. The unconscious patient needs no oral care since he is not eating.

B. Matching. Match Column I with Column II.

Column I	Column II
_e_ 11. bad breath	a. oral hygiene
_a_ 12. mouth care	b. caries
_b_ 13. tooth cavities	c. dentures
_d_ 14. means of relieving pressure	d. bridging
	e. halitosis
_c_ 15. artificial teeth	f. footdrop

C. Multiple Choice. Choose the phrase that best completes each of the following sentences by circling the proper letter.

16. Which of the following patients should be given special mouth care?
    a. One who can brush her own teeth
    b. One who is drinking water ad lib
    c. One who has a broken leg
    d. One who has a high fever

17. To warm lotion before giving a back rub,
    a. hold it under running water.
    b. soak it in a basin of warm water.
    c. let the patient hold the bottle for a few minutes.
    d. None of the above.

18. The best way to support a patient in a side-lying position is to
    a. use a footboard to keep the feet aligned.
    b. place a pillow doubled under the head.
    c. place two pillows lengthwise between the legs.
    d. double a pillow lengthwise behind the back.

19. When brushing a patient's teeth, the best technique includes
    a. inserting the toothbrush with the bristles in a downward position.
    b. brushing in a circular motion.
    c. inserting the toothbrush with bristles facing the teeth.
    d. brushing the teeth in a downward motion only.

20. Back rubs are given
    a. routinely as part of the cleansing bed bath.
    b. following the use of the bedpan.
    c. when changing the position of the helpless patient.
    d. All of the above.

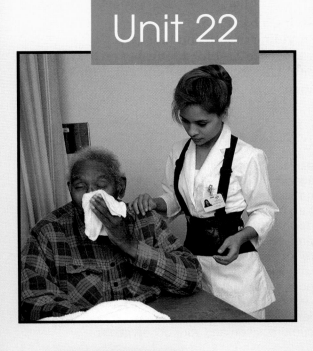

Unit 22

Early Morning and Bedtime Care

As a result of this unit, you will be able to:

- Spell and define terms.
- Demonstrate the procedures for early morning care.
- Demonstrate the procedures for bedtime care.
- Discuss the reasons for early morning and bedtime care.

Learn the meaning and the correct spelling of the following words:

AM care
PM care

Early Morning (AM) Care

This initial care is called early morning or AM care. It helps to set the tone for the entire day. If the patient is refreshed and comfortable before eating breakfast, the day is off to a good start.

The patient is:
- Awakened gently, never abruptly, by placing your hand on the patient's arm and saying patient's name.
- Awakened before breakfast.
- Given the opportunity to use the bathroom if allowed up, or to use a bedpan or urinal.
- Helped to wash his face and hands.

The patient is not awakened early if:
- Going to surgery. ← *NPO*
- Having tests that prohibit eating.

Bedtime (PM) Care

The care given to the patient just before bedtime is similar to that given in the early morning. Bedtime care is called PM care (or HS care).

PM care is given:
- In a quiet, unrushed manner, which will help the patient settle down more easily for sleep.

■ Before medication for sleep is given by the nurse.

Other routine procedures may be carried out during the AM and PM care. These include:

■ Measuring vital signs.

■ Giving a back rub.
■ Providing mouth and hair care.

Refer to Figure 22–1 for a refresher on the routines to be completed at the beginning and completion of each patient care procedure.

BEGINNING PROCEDURE ACTIONS	PROCEDURE COMPLETION ACTIONS
■ Wash your hands. ■ Assemble equipment. ■ Go to the patient's room, knock, and pause before entering. ■ Introduce yourself and identify the patient by checking the identification bracelet. ■ Ask visitors to leave and inform them where they can wait. ■ Provide privacy. ■ Explain what will happen. Answer questions. ■ Raise bed to comfortable working height.	■ Position patient comfortably. ■ Leave signal cord, telephone, and fresh water close at hand. ■ Return bed to lowest position. ■ Perform general safety check of patient and environment. ■ Care for equipment according to facility policy. ■ Wash your hands. ■ Report completion of task. ■ Let visitors know when they may reenter the patient's room. ■ Document action and your observations.

NOTE: Where there are open lesions, wet linen, or possible contact with patient body fluids or blood, disposable gloves are worn during the procedure. Put on gloves before contact with the patient or linen. Properly dispose of gloves after they are removed. ALWAYS APPLY UNIVERSAL PRECAUTIONS.

FIGURE 22–1.   Beginning procedure actions and procedure completion actions

PROCEDURE 76   OBRA

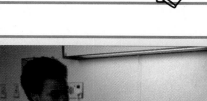

PROVIDING EARLY MORNING (AM) CARE

1. Carry out each beginning procedure action.
2. Remember to wash your hands, identify the patient, and provide privacy.
3. Assemble equipment needed:
   - ■ Wash water
   - ■ Toilet articles
   - ■ Lotion
   - ■ Equipment to measure vital signs
   - ■ Bedpan/urinal
4. Awaken patient gently by placing a hand on the patient's arm and saying patient's name.
5. Offer the bedpan or urinal. Save specimens if ordered.
6. Take routine vital signs (temperature, pulse, blood pressure, and respiration).
7. Provide wash water and toilet articles, Figure 22–2. Assist patient if necessary.
8. Provide for care of mouth and hair. Assist as necessary.
9. Give back rub. Give special attention to pressure areas.

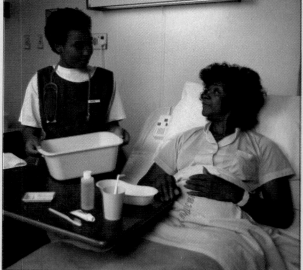

FIGURE 22–2.   Provide the patient with wash water and toilet articles.

10. Tighten the lower sheet and straighten the top linen. Change linens if soiled.

11. Change the patient's gown if soiled.

    Some patients may request to wear their own pajamas or to dress in street clothing. For these situations follow this procedure:

    a. Place all clothing together in the order in which it will be put on.

    b. If a female patient wishes to wear a bra:
       - Fold bath blanket down to waist.
       - Slide the straps up over both arms and up over the shoulders.
       - Bring the bra cups down over the breasts for a comfortable fit.
       - Have the patient lean forward while you hook the bra.

    c. Put the shirt, blouse, or pajama top on next. Remember, if the patient has a weak arm, put this arm in first as described in Unit 20.
       - Gather up one sleeve and place it over the patient's hand.
       - Draw the sleeve up the arm and shoulder as far as possible.
       - Ask the patient to lean forward while you bring the garment across the patient's back.
       - Bend the patient's elbow and bring the sleeve down over the patient's hand and then draw it up the arm.
       - Adjust the garment so it is comfortable and button or snap.

    d. If the patient is wearing shorts or panties:
       - Fold the bath blanket to above the patient's knees.
       - Place both of the patient's feet through the openings of the shorts or panties.
       - Draw the garment up over both legs, to the hips.
       - Ask the patient to raise her hips as you slide the garment up over the hips.
       - If the patient is unable to raise her hips, ask her to turn to the side as you bring the garment up as far as possible—then have the patient turn to the opposite side as you bring the garment up as far as possible.

    e. If the patient can sit on the edge of the bed and then stand, it is easier to put the top garment on with the patient in this position.
       - Put the shorts or panties on, bringing them up as far as the knees.
       - Put the slacks or pajama bottoms on next, bringing them up as far as the knees.
       - Have the patient stand and bring the garments up, one at a time, over the patient's hips.
       - Snap, button, or buckle the belt.

    f. Put the socks on the patient:
       - Roll them to the toe
       - Place a sock over the patient's toes and smooth it down over the foot and up over the heel.
       - Adjust sock for smooth fit.
       - Repeat with other sock.

    g. Put shoes on the patient:
       - Place shoe over toes and then up over heel.
       - Use shoehorn if necessary.
       - Fasten shoe.

    To undress patient, reverse procedure.

12. Clear the over-bed table and adjust the backrest of the bed, if permitted, so that breakfast may be served to the patient.

13. Carry out each procedure completion action. Remember to wash your hands, report completion of task, and document time, AM care, and patient reaction.

PROCEDURE 77 | OBRA

PROVIDING BEDTIME (PM) CARE

1. Carry out each beginning procedure action.
2. Remember to wash your hands, identify the patient, and provide privacy.
3. Assemble equipment needed:
   - Nourishment as permitted
   - Wash water
   - Bedpan/urinal
   - Toilet articles
   - Lotion
4. If permitted, offer nourishment.
5. Offer bedpan or urinal.
6. Provide wash water and toilet articles. Assist with hair and mouth care as necessary.
7. Give back rub. Give special attention to pressure areas.
8. Tighten lower sheet. Then straighten the top linen. Change linens if soiled.
9. Change patient's gown if soiled.
10. Push over-bed table to foot of bed or place it parallel to the bed with water within reach. Put bed in lowest horizontal position and side rails up, Figure 22–3.
11. Remove dish/glass from nourishment and any unnecessary equipment from room according to hospital policy.
12. Leave fresh water and signal cord within reach of patient.
13. Once you have completed PM care and patient is comfortable turn off over-bed light, Figure 22–4.
14. Carry out each procedure completion action. Remember to wash your hands, report completion of task, and document time, bedtime care, side rails up, and patient reaction.

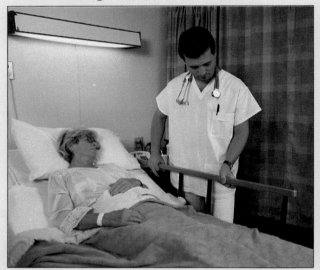

FIGURE 22–3. Side rails must be positioned according to facility policy. Make sure the call bell is close at hand.

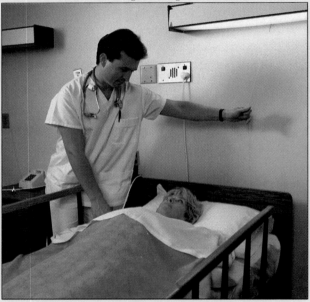

FIGURE 22–4. When you are sure patient is settled and comfortable, turn off light.

SUMMARY

Early morning or AM care:
■ Refreshes the patient before breakfast.
■ Prepares the patient for the day.
Bedtime care is a similar procedure that is followed in the evening before sleep. It helps the patient to:
■ Relax.
■ Prepare for sleep.

Other procedures may be combined during AM and PM care. They include:
■ Serving nourishment.
■ Mouth care.
■ Hair care.
■ Routine vital signs.
■ Back care.
■ Dressing/undressing.

UNIT REVIEW

A. True/False. Answer the following true or false by circling T or F.

T F 1. Patients should never be awakened abruptly.

T F 2. When giving bedtime PM care, the bottom sheet should be tightened and the top linen straightened.

T F 3. After PM care, the bed should be left with the backrest up.

T F 4. The best way to awaken a patient is to stand at the door of the room and call the patient's name.

T F 5. PM care should be completed before sleep medication is given.

T F 6. Mouth and hair care are part of early AM care.

T F 7. AM care is given immediately after breakfast trays are served.

T F 8. All unnecessary equipment should be removed from the patient's room after PM care.

T F 9. If permitted, nourishments should be offered as part of AM care.

T F 10. Side rails must be up at the completion of PM care.

SELF-EVALUATION   Section 7

A. Choose the phrase that best completes each of the following sentences by circling the proper letter.

1. When making an occupied bed, remember
   a. the unit need not be screened.
   b. toepleats may be omitted.
   c. one side of the bottom is made at a time.
   d. one complete side of the bed is made at a time.

2. During the patient's bed bath
   a. the patient is completely uncovered.
   b. the water is changed to maintain warmth.
   c. the unit is not screened.
   d. the top linen remains in place.

3. If a patient tells you he plans to leave the hospital without his doctor's permission, you should
   a. notify the supervising nurse at once.
   b. discuss the problem with other assistants.
   c. try to talk the patient out of it.
   d. call his family and tell them of the patient's plans.

4. When admitting a patient, remember
   a. allow the patient to keep large amounts of money at the bedside.
   b. tell the family to leave because you have work to do.
   c. be courteous and helpful to both the patient and family.
   d. None of the above.

5. During the admission procedure, you will
   a. observe the patient carefully.
   b. take vital signs.
   c. help the patient undress and get into bed.
   d. All of the above.

6. What type of bed is made after a patient is discharged?
   a. Open bed
   b. Surgical bed
   c. Closed bed
   d. Circle bed

7. An open bed is made by
   a. fanfolding the top bedclothes to the foot of the bed.
   b. adding an extra pillow.
   c. leaving the top bedding off.
   d. padding the bottom linen.

8. When gathering linen to make a bed
   a. put the spread on the top of the pile.
   b. include a bath blanket.
   c. include a drawsheet.
   d. put linen in order of use.

9. When making an unoccupied bed
   a. make the entire bottom of the bed first.
   b. change the pillowcase first.
   c. make one entire side first.
   d. place the bottom sheet even with the head of the mattress.

10. Pillowcases should
    a. face the open doorway.
    b. face away from the open doorway.
    c. face in any direction since it doesn't matter.
    d. face the foot of the bed.

11. Before leaving the patient after making an occupied bed, be sure that
    a. the bed is in the highest horizontal position.
    b. the top bedding has been tucked in with a square corner.
    c. the head of the bed is elevated.
    d. the side rails are up.

12. Documentation related to admission should include
    a. date.
    b. time.
    c. pertinent observations.
    d. All of the above.

13. Documentation related to discharge should include
    a. presence of visitors.
    b. method of transport.
    c. report of final urine specimen.
    d. response of other patients.

14. After discharge
    a. return wheelchair if used.
    b. strip unit.
    c. clean and replace all used equipment.
    d. All of the above.

15. When a patient is admitted, you should
    a. determine the proper transportation.
    b. check on the need for special equipment.
    c. observe the patient carefully.
    d. All of the above.

16. When asking visitors to leave
    a. tell them abruptly they can't stay.
    b. let them know how long you will be.
    c. don't take the time to tell them about a refreshment area or lounge.
    d. All of the above.

17. When discharging a patient
    a. allow the patient to walk from the unit to the outside.
    b. throw all disposables away.
    c. call the doctor to check the patient's order.
    d. gather all the patient's belongings and assist with packing.

18. If a patient says she intends to leave without permission, you should
    a. do nothing. It is the patient's decision.
    b. report immediately to your supervisor.
    c. start gathering the patient's belongings.
    d. call the doctor.

19. A good back rub should take about
    a. 1 minute.
    b. 3–5 minutes.
    c. 10 minutes.
    d. 20 minutes.

20. When not in the patient's mouth, dentures should be
    a. left on the bed.
    b. placed on the bedside table.
    c. placed in a container on the bedside table.
    d. left on the bathroom shelf.

21. When giving a bedpan or urinal always
    a. pad the receptacle.
    b. provide privacy.
    c. allow visitors to remain.
    d. disconnect the call bell.

22. To wake a patient
    a. rap loudly on the door.
    b. call the patient's name loudly.
    c. gently place your hand on the patient's arm.
    d. shake the patient vigorously.

23. Bedtime care includes
    a. offering the bedpan.
    b. washing hands and face.
    c. giving a back rub.
    d. All of the above.

24. On admission, the patient should have his
    a. temperature taken.
    b. pulse determined.
    c. weight determined.
    d. All of the above.

25. Identify the patient by asking her name and
    a. checking her chart.
    b. asking a visitor.
    c. asking the charge nurse.
    d. checking the identification bracelet.

26. Valuables brought with the patient to the hospital should be listed and left
    a. in the patient's locker.
    b. at the bedside.
    c. in the hospital safe.
    d. on the patient.

27. The proper temperature of bath water is
    a. 90°F.
    b. 105°F.
    c. 115°F.
    d. 120°F.

28. Nursing assistants are responsible for seeing to the completion of the patient's bathing if
    a. they feel like it.
    b. the supervisor tells them.
    c. the patient cannot.
    d. the patient asks.

29. When giving a bed bath, expose
    a. the entire body at one time.
    b. the part to be washed.
    c. both legs at one time.
    d. one whole side of the body.

30. A female nursing assistant may refuse to wash the genitals of a helpless male patient
    a. because she doesn't want to be embarrassed.
    b. because someone else will do it.
    c. because no one will know.
    d. None of the above.

31. If the patient is receiving an IV and his gown needs to be changed, the assistant will
    a. discontinue the IV.
    b. call the team leader to disconnect the IV.
    c. remove the patient's gown using the proper technique, keeping the IV flowing.
    d. cut off the patient's gown.

32. Patients should be encouraged to help as much as possible during morning care because
    a. the assistant has many patients and the work will be done faster.
    b. it stimulates the patient's general physiology.
    c. you don't want the patient to get too tired.
    d. None of the above.

33. Before the bath procedure
    a. tighten the bottom bedding.
    b. loosen the top bedding.
    c. place two pillows under the patient's head.
    d. remove the laundry hamper from the room.

34. When preparing to give a bed bath, include in your supplies
    a. bed linen and gown.
    b. bath basin.
    c. lotion or powder.
    d. All of the above.

B. **Match Column I with Column II.**

Column I	Column II
_____ 35. caries	a. artificial teeth
_____ 36. halitosis	b. toes involuntarily point down
_____ 37. dentures	
_____ 38. footdrop	c. dental cavities
_____ 39. early (AM) care	d. care given before breakfast
	e. care given before bedtime
	f. unpleasant breath

C. **Answer the following statements true or false by circling T or F.**

T F 40. Nail care is not part of the routine morning care.

T F 41. If a patient feels faint while taking a shower, stay and signal for help.

T F 42. The bathtub need only be rinsed between patients.

T F 43. Bed shampoos may be given without a physician's order.

T F 44. A patient going to surgery at 8 AM should be wakened for breakfast.

T F 45. Adjust bed to comfortable working height before starting an in-bed procedure.

T F 46. Daily shaving of the face is a routine for most male patients.

T F 47. Handwashing need only be performed after completing a patient care procedure.

T F 48. A used bedpan need not be covered when carrying it to the patient's bathroom.

T F 49. When placing a bedpan under a patient, the buttocks should rest on the rounded shelf of the pan.

T F 50. Bed cradles do not need to be padded since their only purpose is to keep the weight of the bedding from the patient's feet.

T F 51. Gloves should be worn when shaving a patient.

T F 52. A trochanter roll should extend from above to below the waist of the patient.

T F 53. Unconscious patients do not require oral care.

T F 54. If a person is dehydrated, oral care is especially important.

T F 55. Gloves should be worn when giving male or female perineal care.

T F 56. Perineal care should be performed each time a patient is incontinent.

T F 57. It is important to provide privacy during perineal care.

T F 58. The washcloth should be rinsed after each side of the labia has been washed.

D. Provide short answers to the following.

59. How might a female patient who cannot separate her legs sufficiently for perineal care be positioned? _____

_____

60. When a male patient has not been circumcised, what special precaution must you take with respect to the foreskin during perineal care?

_____

_____

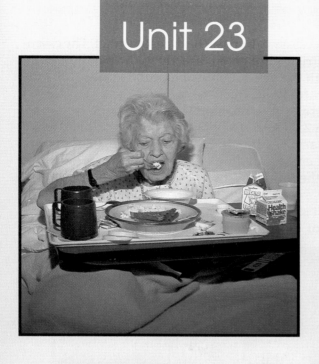

Unit 23

Nutritional Needs and Diet Modifications

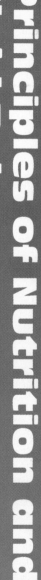

OBJECTIVES

As a result of this unit, you will be able to:

- Spell and define terms.
- Define normal nutrition.
- List types of alternative nutrition.
- List the essential nutrients.
- Name the six food groups and list the foods included in each group.
- State the liquids/foods allowed on the five basic facility diets.
- Describe the purposes of the following diets:
  —clear liquid
  —full liquid
  —soft
  —light
- State the purposes of therapeutic diets.
- Describe the nursing assistant actions when patients are unable to drink fluids independently.
- Feed the helpless patient.

VOCABULARY

Learn the meaning and the correct spelling of the following words:

amino acids
carbohydrates
cellulose
defecation
digestion
enteral feeding
essential nutrients
exchange list
fats
forcing fluids
gastrostomy tube
gavage

hyperalimentation
intravenous infusion (IV)
minerals
nasogastric tube
nutrients
nutrition
protein
total parenteral nutrition (TPN)
therapeutic diets
vitamins

Nutrition is the entire process by which the body takes in food for growth and repair and uses it to maintain health. The signs of good nutrition include:

- Shiny hair
- Clear skin and eyes
- A well-developed body
- An alert expression
- A pleasant disposition
- Healthy sleep patterns
- Appropriate appetite
- Regular bowel habits
- Body weight appropriate to height

98.6

Normal Nutrition

Food is normally taken into the body through the mouth. The mouth is the beginning of the digestive tract. Digestion is the process of breaking down foods into simple substances that can be used by the body cells for nourishment. These substances are called essential nutrients

Alternative Nutrition

When there is disease of the digestive tract or other reasons why food cannot be taken in the normal way, it is necessary to bypass the digestive tract. The essential nutrients are given directly to the patient's body through the veins. Remember, this is called intravenous infusion (IV).

Nurses start and monitor intravenous infusions, Figure 23–1A–E. They change bottles or bags when necessary. You must be alert to bottles or bags that are nearly empty. Call this to the attention of the nurse *before* the fluid runs out.

The speed at which the IV solution enters the patient's body is called the flow rate. The flow rate (rate of flow measured in drops per minute) is

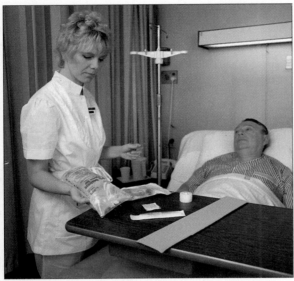

FIGURE 23–1A. Following the nurse's instructions, assemble the necessary equipment and solution for the infusion of nutrients.

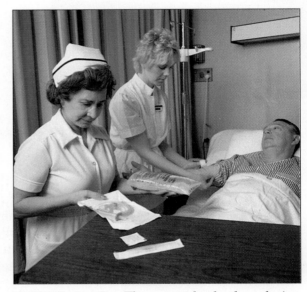

FIGURE 23–1B. The nurse checks the solution to be given.

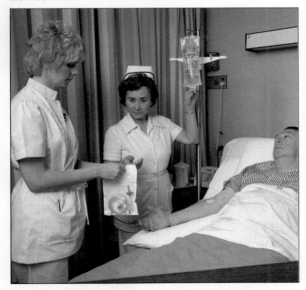

FIGURE 23–1C. Carefully open the tubing package using the proper technique. The nurse then sets up the rest of the equipment.

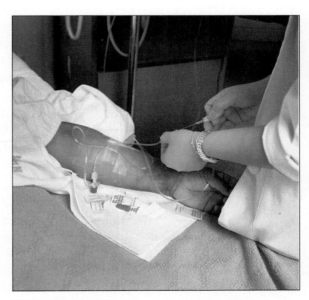

FIGURE 23–1D. The nurse starts the intravenous infusion and adds medication.

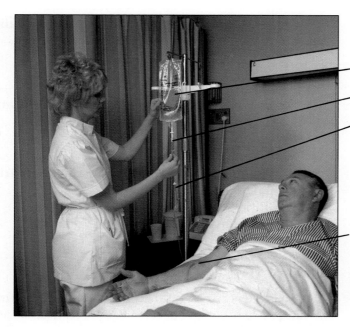

Fluid level in plastic container

Drip chamber

Tubing

Infusion site

FIGURE 23–1E. The nursing assistant may monitor the level of fluid in the container, the drip chamber, the tubing, and the infusion site. The nursing assistant makes *no* adjustments to the IV setup.

ordered by the physician. Actual determination of the flow rate is the responsibility of the nurse. To assist the nurse, you must:

- Know and check how fast the IV fluid is flowing. If the patient is receiving fluid through an infusion pump, notify the nurse if the alarm sounds.
- Report to the nurse if the drip chamber is full.
- Report to the nurse if the flow rate is faster or slower than ordered, or if there is blood in the tubing.
- Report to the nurse if the drip has stopped or the IV drops are continuous.
- Check the infusion site frequently and report signs of redness, swelling, pain or leaking.

Hyperalimentation, or total parenteral nutrition (TPN), is a technique in which high density (concentrated) nutrients are introduced into a large vein such as the subclavian vein or the superior vena cava.

Specially prepared commercial formulas are used for this purpose.

Nutrients may also be provided through a:

- Nasogastric tube feeding (enteral feeding)—a tube leading through the nose and down into the stomach, Figure 23–2.
- Gastrostomy tube—a tube inserted through the abdominal wall into the stomach.

Gavage, or tube feeding, Figures 23–3A and B, requires special skill to be sure of the correct location of the tube. The nurse will carry out this procedure. A prepared commercial formula is used or foods are

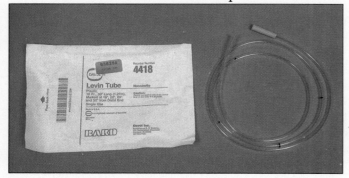

FIGURE 23–2. The nasogastric tube

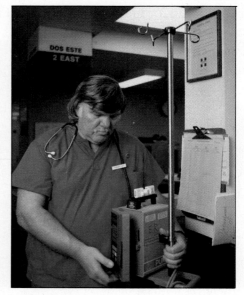

FIGURE 23–3A. Collect the equipment used in your facility to administer an automatic controlled feeding.

73 = 100
220

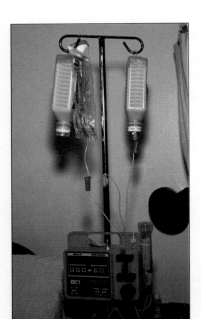

FIGURE 23–3B.
Liquid nutrient ready
for a gavage.

blended into a liquid form and then introduced into the body through the tube.

The nursing assistant has specific responsibilities when patients are on tube feedings. In addition to offering comfort and support, Figure 23–4, the nursing assistant:

- Keeps head of bed elevated 45°–60° during feeding and for 1/2 hour after feeding.
- Checks taping of tubes. If taping is loose, inform the nurse.
- Reports any retching, nausea, or vomiting immediately.
- Checks tubing for kinks. Be sure patient is not lying on tubing.

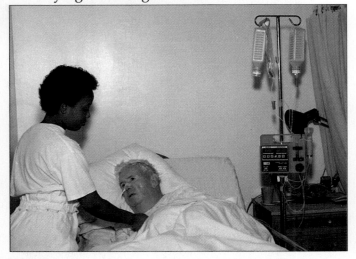

FIGURE 23–4. You can offer comfort and support during the gavage.

- Ensures end of tube is closed between feedings.
- Provides more frequent mouth hygiene.

Essential Nutrients

To be well nourished, we must eat foods that:
- Supply heat and energy.
- Build and repair body tissue.
- Regulate body functions.

These foods are called **nutrients**. The six nutrients essential to maintain health are:

- Proteins
- Carbohydrates
- Fats
- Minerals
- Vitamins
- Water

Protein

Protein is an essential nutrient. It is the basic material of every body cell. It is the only nutrient that can make new cells and rebuild tissue. The foods that contain the greatest amount of protein come from animals. They include:

- Meat
- Poultry
- Eggs
- Milk
- Cheese

Proteins are made of small building blocks (**amino acids**). The body can manufacture some of the amino acids. It cannot manufacture all of them.

- Complete proteins—are proteins that contain all the amino acids the body cannot manufacture. Examples of complete proteins are meat, fish, eggs, and poultry.
- Incomplete proteins—although still important, do not contain all the essential amino acids. Essential amino acids are those that must be obtained through foods. Examples of incomplete proteins are corn, soybeans, peas, and nuts.

Carbohydrates and Fats

Carbohydrates and **fats** are called energy foods because the body uses them to produce heat and energy. When a person eats more energy foods than the body needs, the remainder is stored as fat. Foods that contain the greatest amount of carbohydrates come from plants. They include:

- Fruits
- Vegetables
- Foods that are made from grains such as breads, cereals, and pasta products

Carbohydrate foods also supply the body with roughage (**cellulose**). Cellulose is important in maintaining bowel regularity.

Fats come from both plants and animals. Examples of foods that are rich in fat include:

- Pork
- Butter
- Nuts
- Egg yolk
- Cheese

Vitamins and Minerals

Vitamins and minerals are present in a wide variety of foods. The best way to be sure that you are getting enough vitamins and minerals is to include a variety of foods in the daily diet.

Vitamins are substances that regulate body processes. They help to:

- Build strong teeth and bones.
- Promote growth.
- Aid normal body functioning.
- Strengthen resistance to disease.

You probably know the vitamins by their letter names:

- Vitamin A
- B-complex vitamins
- Vitamin C
- Vitamin D
- Vitamin E
- Vitamin K

Fat-soluble vitamins do not dissolve easily in water. They can be stored in the body. Vitamins A, D, E, and K are fat-soluble vitamins.

Vitamins B and C are water soluble. Water-soluble vitamins dissolve in water. They can be lost in the cooking process. In general, these vitamins are not stored in large amounts. Deficiencies in water-soluble vitamins are more common.

Minerals help to build body tissues, especially the bones and teeth. They also regulate the chemistry of body fluids such as the blood and digestive juices.

Minerals needed in our daily diet include:

- Calcium
- Phosphorus
- Iodine
- Iron
- Copper
- Potassium

Vitamins & Minerals are electrolytes

The Six Food Groups

The U.S. Department of Agriculture has recently revised the recommendations for a balanced food intake. The guidelines include:

- Eat a variety of foods.
- Maintain a healthy body weight.
- Select foods low in fat, saturated fat, and cholesterol.
- Select plenty of vegetables, fruits, and grain products.
- Use sugar in moderation.
- Use salt and sodium in moderation.
- Drink alcoholic beverages in moderation, if at all.

Food Guide Pyramid

Figure 23–5 shows the six food groups. The guide to daily food choices includes:

- 6–11 servings daily from the bread, cereal, rice, and pasta group
- 2–4 servings from the fruit group
- 3–5 servings from the vegetable group
- 2–3 servings from the milk, yogurt, and cheese group
- 2–3 servings from the meat, poultry, fish, dry beans, eggs, and nuts group
- Use fats, oils, and sweets sparingly

The food pyramid is used to represent the need for the foods at the bottom (grain foods) and gives equal importance to fruit and vegetables. Persons eating the lowest number of servings from each group would take in about 1600 calories daily if low-fat foods are chosen. This may be adequate for most older women and some older men. Younger and more active people would need more calories and can obtain them by choosing the larger number of servings.

Average servings of foods include:

- One medium size fruit or its equivalent
- 1/2 cup cooked fruit or vegetable
- 3–4 ounces of meat
- 2–3 ounces of pasta/bread

Figure 23–6 shows average servings for selected foods.

Fruit and Vegetable Group

Select 3–5 servings. Include:

- Dark green or yellow vegetables
- Tomatoes

Food Guide Pyramid
A Guide to Daily Food Choices

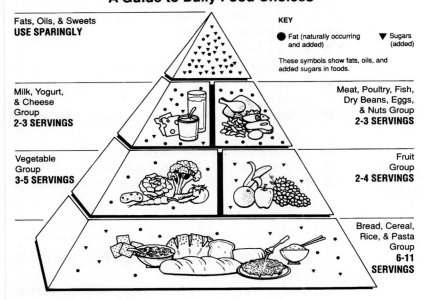

FIGURE 23–5. The food guide pyramid.

- Leafy, green, and yellow vegetables.
- Use vegetables raw, cooked, frozen, or canned.
- This group provides vitamin A, vitamin C, B complex vitamins, calcium, and iron.
- Leafy green vegetables furnish riboflavin and niacin, which are both B vitamins.

Three to Five Servings Daily

asparagus: green
beans: snap, green, lima
broccoli
brussels sprouts
cabbage
carrots
cauliflower
celery
chard
collards
corn
cucumber
endive: green
eggplant
escarole
kale
leeks
lettuce: leaf
other greens including salad greens
mushrooms
mustard greens

okra
onions
parsley
parsnips
peas: green
peppers: green and red
potatoes
pumpkin
radishes
rutabaga
salsify
sauerkraut
spinach
squash: summer
squash: winter
sweet potatoes
tomatoes
turnips
turnip greens
wild greens

Fruit Group

- Select two to four servings daily.
- Use foods in this group raw, cooked, frozen, canned, or dried.
- When eaten in fairly large amounts, foods in this group provide thiamine, vitamins A and C, calcium, and phosphorus.

Two to Four Servings Daily

- apples
- apricots
- artichokes
- avocados
- bananas
- berries
- cantaloupe (muskmelon)
- cherries
- cranberries
- currants
- dates
- figs
- grapefruit
- grapefruit juice
- grapes
- kumquats
- lemons
- limes
- oranges
- peaches
- pears
- persimmons
- pineapple: canned
- pineapple juice: canned
- plums
- prunes
- raisins
- rhubarb
- strawberries
- tangerines

Milk, Yogurt, Cheese Group

- ■ This group provides calcium, phosphorus, riboflavin, protein, vitamin A, and fat.
- ■ People need varying amounts of the nutrients in dairy foods at different periods of their lives.
- ■ Children should have three or four glasses of milk daily.
- ■ Teenagers need four or more glasses.
- ■ Adults should drink two or more glasses.
- ■ Pregnant women should drink at least one quart of milk, or the nutritional equivalent, daily.
- ■ Nursing mothers should increase the amount of milk in their diet to 1-1/2 quarts daily.
- ■ Daily calcium requirement for postmenopausal women is 1500 mg.
- ■ Cheese, ice cream, and other milk-made foods can be substituted for part of the milk requirement. (This increases fat and sodium content.)

Fruit		Vegetables	
Fresh—		Fresh—	3–4 oz.
apple	1 med.	Cooked—	1/2 cup
banana	1 med.	*Milk—*	8 oz.
peach	1 med.		
apricots	2–3	*Eggs—*	1–2 med.
figs	2–3		
		Meat, Fish, Poultry—	
Canned—			3–4 oz. cooked
grapefruit	1/2 can		
pineapple	2 sl.	*Cereal* (dried)—	
peaches	1/2 cup		1 oz. (2/3 cup)
Juice—	6 oz.		
		Bread—	2 slices
		Pasta—	2 oz. (uncooked)

FIGURE 23–6. Average servings for selected foods

The following dairy foods contain calcium equal to that in one cup of milk and may be substituted for milk:

Milk Substitutes
- 1 ounce cheddar-type cheese
- 4 ounces cream cheese
- 12 ounces cottage cheese
- 1-3/4 cups ice cream
- 1 cup yogurt

Milk is available in the following forms:

whole milk	condensed milk
skim milk	buttermilk
evaporated milk	dried milk

Grain Group

- ■ Select six to eleven servings daily.
- ■ This group provides carbohydrates, thiamine, niacin, iron, and roughage.

Six to Eleven Servings Daily

breads: whole wheat, dark rye, enriched cornmeal, whole grain enriched, or oatmeal

rolls or biscuits made with whole wheat or enriched flour

flour: enriched, whole wheat, other whole grain

grits, enriched cereals: whole wheat, rolled oats, brown rice, converted rice, other cereals, if whole grain or restored

noodles, spaghetti, macaroni

Meat Group

- Select two to three servings daily.
- Alternate dried beans, peas, or nuts. These are an incomplete protein.
- This group provides protein, some fat, iron, phosphorus, and B complex vitamins.
- Choose low-fat items.
- Remove skin from poultry and trim fat from meat.

beef	lunch meats, such as
eggs	bologna
lamb	dried beans
game	dried peas
veal	lentils
pork (except bacon and	nuts
fatback)	peanuts
poultry: chicken, duck,	peanut butter
goose, turkey	soybeans
fish, shellfish	soya flour and grits

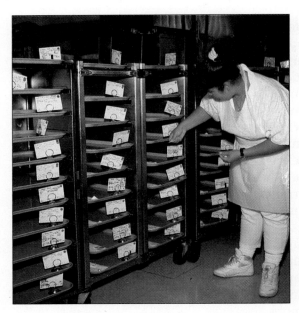

FIGURE 23–7. Patient diets are prepared in the dietary department.

Basic Facility Diets

The food you will serve to patients in the health care facility will be prepared by the dietary department, Figure 23–7. It will include the essential nutrients. The way in which it is prepared and its consistency will depend on the individual patient's condition and needs. Sometimes very strict dietary control is needed.

The trays will usually be delivered to the patient floors in large food containers. Each tray will be labeled with the patient's name and type of diet. You will:

- Prepare the patient for the meal.
- Check the tray card for patient's name.
- Check the tray card against the patient's armband.
- Serve the tray to the patient.
- Assist with feeding as necessary.

Health care facilities usually have many types of diets. Five common diets are:

- Regular or house, sometimes called select, Figure 23–8
- Full liquid
- Clear liquid
- Soft
- Light

Figure 23–9 shows the progression of diets a patient is allowed following surgery. In addition, the dietary department prepares special or **therapeutic** (treatment) **diets**. Therapeutic diets will be discussed later.

Regular Diet

The regular-select or house diet is a normal or full diet, based on the six food groups. The regular diet:

- Includes a great variety of foods.
- Excludes only very rich foods: pastries, heavy cakes, fried foods, and highly seasoned foods, which might be difficult for inactive people to digest.
- Has a lower caloric count because an inactive person doesn't require as many calories as an active person.

In many health care facilities, patients may select foods from a menu.

Liquid Diets

Clear Liquid Diet. This is a temporary diet because it is an inadequate diet. It is made up primarily of water and carbohydrates for energy. Feedings are given every two, three, or four hours as prescribed by the physician. It replaces fluids that may have been lost by vomiting or diarrhea. When a clear liquid diet is held up to the light, you can see through it. The clear liquid diet consists of liquids that do not irritate, cause gas formation, or encourage bowel movements (**defecation**).

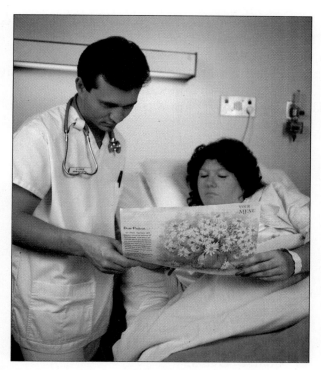

FIGURE 23–8. Patients on a "house diet" can select foods from a menu.

Foods allowed on the clear liquid diet include:

- Tea, coffee with sugar but without cream
- Strained fruit or vegetable juice with gelatin (occasionally)
- Fat-free meat broths
- Ginger ale (usually), 7Up®, Coke®, strained grape or apple juice
- Gelatin (occasionally)

Full Liquid Diet. The full liquid diet does supply nourishment and may be used for longer periods of time than the clear liquid diet. Six to eight ounces are usually given every two to three hours.

The full liquid diet is given to:

- Those with acute infections.
- Patients who have difficulty chewing.

Post-Operative Dietary Regime (Routine)
1. Ice chips/sip of water
2. Clear liquids
3. Full liquids
4. Soft diet
5. Regular diet

FIGURE 23–9. Following surgery, intake is restricted until full recovery from anesthesia is made. Then the intake is gradually changed as tolerance increases.

- Those who have conditions that involve the digestive tract.

The diet includes all of the foods allowed on the clear liquid diet in addition to the following:

- Strained cereal (gruel)
- Strained soups
- Sherbet
- Gelatin
- Eggnog
- Malted milk
- Milk and cream
- Plain ice cream
- Strained vegetables and fruit juices
- Junket
- Solids that liquefy at room temperature
- Yogurt

Soft Diet

The soft diet usually follows the full liquid diet. Although this diet nourishes the body, between-meal feedings are sometimes given to increase calorie count. Foods allowed on the soft diet are:

- Low-residue, which are almost completely used by the body.
- Mildly flavored, slightly seasoned or unseasoned.
- Prepared in a form that requires little digestion.

The diet includes liquids and semi-solid foods that have a soft texture and are easily digested, Figure 23–10. It is given to patients who:

- Have infections and fevers.
- Have difficulty chewing.
- Have conditions that involve the digestive tract.
- Are on a progressive post-operative dietary regime.

The following foods are usually allowed on the soft diet:

- Soups
- Cream cheese and cottage cheese
- Crackers, toast
- Fish
- White meat of chicken or turkey (boiled or stewed)
- Fruit juices
- Cooked fruit (sieved)
- Tea, coffee
- Milk, cream, butter
- Cooked cereals
- Eggs (not fried)

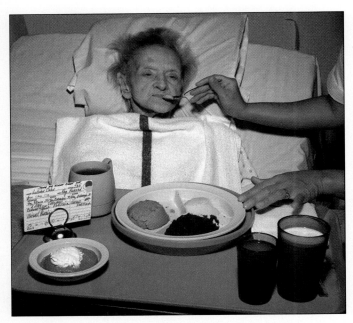

FIGURE 23–10. Soft diets include foods that require little chewing.

- Beef and lamb (scraped or finely ground)
- Cooked vegetables (mashed or sieved)
- Angel or sponge cake
- Small amounts of sugar
- Gelatin, custard
- Pudding
- Plain ice cream

Foods to be avoided include:
- Coarse cereals
- Spices
- Gas-forming foods (onions, cabbage, beans)
- Rich pastries and desserts
- Foods high in roughage
- Fried foods
- Raw fruits and vegetables
- Corn
- Pork (except bacon)

Light Diet

The light or convalescent diet is an intermediate diet between the soft and the regular diets.

This diet differs from the regular diet only in the method of preparing the food. Because digestibility of food is of prime importance, foods should not be fried. They should be:
- Baked
- Boiled
- Broiled

Rich, spicy, and coarse foods should be avoided. The light diet is used for:
- Convalescent patients
- Those who are pre-operative or post-operative
- Patients with minor illnesses

The following foods are allowed on the light diet:
- Soft diet foods
- Broiled or baked lean meat
- Fruits, except those high in cellulose
- Vegetables, except those high in cellulose
- Refined cereals
- Any bread, except bran
- Desserts, except rich pastries
- Butter, cream, bacon
- Small amounts of sweets
- Tea, coffee

Foods to be avoided include:
- Rich pastries
- Heavy salad dressings
- Fried foods
- Coarse cereals
- Pork (except bacon)
- Vegetables and fruits high in cellulose

Special Diets

Special diets are planned to meet specific patient needs. Patients may need special diets because of religious preferences or health needs.

Religious Restrictions

Religious practice requires changes in diet for some patients. For example, persons of the conservative Jewish faith have strict food laws to be followed.
- There are strict prohibitions against shellfish and nonkosher meats such as pork.
- Certain fish such as tuna and salmon are permitted.
- Foods may not be prepared in utensils that have been used for nonkosher food preparation.
- There are strict rules regarding the sequence in which milk products and meat may be consumed.

Some other faith restrictions are summarized in Figure 23–11.

Therapeutic Diets

Standard diets can be changed to conform with special dietary requirements. For example, an order might be written for a low-sodium soft diet when a

Faith ⟹	Christian Science	Roman Catholic	Muslim Moslem	Seventh Day Adventist	Some Baptists	Greek Orthodox (on fast days)
Restricted Food						
Coffee	●			●	●	
Tea	●			●	●	
Alcohol	●		●	●	●	
Pork/pork products			●	●		
Caffeine-containing foods				●		
Dairy products						●
All meats		1 hour before communion; Ash Wed., Good Friday		Some groups		●

In addition, the Jewish Orthodox faith:
- ■ forbids the serving of milk and milk products with meat.
- ■ forbids cooking of food on the Sabbath.

- ■ forbids eating of leavened bread during Passover.
- ■ observes specific fast days.

FIGURE 23–11. Religious dietary practices

patient has poor dentures and heart disease. These therapeutic diets are prepared for patients with individual health problems.

Commonly prescribed therapeutic diets include the diabetic diet, sodium-restricted diet, and low-fat diet.

The Diabetic Diet

Diet is an integral part of the therapy of the patient with *diabetes mellitus*. The diet is nutritionally adequate. It provides enough energy in the form of calories for a 24-hour period. Sometimes a proper diet is all that is needed to control the disease. Usually, however, the food intake is balanced by the administration of insulin or hypoglycemic drugs.

It is important for you to accurately evaluate and report the patient's intake. Foods and liquids have a major impact on diabetes management. Illness increases the need for insulin since the liver releases more glucose in response to the stress. Dehydration is a particularly serious problem for the diabetic. This can occur when insufficient foods and fluids are taken in. Insulin administration may be dependent upon your observations. Not all physicians prescribe dietary intake in the same way.

- ■ Some physicians prescribe a very carefully balanced diet and insulin to maintain the level of blood sugar (glucose) within normal limits. All foods must be weighed and repeated injections of insulin are required.

- ■ Other physicians are much more liberal in their approach. They permit an unmeasured diet, limiting only sugar and high-sugar foods. This diet is known as a low-concentrated sweets diet. It may be balanced by insulin or hypoglycemic drugs.
- ■ Many physicians treat diabetes with an approach that is midway between the former two methods. They prescribe the American Dietetic Association diets with specific calorie levels, such as the 1200-calorie diet or the 1500-calorie diet. The dietician teaches the patient about the diet and acts as a major resource for health care providers. The diet is balanced by insulin or hypoglycemic drugs.

The Exchange List. The **exchange list** method of balancing the diabetic diet:
- ■ Is based on standard household measurements to make it easier to measure.
- ■ Excludes sugar or high-sugar-content foods to prevent rapid swings in blood sugar.
- ■ Divides foods into six groups.
- ■ Allows equivalent exchanges to be made within a group but not from group to group.

The six groups are:
- ■ Milk exchanges
- ■ Vegetable exchange: Group A, Group B
- ■ Fruit exchange

- Bread exchange
- Meat exchange
- Fat exchange

Sodium-restricted Diet (Solt) NA -2.6 m NA.

Sodium-restricted diets may be ordered for patients with chronic renal failure and cardiovascular disease. Diets that are moderately, mildly, or severely restricted in sodium content may be prescribed. This latter diet is one of the most difficult for patients to follow. Processing foods may add significant levels of sodium. This factor is considered in planning and selecting foods for the sodium-restricted diet. It is important to carefully read the label for the contents of all commercially prepared foods.

Some foods naturally contain relatively large amounts of sodium. These foods may be somewhat restricted. They include:

- Meat
- Fish
- Poultry
- Milk and milk products
- Eggs

Avoid:

- Pork
- Potato chips
- Pop (soda)
- Pickles
- Processed meats
- Canned foods, such as vegetables and soups

Some foods are naturally low in sodium. They can be used more liberally. They are:

- Some cereals such as shredded wheat
- Vegetables
- Fruits

Calorie-restricted Diet

Providing activity remains constant, a person must take in approximately 500 calories a day less than usual (3500 calories deficit per week) to lose one pound).

Calorie-restricted diets are prescribed for patients who are overweight. They are planned to meet general nutritional needs. They take into consideration the patient's energy output, general nutritional state, and weight goal.

In planning the calorie-restricted diet, the dietician tries to create a realistic balance between fats, proteins, and carbohydrates. This type of diet is considered to encourage the patient to form better, more consistent food intake habits.

Exact amounts of the three nutrients are not uniformly prescribed, but they may be included as follows:

- Proteins   20%
- Fats   25–35%
- Carbohydrates   45–65%

Some physicians use a factor of ten calories multiplied by the desired weight in calculating the daily calorie requirements. For example:

- Desired weight 120 lb. × 10 = 1200 calories per day.
- Desired weight 160 lb. × 10 = 1600 calories per day.

Low-Fat/Low-Cholesterol Diet

Low-fat/low-cholesterol diets are prescribed for patients who suffer from vascular, heart, liver, or gallbladder disease, and for those who have difficulty with fat metabolism. Fats are limited and calories are balanced by increasing proteins and carbohydrates. Foods are baked, roasted, or broiled, and the skin is removed from chicken.

Foods include:

- Low-fat cottage cheese (no other allowed)
- Skim milk, buttermilk, yogurt, and margarine
- Lean meats, fish, chicken
- Vegetables and fruits
- Jams, jellies, ices
- Cereals, pasta, bread, potatoes, rice
- Carbonated beverages, tea, coffee

Supplementary Nourishments

Serving between-meal nourishments is an important function of the assistant, Figure 23–12. Between-meal nourishments are usually served:

- Midmorning—between 9:30–10:00 AM
- Midafternoon—between 2:30–3:00 PM
- At bedtime—between 8:00–10:00 PM

Snacks served include:

- Milk
- Juices
- Gelatin
- Custard
- Ice cream
- Sherbet
- High-protein drinks
- Fruits

To serve nourishments:

- Wash your hands.
- Check the nourishment list of each patient for any limitations or special dietary instructions.
- Allow patients to choose from the available nourishments whenever possible.

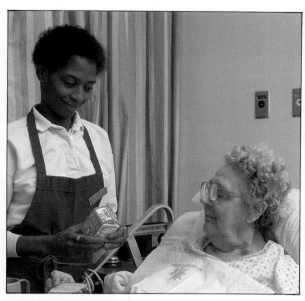

FIGURE 23–12. Supplementary nourishments are served between meals.

- Assist those who are unable to take their nourishment alone.
- Remember to pick up used glasses and dishes after the patient has finished and return them to the proper area.
- Notice what the patient was or was not able to take.
- Record on I & O sheet if required.

Changing Water

It is important to provide fresh water for patients since water is essential to life. In all cases, you should know whether a patient is allowed ice or tap water and if water is to be especially encouraged. Even without an order to force fluids, you must encourage patients to take 6–8 glasses of fluids daily, unless the patient is NPO (nothing by mouth) or on restricted fluids. Give special attention to confused patients, patients who may be removed from a source of water, and the elderly. The need for adequate water intake cannot be overstressed. Because patients often do not drink enough water, sometimes the physician will leave orders that fluids are to be forced to a

BEGINNING PROCEDURE ACTIONS	PROCEDURE COMPLETION ACTIONS
■ Wash your hands.	■ Position patient comfortably.
■ Assemble equipment needed.	■ Leave signal cord, telephone, and fresh water close at hand.
■ Go to the patient's room, knock, and pause before entering.	■ Return bed to lowest position.
■ Introduce yourself and identify the patient by checking the identification bracelet.	■ Perform general safety check of patient and environment.
■ Provide privacy.	■ Care for equipment according to facility policy.
■ Explain what foods are on the tray.	■ Wash your hands.
■ Allow patient to assist in procedure as much as possible.	■ Report completion of task.
■ Raise bed to comfortable working height.	■ Let visitors know when they may reenter the patient's room.
■ Position patient comfortably.	■ Document action and your observation.

NOTE: Where there are open lesions, wet linen, or possible contact with patient body fluids or blood, disposable gloves are worn during the procedure. Put on gloves before contact with the patient or linen. Properly dispose of gloves after they are removed. ALWAYS APPLY UNIVERSAL PRECAUTIONS.

FIGURE 23–13. Beginning procedure actions and procedure completion actions

specific number of cc per day. **Forcing fluids** means that the patient must be encouraged to take as much fluid as possible. Providing fresh water is one way to encourage the patient to increase intake of fluids. The procedure for providing fresh water varies greatly.

■ In some hospitals, the water pitcher and glass are replaced with a new sterilized set each time water is provided.

■ In others, the pitcher and glass are washed, refilled, and returned to the patient's bedside table.

In all cases, be sure you know whether a patient is allowed ice or tap water.

Feeding the Patient

Eating should be an enjoyable experience. Prepare the patient for his tray before it arrives by:

■ Offering the bedpan.
■ Assisting him to wash hands and face.
■ Assisting with oral hygiene.
■ Raising head of bed, if permitted.
■ Assisting patient out of bed and into a chair, if permitted.

■ Adjusting the in-bed patient's position with pillows.
■ Clearing away anything that is unpleasant, such as emesis basin and bedpan.
■ Clearing the over-bed table.
■ Allowing the patient to do as much as possible.

When you have served the tray and after you have washed your hands, assist the patient as needed by:

■ Being unhurried and pleasant.
■ Opening pre-packaged items.
■ Cutting meat.
■ Pouring liquids.
■ Buttering bread.
■ Explaining the arrangement of the tray as items relate to the face of a clock if patient cannot see.

There are times when you will be responsible for the entire feeding procedure.

NOTE: Carry some extra straws with you during meal times. It can save you steps.

Refer to Figure 23–13 for the beginning procedure actions and the procedure completion actions to be performed for each patient care procedure.

PROCEDURE 78   **OBRA**

ASSISTING THE PATIENT WHO CAN FEED SELF

1. Carry out each beginning procedure action.
2. Remember to wash your hands, identify the patient, and provide privacy.
3. Assemble equipment needed:
   ■ Bedpan/urinal
   ■ Wash water
   ■ Oral hygiene items
   ■ Tray of food
4. Offer bedpan/urinal. (If used, follow procedure in Unit 21—"Giving and Receiving the Bedpan.")
5. If permitted, elevate head of bed or assist patient out of bed.
6. Provide water, soap, and towel to wash patient's hands and face, Figure 23–14A and B.
7. Assist with oral hygiene or assist with dentures.
8. Clear over-bed table and position in front of patient. Remove unpleasant equipment from sight, Figure 23–14C.
9. Wash your hands. Obtain tray from dietary area, Figure 23–14D.

10. Check dietary name tag against patient's identification, Figure 23–14E.

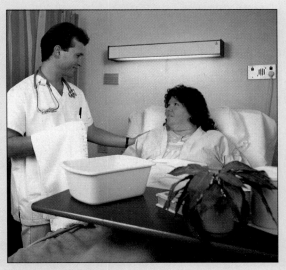

FIGURE 23–14A.   Give patient water to wash hands.

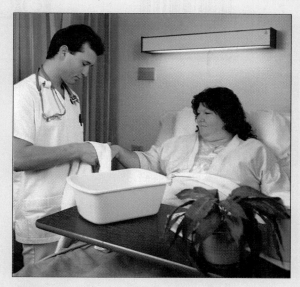

FIGURE 23–14B. Assist patient if necessary.

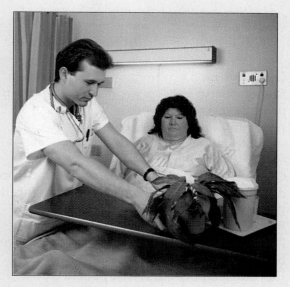

FIGURE 23–14C. Patients eat better when properly prepared for their meal. Prepare over-bed table to make room for tray.

11. Place tray on over-bed table and arrange food in a convenient manner.
12. Assist in food preparation as needed, Figure 23–14F. Encourage patient to do as much for self as permitted.
13. Remove tray as soon as patient is finished. Make sure to note what the patient has and has not eaten.

14. Record fluids on intake record, if necessary.
15. Push over-bed table out of the way.
16. Carry out each procedure completion action. Remember to wash your hands, report completion of task, and document time, amount and type of food consumed, and patient reaction.

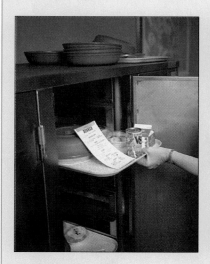

FIGURE 23–14D. Obtain the proper tray from food conveyor or cart.

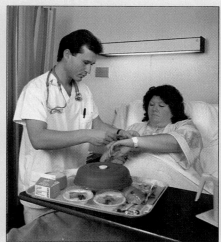

FIGURE 23–14E. Check patient's arm band against tray card.

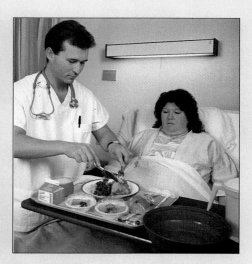

FIGURE 23–14F. Assist patient in food preparation as needed.

PROCEDURE 79   OBRA

FEEDING THE HELPLESS PATIENT

1. Carry out each beginning procedure action.
2. Remember to wash your hands, identify the patient, and provide privacy.
3. Assemble equipment needed:
   - Bedpan/urinal
   - Wash water
   - Oral hygiene items
   - Tray of food
4. Offer bedpan or urinal. (If used, follow procedure in Unit 21—"Giving and Receiving the Bedpan.")
5. Provide oral hygiene.
6. Remove unnecessary articles from the over-bed table.
7. Elevate head of bed. Assist patient into a high Fowler's position with head slightly bent forward.
8. Place towel or protector under patient's chin, Figure 23–15A.
9. Obtain tray and check against patient's identification band.
10. Place tray on over-bed table, Figure 23–15B.
11. Butter bread and cut meat. Do not pour hot beverage until patient is ready for it.
12. Use different drinking straws to give each fluid or use a cup. Thick fluids are more easily controlled by using a straw.

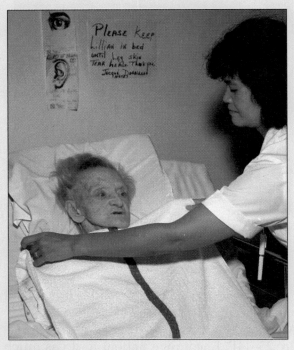

FIGURE 23–15A. Place a towel or bed protector over patient.

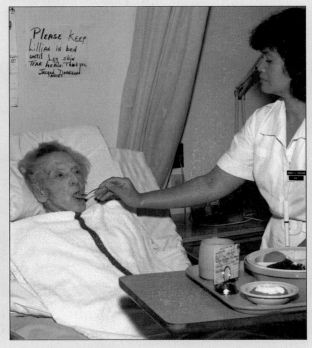

FIGURE 23–15C. Give solid foods from tip of spoon.

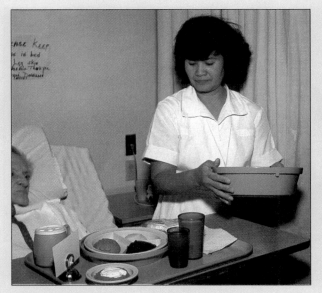

FIGURE 23–15B. Uncover food and arrange on bedside table.

13. Sit down if you can, while you are feeding the patient, so you are at eye level.
14. Holding spoon at a right angle:
    ■ Give solid foods from point of spoon, Figure 23–15C.
    ■ Alternate solids and liquids.
    ■ Ask the patient in what order you should offer the food.
    ■ Describe or show patient what kind of food you are giving, Figure 23–15D.
    ■ If patient has had stroke, direct food to unaffected side and check for food stored in affected side. Watch the patient's throat to check for swallowing.
    ■ Test hot foods by dropping a small amount on the inside of your wrist before feeding them to the patient.
    ■ Never blow on the patient's food to cool it.
    ■ Never taste the patient's food.
15. Allow patient to hold bread or assist to the extent that patient is able.
16. Use napkin to wipe patient's mouth as often as necessary.
17. Remove tray as soon as patient is finished. Make sure you note what the patient has or has not eaten.

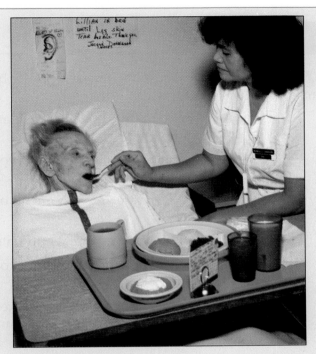

FIGURE 23–15D. Describe food as you feed patient.

18. Carry out each procedure completion action. Remember to wash your hands, report completion of task, and document time, amount and type of food consumed, and patient reaction.

SUMMARY

Food is usually taken into the body through the mouth. Sometimes, however, alternative ways of meeting dietary needs must be found. For example:
■ Intravenous infusions
■ Gastrostomy feedings
■ Gavage

The nutritional needs are best met when selections are made properly from the six food groups:
■ Meat
■ Dairy
■ Vegetables
■ Fruits
■ Breads, cereals, and pastas
■ Fats, oils, and sweets

Foods for facility diets are selected from the six food groups. They are prepared in special ways. There are five routine facility diets:

■ House, regular or select
■ Liquid, clear
■ Liquid, full
■ Soft
■ Light

Many special or therapeutic diets are also prescribed. The patient's dietary intake is based on:
■ Personal preference
■ Health requirements
■ Religious preferences

The assistant helps meet the patient's nutritional needs by:
■ Serving trays.
■ Serving special nourishments.
■ Providing fresh drinking water.
■ Assisting patients with feeding.
■ Feeding patients who are unable to feed themselves.

UNIT REVIEW

A. True/False. Answer the following true or false by circling T or F.

T F   1. Vitamins are nutrients that help regulate body activities.

T F   2. When a patient is receiving an IV, you must check the infusion site regularly.

T F   3. The exchange lists are used by patients on low-salt diets.

T F   4. Fats are one of the six essential nutrients.

T F   5. Ice cream would be served to a patient on a clear liquid diet.

T F   6. Labels of canned foods must be checked when planning their use in low-sodium diets.

T F   7. A gastrostomy tube introduces nutrients directly into the stomach.

T F   8. Carbohydrate foods are used to make new body cells and build tissues.

T F   9. Green leafy vegetables are a good source of calcium, iron, and B vitamins.

T F 10. Complete protein foods like poultry contain all of the essential amino acids.

B. Matching. Match Column I with Column II.

Column I	Column II
_____ 11. calcium	a. therapeutic
_____ 12. roughage	b. mineral
_____ 13. encourage liquid intake	c. nutrition
	d. forcing fluids
_____ 14. all the processes involved in taking in food and building and repairing the body	e. cellulose
	f. vitamin
_____ 15. treatment	

C. Multiple Choice. Choose the answer that best completes each of the following sentences by circling the proper letter.

16. Feeding the patient through a nasogastric tube is known as a/an
    a. intravenous infusion.   c. gavage.
    b. gastrostomy feeding.   d. lavage.

17. Which of the following is an example of a water-soluble vitamin?
    a. Vitamin C   c. Vitamin A
    b. Vitamin E   d. Vitamin D

18. An example of a fat-soluble vitamin is
    a. vitamin C.   c. vitamin D.
    b. vitamin B-complex. d. vitamin N.

19. An average serving of meat is
    a. 1 ounce.   c. 8 ounces.
    b. 3–4 ounces.   d. 16 ounces.

20. Which of the following is part of the meat group?
    a. Peas   c. Poultry
    b. Nuts   d. All of the above

21. Foods naturally high in sodium include
    a. milk.   c. vegetables.
    b. cereals.   d. fruits.

22. Supplemental nourishments might include
    a. hot fudge sundaes.   c. scrambled eggs.
    b. mashed potatoes.   d. cranberry juice.

23. A serving of cooked vegetables would be approximately
    a. 1/2 cup.   c. 1 cup.
    b. 3/4 cup.   d. 1-1/2 cups.

24. You notice the last bottle of an IV infusion is almost empty. You should
    a. discontinue the IV by clamping the tubing.
    b. inform the nurse right away.
    c. wait until it is completely empty and then inform the nurse.
    d. let it run through since it's the last bottle anyway.

25. It is especially important to report to the nurse that the patient only ate two-thirds of her meal when the patient is on a
    a. low-salt diet.
    b. calorie-restricted diet.
    c. diabetic diet.
    d. house diet.

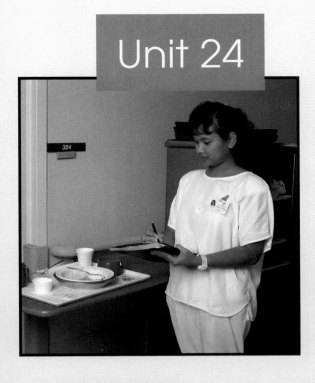

Recording Intake and Output and Collecting and Testing Routine Specimens

OBJECTIVES

As a result of this unit, you will be able to:

■ Spell and define terms.

■ Describe patient conditions that require a record of intake and output.

■ Use the metric system of measurement.

■ Explain the importance of accurate measurements in health care facilities.

■ Describe the importance of wearing gloves while collecting and handling specimens.

■ Calculate and record intake and output.

■ Collect and label specimens.

VOCABULARY

Learn the meaning and the correct spelling of the following words and phrases:

catheter
clean-catch urine
    specimen
dehydration
diaphoresis
diuresis
edema
emesis
expectorate
fecal

intake and output
    (I & O)
labia
meatus
occult blood
specimen
sputum
urinalysis
void
vulva

Because two-thirds of the body weight is water, there must be a careful balance between the amount of fluid taken into the body and the amount that is lost under normal conditions. Generally, we do not need to concern ourselves about this balance. It usually takes care of itself.

Intake and Output

Intake

We take in approximately 2-1/2 quarts (2500 ml) of fluid daily:

- As liquids such as water, tea, and soft drinks.
- As foods such as fruits and vegetables.
- Artificially, such as by intravenous infusions or gavage.

Most adult patients will need to consume an average 600–800 ml of fluid during each eight-hour shift. Since patients may sleep during most of the night shift, additional fluids need to be provided during waking hours to keep the body in balance. Excessive fluid retention is called edema. Inadequate fluid results in dehydration, or the lack of sufficient fluid in body tissues. Some disease conditions may change the amounts of fluid the patient is allowed to have.

Output

Typical output equals about 2-1/2 quarts daily in the form of:

- Urine—1-1/2 quarts (1500 ml)
- Perspiration
- Moisture from the lungs
- Moisture from the bowel

Excessive fluid loss results in dehydration. This can occur through:

- Diarrhea
- Vomiting
- Excessive urine output (diuresis)
- Excessive perspiration (diaphoresis)

Recording Intake and Output

An accurate recording of intake and output (I & O), or fluid taken in and given off by the body, is basic to the care of many patients. Intake and output records are kept when specifically ordered by the physician and when patients:

- Are dehydrated.
- Receive intravenous infusion.
- Have recently had surgery.
- Have a urinary catheter.
- Are perspiring profusely or vomiting.
- Have specific diagnoses such as congestive heart failure or renal disease that require accurate monitoring of I & O.

U.S. Customary Units	Metric Units
1 minim	0.06 milliliter (ml)
16 minims	1 ml
1 ounce	30 ml
1 pint	500 ml
1 quart	1000 ml (1 liter)
2.2 pounds	1 kilogram (kg)
1 inch	2.5 centimeters (cm)
1 foot	30 cm

FIGURE 24–1. Comparison of U.S. customary and metric measurements

Metric System

A knowledge of metric measurement, Figure 24–1, is essential in measuring intake and output because:

- Most of the scientific work in the United States and Canada is done with the metric system.
- The containers used in hospitals for measuring fluids such as urine are marked in metric measurements. For example, containers may be labeled in cubic centimeters (cc) or milliliters (ml) (1 cc = 1 ml).

NOTE: Disposable gloves are required when handling body excretions, since all excretions are considered potentially infectious. For this reason, disposable gloves are listed with each procedure in which there may be contact with body excretions.

Refer to Figure 24–2 for a summary of the beginning procedure actions and procedure completion actions to be performed for each patient care procedure.

Routine Specimens

Laboratory tests are frequently performed on body fluids such as blood and spinal fluid and on body discharges such as urine, feces, and sputum. All specimens are considered potentially infectious and gloves must be worn when obtaining and handling them.

- Results of these tests give the physician much information about the patient's condition.
- All specimens must be carefully cared for, labeled, and sent to the lab as soon as possible.
- Mistakes in labeling and preparing the specimens can make the test results inaccurate and they can endanger your patients.

BEGINNING PROCEDURE ACTIONS	PROCEDURE COMPLETION ACTIONS
■ Wash your hands. ■ Assemble equipment needed. ■ Go to the patient's room, knock, and pause before entering. ■ Introduce yourself and identify the patient by checking identification bracelet. ■ Ask visitors to leave and inform them where they can wait. ■ Provide privacy. ■ Explain what will happen and answer questions. ■ Allow patient to assist in procedure as much as possible. ■ Raise bed to comfortable working height.	■ Position patient comfortably. ■ Leave signal cord, telephone, and fresh water close at hand. ■ Return bed to lowest position. ■ Perform general safety check of patient and environment. ■ Care for equipment according to facility policy. ■ Wash your hands. ■ Report completion of task. ■ Let visitors know when they may reenter the patient's room. ■ Document action and your observations.

NOTE: Where there are open lesions, wet linen, or possible contact with patient body fluids or blood, disposable gloves are worn during the procedure. Put on gloves before contact with the patient or linen. Properly dispose of gloves after they are removed. ALWAYS APPLY UNIVERSAL PRECAUTIONS.

FIGURE 24–2. Beginning procedure actions and procedure completion actions

PROCEDURE 80 | OBRA

SIDE 7

MEASURING AND RECORDING FLUID INTAKE

1. Carry out each beginning procedure action.
2. Remember to wash your hands, identify the patient, and provide privacy.
3. Assemble equipment needed:
   ■ Intake and output record at bedside
   ■ Containers that hold the liquids
   ■ Pen for recording
4. Explain how the patient may help record the amount of fluid taken by writing down the amounts and kinds of fluids consumed by mouth, Figure 24–3. The record is kept on the bedside intake-output sheet.
5. To calculate oral liquid intake:
   ■ Know what the container held when it was full—for example, a carton of milk holds 240 ml when full, or a glass of water holds 200 ml when full.
   ■ Estimate how much the patient has drunk from the container—for example 1/4 of the container, 1/2 of the container, or 3/4 of the container.
   ■ Convert this to ml. For example, if the patient drinks 1/2 of the carton of milk, the intake is recorded as 120 ml of milk. If the patient drinks 3/4 of the glass of water, the intake is recorded as 150 ml of water.

Coffee/tea cup, 8 oz	240 ml
Water carafe, 16 oz	480 ml
Foam cup, 8 oz	240 ml
Water glass, 8 oz	240 ml
Soup bowl, 6 oz	180 ml
Jello, 1 serving	120 ml
Ice chips, full 4 oz glass	120 ml

FIGURE 24–3. Approximate liquid amounts of common containers and servings. Note: Sizes of containers vary. Learn the fluid content of the containers used at your facility. Remember that there are 30 ml per ounce (240 ml ÷ 30 ml = 8 oz).

INTAKE	
I.V.	3000 ml
By mouth	2000 ml
Total	5000 ml
OUTPUT	
Urine	2000 ml
Vomitus	500 ml
Drainage	600 ml
Total	3100 ml

FIGURE 24–4. Computing intake and output

continues

- Remember: you are calculating what is gone from the container (what the patient has taken in).
6. Record intake on the intake-output record at the bedside by listing all fluids taken in. Total intake includes:
  - The amount of liquid the patient takes with meals.
  - The amount of water and other liquids taken between meals.

- All other fluids given by mouth, intravenously, or by tube feeding. How these fluids are taken should also be recorded.
7. Copy information to the patient's chart from the bedside intake and output record, according to facility policy.
  - Remember, intake and output (I & O) are recorded in milliliters (ml), which are the same as cubic centimeters (cc).
  - The total is recorded at the end of each shift and at the end of 24 hours, Figure 24–4.

PROCEDURE 81 | **OBRA**   SIDE 7

MEASURING AND RECORDING FLUID OUTPUT

1. Carry out each beginning procedure action.
2. Remember to wash your hands, identify the patient, and provide privacy.
3. Assemble equipment needed:
   - Intake and output record
   - Graduated container to hold liquid
   - Pen for recording
   - Disposable gloves
4. Put on disposable gloves.
5. Save urine **specimen** (amount collected) and take to utility room or patient's bathroom.

6. Instruct the patient who is able to ambulate to the bathroom to use the "hat-shaped" specimen collection container.
7. Pour urine from bedpan or urinal into gradu-

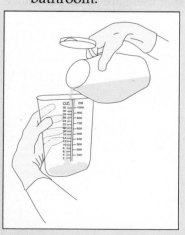

Date	Time	Method of Admin.	Solution	Intake Amounts Rec'd	Time	Output Urine Amount	Others Kind	Others Amount
7/16	0700	P.O.	water	120 ml		500 ml		
	0830	P.O.	water or. ju.	240 ml 120 ml				
	1030	P.O.	cran. ju.	120 ml				
	1100					300 ml		
	1230	P.O.	tea	240 ml				
	1400	P.O.	water	150 ml				
Shift Totals	1500			990 ml		800 ml		
	1530	P.O.	gelatin	120 ml				
	1700	P.O.	tea	120 ml				
			soup	180 ml				
	2000					512 ml		
	2045						vomitus	500 ml
	2205						vomitus	90 ml
Shift Totals	2300			420 ml		512 ml		590 ml
	2345						vomitus	80 ml
	0130	IV	D/W	500 ml				
	0315					400 ml		
Shift Totals	0700			500 ml		400 ml		80 ml
24 Hour Totals				1910 ml		1712 ml		670 ml vomitus

FIGURE 24–5. Measuring the urine specimen

FIGURE 24–6. Sample intake and output sheet (bedside)

ated container, Figure 24–5. Measure amount.

8. Record amounts immediately under output column on bedside intake and output record, Figure 24–6. All liquid output should be recorded. Output includes:
   - Urine
   - Vomitus—also called *emesis*
   - Drainage from a wound or the stomach
   - Liquid stool—record an estimated amount
   - Blood loss—record an estimated amount if on sheets or dressings, otherwise measure with a graduate
   - Perspiration—record an estimated amount

   NOTE: Fluids used to irrigate the bladder or for an enema are not included in calculating the output.

9. Empty urine into toilet.
   - If specimen is accidentally lost, estimate amount and make notation that it is an estimate.
   - In some cases, the physician will request that the totally incontinent patient's diapers be weighed to determine output.

NOTE: Some health care facilities have guidelines for the amount of urine or blood on pads or linen by the diameter of the wet area.

10. Rinse fluid container with cold water. Clean according to facility policy.

11. Clean bedpan or urinal and return it to proper place, according to facility policy.

12. Remove and dispose of gloves according to facility policy.

13. Carry out each procedure completion action. Remember to wash your hands, report completion of task, and document time, urine output—amount/character—and patient reaction.

14. Copy information to chart from intake and output record according to facility policy.
   - Perspiration and blood loss may be described as *little*, *moderate*, or *excessive*.
   - Also record on the chart the number of times linens or dressings have been changed or reinforced because of such fluid losses.
   - Blood loss is measured by marking dressings and measuring amounts in Hemovac containers.

Urine Specimens

Routine Urine Specimen. Urinalysis is the most common laboratory test. The specimen is usually taken when the patient first **voids** (urinates) in the morning. Properties of fresh urine begin to change after 15 minutes. Therefore, it is important that you take the sample immediately to the laboratory or refrigerate the sample until delivery can be made.

PROCEDURE 82

COLLECTING A ROUTINE URINE SPECIMEN

1. Carry out each beginning procedure action.
2. Remember to wash your hands, identify the patient, and provide privacy.
3. Assemble equipment needed:
   - Bedpan/urinal
   - Bed protector or paper towels
   - Container and cover for specimen
   - Label including:
     — Patient's full name
     — Room number
     — Facility number
     — Date and time of collection
     — Physician's name
     — Examination to be done
     — Other information as requested
   - Biohazard bag
   - Graduate pitcher
   - Disposable gloves
   - Laboratory requisition slip, properly filled out
4. Completely fill out the label of the specimen container, Figure 24–7A and attach to container.
5. Put on disposable gloves.

continues

6. Offer bedpan or urinal.
7. Instruct the patient not to discard toilet tissue in the pan with the urine. Provide paper towels or a small plastic bag in which to place the soiled tissue.
8. After patient has voided, cover pan and place on protector on chair. Offer wash water to patient.
9. If patient can ambulate to bathroom, place specimen collector in toilet.
10. Assist patient to bathroom. Ask patient to void into specimen collector. Instruct patient to discard soiled toilet tissue in paper or plastic bag provided. Tissue must not be placed in collector.

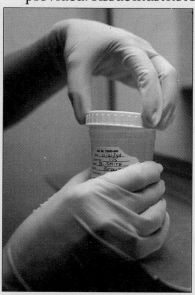

FIGURE 24–7A. Fill out label of urine specimen container completely before collecting specimen.

11. Remove specimen collector from toilet. If patient is on I & O, note amount of urine voided against scale in the collector, Figure 24–7B. Record amount. If patient used bedpan, pour urine into graduate to measure. Record amount.
12. Remove cap from specimen container, and place it (inside up) on top of shelf in bathroom or utility room, Figure 24–7C. Do not touch inside of cap or container.
13. To obtain specimen from collector, carefully pour urine into specimen container, Figure 24–7D. Pour about 120 ml of urine into specimen container without touching lip of container.
14. Remove and dispose of gloves according to facility policy.
15. Wash your hands. Do not contaminate outside of container.
16. Cover container. Attach completed label and requisition slip to container. Place specimen in protective biohazard bag for transport.
17. Carry out each procedure completion action. Remember to wash your hands, report completion of task, and document time, urine specimen to laboratory, and patient reaction.
18. Take specimen to laboratory if this is your responsibility.

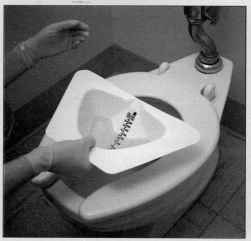

FIGURE 24–7B. Remove specimen collector from toilet. Note amount of voiding if patient is on I & O.

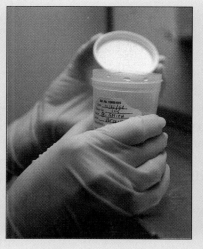

FIGURE 24–7C. Remove cover and place it on shelf. Do not touch inside of lid or container.

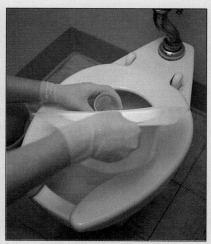

FIGURE 24–7D. Carefully pour specimen from collector into container.

PROCEDURE 83

COLLECTING A ROUTINE URINE SPECIMEN FROM AN INFANT

1. Carry out each beginning procedure action.
2. Remember to wash your hands, identify the patient, and provide privacy.
3. Assemble equipment needed:
   - Clean diapers (2)
   - Disposable urine collection bag
   - Sterile cotton balls
   - Wash basin
   - Biohazard bag
   - Specimen container/labels
   - Disposable gloves
4. Put on disposable gloves.
5. Fill the basin with warm water and take to bedside.
6. Screen unit and lower crib side.
7. Place child on back and remove diaper. Dispose according to facility policy.
8. Flex knees to expose perineum.
9. Using cotton balls, cleanse the perineal area.
   a. Each cotton ball should be used only once for a single stroke from front to back.
   b. Clean directly over the urinary meatus (opening) last.
   c. Rinse and dry area.
   NOTE: In male child, wipe around base of penis with alcohol. Let skin dry. This removes oils and permits the bag to stick better.
10. Remove paper cover from adhesive portion of collection bag, Figure 24–8A.
    - If female child, bending the adhesive area slightly on the bottom will help it fit more snugly against the perineum, Figure 24–8B. Position this section first, bringing up against vulva, Figure 24–9A.
    - If male child, position penis in opening of bag and secure adhesive area to skin, Figure 24–9B.
11. Remove and dispose of gloves according to facility policy.
12. Apply clean diaper.
13. Offer fluids, if permitted, to encourage voiding.
14. Make sure child is secure in crib, with side rails up before leaving unit.
15. Wash your hands.
16. Check child frequently until voiding has been achieved.
17. Wash your hands and screen unit.
18. Put on disposable gloves.
19. Fill the basin with warm water and take to bedside. Lower side rail.
20. Remove diaper and dispose of properly.
21. Gently remove collection bag by lifting the

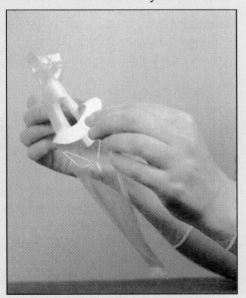

FIGURE 24–8A. Remove paper covering adhesive portion before applying infant urine collection bag.

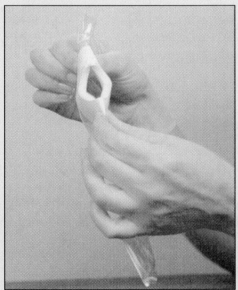

FIGURE 24–8B. Slightly bending the opening will help it fit more snugly against female perineum.

continues

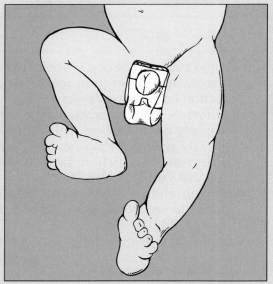
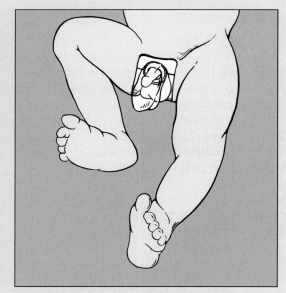

A. female   **B.** male

FIGURE 24–9.   Infant urine collection bag in place.

edges and pulling toward perineum. Be careful not to spill urine.

22. Put adhesive edges together and pour urine into the specimen container through drainage port. Be very careful not to lose specimen.

23. Wash and dry perineal area using the same technique as in Step 9. Be sure all adhesive is removed. Observe and report any skin irritation.

24. Apply a fresh diaper.

25. Raise side rails, unscreen unit, and be sure child is secure in crib before leaving.

26. Take equipment to patient's bathroom or utility room and clean according to facility policy.

27. Remove and dispose of gloves according to facility policy.

28. Wash your hands. Label specimen properly.

29. Care for specimen per instruction. Place specimen in protective biohazard bag for transport.

30. Carry out each procedure completion action. Remember to wash your hands, report completion of task, and document time, urine specimen to laboratory, and patient reaction.

PROCEDURE 84   SIDE **7**

COLLECTING A CLEAN-CATCH URINE SPECIMEN

1. Carry out each beginning procedure action.
2. Remember to wash your hands, identify the patient, and provide privacy.
3. Assemble equipment needed:
   - Sterile urine specimen container
   - Disposable gloves
   - Bedpan, urinal
   - Label for container with:
     — Patient's full name
     — Room number
     — Date and time of collection
     — Physician's name
     — Type of specimen/test to be performed
     — Any other information requested
   - Biohazard bag
   - Gauze squares or cotton
   - Antiseptic solution
4. Put on disposable gloves.
5. Wash the patient's genital area properly or

instruct the patient to do so. If highly soiled due to incontinence, perform perineal care first.

a. For female patients:
1. Using the gauze or cotton and the antiseptic solution, cleanse the outer folds of the vulva (folds are also called labia or lips) with a front-to-back motion, Figure 24–10. Use separate cotton/gauze for each side.
2. Discard the gauze/cotton. Then cleanse the inner folds of the vulva with two pieces of gauze and antiseptic solution, again with a front-to-back motion. Discard gauze/cotton.
3. Finally, cleanse the middle, innermost area (meatus or urinary opening) in the same manner. Discard the gauze/cotton.
4. Keep the labia separated so that the folds

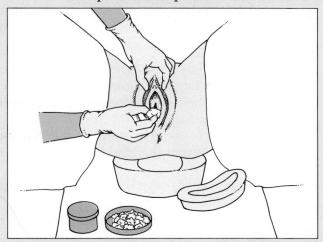

FIGURE 24–10. Wipe each side of vulva with cotton balls. Wipe directly over meatus from top to bottom (front to back). Discard cotton balls. Rinse using clean cotton balls or gauze and antiseptic. Repeat procedure with clean cotton balls and antiseptic on inner folds. Note that gloves are worn for this procedure.

do not fall back and cover the meatus.
b. For male patients:
1. Using the gauze/cotton and the antiseptic solution, cleanse the tip of the penis from the urinary meatus down, using a circular motion.
2. Discard gauze/cotton.
6. Instruct the patient to void, allowing the first part of the urine to escape. Then:
a. Catch the urine stream that follows in the sterile specimen container.
b. Allow the last portion of the urine stream to escape.
NOTE: If the patient's I & O is being monitored, or if the amount of urine passed must be measured, catch the first and last part of the urine in a bedpan or urinal.
7. Place the sterile cap on the urine container immediately to prevent contamination of the urine specimen.
8. Allow the patient to wash hands.
9. With the cap securely tightened, wash the outside of the specimen container.
10. Remove and dispose of gloves according to facility policy.
11. Wash your hands.
12. Label the container as instructed previously. Attach requisition slip for appropriate test.
13. Place specimen container in a protective biohazard bag for transport.
14. Carry out each procedure completion action. Remember to wash your hands, report completion of task, and document time, clean-catch urine specimen to laboratory, and patient reaction.
15. Take or send specimen to laboratory immediately if transportation is your responsibility.

PROCEDURE 85

COLLECTING A FRESH FRACTIONAL URINE SPECIMEN

1. Carry out each beginning procedure action.
2. Remember to wash your hands, identify the patient, and provide privacy.
3. Assemble equipment needed:
   - Two specimen containers
   - Urinal or bedpan

- Testing materials if urine testing is to be performed (Ketostix)
- Small plastic bag for used toilet tissue
- Disposable gloves
- Biohazard bag

continues

4. About one hour before testing is to be done, wash your hands and take equipment to bedside. Instruct patient that two samples will be taken: an initial sample now and a smaller sample in about one hour or less.
5. Screen unit and offer bedpan or urinal (patient may be assisted to the commode, if permitted).
6. Put on disposable gloves.
7. Encourage patient to empty bladder.
8. Do not permit tissue to be placed in receptacle. Place in plastic bag and discard.
9. Take receptacle to bathroom or utility room.
10. Pour sample into one specimen container. Test this sample in case patient fails to void second specimen.
11. Make a note of the test result but do not officially record it.
12. Clean equipment according to facility policy and return to the proper area. Measure and record urine if patient is on I & O.
13. Remove and dispose of gloves according to facility policy.
14. Wash your hands.
15. Offer wash water for the patient to wash own hands.
16. If permitted, encourage patient to drink water. Be sure to record intake on I & O sheet.
17. Tell patient when you will return for the second sample. Return to the patient's unit at the proper time.
18. Wash your hands and identify the patient. Explain what you plan to do, and how the patient can help.
19. Repeat Steps 5–15.
20. Place specimen in protective biohazard bag for transport.
21. Carry out each procedure completion action. Remember to wash your hands, report completion of task, and document time, fractional urine specimen to laboratory, and patient reaction.

Catheterized Urine Specimen. When a urine specimen is needed that is free of contamination from organisms that are found in areas near the urinary meatus (opening), the specimen may be collected by inserting a sterile tube (catheter). The nurse will perform this procedure.

Twenty-four Hour Specimen. If a 24-hour urine specimen is ordered, all urine excreted by the patient in a 24-hour period is collected and saved, Figure 24–11. A 24-hour urine specimen requires that the patient start the 24-hour time period with an empty bladder. For this reason, the first specimen is discarded.

■ All urine is saved in a large, carefully labeled container that is supplied by the laboratory and may contain a preservative.
■ The container is usually surrounded by ice. If the patient has an indwelling catheter, place the catheter bag in a container surrounded by ice. Empty the bag into the container supplied by the laboratory.
■ The patient is asked to void. This first urine is discarded so that the bladder is empty at the time the test begins.
■ All other urine is saved, including that voided as the test time finishes.
■ No toilet tissue should be allowed to enter the container.
■ If you or the patient forget to save a specimen during the test period, report it immediately to the nurse. The test must be discontinued and started again for another 24 hours.

Remember to put on disposable gloves and remove and dispose of them properly each time you collect a specimen.

PROCEDURE 86

SIDE **7**

COLLECTING A 24-HOUR URINE SPECIMEN

1. Carry out each beginning procedure action.
2. Remember to wash your hands, identify the patient, and provide privacy.
3. Assemble equipment needed:
   ■ 24-hour specimen container (supplied by health care facility)
   ■ Label
   ■ Bedpan, urinal, or commode or specimen collector for toilet
   ■ Sign for patient's bed

- Disposable gloves
- Biohazard bag

4. Label the container with the:
   - Patient's name
   - Room number
   - Test ordered
   - Type of specimen
   - Time started
   - Time ended
   - Date
   - Physician's name

5. Emphasize to the patient the necessity of saving all urine passed.

6. Place the specimen collection container in the bathroom in a pan of ice, Figure 24–11A and B. The ice will keep the specimen cool for 24 hours.

7. Put on disposable gloves.

8. Allow the patient to void.
   a. Assist with the bedpan/urinal as needed.

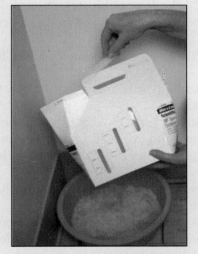

A. Place the 24-hour specimen container in patient's bathroom. A plastic fastener holds the top secure. Place specimen container in pan of ice.

   b. Measure the amount of urine passed if the patient's I & O is being monitored.
   c. Discard the urine specimen.
   d. Note the date and time of voiding. This time will mark the start of the 24-hour collection.

9. Place a sign on the patient's bed to alert other health care team members that a 24-hour urine specimen is being collected. (The sign may read: *Save all urine—24-hour specimen.*)

10. From this time on, all urine voided is added to the specimen container for a period of 24 hours, Figure 24–11C and D. The container is kept on ice when not in use. Check facility policy regarding handling of the specimen container.

11. At the end of the 24-hour period:
    a. Put on disposable gloves.
    b. Ask patient to void one last time.
    c. Add this urine to the specimen container.

12. Remove sign from patient's bed. Check container label for accuracy and completeness. Attach the appropriate requisition slip.

13. Remove and dispose of gloves according to facility policy.

14. Place specimen in protective biohazard bag for transport.

15. Carry out each procedure completion action. Remember to wash your hands, report completion of task, and document time, 24-hour urine specimen to lab, and patient reaction.

16. Clean and replace all equipment used, according to facility policy.

17. Take or send specimen to laboratory immediately.

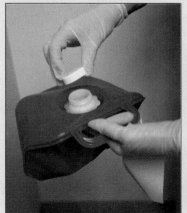

B. Some facilities use plastic containers with screw tops when collecting a 24-hour urine specimen.

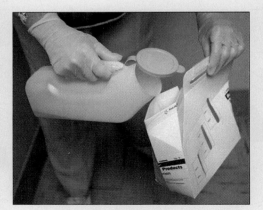

C. Open mouth of container wide to avoid spilling specimen.

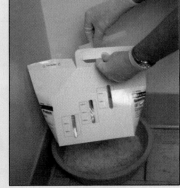

D. Reseal container and return to pan of ice after each voiding until entire specimen has been collected.

FIGURE 24–11. Many facilities use disposable containers for 24-hour urine specimen collection. The urine is preserved by the use of chemicals or cold storage.

Stool Specimens

A specimen of stool is a sample of *fecal* material (solid body waste or bowel movement) collected in a special container. The specimen is then sent to the laboratory for examination. In the laboratory, stool may be examined for:

■ Pathogenic microorganisms (germs)
■ Parasites
■ Occult blood (hidden blood or blood that cannot be seen by the naked eye)
■ Chemical analysis

PROCEDURE 87

SIDE 8

COLLECTING A STOOL SPECIMEN

1. Carry out each beginning procedure action.
2. Remember to wash your hands, identify the patient, and provide privacy.
3. Assemble equipment needed:
   ■ Bedpan and cover
   ■ Specimen container and cover
   ■ Label including:
      — Patient's full name
      — Room number
      — Date and time of collection
      — Physician's name
      — Examination to be performed
      — Other information as it is requested
   ■ Toilet tissue
   ■ Tongue blades
   ■ Disposable gloves
   ■ Biohazard bag
4. Put on disposable gloves.
5. Collect stool from daily bowel movement in the bedpan or diaper. Offer wash water to patient. Take covered pan to utility room.
6. Use tongue blades to remove specimen from bedpan or diaper and place in specimen container, Figure 24–12. If possible, take a sample (about 1 teaspoon) from each part of the specimen.
7. Remove and dispose of gloves according to facility policy.
8. Wash your hands. Do not contaminate the outside of the container.
9. Cover container and attach completed label. Make sure cover is on container tightly. Label the container appropriately. Place specimen in protective biohazard bag for transport.
10. Take or send specimen to laboratory promptly. (Stool specimens are never refrigerated.)
11. Carry out each procedure completion action. Remember to wash your hands, report completion of task, and document time, stool specimen to lab, and patient reaction.

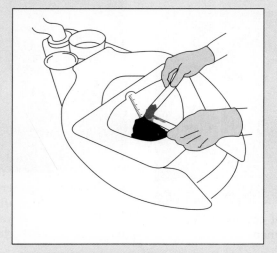
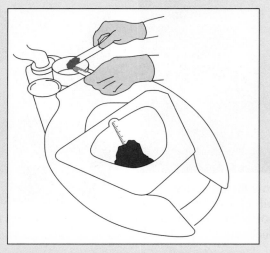

FIGURE 24–12. Use tongue blades to transfer the stool specimen from the collection container to the specimen container.

The following advanced procedures are included in Unit 42:

- Testing for Occult Blood Using Hemoccult® and Developer
- Testing for Occult Blood Using Hematest® Reagent Tablets
- Testing Urine with the Hemacombostix®

Sputum Specimens

Sputum refers to mucus that is brought up into the mouth, usually after coughing.

- Specimens are taken early in the morning since secretions have pooled during the night.
- This matter is not just saliva but comes from the lungs.
- Sputum specimens are frequently taken from patients who have chest conditions.

SIDE
8

PROCEDURE 88

COLLECTING A SPUTUM SPECIMEN

1. Carry out each beginning procedure action.
2. Remember to wash your hands, identify the patient, and provide privacy.
3. Assemble equipment needed:
   - Container and cover for specimen
   - Glass of water
   - Label including:
     — Patient's full name
     — Room number
     — Hospital number
     — Date and time of collection
     — Physician's name
     — Examination to be done
     — Other information as it is requested
   - Disposable gloves
   - Tissues
   - Emesis basin
   - Biohazard bag
4. Put on disposable gloves.
5. Have the patient rinse mouth. Use emesis basin for waste.
6. Ask patient to cough deeply to bring up sputum and expectorate (spit) into the container, Figure 24–13.
   - Have patient cover mouth with tissue to prevent spread of infection.
   - Collect 1 to 2 tablespoonsful of sputum unless otherwise ordered.
   - Do not contaminate the outside of the container.
     NOTE: If a 24-hour specimen is being collected, the container will be left at the patient's bedside.
7. Remove and dispose of gloves according to facility policy.

8. Wash your hands.
9. Cover container tightly and attach completed label. Place specimen in protective biohazard bag for transport.
10. Carry out each procedure completion action. Remember to wash your hands, report completion of task, and document time, sputum specimen to lab/color and character, and patient reaction.
11. Take or send specimen to laboratory promptly.

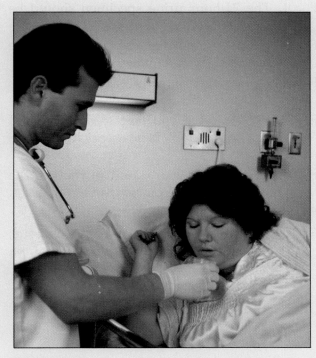

FIGURE 24–13. After coughing deeply, the patient deposits the sputum specimen directly into the container.

SUMMARY

Careful measurement and monitoring of intake and output is basic to the care of patients who have
- Renal or cardiac disease.
- Lost excessive fluids.
- Retained fluids abnormally.
- Intravenous therapy.
- Catheters.
- Had recent surgery.

Intake and output are measured in containers graduated in metric increments. Therefore, a knowledge of metric measurements and their common equivalents is important.

Laboratory tests are made on body excretions and secretions. These include, but are not limited to, samples of:
- Urine   - Feces   - Sputum

Careful collecting, handling, and labeling of these specimens protect your patient and assure accuracy in results. The use of disposable gloves when handling patient discharges and excretions is required to protect the care giver.

UNIT REVIEW

A. True/False. Answer the following true or false by circling T or F.

T F 1. Perspiration and blood loss are usually described in actual ml amounts.

T F 2. Eight specimens are needed to collect a fractional sample.

T F 3. Urine output is the only way fluid is lost from the body.

T F 4. The 24-hour urine specimen should be kept refrigerated or on ice.

T F 5. Fluid used to irrigate a bladder would be included in total intake.

T F 6. Urine output is approximately 3 quarts (3000 cc) daily.

T F 7. Explain what you plan to do to a child even if you don't believe the child understands.

T F 8. Tongue blades are used to transfer the stool specimen from bedpan to container.

T F 9. Fruits can be a source of liquid intake.

T F 10. Since it is such a complicated technique, patients are never permitted to obtain a midstream specimen from themselves.

B. Multiple Choice. Choose the answer that best completes each of the following sentences by circling the proper letter.

11. Average fluid intake is
    a. 500 ml.   c. 2500 ml.
    b. 1000 cc.   d. 3 quarts.

12. Monitoring I & O is especially important when the patient
    a. has a rash.   c. drinks normal
    b. has a urinary   amounts of fluid.
       catheter.   d. is not sleeping well.

13. When computing total output, you must consider
    a. vomitus.   c. blood loss.
    b. perspiration.   d. All of these.

14. An 8-ounce water glass holds approximately
    a. 240 ml.   c. 60 ml.
    b. 120 ml.   d. 30 ml.

15. When collecting a 24-hour urine specimen,
    a. save all urine.
    b. discard the last urine when time is up.
    c. discard the first urine at beginning of test.
    d. take each urine obtained to the lab.

C. Matching. Match the words in Column II with the statements in Column I.

Column I	Column II
_____ 16. approximate equivalent of an ounce	a. one milliliter
_____ 17. matter brought up from the lungs	b. specimen
_____ 18. fluid retention in the tissues	c. dehydration
_____ 19. vomitus	d. void
_____ 20. opening	e. sputum
_____ 21. approximate equivalent to 1 cc	f. emesis
_____ 22. urinate	g. feces
_____ 23. solid waste from bowel	h. 30 ml
_____ 24. sample of body fluid	i. edema
	j. meatus

D. Completion. Do the following practical application.

25. The patient kept this record in the bedside stand. Convert each amount to milliliters. Determine the total intake.

Time	Liquid and Amount	Milliliter Equivalent
0715	1/2 glass water	_120_ ml
0800	1 glass orange juice, 1 cup of coffee and 1/2 cup milk	_600_ ml
0900–1000	Sips of water, about 1/2 glass	____ ml
1030	1 glass cranberry juice	____ ml
1215	1 jello	____ ml
	1 bowl of soup	____ ml
	1 glass milk	____ ml
1345	1 glass water	____ ml
1430	1/2 foam cup apple juice	____ ml
		Total

SELF-EVALUATION   Section 8

A. Match Column I with Column II.

Column I

_____ 1. gastrostomy tube

_____ 2. carbohydrates

_____ 3. proteins

_____ 4. roughage

_____ 5. f.f.

_____ 6. gavage

_____ 7. feces

_____ 8. fats

Column II

a. tube feeding

b. important nutrient for body building and repair

c. stored form of energy

d. solid body wastes

e. artificial tube leading directly into the stomach

f. encourage fluid intake

g. called "energy" foods

h. cellulose

B. Choose the phrase that best completes each of the following sentences by circling the proper letter.

9. Foods that contain the greatest amount of carbohydrates come from
   a. eggs.
   b. milk.
   c. fruits.
   d. nuts.
   e. pork.

10. Your patient has an order for a regular diet. This means
    a. rich pastries will be included.
    b. more calories than usual must be supplied.
    c. only liquids may be consumed.
    d. a basic normal diet will be provided.
    e. salt must be omitted.

11. Your patient has been nauseated and has been placed on a clear liquid diet. You would
    a. feed your patient once a day.
    b. offer coffee with cream and sugar.
    c. offer 7Up or ginger ale.
    d. offer tomato juice.
    e. offer vegetable soup.

12. Your patient has dentures that fit poorly. His nutritional needs would best be met with a
    a. regular diet.
    b. full liquid diet.
    c. salt-free diet.
    d. clear liquid diet.
    e. soft diet.

13. Your patient is on a full liquid diet. When the tray arrives and you check it, you discover one of the following which does not belong:
    a. soup (strained).
    b. sherbet.
    c. eggnog.
    d. crackers.
    e. strained grape juice.

14. You are assigned to pass nourishments. One patient's name has a "withhold." You will
    a. offer only solids.
    b. remember to measure intake.
    c. offer an extra portion of juice.
    d. refuse to give juice.
    e. give a choice of nourishments.

15. Your patient is blind but able to feed himself. You will
    a. feed him; it's faster.
    b. explain the tray arrangement related to the face of a clock.
    c. place all food in a straight line across the over-bed table.
    d. place the tray with no explanation.
    e. explain the tray arrangement by putting all hot foods toward the tray top and cold toward the tray bottom.

16. You're assigned to record your patient's I & O. Which of the following should be counted?
    a. 500 ml IV D/W
    b. 700 ml urine
    c. 200 ml vomitus
    d. 300 ml gavaged nutrients
    e. All of the above

17. Your patient has had a 24-hour specimen collected. You know you will
    a. collect the first specimen after 24 hours of hospitalization.
    b. send each individual specimen of urine to the lab immediately after the patient voids.
    c. collect the first specimen of urine every 24 hours for three days.
    d. report immediately to your nurse if a specimen is lost, since the test will be discontinued.
    e. leave the urine collection jar on the open table in the dirty utility room.

18. Your patient took in 240 ml of juice and 180 ml of sherbet. The total intake would be
    a. 8 ounces.
    b. 320 ml.
    c. 10 ounces.
    d. 410 ml.
    e. 14 ounces.

19. Your patient put out 16 ounces of urine. You might record this as
    a. 460 ml.
    b. 480 ml.
    c. 500 ml.
    d. 520 ml.
    e. 556 ml.

20. When cleansing a female patient in order to collect a midstream urine specimen, you should
    a. cleanse only the meatus.
    b. always cleanse from front to back.
    c. allow the labia to gently close after cleansing.
    d. cleanse from back to front.
    e. cleanse the inner thighs.

21. When collecting a sputum specimen
    a. ask the patient to cough deeply.
    b. rinse the mouth out first.
    c. do not allow expectorant to contaminate the outside of the container.
    d. use disposable gloves.
    e. All of the above.

C. The daily servings from each of the food groups should include:

Group		Servings
22. fruits	b	a. sparingly
23. vegetables	c	b. 2–4 or more
24. breads, cereals, pastas, rice	e	c. 3–5 or more
		d. 1–2
25. fats, oils, sweets	d	e. 6–11

D. Provide short answers to the following.

26. List four observations about a patient receiving an IV that should be reported to the nurse.
    a. _____
    b. _____
    c. _____
    d. _____

27. Name five foods permitted on a low-fat/ cholesterol diet.
    a. _____
    b. _____
    c. _____
    d. _____
    e. _____

28. Explain why elderly patients may be at risk for dehydration. _____
    _____

29. Explain how a patient may assist in accounting for fluid intake. _____
    _____

30. List five patients who might require more careful monitoring of their intake and output.
    a. Dibetics _____
    b. _____
    c. _____
    d. _____
    e. _____

Unit 25

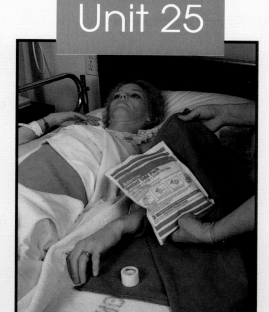

Heat and Cold Applications

OBJECTIVES

As a result of this unit, you will be able to:

■ Spell and define terms.

■ List the physical conditions requiring the use of heat and cold.

■ Name types of heat and cold applications.

■ Describe the effects of local cold applications.

■ Describe the effects of local heat applications.

■ Demonstrate local cold application procedures.

■ Demonstrate local heat application procedures.

■ List safety concerns related to application of heat and cold.

VOCABULARY

Learn the meaning and the correct spelling of the following words:

diathermy
hemorrhage
hypothermia-
   hyperthermia blanket

vasoconstriction
vasodilation

Heat and cold applications are used only on written orders from the physician or nurse for a specific length of time. Some facilities allow only professional personnel to apply heat and cold. Some states have laws against nursing assistants applying heat or cold in a home health setting. In other facilities, nursing assistants who have been specially trained are permitted to carry out these procedures under the supervision of the nurse. Be sure you know and follow the policy of your facility and are adequately prepared and *supervised*.

Therapy with Heat and Cold

The physician orders the use of heat or cold applications to:

■ Relieve pain.

■ Combat local infection, swelling, or inflammation.

■ Control bleeding (hemorrhage).
■ Reduce body temperature.

Local applications of heat and cold are made with:
■ Ice bags.
■ Electronically operated Aquamatic K-Pads®. K-Pads® come in many shapes and sizes. They can be used to apply dry heat. By using an attachment, they can also be used for cooling.
■ Prepackaged, single-use units for the application of hot and cold. A single blow to the surface activates the contents, providing a controlled temperature.
■ Gel packs that can be cooled or heated as needed.

General treatments of heat and cold consist of:
■ Thermal mattresses known as hypothermia-hyperthermia blankets These are widely used to:
  — Lower body temperature when there is fever.
  — Elevate body temperature in cases of hypothermia.

Types of Heat and Cold

Moisture intensifies heat or cold. When it is used, extra care must be taken. Cold applications may be applied dry or moist.
■ Dry cold is provided by:
  — Ice bags
  — Ice caps
  — Ice collars
  — Prepackaged units
  — Gel packs
■ Moist cold is applied with:
  — Compresses
  — Soaks
  — Packs

Heat applications may be applied dry or moist.
■ Dry heat is produced by:
  — Hot water bottles
  — Electric heating pads/units
  — Single-use units
  — Gel packs
■ Moist heat is produced with:
  — Soaks
  — Compresses
  — Packs

Cold and heat applications affect the body in different ways.
■ Cold affects the body by:
  — Causing blood vessels to become smaller (vasoconstriction).
  — Reducing edema by decreasing the blood flow to the area.
  — Numbing the sensation of pain.
  — Slowing life processes.
  — Slowing inflammation.
  — Reducing itching.
■ Heat (diathermy)
  — Makes blood vessels larger (vasodilation).
  — Provides added nourishment and oxygen to cells and removes wastes.
  — Increases the blood supply to the area.
  — Promotes healing.
  — Can be soothing.

CAUTIONS

You must be very watchful when applying cold or warm treatments. When assigned to this task, keep in mind the following:
■ The age and condition of the patient should be considered. Give extra care to:
  — Young children
  — The aged
  — Patients who are uncooperative
  — Patients who are unconscious
  — Patients who are paralyzed
  — Patients with tissue damage
  — Patients with poor circulation
■ An electric heating pad must not be used with moist dressings unless a rubber cover is placed over the pad. If the wires become damp, a short circuit may result. The patient must not lie on the pad since severe burns can result. Sensitivity to heat varies, so patients receiving heat treatments must be checked frequently. Although heating pads are not used in health care facilities, they are used by individuals in homes.

- Heat cradles are used to stimulate the circulation in the legs, feet, and perineal areas. The heat cradle must be used with care so that the patient is not burned. A bed cradle is equipped with ordinary light bulbs of 25 watts placed three feet from the area to be treated to provide continuous dry heat. The bulbs are hung under the top of the cradle and encased in wire frames to avoid burning the patient.

- Other lamp treatments, such as infrared and ultraviolet, are given by experts because of the danger involved since these produce penetrating heat.

- Heat is not applied to the head since it could cause blood vessels in the area to dilate, causing headaches.

- Heat should not be applied to the abdomen if there is any question of appendicitis because it would increase the chance of the appendix rupturing.

- Areas where cold treatments are used should be carefully and frequently checked for discoloration and numbness. If the area is discolored or numb, discontinue the treatment and report to the nurse.

- Rubber or plastic should never touch the patient's skin. Be sure all appliances are covered with cloth.

Refer to Figure 25–1 to refresh your memory of the beginning procedure actions and procedure completion actions that must be carried out for all patient care procedures.

BEGINNING PROCEDURE ACTIONS

- Wash your hands.
- Assemble equipment.
- Go to the patient's room, knock, and pause before entering.
- Introduce yourself and identify the patient by checking the identification bracelet.
- Ask visitors to leave and inform them where they can wait.
- Provide privacy.
- Explain what will happen and answer questions.
- Raise bed to comfortable working height.

PROCEDURE COMPLETION ACTIONS

- Position patient comfortably.
- Leave signal cord, telephone, and fresh water close at hand.
- Return bed to lowest position.
- Perform general safety check of patient and environment.
- Care for equipment according to facility policy.
- Wash your hands.
- Report completion of task.
- Let visitors know when they may reenter the patient's room.
- Document action and your observations.

NOTE: Where there are open lesions, wet linen, or possible contact with patient body fluids or blood, disposable gloves are worn during the procedure. Put on gloves before contact with the patient or linen. Properly dispose of gloves after they are removed. ALWAYS APPLY UNIVERSAL PRECAUTIONS.

FIGURE 25–1. Beginning procedure actions and procedure completion actions

PROCEDURE 89

SIDE
8

APPLYING AN ICE BAG

1. Wash your hands.
2. Go into utility room and assemble the needed equipment:
   - Ice cap or collar
   - Cover (usually muslin)
   - Paper towels
   - Spoon or similar utensil
   - Ice cubes or ice chips
3. Prepare ice cap as follows:
   a. If ice cubes are used, rinse them in water to remove sharp edges.
   b. Fill ice cap half full, using ice scooper or

continues

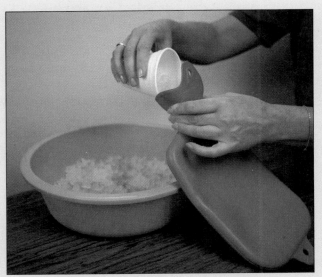

FIGURE 25–2. The ice bag is filled half full and the air is expelled.

5-15 MIN

large spoon, Figure 25–2. Avoid making ice bags too heavy.
c. To expel air from the ice bag:
  1. Rest ice bag on table in horizontal position with top in place.
  2. Do not screw top on.
  3. Squeeze bag until air has been removed.
d. Fasten top securely.
e. Test for leakage.

f. Wipe dry with paper towels. A paper towel placed between bag and muslin keeps the muslin from becoming wet.

NOTE: If available, frozen gel pack may be taken from the freezer. Proceed as with an ice bag.

4. Take equipment to bedside on tray.
5. Carry out each beginning procedure action.
6. Remember to wash your hands, identify the patient, and provide privacy.
7. Apply ice bag to the affected part with the metal cap away from patient.
8. Refill bag before all ice is melted.
9. Check skin area with each application. Report to supervising nurse immediately if skin is discolored or white or if patient reports skin is numb.
10. Carry out each procedure completion action. Remember to wash your hands, report completion of task, and document time, ice pack applied (area of application), length of application, and patient reaction.
11. When ice bag is removed after use, wash it with soap and water, rinse, dry, and screw top on. Leave air in ice bag to prevent sides from sticking together.
12. If a reusable cold pack is used, wash it thoroughly with soap and water and return it to the refrigerator. Discard a disposable pack.

PROCEDURE 90

SIDE 8

APPLYING A DISPOSABLE COLD PACK

1. Carry out each beginning procedure action.
2. Remember to wash your hands, identify the patient, and provide privacy.
3. Assemble equipment needed:
   ■ Disposable cold pack (commercially prepared). Read directions.
   ■ Cloth covering (towel, hot water bag cover)
   ■ Tape or rolls of gauze
4. Expose area to be treated. Note condition of area.
5. Place cold pack in cloth covering, Figure 25–3.
6. Strike or squeeze cold pack to activate chemicals.

7. Place covered cold pack on proper area and enclose with a towel, Figure 25–4. Note time of application.
8. Secure with tape or gauze.
9. Leave patient in comfortable position with signal cord within easy reach.
10. Return to bedside every 10 minutes. Check area being treated for discoloration or numbness. If these signs and symptoms occur, discontinue treatment and report them to your supervisor.
11. If no adverse symptoms occur, remove pack in 30 minutes. Note condition of area. Continu-

ous treatment requires application of a fresh pack.

12. Remove pack from cover and discard according to facility policy. Return unused gauze and tape.

13. Put cover in laundry.

14. Carry out each procedure completion action. Remember to wash your hands, report completion of task, and document time, application of disposable cold pack to (area of application), length of treatment, and patient reaction.

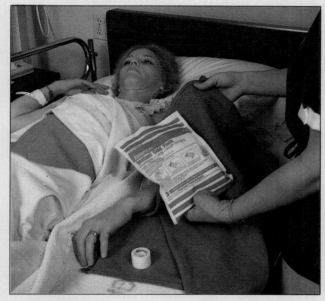

FIGURE 25–3. Cover the disposable cold pack with a towel before applying it to the patient.

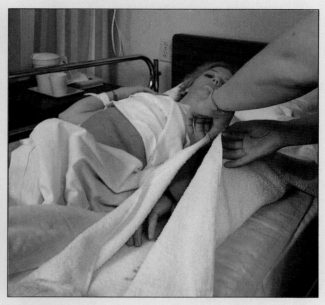

FIGURE 25–4. Cover the cold pack application with another towel.

PROCEDURE 91

APPLYING A WARM WATER BAG

NOTE: Water bottles are no longer used in health care facilities. Because of their widespread use in homes, the procedure has been included.

1. Wash your hands, Figure 25–5A.
2. Assemble equipment needed, Figure 25–5B.
   - Hot water bag
   - Paper towels
   - Thermometer
   - Container for hot water, or use sink
   - Cover
3. Prepare the hot water bottle as follows:
   a. Fill container with water and test for correct temperature, Figure 25–5C. The temperature should be approximately 115°F.
   b. Fill hot water bag one-third to one-half full to avoid unnecessary weight, Figure 25–5D.

   c. Expel air by:
      1. Placing hot water bag horizontally on flat surface, Figure 25–5E.
      2. Holding neck of bag upright until water reaches neck.
      3. Closing the top when all air has been expelled.
   d. Wipe hot water bag dry with paper towels, Figure 25–5F. Turn bag upside down to check for leakage, Figure 25–5G.
   e. Place cover on hot water bag so that patient's skin does not come in contact with rubber or plastic, Figure 25–5H.
4. Take equipment to bedside on tray.
5. Apply bag to the affected area. Never allow patient to lie on the hot water bag.
6. Check condition of skin.

continues

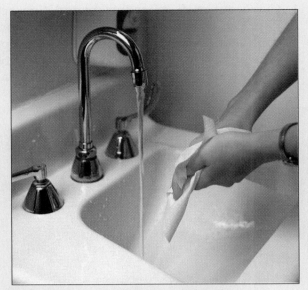

FIGURE 25–5A. Wash your hands.

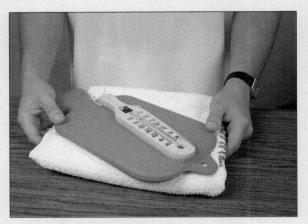

FIGURE 25–5B. Assemble equipment.

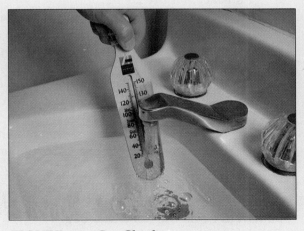

FIGURE 25–5C. Check water temperature.

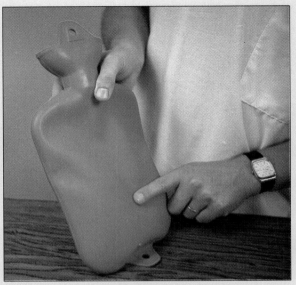

FIGURE 25–5D. Fill bag one-third to one-half full.

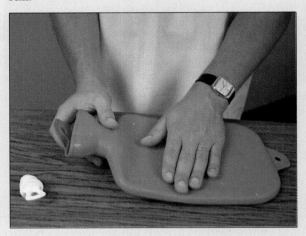

FIGURE 25–5E. Expel air by placing bag flat and compressing it with the flat of your hand.

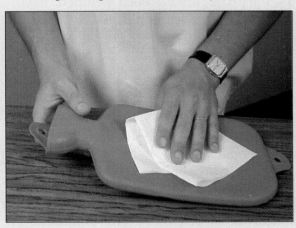

FIGURE 25–5F. Dry bag with paper towel.

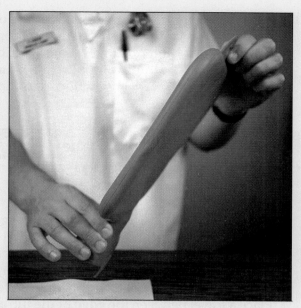

FIGURE 25–5G. Test for leaks after securing cap.

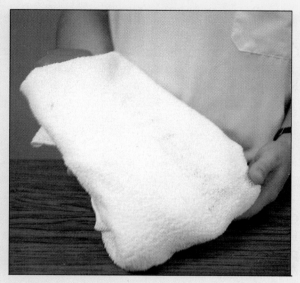

FIGURE 25–5H. Cover bag before applying.

PROCEDURE 92

SIDE
8

APPLYING AN AQUAMATIC K-PAD®

1. Carry out each beginning procedure action.
2. Remember to wash your hands, identify the patient, and provide privacy.
3. Assemble equipment needed:
   - K-Pad® and control unit
   - Distilled water
   - Covering for pad
4. Place the control unit on the bedside stand, Figure 25–6.
5. Remove the cover and fill the unit with distilled water to the fill line.
6. Screw the cover in place and loosen it one-quarter turn. Plug unit into electric socket.
7. Note time of application. In most facilities, the temperature is preset by the central service department. If this has not been done, turn on the unit. The temperature, usually 95–100°F, is set by a key. The key is removed after setting.
8. Cover pad and place it on the patient.
   - Secure with tape.
   - Never use pins.
   - Be sure that the tubing is coiled on the bed to facilitate the flow.

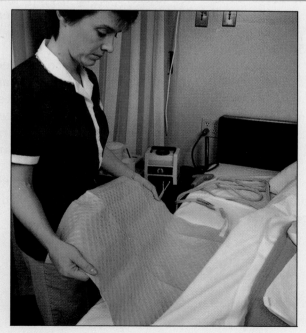

FIGURE 25–6. The disposable Aquamatic K–Pad® and control unit maintain an even temperature.

continues

- ■ Do not allow the tubing to hang below the level of the bed.
9. Check the control unit periodically. Refill the unit if the water drops below the fill line.
10. Remove pad after prescribed period of time.

11. Carry out each procedure completion action. Remember to wash your hands, report completion of task, and document time, application of K-Pad® to (area of application), time applied and removed, and patient reaction.

SIDE 8

PROCEDURE 93

PERFORMING THE WARM FOOT SOAK

1. Carry out each beginning procedure action.
2. Remember to wash your hands, identify the patient, and provide privacy.
3. Assemble equipment needed:
   - ■ Bath thermometer
   - ■ Extra pitcher of 105°F water
   - ■ Solution, as ordered, in container

   Place the tray on the over-bed table. Also bring the following equipment to the bed:
   - ■ Large rubber or plastic sheet
   - ■ Tub or basin of appropriate size
   - ■ 2 bath blankets
   - ■ 2 bath towels
4. Have patient flex knees. Loosen the top bedclothes at the foot of the bed and fold them back, just below patient's knees.
5. To make bed protector:
   a. Place rubber sheet across the foot of the bed.
   b. Place bath blanket folded in half, top half fanfolded toward foot of bed, over rubber sheet.
6. Raising patient's feet, draw rubber sheet, blanket, and bath towel up under the legs and feet of patient. Bring upper half of bath blanket over feet.

NOTE: This procedure may be carried out with the patient sitting in a chair and the foot soak tub on the protected floor.

7. Fill tub half full of water and place it lengthwise at foot of bed. Temperature should be 105°F unless otherwise ordered.
8. Raising the patient's feet with one hand, draw tub under them and gradually immerse feet. Place a towel between the edge of the tub and the legs.
9. Draw the bath blanket up over the knees and fold it over from each side. Bring top covers over foot of bed to retain heat.
10. Replenish water as necessary to maintain desired temperature. Remove feet each time water is added.
11. Discontinue treatment within 15 or 20 minutes.
12. Remove the patient's feet from tub and move them to the towel. Cover feet.
13. Remove tub to table or chair.
14. Dry feet. Apply lotion if needed.
15. Remove bath blanket, rubber sheet, and towel.
16. Draw down top covers and tuck in at foot.
17. Carry out each procedure completion action. Remember to wash your hands, report completion of task, and document time, (left/right) warm foot soak, temperature of water, length of treatment, and patient reaction.

PROCEDURE 94

PERFORMING THE WARM ARM SOAK

1. Carry out each beginning procedure action.
2. Remember to wash your hands, identify the patient, and provide privacy.
3. Assemble equipment needed:
   - ■ Bath thermometer
   - ■ Arm-soak basin
   - ■ Pitcher
   - ■ Large plastic sheet

- Bath towel
- Bath blanket

4. Bring equipment to bedside.
5. Cover patient with bath blanket.
6. Fanfold bedding to foot of bed.
7. Expose arm to be soaked.
8. Elevate head of bed to a sitting position, if permitted.
9. Help patient to move to far side of bed, opposite the arm to be soaked. Be sure side rail is up and secure.
10. Cover bed with plastic sheet and towel.
11. Fill arm-soak basin half full with water at prescribed temperature (usually 100°F). Check temperature with bath thermometer.
12. Take arm-soak basin from over-bed table and position on bed protector.
13. Assist patient to gradually place arm in basin.
14. Check temperature every 5 minutes. Use pitcher to get additional water and add to arm-soak basin to maintain temperature.

15. Discontinue procedure at end of prescribed time.
    a. Lift patient's arm out of basin.
    b. Slip basin forward and allow arm to rest on bath towel.
    c. Place basin on over-bed table. Gently pat arm dry with towel.
16. Remove plastic sheet and towel.
17. Adjust bedding and remove bath blanket. If treatment is to be repeated, fold bath blanket and place in bedside table. Leave unit tidy and call bell within reach.
18. Lower head of bed and make patient comfortable.
19. Take equipment to utility room. Clean and store according to facility policy.
20. Carry out each procedure completion action. Remember to wash your hands, report completion of task, and document time, (left/right) warm arm soak, temperature of water, length of treatment, and patient reaction.

PROCEDURE 95

APPLYING A MOIST COMPRESS

1. Carry out each beginning procedure action.
2. Remember to wash your hands, identify the patient, and provide privacy.
3. Assemble equipment needed:
    - Disposable gloves
    - Asepto syringe
    - Bed protector
    - Compresses
    - Bath thermometer
    - Binder or towel
    - Pins or bandage
    - Basin with prescribed solution at temperature ordered
4. Bring equipment to bedside.
5. Expose only the area to be treated.
6. Protect bed and patient's clothing with bed protector (Chux®), Figure 25–7A.
7. Put on disposable gloves.
8. Moisten the compresses; remove excess liquid, Figure 25–7B. Apply to treatment area, Figure 25–7C.

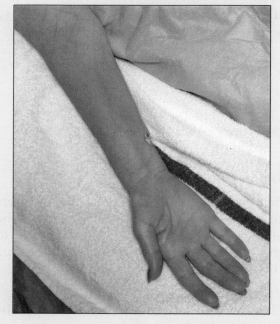

FIGURE 25–7A. Protect bed with a towel or other protector.

continues

9. Secure the dressings with bandage or binder. Dressing must be in contact with skin.
10. Help patient to maintain a comfortable position throughout the treatment.
11. Unscreen unit. Leave unit neat and tidy with signal cord within easy reach.
12. Maintain proper temperature and moisture.
    - ■ If dressings are to be kept hot, a hot water bag or K-Pad® may be applied.
    - ■ If dressings are to be kept cool, an ice bag may be applied.
    - ■ A syringe may be used to apply the solution to keep dressings wet.
13. Remove dressings when ordered. Change as ordered or once in 24 hours. Check skin several times each day.

14. Discard compresses.
15. Remove and dispose of gloves according to facility policy.
16. Carry out each procedure completion action. Remember to wash your hands, report completion of task, and document time, moist compresses (temperature) to (area of application), length of treatment, and patient reaction.

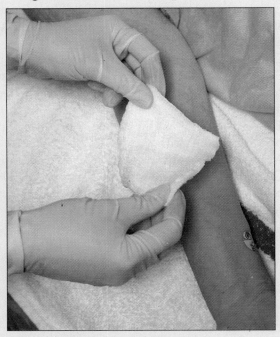

FIGURE 25–7C. Apply open compress to inflamed area.

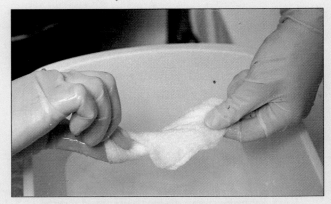

FIGURE 25–7B. Dip compress into basin of hot water. Grasping edges, squeeze out excess water.

Temperature Control Measures

Cooling Baths

Cooling baths are ordered when a patient's temperature is very elevated and nonresponsive to other treatments. The procedure may be too drastic for some children and some elderly. This procedure should be supervised by the nurse.

General Precautions.
- ■ Check with nurse to see if ice cubes or alcohol are to be added to the solution.
- ■ Take temperature at the beginning of the procedure, immediately after, and 30 minutes later.

- ■ Bathe only one part of the body at a time, keeping the rest of the body covered.
- ■ Use long, smooth strokes, bathing each part for approximately 5 minutes. Do not dry.
- ■ Do not bathe eyes or genitals.
- ■ Add water as needed to maintain proper temperature, which is usually 68–86°F.
- ■ End bath and report to nurse if the:
    - — Temperature drops to 1–2°F above desired temperature.
    - — Patient chills, begins to shiver, or becomes cyanotic.
    - — Pulse becomes rapid or irregular.
    - — Patient shows signs of shock.
- ■ Take a rectal temperature for greater accuracy.

Hypothermia-Hyperthermia Blankets

In acute care facilities excessively high or low body temperatures are treated by placing hypothermia-hyperthermia blankets over and under the patient. These blankets are units filled with water. The tem-perature of the water can be adjusted higher or lower depending on the individual patient's need to either raise or lower the temperature. This is a professional nursing responsibility.

SUMMARY

Treatments with warmth and cold are sometimes performed by nursing assistants. They must be performed with great caution to prevent injury to the patient. The procedures must be performed following the facility policy and be nursing assistant functions as permitted by state law.

These treatments:

- Require a physician's or registered nurse's order which specifies type, length, and temperature of treatment.
- Are supervised by a nurse.
- Must be done in a way that protects the patient against contact with light bulbs, metal, plastic, or rubber.

- Include applying:
  — Disposable cold packs
  — Hot water bottles
  — Aquamatic K-Pads®
  — Moist compresses
  — Gel packs
- Include performing:
  — Warm foot soaks
  — Warm arm soaks
  — Hypothermia-hyperthermia blankets

UNIT REVIEW

A. True/False. Answer the following statements true or false by circling T or F.

T F 1. Heat and cold treatments should be supervised by the nurse.

T F 2. If a patient has a possible diagnosis of appendicitis, heat should not be applied to the abdomen.

T F 3. The temperature of a warm-arm-soak solution should be approximately 100°F.

T F 4. Special blankets used to alter patient's temperature are called infrared blankets.

T F 5. A heat lamp with a 40-watt bulb should be placed approximately 6 inches from the patient's body.

T F 6. A patient who is unconscious must receive special attention during a heat treatment.

T F 7. A hot water bag need not be covered before applying.

T F 8. Heat is frequently applied to the head.

T F 9. When charting an application of cold, always include the length of time of the application.

T F 10. Aquamatic K-Pads® are usually set at 115°F.

B. Multiple Choice. Choose the phrase that best completes each of the following sentences by circling the proper letter.

11. Heat affects the body by
    a. causing vasodilation.
    b. increasing blood supply to the area.
    c. promoting healing.
    d. All of the above.

12. Special care with heat and cold treatments must be taken when the patient is
    a. aged.
    b. very young.
    c. uncooperative.
    d. All of the above.

13. Dry cold is provided by
    a. compresses.
    b. hyperthermia blanket.
    c. ice caps.
    d. soaks.

14. Cold affects the body by
    a. reducing pain sensations
    b. stimulating life processes.
    c. promoting inflammation.
    d. promoting healing.

15. Moist cold is applied with
    a. ice bags.
    b. ice caps.
    c. ice collars.
    d. soaks.

C. Matching. Match the words in Column II with the statements in Column I.

Column I		Column II
_e_ 16.	excessive blood loss	a. diathermy
_c_ 17.	increase in size of blood vessel	b. vasoconstriction
_f_ 18.	heat treatment	c. vasodilation
_a_ 19.	heat treatment given only by persons specially trained in the procedure	d. hypothermia blanket
		e. hemorrhage
_d_ 20.	used to lower body temperature	f. infrared

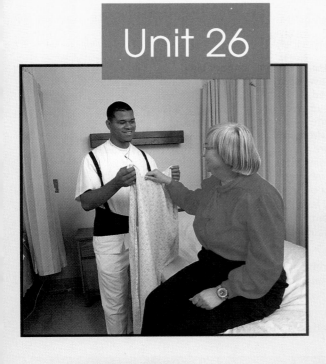

Assisting with the Physical Examination

VOCABULARY

Learn the meaning and the correct spelling of the following words:

apprehensive
dorsal lithotomy
  position
dorsal recumbent
  position
horizontal recumbent
  position (supine)
knee-chest position
ophthalmoscope

otoscope
percussion hammer
prone position
semi-Fowler's position
Sims' position
speculum
Trendelenburg
  position

OBJECTIVES

As a result of this unit, you will be able to:

■ Spell and define terms.

■ Describe the responsibilities of the nursing assistant during the physical assessment.

■ Name the positions for the various physical examinations.

■ Drape patient for the various positions.

■ Name the basic instruments necessary for physical examinations.

Physical examinations are done in the physician's office, in clinics, after the patient's admission to the facility, and in the patient's home. Remember to carry out each beginning procedure action and procedure completion action as you assist, Figure 26–1.

The physical examination helps the physician:

■ Evaluate the patient's current status.

■ Establish a diagnosis.

■ Determine the patient's progress and response to therapy.

Nursing physical assessments will be performed by the nurse in the facility after the patient is admitted. This information is used by the nurse to establish a nursing diagnosis.

Both of these procedures are carried out in a similar manner. The responsibilities of the nursing assistant include:

■ Providing for the comfort of the patient.

■ Trying to anticipate the examiner's needs.

■ Draping and positioning patients.

■ Using proper body mechanics and exposing only the part being examined.

■ Preparing equipment that might be needed.

■ Reassuring the patient.

■ Handing equipment as needed.

BEGINNING PROCEDURE ACTIONS	PROCEDURE COMPLETION ACTIONS
■ Wash your hands. ■ Assemble equipment needed. ■ Go to the patient's room, knock, and pause before entering. ■ Introduce yourself and identify the patient by checking the identification bracelet. ■ Ask visitors to leave and inform them where they can wait. ■ Provide privacy. ■ Assist patient to undress (in office or clinic). ■ Explain what will happen and answer questions. ■ Allow patient to assist in procedure as much as possible. ■ Raise bed or table to comfortable working height.	■ Position patient comfortably. ■ Leave signal cord, telephone, and fresh water close at hand. ■ Return bed or table to lowest position. ■ Perform general safety check of patient and environment. ■ Care for equipment according to facility policy. ■ Assist patient to dress (if in office or clinic). ■ Wash your hands. ■ Report completion of task. ■ Let visitors know when they may reenter the patient's room. ■ Document action and your observations.

NOTE: Where there are open lesions, wet linen, or possible contact with patient body fluids or blood, disposable gloves are to be worn during the procedure. Put on gloves before contact with the patient or linen. Properly dispose of gloves after they are removed. ALWAYS APPLY UNIVERSAL PRECAUTIONS.

FIGURE 26–1. Beginning procedure actions and procedure completion actions

■ Cleaning equipment after use.
■ Adjusting lighting.
■ Remaining available during the examination.

Positioning the Patient

Office Examination

When the examination takes place on an examination table, extra attention must be given to safety. The examination table may be raised or lowered in sections and stirrups and shoulder braces applied to assist in positioning. Be sure you know how to properly operate the examination table before positioning a patient on it.

Modifications

Some of the positions discussed may be modified and used for other purposes. For example, they might be used to change the position of a patient confined to bed or to perform specific procedures. Pillows must be used to support a patient who is to be kept in position for a period of time. Remember, the patient who "feels" covered and comfortable will be able to cooperate more fully. Providing privacy for the patient is one of your tasks, Figure 26–2.

Dorsal Recumbent Position

This is the basic examination position.
■ Assist the patient to be flat on the back with knees flexed and slightly

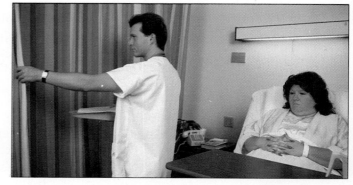

FIGURE 26–2. You assist the examination by drawing the curtains to provide privacy.

separated. The feet should be flat on the bed, Figure 26–3.
■ Place a small pillow under the patient's head.
■ Loosen the gown at the neck.
■ Cover the patient with a sheet.

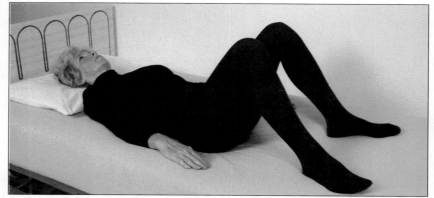

FIGURE 26–3. The dorsal recumbent position. (Draping and side rails have been omitted for clarity.)

Horizontal Recumbent Position

- Assist the patient to lie flat on the back. The legs are extended and slightly separated, Figure 26–4.
- Place a pillow under the patient's head.
- Cover the patient with a sheet.
- Loosen the gown at the neck.

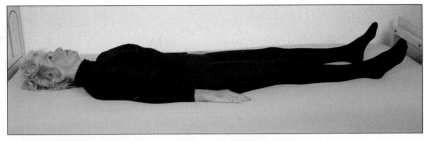

FIGURE 26–4. The horizontal recumbent position (supine)

Knee-chest Position

This position may be used to examine the rectal or vaginal areas and to relieve pain following childbirth. This is a difficult position to maintain, so never leave the patient alone. Position the patient in a prone position until the examiner is ready.

- Draping may be done with one or two sheets.
- Place a small pillow under the patient's head.
- Assist the patient to turn and lie on the abdomen with head turned to one side.
- Have the patient flex her arms and bring them up on either side of the head.
- Assist the patient to flex the knees and draw them up to meet the chest, Figure 26–5.

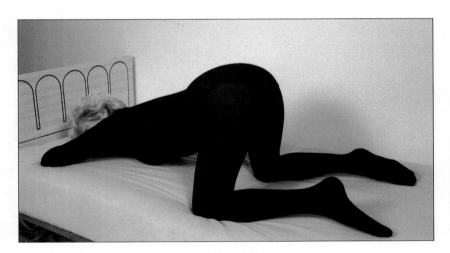

FIGURE 26–5. The knee-chest position

Prone Position

This position is used to examine the patient's back.

- Assist patient to lie on the abdomen with head turned to one side.
- Place a small pillow under the patient's head.
- Arms may be extended at the patient's side or flexed and brought up on either side of the head, Figure 26–6.
- One sheet is used for draping.

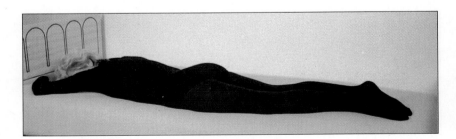

FIGURE 26–6. The prone position

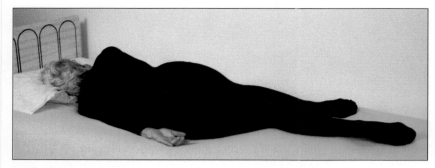

FIGURE 26–7.   Sims' position

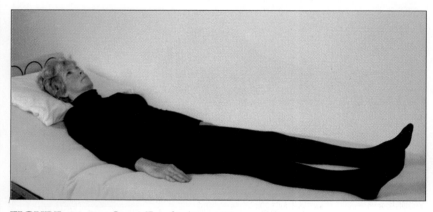

FIGURE 26–8.   Semi-Fowler's position

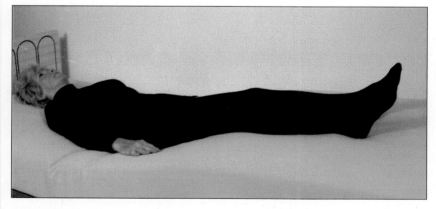

FIGURE 26–9.   Trendelenburg position. The bottom of the bed is raised.

Sims' Position

This position is used for vaginal and rectal procedures, including enema administration.

- Assist patient to turn on the left side with head turned to the same side on a small pillow.
- Position the left arm extended behind the body.
- Flex the right arm and position it in front of the patient.
- The left leg is slightly bent while the right leg is sharply flexed, Figure 26–7.
- One drape is usually adequate.

Semi-Fowler's Position

This is a common position for head and neck examinations of the in-bed patient.

- Assist patient to a semi-sitting position with backrest elevated at a 30-degree angle to the bed.
- The knees are supported in a slightly flexed position, Figure 26–8.
- The arms rest at the sides.
- One drape is usually enough.

Trendelenburg Position

This position encourages circulation to the patient's heart and brain. It is used when the patient is in shock.

- Assist patient to lie flat on the back with the head lower than the rest of the body.
- If possible, the lower half of the bed or table is broken so the legs are slightly flexed.
- In an emergency, the entire bed frame may be supported on blocks, tilting the bed to a 45-degree plane, Figure 26–9.
- Beds that are electrically powered may be adjusted to this position.
- Shoulder braces may be needed to prevent the patient from slipping.
- One drape is usually sufficient.

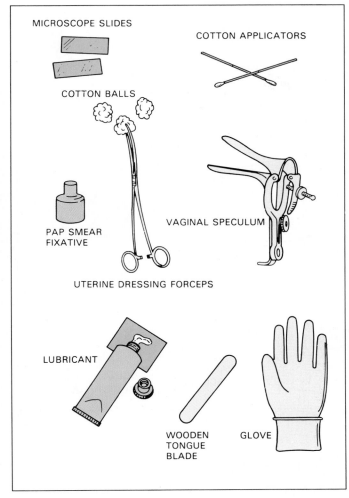

FIGURE 26–10. Equipment for pelvic examination

Dorsal Lithotomy Position

This position is frequently used for the pelvic examination of female patients. The special equipment you will assemble for the pelvic examination is shown in Figure 26–10. This is a difficult examination for most women, so make sure your draping makes the patient feel covered.

■ Make sure the patient voids prior to the examination.

■ The patient is positioned on her back.

■ The knees are well separated and flexed.

■ Usually, this position is achieved by placing the feet in stirrups, Figure 26–11.

■ One or two drapes may be used to cover the patient. The draping may be similar to draping for the knee-chest position.

Equipment for Physical Examination

Some health care facilities have examining instruments and equipment collected on trays. At other facilities, you will gather the necessary equipment and assemble it, Figure 26–12. The basic equipment includes:

■ Flashlight

■ Gloves

■ Percussion hammer (tests nerve reflex)

■ Tongue depressors

■ Cotton balls in antiseptic solution

■ Emesis basin (lined with paper towel)

■ Vaginal speculum

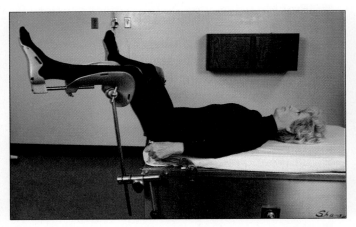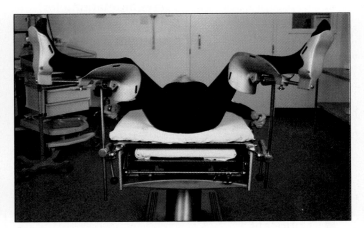

FIGURE 26–11. The patient's feet are placed in stirrups for the dorsal lithotomy position so that the knees are well-flexed and separated.

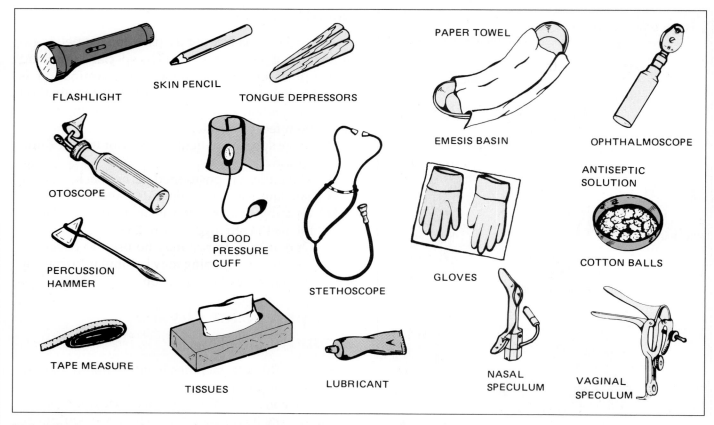

FIGURE 26–12. Basic equipment for the physical examination

- Tissues
- Lubricant
- Skin pencil
- Tape measure
- Nasal speculum
- Otoscope (used to examine ears)
- Ophthalmoscope (used to examine eyes)
- Blood pressure cuff (sphygmomanometer)
- Stethoscope

NOTE: A speculum is an instrument used to spread a body opening.

If only a female pelvic examination is to be performed, the following equipment will be needed:

- Microscope slides
- Cotton balls
- Pap smear fixative
- Uterine dressing forceps
- Cotton applicators
- Vaginal speculum
- Wooden tongue blades
- Lubricant
- Glove

SUMMARY

Another member of the staff must be present during a physical examination. The nursing assistant may assist the physician during the physical examination and as the nurse performs a nursing assessment. You do this successfully when you:

- Provide privacy while the patient's history is discussed.
- Are ready to assist during the examination and to provide proper lighting.
- Avoid overexposing the patient as you adjust the drapes.
- Remember that most patients feel apprehensive (frightened) about physical examinations. Be reassuring.
- Drape and position patients safely while maintaining proper body mechanics.
- Know and prepare the proper equipment for the examination.
- Assist patients during the examination and after the examination is completed.
- Properly clean up the room and equipment after the examination is completed.

UNIT REVIEW

A. True/False. Answer the following true or false by circling T or F.

T F 1. The physical examination helps the physician establish a nursing assessment.

T F 2. A patient who "feels" covered is able to cooperate more fully.

T F 3. Positions used for the physical examination can only be used for that purpose.

T F 4. The nursing assistant performs the actual physical exam.

T F 5. When a patient is placed in the Trendelenburg position, the feet must be at the same level as the knees.

T F 6. When positioning a patient for a physical examination, you must maintain proper body mechanics.

T F 7. Once you have the patient positioned for a physical examination, you should leave the room.

T F 8. The nursing assistant assists the physical assessment by draping and positioning the patient.

T F 9. Lighting may need to be adjusted during the examination.

T F 10. The semi-Fowler's position encourages blood flow to the head and heart.

B. Multiple Choice. Choose the phrase that best completes each of the following sentences by circling the proper letter.

11. The basic examination position is
    a. Sims'.
    b. dorsal recumbent.
    c. dorsal lithotomy.
    d. Trendelenburg.

12. Which of the following positions might best be selected to administer an enema?
    a. Sims'
    b. Semi-Fowler's
    c. Trendelenburg
    d. Dorsal recumbent

13. Your female patient is to have a pelvic examination. Which instrument would you be sure to have ready?
    a. Otoscope
    b. Vaginal speculum
    c. Nasal speculum
    d. Ophthalmoscope

14. The patient has vaginal bleeding and the physician orders a change of position. Which position would you prepare for?
    a. Sims'
    b. Semi-Fowler's
    c. Trendelenburg
    d. Lithotomy

15. Stirrups are of use in which position?
    a. Dorsal lithotomy
    b. Semi-Fowler's
    c. Sims'
    d. Trendelenburg

C. Matching. Match the word in Column II with the word or phrases in Column I.

Column I	Column II
_____ 16. instrument to examine the ear	a. apprehensive
_____ 17. instrument to examine the eye	b. drape
	c. ophthalmoscope
_____ 18. instrument to dilate a body opening	d. otoscope
_____ 19. full of fear	e. speculum
_____ 20. covering	f. percussion hammer

The Surgical Patient

As a result of this unit, you will be able to:

■ Spell and define terms.

■ Describe the concerns of patients who are about to have surgery.

■ List the various types of anesthesia.

■ Assist patients in preoperative care.

■ Shave the operative area.

■ Prepare the patient's unit for the patient's return from the operating room.

■ Prepare a recovery bed.

■ Assist patients in postoperative care.

Learn the meaning and the correct spelling of the following words and phrases:

ambulation
anesthesia
anti-embolism hose
aspirate
atelectasis
dangling
depilatory
disruption
distention
drainage
embolus
general anesthetic
hypoxia
incentive spirometer
local anesthetic
nosocomial
NPO
outpatient surgery
operative
orifice

perioperative
postanesthesia care
    unit (PACU)
postoperative
preoperative
prosthesis
recovery room (post-
    anesthesia care unit)
short-term surgery
singultus
spinal anesthesia
stable
surgical bed
T-binder
TED hose
thrombophlebitis
thrombus
umbilicus
vertigo

Patients facing any surgical procedure tend to be fearful. It is well to remember that these patients require great emotional as well as physical support, Figure 27–1. Such support should be given from the time the patient is admitted through the discharge.

Patients are concerned with:

■ Disfigurement

■ Pain

■ Loss of control as they undergo anesthesia

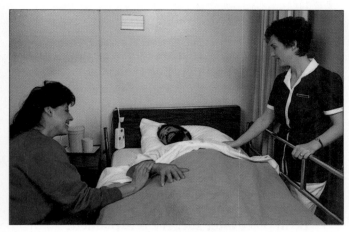

FIGURE 27–1.   Patients and their families need support during the preoperative period.

- What serious conditions might be found
- Length and cost of recovery
- Possibility of death

Surgery is often associated with anxiety, pain, and discomfort. For this reason, medications are given before, during, and after surgery.

Pain Perception

In order for a person to realize pain sensations the:
- Pain receptors record the sensation.
- Sensation is sent by the spinal nerves to the spinal cord and then to the brain.
- Sensation is received and interpreted in the brain.

Before surgery, the patient is given medication to

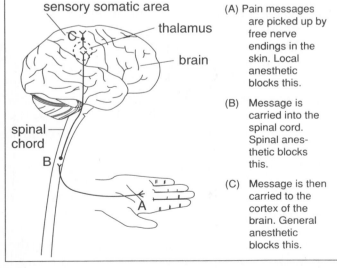

sensory somatic area
thalamus
brain
spinal chord
B
A
C

(A) Pain messages are picked up by free nerve endings in the skin. Local anesthetic blocks this.

(B) Message is carried into the spinal cord. Spinal anesthetic blocks this.

(C) Message is then carried to the cortex of the brain. General anesthetic blocks this.

FIGURE 27–2.   Pain may be blocked through the action of anesthetics at points A, B, or C.

promote relaxation. During surgery, anesthetics are given to prevent pain, Figure 27–2. After surgery, medications are given to reduce discomfort.

Anesthesia

Anesthesia is given to prevent pain, to relax muscles, and to induce forgetfulness. The choice of anesthetic agent (drug) and method of administration are determined by the location and type of surgery to be performed, the length of time needed for surgery, and the patient's physical condition.

There are two main types of anesthetics:
1. General anesthetics—These induce the patient to become unconscious.
2. Local anesthetics—These induce loss of feeling in a specific area.

General Anesthetics

General anesthetics block reception of pain in the brain. They are usually given in one of two ways:
1. Inhalation—Some gases that are used as anesthetics include ether, nitrous oxide, and cyclopropane.
   a. Inhaled anesthetics are apt to make the patient secrete more mucus and to experience nausea.
   b. Special attention must be given after surgery to keep the respiratory tract clear.
   c. There is a real danger that the patient may aspirate (draw) vomitus into the respiratory tract.
2. Intravenously—Drugs are introduced directly into the veins.
   a. These drugs, such as sodium pentathol, act rapidly.
   b. The patient quickly loses consciousness.
   c. IV anesthetics are often used with other types of anesthesia for short operations.

Local Anesthetics

Local anesthetics act by:
1. Blocking pain receptors in the operative area.
   a. Drugs such as procaine hydrochloride may be injected into the area around the operative area.
   b. These drugs stop the sensation of pain only in that area.
   c. The patient remains awake but free from pain during the operation.

2. Blocking transmission of the pain sensation at the level of the spinal cord.
   a. A drug is injected into the spinal canal that prevents feeling from any point below the level of the injection.
   b. The patient remains awake.
   c. This type of anesthesia is commonly used for abdominal surgery because it produces good relaxation of the muscles.
   d. This technique is called spinal anesthesia.

Following this type of anesthetic, the patient is unable to feel or move the legs for a period of time. If not prepared ahead of time, the patient may be frightened by this experience.

Surgical Care

The care of the surgical patient (perioperative) can be divided into three parts:
- Preoperative (before surgery)
- Operative (in the operating room)
- Postoperative (after surgery)

Preoperative Care

Preoperative care begins at the moment when surgery is planned by the physician with the patient. Your responsibilities begin when the patient is admitted to the hospital. Remember that you may answer general questions that the patient asks but you must refer specific questions about the surgery, its possible outcome, and anesthesia to your team leader.

Although it is the responsibility of the physician and nurse to answer questions and give explanations, it is helpful if you are aware of the information that has been given.

Teaching

Time spent with the patient in the preoperative period is well spent. Patients who are prepared are able to cooperate in their recovery more successfully. Ideally, this time is spent shortly after the patient's admission. Sometimes much of the information is given in the doctor's office or clinic.

During the preoperative period, the nurse will determine the patient's specific needs. The nurse also does preoperative teaching. The other staff members support this effort.
- Tests, medications, and preoperative procedures are explained.

- Questions regarding the postoperative period are answered.
- The patient is taught and given an opportunity to practice postoperative exercises, such as leg exercises and respiratory exercises.
- The events of the preoperative period and what the patient may experience while being taken to the operating room and given anesthesia are discussed.
- The recovery period is outlined and the purpose of special equipment or procedures such as tubes or intravenous fluid lines which may be in place after surgery is explained.
- Play therapy may be used to explain to children.
- Every effort is made to teach ways of decreasing discomfort and to assure the patient that the means for pain relief will be available.
- Planning for the discharge period begins now.

Psychological Preparation

The nursing staff spends as much time as possible helping patients deal with their emotional stress.

All members of the health team need to be sensitive and responsive to the psychological needs of the patient. Being in frequent contact with the patient, you may be the first person to recognize signs of fear or concern. Listen to what the patient says and observe the patient's body language carefully. Report your observations to the nurse so that appropriate nursing intervention may be carried out.

Build patient confidence by:
- Performing your work in an efficient, calm manner.
- Being available to listen.
- Explaining what you plan to do before carrying out any procedure.
- Encouraging the patient to participate in his own care as much as possible. This helps the patient feel he still has a measure of control over his life.
- Immediately transmitting requests for clergy visits.

Physical Preparation

The Evening Before Surgery. If the patient is in the hospital the evening before surgery, part of the surgical preparation may be done then. It usually includes:
- Bath or shower with surgical soap

- Enema
- Surgical prep (shaving of the operative site)
- Special tests
- Medication to ensure a good night's rest when indicated
- Insertion of special tubes for draining body cavities
- Being placed on NPO (nothing by mouth) after midnight
- Removal of the water pitcher from the bedside table and having the NPO notice posted over the bed, bedside table, on the door, on the patient's chart, and on the Kardex.

Nosocomial infections are those acquired during the hospital stay. It is known that such infections:

- Occur with greater frequency the longer the patient is in the hospital.
- Add days to the hospital stay.
- Increase the cost of hospitalization.
- Can be life-threatening.

To decrease costs and the potential for nosocomial infections, patients are often admitted the morning of surgery and are sometimes discharged the day of surgery or the day after. In this circumstance, much of the preoperative care must be done at home or immediately upon admission. This is called outpatient or "short-term" surgery.

The Surgical Prep Area. Skin preparation prior to surgery may or may not include hair removal. There is a trend away from removing the hair unless its thickness will interfere with the surgery. In fact, some studies have shown more infections among shaved patients compared with unshaved patients.

If shaving is ordered, it must follow the procedure provided. It must be performed skillfully in a well-lighted area. Also, the area to be washed and shaved will be greater than the surgical incision area, Figure 27–3. In some cases, a depilatory (hair removing) cream will be ordered for use the night before surgery. If a depilatory is used, check the skin for sensitivity by applying a small amount to the skin of the forearm. Wait 10 minutes. If redness occurs, do not continue but report to the nurse.

Skin preparation may be performed by:

- Special surgical prep team
- Operating room staff in the OR

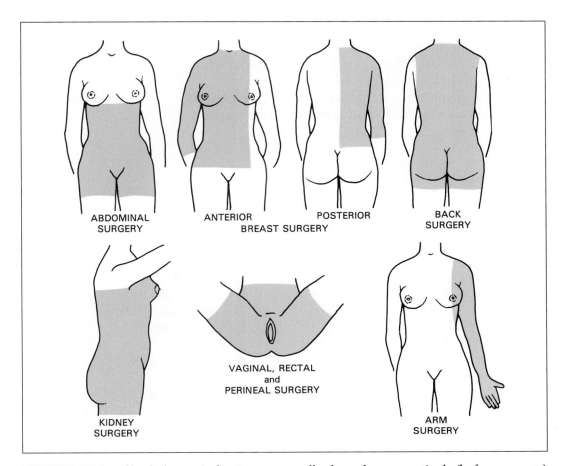

ABDOMINAL SURGERY

ANTERIOR BREAST SURGERY

POSTERIOR

BACK SURGERY

KIDNEY SURGERY

VAGINAL, RECTAL and PERINEAL SURGERY

ARM SURGERY

FIGURE 27–3. Shaded areas indicate areas usually shaved preoperatively (before surgery).

BEGINNING PROCEDURE ACTIONS	PROCEDURE COMPLETION ACTIONS
■ Wash your hands. ■ Assemble equipment needed. ■ Go to the patient's room, knock, and pause before entering. ■ Introduce yourself and identify the patient by checking identification bracelet. ■ Ask visitors to leave and inform them where they can wait. ■ Provide privacy. ■ Explain what will happen and answer questions. ■ Allow patient to assist in procedure as much as possible. ■ Raise bed to comfortable working height.	■ Position patient comfortably. ■ Leave signal cord, telephone, and fresh water close at hand. ■ Return bed to lowest position. ■ Perform general safety check of patient and environment. ■ Care for equipment according to facility policy. ■ Wash your hands. ■ Report completion of task. ■ Let visitors know when they may reenter the patient's room. ■ Document action and your observations.

NOTE: Where there are open lesions, wet linen, or possible contact with patient body fluids or blood, disposable gloves are worn during the procedure. Put on gloves before contact with the patient or linen. Properly dispose of gloves after they are removed. ALWAYS APPLY UNIVERSAL PRECAUTIONS.

FIGURE 27–4.   Beginning procedure actions and procedure completion actions

■ Nursing staff in the patient's unit just prior to surgery.

To prepare the surgical area by shaving:

■ Make sure you know exactly what area is to be shaved. Most hospitals have routine prep areas.

■ Do not shave the neck or face of a female patient. If in doubt, check with the nurse.

■ Be aware that the preparations for cranial surgery are usually performed after the patient has been medicated and taken to the operating suite.

Doctors have special preferences in this regard.

■ Remember that if a spinal anesthesia is to be given, the back may also be shaved.

Calm the fears of the patient by explaining that the area prepared is much larger than the actual incision area. This is to prevent contamination of the surgical site which may lead to possible complications after surgery.

Refer to Figure 27–4 to review the beginning procedure actions and the procedure completion actions.

PROCEDURE 96

SHAVING THE OPERATIVE AREA

1. Carry out each beginning procedure action.
2. Remember to wash your hands, identify the patient, and provide privacy.
3. Assemble equipment needed:
   ■ Bath blanket
   ■ Individual prep pack, OR
   ■ Tray with razor and new razor blades, OR
   ■ Electric clipper—make sure heads are disposable or, if reusable, that they have been sterilized.
   ■ 2 small bowls

   ■ Applicators
   ■ Cleansing soap
   ■ Lighting—for example, a spotlight or gooseneck lamp
   ■ Disposable gloves
   ■ 4 × 4 sponges
   ■ Paper towels
   ■ Towels or disposable Chux® (bed protector)
4. Determine exact area to be prepped.
5. In utility room:

a. Fill small bowls with warm water.

b. Add cleansing soap to one.

c. Adjust razor and blade.

d. Make sure razor and blade are tight.

6. Cover tray and take to bedside.

7. Drape patient with bath blanket. Place towel or bed protector under area to be shaved.

8. Put on disposable gloves.

9. If a safety razor and blade are used, soften hairs with soapy solution and wait 1 minute. This makes hair removal easier and helps avoid skin injury.

10. Holding skin taut with one hand, lather area to be shaved. If hair is very long, such as on the pubis and axilla, it may be clipped with scissors before shaving. Take care when clipping—do not nick the skin. If an electric clipper is used, attach heads and check for security.

11. Shave area with strokes in same direction as the hair grows. Be careful not to cut the skin or to remove any warts or moles. Work carefully around this area.

12. Using the applicators, clean the umbilicus (navel) and shave it if it is in the operative area.

13. Check carefully for hairs after shaving is complete.

   ■ Unattached hairs are easily removed by gently pressing a piece of tape against the area.

   ■ Discard hair in paper towel.

14. Cleanse the skin with warm, soapy water. Rinse and dry thoroughly.

15. Dispose of equipment according to facility policy.

16. Remove the towel from under patient.

   ■ Make sure side rails are up.

   ■ Make sure linen is dry.

   ■ Change, if necessary.

17. Remove and dispose of gloves according to facility policy.

18. Carry out each procedure completion action. Remember to wash your hands, report completion of task, and document time, surgical skin prep (area shaved), and patient reaction.

Immediate Preoperative Care. Approximately one hour before surgery, the patient will be given additional medication by the nurse. All your responsibilities regarding the patient must be completed before this time. You may be asked to do the following:

■ Take and record vital signs, Figure 27–5 (see Section 6).

■ Take care of valuables according to hospital policy. Remove dentures and any other prosthesis (artificial part) such as a hearing aid and glasses. See that they are safely marked with the patient's name and cared for.

■ Remove nail polish, makeup, hairpins, and jewelry. Long hair should be neatly braided or capped. Plain wedding bands may be taped in place.

■ Dress the patient in a gown and cover the hair with surgical cap.

■ See that the patient voids and measure the urine. Drain Foley bag, if present.

■ Make sure that the room is quiet and comfortable, with television off.

As soon as the nurse gives the preoperative medication:

■ Elevate the bed to stretcher level.

■ Be sure the side rails are in place for safety.

■ Remove all unnecessary equipment.

■ Push the bedside table, over-bed table, and chair out of the way to make room for the stretcher when it arrives from surgery.

■ Complete the surgical checklist, Figure 27–6:

   — Check off those duties to which you were assigned.

   — Note the time your patient leaves for surgery.

■ Follow facility policy regarding visitors. Sometimes they are allowed to wait quietly with the

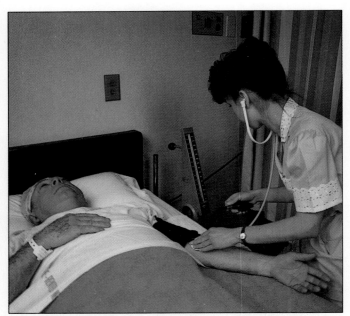

FIGURE 27–5. Immediate preoperative care includes taking vital signs.

☐ Admission sheet
☐ Surgical consent
☐ Sterilization consent (if necessary)
☐ Consultation sheet (if necessary)
☐ History and physical
☐ Lab reports (pregnancy test also if necessary)
☐ Surgery prep done and charted, if required
☐ Latest TPR and blood pressure charted
☐ Preoperative medication has been given and charted (if required)
☐ Name tape on patient
☐ Fingernail polish and makeup removed
☐ Metallic objects removed (rings may be taped)
☐ Dentures removed
☐ Other prostheses removed (such as artificial limb or eye)
☐ Bath blanket and head cap in place
☐ Bed in high position and side rails up after preop medication is given
☐ Patient has voided

FIGURE 27–6. Surgical checklist

patient. Sometimes they need to be directed to the visitors' waiting room.

The nurse and surgical attendant will check the patient's identification and surgical checklist before the patient is moved. A staff member, and sometimes a family member, accompanies the patient to the doors of the operating room. You will probably be asked to assist in transferring the patient from the bed to the stretcher and after surgery, from the stretcher to the bed. Review procedure in Unit 13.

During the Operative Period

While the patient is in the operating room, you will prepare the room for the patient's return.

■ A special surgical bed will be prepared. This was described in Unit 19. The surgical bed is also called a postop bed or recovery bed.

■ Everything should be removed from the bedside stand except an emesis basin, tissue wipes, tongue depressors, and equipment to check vital signs.

■ A pencil and small pad to record the signs should also be available.

■ Check with your team leader for any special equipment such as oxygen, IV poles, suction, or drainage bags that might be necessary for your patient.

■ Be watchful while carrying out your other assignments for the return of your patient from surgery.

■ Follow facility policy regarding the location of visitors and family during surgery. They are sometimes permitted to wait in the patient's room. In most cases they are directed to a special waiting area.

Postoperative Care

During the immediate postoperative period, the patient recovers from anesthesia. For this period, the patient is placed in a special area called the recovery room, Figure 27–7. The recovery room is located next to the operating room and is sometimes called the postanesthesia care unit (PACU)

When the patient's condition is stabilized, the patient is returned to the unit. Upon the patient's return from the recovery room, you should:

■ Identify the patient.

■ Assist in the transfer from stretcher to bed, Figures 27–8A and B (see Unit 13).

■ Never leave the unconscious patient alone at any time.

■ Learn from your team leader any special instructions to be followed.

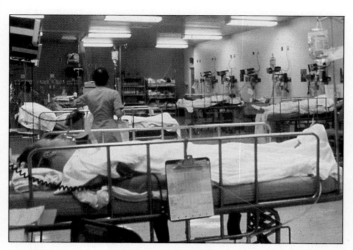

FIGURE 27–7. Following surgery, the patient remains in recovery room until vital signs are stable. (*Photo courtesy of Memorial Medical Center of Long Beach, CA*)

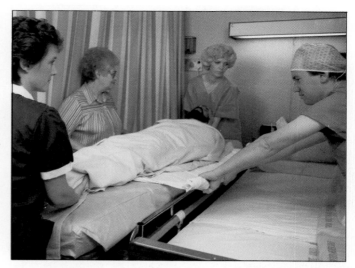

FIGURE 27–8A. Use lift sheet to transfer patient from gurney to bed. One person should support patient's head, neck, and shoulders.

- Realize that the patient may be drowsy for several hours after return.
- Have an extra blanket available since many patients complain of feeling cold upon return.

The following are routine instructions to be followed unless otherwise ordered.

- Take vital signs of the patient upon arrival on the unit, Figure 27–9, and every 15 minutes for four readings (see Section 6). The patient's temperature may not always be taken at this time. If signs are stable (approximately the same) at the end of this time, repeat in one hour. Note the patient's state of consciousness (unresponsive, drowsy, alert).
- Check dressings for amount and type of any drainage. The nurse may reinforce them as necessary.
- Check IV solution for flow rate. Restrain infusion site whenever ordered by the physician and report to the charge nurse. Remember the flow rate is ordered by the physician.
- Encourage the patient to breathe deeply, cough, and move in bed. Position should be changed every 2 hours.
- Turn the patient's head to one side and support if vomiting. Have emesis basin ready, as well as tissues and wet cloth. If patient is conscious, allow patient to rinse mouth with water after vomiting. Note type and amount of vomitus.
- Check pulses distal to operative site. Inform the nurse if the pulse is weak or cannot be felt.

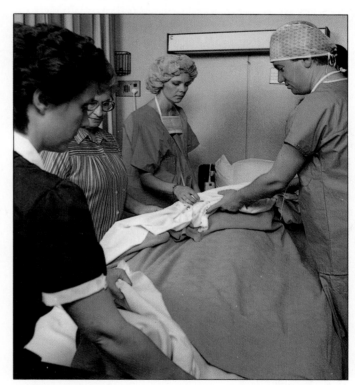

FIGURE 27–8B. Cover patient with bedding to prevent chilling.

- If the patient was given a spinal anesthesia:
  — Give extra care in turning frequently and maintaining proper alignment.
  — Remember the patient will be unable to move independently until sensation and

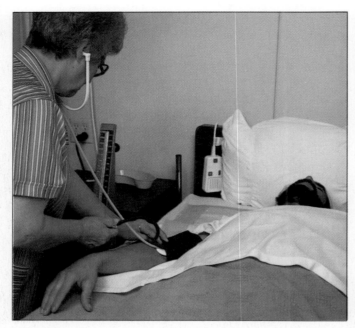

FIGURE 27–9.   Check vital signs carefully until they are stable.

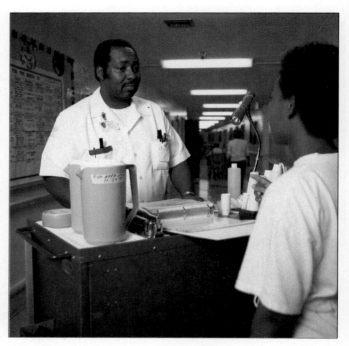

FIGURE 27–10.   Report complaints of discomfort and pain to the nurse.

motor functions return. Make sure to calm the patient's fear about this.

— Some physicians require that the patient remain flat on the back and without a pillow for 8–12 hours following spinal anesthesia to avoid headaches.

— Any complaints of a headache following spinal anesthesia should be reported promptly.

— Provide extra blankets if patient is cold.

■ Be sure all drainage tubes have been connected (the nurse will usually attend to this). If you notice a tube clamped shut, check with your team leader.

■ Measure and record the first postoperative voiding. Inform nurse.

■ Report any patient complaints of discomfort and pain to the nurse, Figure 27–10.

Tubes

Patients often return from surgery with a variety of tubes and drains in place.

■ Some tubes may deliver materials into the patient. Examples of these are oxygen tubes or intravenous tubes.

■ Other tubes may have been placed in the patient to provide drainage from wounds or body cavities. Examples of these are drains in the incision or urinary catheters.

The following are some special precautions to be taken:

■ Learn the type, purpose, and location of each tube.

■ Check drainage for character and amount.

■ Check for obstructions to the tube system.

■ Check flow rate of infusions from intravenous lines.

■ Keep orifices (body openings) clear of secretions and discharge.

■ Never disconnect tubes or raise drainage bottles above the level of the drainage site.

■ Never lower infusion bottles below the level of the infusion site.

■ Never put stress on the tubes when moving the patient or giving care.

■ Restrain infusion sites with a physician's order as necessary to prevent dislocation.

■ Monitor levels of infusions and report to the nurse before they run out.

■ Report any signs of leakage or disconnected tubes at once.

■ Report pain, discoloration, or swelling at sites of drainage and infusion.

Drainage

When a body cavity is the operative site, it may be necessary to drain fluid such as blood, pus, serous drainage caused by tissue trauma, or gastric contents from it before or after surgery. The **drainage** outlet may be a:

- Catheter
- Penrose drain
- T-tube
- Cigarette drain
- Jackson–Pratt (J–P)® drain

When such a drain is in place, the drainage accumulates on the dressing, Figures 27–11A and B. You should:

- Note the amount and character of the drainage.
- Inform the nurse when the dressing needs to be changed or reinforced.

At times, the withdrawal of fluids is controlled by attaching the drainage tube to a connecting tube and then a suction apparatus. The drainage accumulates in a container. The container is emptied and the contents measured at the end of each shift. The Jackson-Pratt® or Hemovac drains are closed drainage systems. The drains are placed directly in the wound, and drainage goes directly into an expandable container. A record of the amount and character of the drainage is entered in both the output chart and the nurses' notes.

It is your responsibility to:

- Report either heavy or light drainage.
- Report a change in the character and amount of the drainage.
- Make sure that the flow of drainage is not blocked by kinking of the tube, Figure 27–12.
- Never assume responsibility for chest drainage or attempt to empty chest bottles. Chest bottles and irrigations require the nurse's or physician's attention.

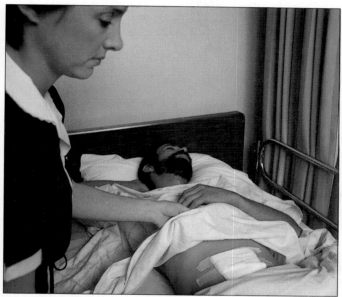

FIGURE 27–11A.   Check dressing for drainage.

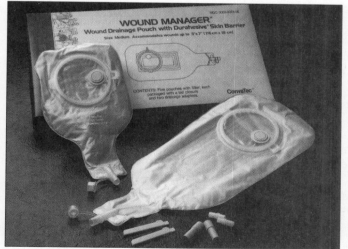

FIGURE 27–11B.   When much drainage is expected, a drainage pouch may be applied to the wound and attached to a drainage bag. *(Photo courtesy of ConvaTec)*

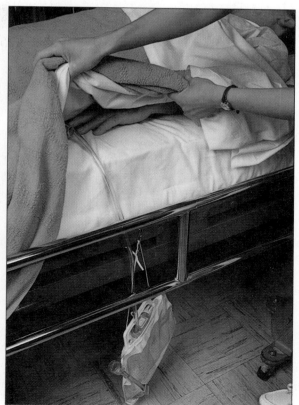

FIGURE 27–12.   Check to be sure all drainage tubes are unobstructed.

Careful preoperative preparation and postoperative care can help limit the extent of postoperative discomfort and complication.

The patient must be carefully observed, especially during the first 24 hours, for possible complications. Possible postoperative discomfort and complications and appropriate nursing assistant actions are summarized in Figure 27–13.

When the patient has responded sufficiently and vital signs are stable, the patient may be refreshed by:
- Washing the hands and face.
- Changing the linen.
- Being given a light back rub.

Possible Discomfort	Report	What You Can Do*
Thirst	Patient complaints of dryness of lips, mouth, and skin	Carefully check I & O. Increase fluid intake by mouth with permission. Monitor IV if ordered. Mouth care. Check BP and pulse. Watch for signs of shock and hemorrhage.
Singultus (hiccups)—intermittent spasms of the diaphragm	Incidence of hiccups	Allow patient to rest; hiccups can be tiring. Support incisional area. Assist patient to breathe into paper bag.
Pain	Location, intensity, type	Change position. Apply warmth if instructed. Monitor carefully for and report effects of medication given by nurse.
Distention (accumulation of gas in bowel)	Distention of abdomen, complaints of pain	Increase mobility. Insert a rectal tube if instructed and permitted.
Nausea, vomiting	Nausea, character of vomitus	Keep emesis basin at bedside. Monitor IV fluids, which are substituted for oral fluids. Mouth care. Limit fluids by mouth. Encourage patient to breathe deeply.
Urinary retention	Amount and time of first voiding. Distention, restlessness, imbalance between I & O	Monitor I & O carefully. Check for distention.
Complication	Report	What You Can Do*
Hemorrhage (excessive blood loss)	Fall in blood pressure; cold, moist skin; weak, rapid pulse; restlessness; pallor/cyanosis; condition of dressing; thirst	Report immediately to nurse. Keep patient quiet. Check vital signs.
Shock	Fall in blood pressure; weak, rapid pulse; cold, moist skin; pallor	Report immediately to nurse. Keep patient quiet. Monitor ordered fluids. Monitor ordered oxygen. Be prepared to follow additional instructions.
Hypoxia (lack of oxygen)	Restlessness, dyspnea, crowing sounds to respirations, pounding pulse, perspiring	Report immediately to nurse. Elevate patient to sitting position, if permitted. Monitor oxygen, if ordered.
Atelectasis (failure of lungs to expand)	Dyspnea; cyanosis/pallor	Report immediately to nurse. Encourage deep breathing. Change position. Encourage use of incentive spirometer.
Wound infection	Increased pain in incisional area; fever; chills, anorexia, increased drainage on dressing	Be observant. Report findings promptly to nurse. Check dressing.
Wound disruption (separation of wound edges)	Pinkish drainage. Complaints by the patient that he "feels open," "broken," "given away"	Report immediately to nurse. Keep patient quiet. Support incisional area.
Pulmonary emboli	Anxiety, difficulty breathing; feelings of "heaviness in chest," cyanosis, chest pain	Keep patient quiet. Report immediately to nurse. Elevate head of bed.

*In all cases, be prepared to follow the nurse's additional instructions.

FIGURE 27–13. Postoperative complications and nursing assistant actions

The patient is now ready to more actively participate in recovery. Exercises taught in the preoperative period are practiced: They include:

- Deep breathing and coughing
- Use of the incentive spirometer
- Leg exercises

Deep Breathing and Coughing

Deep breathing and coughing clear the air passages. This helps to prevent postoperative respiratory complications such as pneumonia and atelectasis, which is the collapse of the alveolar air sacs. This may be an uncomfortable task when the patient has a new incision and feels fatigued. You can best assist the patient by:

- Explaining the value of the exercise and carrying out the following procedure.
- Checking with the nurse to see if medication for pain is to be administered before the exercise. If so, wait for 45 minutes after the medication has been given before carrying out the exercise.
- Learning from the nurse how many deep breaths and coughs should be attempted. The usual number is 5–10 breaths and 2–3 coughs.
- Using a pillow or binder to support the incision during the procedure.

Using the Incentive Spirometer

The physician may write orders for an incentive spirometer, Figure 27–16, to help the lungs to expand fully. This prevents atelectasis and also helps prevent pneumonia.

This procedure may be carried out with the patient in bed, with head and shoulders well-supported, if permitted. The procedure usually is taught before surgery.

- The patient is instructed how to use the incentive spirometer by a respiratory therapist or nurse.
- The idea, in one type of spirometer, is for the patient to exhale normally and then, with the lips placed tightly around the mouthpiece, to inhale through the mouth sufficiently to raise the balls in the chambers.
- The deep breath should be held as long as possible (or as ordered), thereby keeping the balls suspended.
- The patient then removes the mouthpiece and exhales in the normal manner.
- The exercise is repeated as many times as is ordered.

Although this procedure is started by the professional, you too have responsibilities:

- Observe the patient for correctness of procedure.

PROCEDURE 97

ASSISTING PATIENT TO DEEP BREATHE AND COUGH

1. Carry out each beginning procedure action.
2. Remember to wash your hands, identify the patient, and provide privacy.
3. Assemble equipment needed:
   - Disposable gloves
   - A pillowcase-covered pillow or binder, if ordered
   - Tissues
   - Emesis basin
4. Elevate head of bed and assist patient to assume a comfortable semi-Fowler's position.
5. Have patient place hands on either side of his rib cage or over operative site, Figure 27–14. A pillow over operative site can be used to support incision during respiratory exercises.

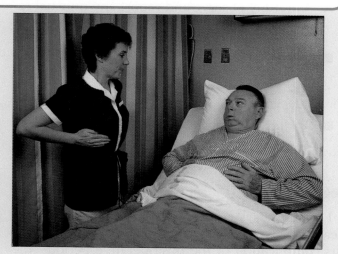

FIGURE 27–14. Encourage patient to perform deep breathing exercises taught before surgery.

continues

6. Ask patient to take as deep a breath as is possible and hold it for 3–5 seconds and then to exhale slowly through pursed lips.
7. Repeat this exercise about five times unless the patient seems too tired. If so, stop procedure and report to nurse.
8. Apply binder (see procedure, this unit) or place the pillow across the incision line as a brace. Have patient hold pillow on either side or have patient interlace fingers across incision to act as a brace.
9. Pass tissues to patient and instruct patient to take a deep breath and cough forcefully twice with mouth open, collecting any secretions that are brought up in tissues, Figure 27–15.
10. Put on disposable gloves to handle tissues.
11. Dispose of tissues in emesis basin.
12. Assist patient to assume a new, comfortable position.
13. Clean emesis basin.
14. Remove and dispose of gloves according to facility policy.
15. Carry out each procedure completion action. Remember to wash your hands, report comple-

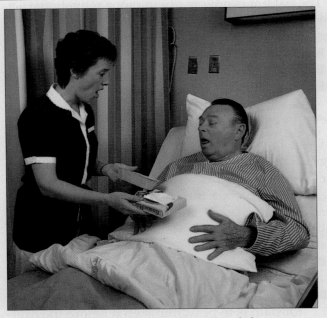

FIGURE 27–15. A pillow across the abdomen supports the incision during deep coughing.

tion of task, and document time, coughed and deep breathed (indicate number of times), and patient reaction.

- Be sure the patient does not become overly fatigued.
- Encourage the patient to cough and clear the respiratory passages.
- Report to your team leader if the patient seems overly fatigued during the procedure.
- Carefully observe and report any unusual responses such as pain, dizziness, or throat and airway irritation.
- When patient has completed the pulmonary exercise, the mouthpiece should be washed in warm water, dried, replaced in the plastic bag, and left at the bedside.
- Patients should be praised for efforts. Many times this encourages greater effort the next time the incentive spirometer is used.

Leg Exercises

Leg exercises following surgery encourage a steady circulation. This helps to prevent another serious complication of the postoperative period—the development of blood clots.

A blood clot or thrombus could develop in the venous system and block the essential blood flow. A small piece of thrombus broken off (embolus) could

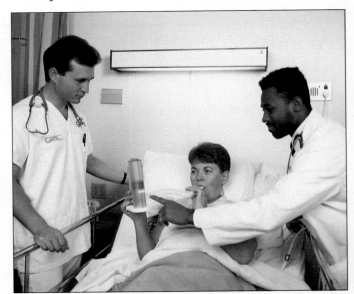

FIGURE 27–16. The nursing assistant may help the respiratory therapist or patient with equipment, but the incentive spirometer is a self-administered treatment.

travel throughout the vascular system and block a vessel in the lungs.

A specific order must be written for leg exercises when there has been surgery on the legs themselves. Otherwise, leg exercises are routinely performed by the patient. If the patient is very weak, you may need to assist.

- Encourage leg exercises and be sure they have been performed.
- Each exercise should be performed 3–5 times at least every one or two hours and at other times as well.
- Carry out leg exercises as you assist position changes.
- Apply or reapply support hose (TED) after exercises if ordered.

Binders

The sutures used in modern surgery require less support. Often, however, patients will complain or express concern that their abdomen feels "heavy" or "weak" following surgery. You can assure them that as they heal their suture line will feel stronger. Sometimes binders are ordered.

Binders are pieces of cotton material that are applied to different parts of the body to hold surgical dressings in place and provide support, Figure 27–18. The binder should:

- Be clean.
- Be applied smoothly to prevent pressure areas.
- Fit snugly, but it should not be so tight that it causes discomfort.

PROCEDURE 98

PERFORMING POSTOPERATIVE LEG EXERCISES

1. Carry out each beginning procedure action.
2. Remember to wash your hands, identify the patient, and provide privacy.
3. Explain how the exercise is to be performed. Have patient:
   - Brace the incisional area with laced hands.
   - Rotate each ankle by drawing imaginary circles.
   - Dorsiflex (bringing toes toward knee) and plantar flex (pointing toes and foot down) each ankle, Figure 27–17.
   - Flex and extend each knee.
   - Flex and extend each hip.
   - Repeat each exercise 3–5 times. Assist as needed.
4. Lower side rail.
5. Cover with bath blanket and draw top bedding to the foot of bed.
6. Supervise exercises or assist. Apply or reapply support hose (TED hose) as ordered after exercises.
7. Draw bedding up and remove bath blanket.
8. Fold bath blanket and place in bedside stand for reuse.
9. Carry out each procedure completion action. Remember to wash your hands, report com-

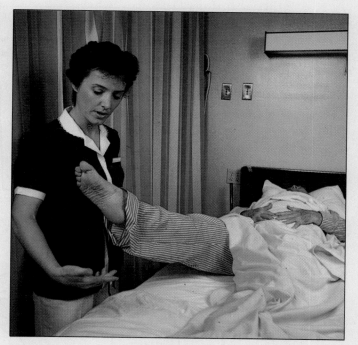

FIGURE 27–17. Help the patient perform leg exercises, which encourage circulation.

pletion of task, and document time, leg exercises, and patient reaction.

Two kinds of binders may be used:

■ The straight abdominal binder or a special halter type may be used to support the breasts of a female patient.

■ Single and double T-binders. T-binders are used to hold dressings on the rectal and perineal areas in place.

— The single T-binder is usually used for female patients.

— The double T-binder is usually used for male patients.

— The binder is placed around the patient's waist, and the tail is passed between the patient's legs and fastened at the waist with a pin.

— The split tails of the double T-binder are brought up on either side of the scrotum.

Elasticized Stockings

Elasticized stockings, called TED hose or anti-embolism hose, or Ace bandages that extend from the ankle or foot to calf or mid-thigh are often applied during the preoperative and postoperative periods to support the veins of the legs. This reduces the incidence of thrombophlebitis, which is inflammation of the veins that can lead to blood clots. The stockings must be applied smoothly and evenly before getting the patient out of bed. They should be removed and reapplied at least every eight hours—more often if necessary or as ordered.

Initial Ambulation

Some time after surgery, a patient is permitted to sit up with the legs over the edge of the bed. This position is called dangling. *болтать ногами в воду*

■ Watch carefully for signs of fatigue or dizziness (vertigo).

■ Assist the patient to assume the position slowly.

The first ambulation (walk) is usually short. The patient usually dangles for a short time before ambulating. Dangling is an important part of postoperative care since it stimulates circulation and helps prevent the formation of blood clots (thrombi).

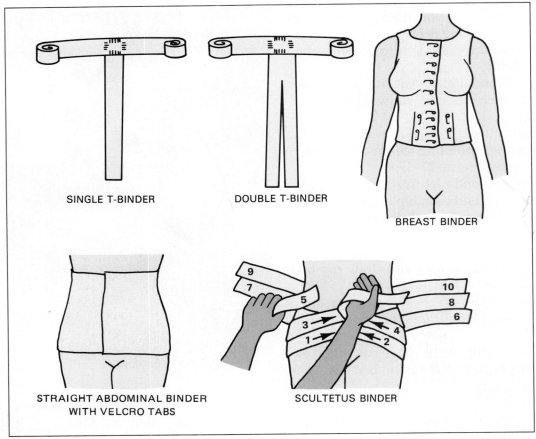

SINGLE T-BINDER   DOUBLE T-BINDER   BREAST BINDER

STRAIGHT ABDOMINAL BINDER WITH VELCRO TABS   SCULTETUS BINDER

FIGURE 27–18. Types of binders

SIDE
8

PROCEDURE 99   OBRA

APPLYING ELASTICIZED STOCKINGS

1. Carry out each beginning procedure action.
2. Remember to wash your hands, identify the patient, and provide privacy.
3. Assemble equipment needed:
   ■ Elasticized stockings of proper length and size

4. With patient lying down, expose one leg at a time.
5. Grasp stocking with both hands at the top and roll toward toe end, Figure 27–19A.

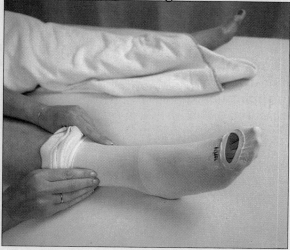

FIGURE 27–19C. Draw stocking smoothly toward knee.

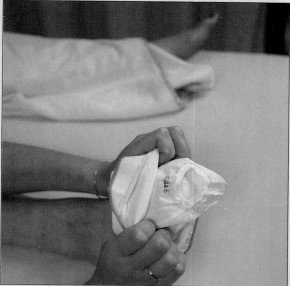

FIGURE 27–19A. Grasp stocking with both hands at stocking top, gather, and slip over toes.

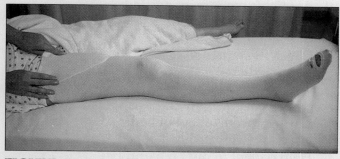

FIGURE 27–19D. Then draw stocking to upper thigh.

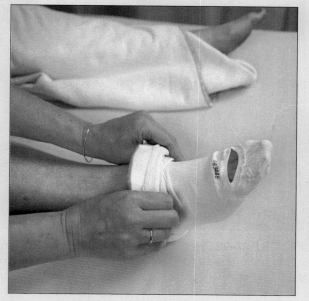

FIGURE 27–19B. Position opening on top of foot at base of toes.

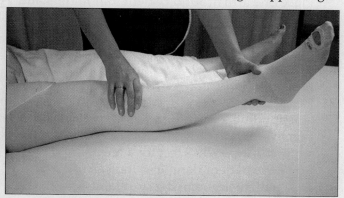

FIGURE 27–19E. Check to be sure stocking has no wrinkles.

continues

6. Adjust over toes, positioning opening at base of toes (unless toes are to be covered), Figure 27–19B. Remember that the raised seams should be on the outside.
7. Apply stocking to leg by rolling upward toward body, Figure 27–19C and D.
8. Check to be sure stocking is applied evenly and smoothly and there are no wrinkles, Figure 27–19E and F.
9. Repeat procedure on opposite leg.
10. Carry out each procedure completion action. Remember to wash your hands, report completion of task, and document time, application or reapplication of elasticized hose, and patient reaction.

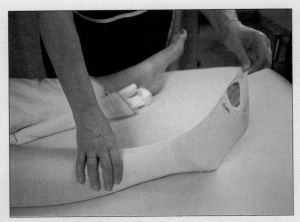

FIGURE 27–19F. Check material on toes to be sure it is not too tight.

PROCEDURE 100   OBRA

SIDE
8

ASSISTING THE PATIENT TO DANGLE

1. Carry out each beginning procedure action.
2. Remember to wash your hands, identify the patient, and provide privacy.
3. Assemble equipment needed:
   - Bath blanket
   - Pillow
4. Check the pulse (see Unit 15).
5. Lower side rail nearest to you. Lock bed at the lowest position.
6. Drape patient with bath blanket and fanfold top bedcovers to foot of bed.
7. Gradually elevate head of bed.
8. Help patient to put on bathrobe.
9. Place one arm around patient's shoulders and the other under the knees.
10. Gently and slowly turn patient toward you, Figure 27–20. Allow patient's legs to hang over the side of the bed.
11. Roll pillow and tuck firmly to patient's back for support.
12. After putting slippers on patient, give an instruction to swing the legs. A chair may be placed to support the patient's feet for a few minutes.
13. Have the patient dangle as long as ordered.
    - If patient becomes dizzy or faint, assist to lie down.
    - Report to the supervising nurse immediately.

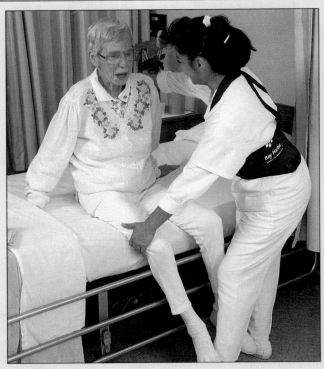

FIGURE 27–20. Help patient to a sitting position and allow patient to sit for a few minutes before putting on robe and slippers.

14. Check the patient's pulse.
15. Rearrange pillow at head of bed. Remove patient's bathrobe and slippers.
16. Place one arm around patient's shoulders and the other under the knees. Gently and slowly swing patient's legs onto the bed.

17. Check patient's pulse. Lower head of bed and raise side rails.
18. Carry out each procedure completion action. Remember to wash your hands, report completion of task, and document time, dangled (duration), pulse, and patient reaction.

PROCEDURE 101 OBRA

ASSISTING THE PATIENT IN INITIAL AMBULATION

1. Follow the procedure for dangling. Make sure bed is in low position. Have a chair available in case patient becomes fatigued.
2. After patient has dangled without ill effects, assist to stand, Figure 27–21. Check pulse.
   - ■ If pulse has increased more than 10 points, return to bed and inform nurse.
   - ■ If patient becomes dizzy or faint, return to bed.
   - ■ Have patient take deep breaths and look around the room. Patient is to keep head up and eyes open.
   - ■ Talk to and reassure the patient.

NOTE: If there has been no abdominal surgery and there is no other counterindication, use a transfer belt to assist during the initial ambulation.

3. Transfer your arm behind the patient's waist and turn so you face the same direction.
4. Walk slowly for a short distance and return to bedside. If patient appears tired or faint or if there is a marked change in the pulse, allow to rest.
5. Remove transfer belt if used. Assist patient back to bed and make him comfortable.
6. If patient should faint during procedure:
   - ■ Gently lower patient to the floor.
   - ■ Protect patient's head.

   - ■ Do not attempt to hold patient up.
   - ■ Signal for help.
7. Carry out each procedure completion action. Remember to wash your hands, report completion of task, and document time, initial ambulation (duration), pulse (rate), and patient reaction.

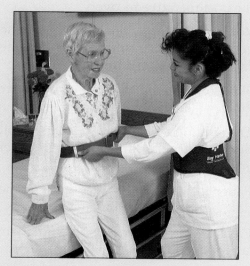

FIGURE 27–21. Allow the patient to stand for a few minutes beside the bed before trying to walk.

SUMMARY

The surgical patient requires continuous care before, during, and after surgery. The nursing assistant helps in preoperative and postoperative care.

Nursing assistant responsibilities in the preoperative period include:

- ■ Preparing the operative site.
- ■ Readying the patient on the morning of surgery.
- ■ Helping in the transfer of the patient to and from the stretcher.
- ■ Providing emotional support.

Nursing assistant responsibilities during the operative period include:
- Preparing a surgical (postoperative) bed.
- Securing equipment needed for the postoperative period.

Nursing assistant responsibilities in the postoperative period include:
- Assisting in the transfer from stretcher to bed.
- Carefully observing and reporting.
- Assisting the patient with postoperative exercises, including:
  — Position changes
  — Leg exercises
  — Respiratory exercises
- Applying elasticized stockings.
- Assisting in dangling and initial ambulation.

UNIT REVIEW

A. True/False. Answer the following statements true or false by circling T or F.

T F 1. Patients receiving local anesthetics lose consciousness during the surgery.

T F 2. When spinal anesthetics are used, patients may lose feeling and movement in their legs.

T F 3. Preoperative teaching has little effect on the postoperative recovery.

T F 4. You help build patient confidence when you explain what you plan to do when carrying out procedures.

T F 5. Skin preparation involves shaving an area greater than the size of the incision.

T F 6. The nursing assistant has no responsibilities related to the patient while the patient is in surgery.

T F 7. Patients should be dangled without incident before initial ambulation.

T F 8. Patients who are unconscious following surgery should not be left alone.

T F 9. Nosocomial infections do not affect the cost or length of hospital stay.

T F 10. Patients who are faced with surgery are often filled with apprehension and fears.

B. Matching. Match the word in Column II with the phrases in Column I.

Column I

_____ 11. inflammation of a vein with clot formation

_____ 12. period before surgery

_____ 13. medicine given to prevent pain

_____ 14. hospital-acquired

_____ 15. opening

_____ 16. walking

_____ 17. dizziness

_____ 18. lung collapse

_____ 19. blood clot

_____ 20. area where immediate postoperative care is given

Column II

a. ambulation

b. orifice

c. nosocomial

d. recovery room

e. umbilicus

f. vertigo

g. anesthesia

h. preoperative

i. aspiration

j. emboli

k. atelectasis

l. thrombophlebitis

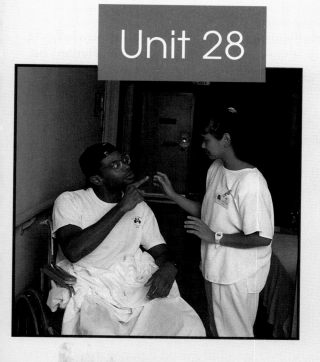

Unit 28

Caring for the Emotionally Stressed Patient

OBJECTIVES

OBJECTIVES

As a result of this unit, you will be able to:

- Spell and define terms.
- Define mental health.
- Explain the interrelatedness of physical and mental health.
- Understand mental health as a process of adaptations.
- Recognize commonly used defense mechanisms.
- Describe ways to help patients cope with stressful situations.
- Recognize the signs and symptoms of maladaptive behaviors that need to be documented and reported.
- List nursing assistant measures in providing care for patients with adaptive and maladaptive reactions.

VOCABULARY

Learn the meaning and the correct spelling of the following words and phrases:

adaptation
agitation
alcoholism
coping
defense mechanisms
delusions
denial
depression
disorientation
hypochondriasis

maladaptive behavior
mental illness
paranoia
projection
reaction formation
reality orientation
repression
stressors
suicide
suppression

There are varying degrees and differing aspects of health. A person who is in poor physical health may be mentally healthy. Because of good mental health, the person may be self-reliant and able to make decisions and to live an effective, productive life.

On the other hand, a person with good physical health may not be able to cope with and adapt to changes. This inability limits the person's chances to participate successfully in society.

Mental Health

Mental health means exhibiting those behaviors that reflect a person's adaptation or adjust-

- ■ Illness
- ■ Hospitalization
- ■ Loss of a loved one
- ■ Loss of a job
- ■ Loss of status

FIGURE 28–1. Common life stresses

ment to the multiple stresses of life, Figure 28–1. Stresses or stressors are situations, feelings, or conditions that cause a person to be anxious about his or her physical or emotional well-being. Good mental health leads to positive adaptations. Poor mental health is demonstrated by maladaptive behaviors.

Physical and mental health are interrelated. Physical illness is often preceded by stressful life situations. Ill health causes emotional stress. It is easy to understand that each of these factors contributes to the total health pattern of each person.

Ways of coping with (handling) stressful situations, Figure 28–2, are learned early in life. As people grow they find those behaviors that work best for them. They learn to use them to reduce stress and protect self-esteem. These coping patterns become ingrained in the individual's responses, becoming more and more pronounced as the person ages.

Defense Mechanisms

When any person feels unable to cope with stress and the situation threatens self-esteem, the person tends to act in protective ways. These ways are called defense mechanisms. A diagnosis of cancer, for instance, may be so overwhelming that a person must

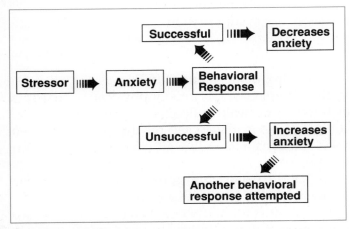

FIGURE 28–2. Individuals learn to cope with stress in different ways. The coping pattern becomes ingrained, but at times alternative responses may be required to deal successfully with the stressor.

temporarily defend himself against acknowledging the truth. Everyone uses these defense-oriented behaviors from time to time to protect themselves. You use them. Patients use them. Your coworkers use them.

You must recognize and understand the need to use defense mechanisms. Do not be critical of their occasional use. Most people do not use one mechanism all the time. They usually rely on a combination of defenses. They may not even be aware that they are behaving in a defensive way.

Defensive behavior becomes harmful only when it is the major means of coping with stress. In such cases, the person continuously avoids recognizing and responding to reality with problem-solving methods. The person's stress is temporarily reduced, but the stressor (feeling or situation) is not resolved. Such a person needs counseling from a trained mental health provider.

Some of the commonly used defense mechanisms include:

- ■ Repression—The involuntary exclusion from awareness of a painful or conflict-creating thought, memory, feeling, or impulse. For example, a woman has a lump in her breast, but refuses to go to a physician for examination and diagnosis. She has recently lost her husband, her house, and her job. She feels that she can't "acknowledge" any other illness or crisis, so she unconsciously represses the knowledge of the lump in her breast. She's not going to take the chance that the lump may be cancer. She can't face the possibility of a "terminal disease."

- ■ Suppression—This mechanism differs from repression since the person is aware of the unacceptable feelings and thoughts but deliberately refuses to acknowledge them. For example, a man becomes immobilized with the fear of rejection by his wife if he tells her he has a diagnosis of AIDS. Therefore, he consciously suppresses the knowledge of the AIDS diagnosis because he can't handle the anxiety associated with telling his wife.

- ■ Projection—A person's own unacceptable feelings and thoughts are attributed to others. The person blames others for his own shortcomings. For example, a person blames his wife or family for his alcoholism and loss of jobs. He projects his "failings" onto his wife and children.

■ Denial—Blocking out painful or anxiety-producing events or feelings. This is one of the most common defenses against the stress of diagnosis and illness. For example, a patient with a very high elevation of blood pressure refuses to remain in bed or to stop smoking. She continues to eat a diet high in fats. She cannot deal with her fear of disability and unemployment so she refuses to accept the seriousness of her condition.

■ Reaction formation—A person using this defense mechanism represses the reality of a situation and then exhibits behaviors that are the exact opposite of the real feelings. For example, a woman who dislikes one nursing assistant but is fearful that if she expresses that feeling, the assistant will be less caring, may be overly friendly and cooperative with the assistant. Other adaptive behaviors are shown in Figure 28–3.

Assisting Patients to Cope

Some ways to help patients become better able to cope and adapt include:

■ Be a good listener.
■ Be sensitive to nonverbal messages that may give clues to the source of stress.
■ Treat the person with respect, recognizing him as a unique individual.
■ Understand the behavior in the same way the patient is viewing it without "labeling" the behavior and passing judgment.
■ Let the patient know you are reliable and you respect her privacy and feelings.
■ Never argue or enter into a "power" struggle or debate with a patient even when you know the patient is "wrong."
■ Try to determine the source of stress so as to find a way to reduce it.
■ Be supportive of the person's own attempts to overcome the stress, Figure 28–4.

Remember that illness, age, and separation from family and home are major stress factors.

The Demanding Patient

In every nursing care situation, you will meet patients who are very demanding. This can be a difficult experience for everyone if it is not handled correctly.

■ Displacement—Substituting an object or person for another and behaving as if it were the original object or person.   *Example:* Being angry with the nursing assistant because another patient is annoying.
■ Identification—Behaving like another person whom one holds as an ideal.   *Example:* Speaking to coworkers with the same tone the supervisor uses with you.
■ Compensation—Excelling in one area to make up for feelings of failure in another.   *Example:* The nursing assistant who overachieves in the skill area because her ability to read written directions is poor.
■ Conversion—Offering a socially acceptable reason to avoid an unpleasant situation.   *Example:* The nursing assistant who calls saying she can't report for duty because she has the "flu" when she is just tired from staying up too late.
■ Fantasy—The use of imagination to solve problems.   *Example:* The supervisor criticizes the nursing assistant who then thinks of a time when she is the head of nursing and can fire the supervisor.
■ Undoing—A method of reversing something wrong that was done.   *Example:* The person who used his hands to hurt another may wash the hands repeatedly to undo the deed.

FIGURE 28–3. Other adaptive behaviors

Being demanding is another way that patients show their frustration. It is a coping behavior. Patients who are very demanding are usually frustrated by their loss of control. To be successful in caring for these patients, the nursing assistant must:

■ Try to learn and appreciate the factors that are causing the demanding behavior.
■ Show that you care about the patient's situation, but maintain control of your emotions.
■ Maintain open communications by listening to the patient's words and by being sensitive to the patient's body language.

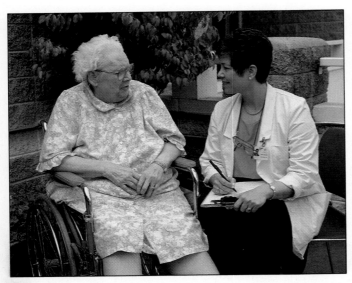

FIGURE 28–4. Working with patients, staff can help emotionally stressed patients find acceptable ways of coping.

- Provide opportunities that allow the patient to regain some control by making choices.
- Be consistent in the manner of care. This builds the patient's sense of security.
- Do not take the patient's demands personally.
- Report observations to the supervisor with suggestions for changes in the care plan.

Alcoholism

Some people turn to the use of alcohol as a means of coping with stress. The National Institute for Alcohol Abuse reports that two-thirds of the senior population uses alcohol. Fifteen percent of them become alcoholics. Alcoholism is regarded as a disease. Factors that contribute to the excessive use of alcohol include:

- Retirement
- Lowered income
- Grief
- Loss of spouse/friends
- Loneliness
- Stress in the family
- Decline in health
- Pain

Alcohol toxicity in the elderly may be associated with an acute onset of:

- Altered levels of awareness
- Mild confusion
- Progressive stupor
- Acute delirium

Drug taken by patient	Effects to report
Narcotics	Increased central nervous system (CNS) depression with acute intoxication
Salicylates	Gastrointestinal bleeding
Sedatives and psychotropic drugs	Increased CNS depression with acute intoxication
Barbiturates	Decreased sedative effect after chronic alcohol abuse
Chloral hydrate	Prolonged hypnotic effects
Chlordiazepoxide (Librium, Librax)	Increased CNS depression
Chlorpromazine (Thorazine)	Increased CNS depression
Diazepam (Valium)	Increased CNS depression
Oxazepam (Serax)	Increased CNS depression
Antihistamines	Increased CNS depression
Antabuse	Flushing, vomiting, excessive sweating, hyperventilation, confusion, and drowsiness

FIGURE 28–5. Common alcohol–drug interactions

- Disorientation similar to that seen in irreversible brain syndrome

Alcohol slows down brain activity. It impairs mental alertness, judgment, physical coordination, and reaction time—increasing the risk of falls and accidents.

Alcohol can affect the body in unusual ways. It can make it difficult to diagnose diseases/conditions of the cardiovascular system. It can mask pain that might otherwise serve as a warning sign of heart attack. Alcohol can also produce:

- Symptoms similar to dementia
- Forgetfulness
- Reduced attention
- Restlessness
- Impatience
- Agitation
- Confusion

Alcohol is a drug. It mixes unfavorably with many other drugs, Figure 28–5. The use of alcohol can cause some drugs to metabolize more rapidly, producing exaggerated responses. Such drugs include:

- Anticonvulsants
- Anticoagulants

- Antidiabetic drugs
- Diuretics

The alcoholic in withdrawal feels depressed and defensive. He needs to identify the stressors that bring on his need for alcohol and to find new ways of coping. This process takes professional skill, but you can:

- Not allow the alcoholic to manipulate you.
- Listen with empathy.
- Reflect the person's ideas and thoughts.
- Be sure alcohol is not available.
- Be consistent in the limits that have been set.

Care of the intoxicated patient includes:

- Caution during feeding to prevent choking or strangling.
- Supervision of activities to prevent injury and falls.
- Safety checks during bathing to prevent burns.
- Close supervision if there is confusion or delirium.

Older problem drinkers and alcoholics have a good chance for recovery. Getting help should start with the family physician, a member of the clergy, the local mental health association, or the local chapter of Alcoholics Anonymous.

Maladaptive Behaviors

Mental illness or maladaptive behavior occurs where the behaviors and responses disrupt the person's ability to function smoothly within the family, environment, or community.

You must be careful about applying the label of mental illness to any patient. Even when an official diagnosis of mental illness has been made, care must be taken not to stereotype the patient.

Remember that stereotypes often contain myths associated with them and that myths are false beliefs. It is far better to view the person as an individual demonstrating poor behavioral responses.

As a nursing assistant, you need to be aware that sometimes signs and symptoms such as fatigue, loss of appetite, insomnia, and pain may reflect either physical or emotional stress. Note and report any unusual behavior or symptoms. Be careful, however, to be objective. Do not make judgments about your findings.

Remember also that confusion, disorientation, and aggressive behavior may only be temporary responses to a fever, drug interaction, or a full bladder and that continuation of such behavior may be the result of organic brain changes.

Assessing the Patient's Behavior

An initial assessment of the person's mental and emotional state will be made by the licensed care provider. Since you make frequent contact with the patient, you can make a valuable contribution to the nursing assessment process by making careful and sensitive objective observations.

Report observations regarding:

- Physical responses related to eating, personal hygiene, sleeping, participation in activities, or any strange or unusual behaviors.
- Emotional responses related to interactions between the patient and yourself or between the patient and other patients, emotional outbursts, or inappropriate responses.
- Patient's behavior as it relates to judgment and affects memory, comprehension, and orientation.

Working in long-term care, you will find many people whose coping ability has failed and so are demonstrating maladaptive behavior. The many losses these people have suffered add to their inability to cope. Physical problems make dealing with reality more difficult.

Common maladaptive responses result in:

- Depression
- Disorientation or delirium
- Agitation
- Paranoia

Depression

Depression is the most common functional disorder in older people, Figure 28–6, but younger people also may experience depression. Depression may be shown in a variety of ways. Figure 28–7 lists some of the more commonly seen responses. You will note that depression is often masked by symptoms that make it seem as though the patient is physically ill.

Some drugs that are used to treat actual physical illness in the elderly may cause depression. They are:

- Digitalis
- Reserpine
- Inderal
- Diuretics
- Most of the antihypertensive drugs

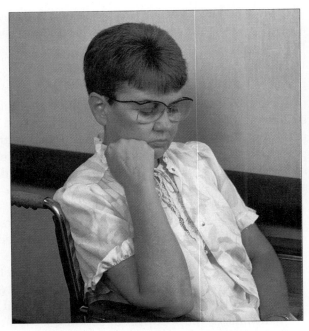

FIGURE 28–6. Be sensitive to body language and withdrawal that are common to the depressed patient.

If your patient is receiving any of these drugs, be on the alert for signs of depression. If the depression is drug-induced, it will be relieved when the drug is withdrawn.

Depression may also be a mental disorder. You can help the depressed patient by:

■ Reinforcing the person's self-concept by stressing a continued value to society and helping the patient to use the support systems that are available, Figure 28–8.

■ Not acting in a pitying way. This only validates the person's depressed feelings.

■ Preoccupation with constipation	■ Loss of appetite
	■ Fatigue
■ Flatulence	■ Headaches
■ Bad taste in the mouth	■ Backaches
■ Burning tongue	■ Stiff joints
■ Vague oral discomforts associated with dentures	■ Apathy
	■ Inability to concentrate
■ Burning on urination	■ Lethargy
■ Pain in lower abdomen	■ Agitation
■ Crying spells	■ Hallucinations
■ Trouble sleeping	■ Suicidal threats

FIGURE 28–7. Signs and symptoms that may indicate depression

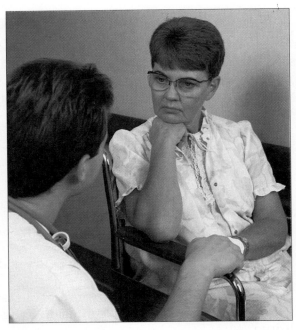

FIGURE 28–8. When talking to the depressed person, try to reinforce the person's sense of value or self-worth.

■ Making sure physical supports such as eyeglasses and hearing aids are in place. These help the person to focus on reality.

■ Reporting all complaints so actual physical problems may be identified and corrected and not attributed to the depression.

■ Providing the person with activities within her limitations to help her think beyond herself. For example, engaging the person in some meaningful activity such as reading, making puzzles, or conversing with others.

■ Avoiding tiring activities.

■ Using simple language and speaking slowly when giving instructions.

■ Monitoring elimination carefully since constipation is common.

■ Providing fluids frequently because the depressed patient may be too preoccupied to drink.

■ Being alert to the potential for suicide (the taking of one's own life).

Depressed patients usually are treated with:

■ Antidepressants

■ Electroshock therapy (in severe cases)

■ Talk therapy

A mental health clinical nurse specialist, psychologist, or psychiatrist will direct and support the staff efforts.

When depression is severe, suicidal thoughts and attempts are a real possibility. You must be sensitive to the possibility of such a situation and report and document the observations. The suicidal patient must be carefully protected. Watch for and report:

- Change in response such as deepening depression or sudden elevation of mood
- Evidence of withdrawal or secretiveness
- Sudden loss of a support system
- Repeated prolonged or sporadic refusal of food (oral or through nasal tubes), care, medications, or fluids
- Hoarding of medication (stockpiling of pills)
- Sudden decision to donate body parts to a medical school
- Changes in behavior, especially episodes of depression, screaming, hitting, throwing things, or a sudden failure to get along with family, friends, or peers
- Sudden interest or disinterest in religion
- Purchasing of a gun
- Purchasing of razor blades and hiding them
- Statements such as: "I just want out," "I want to end it all," "I'll never get well," "I'm going to kill myself," or "You would be better off without me."
- Increased use of alcohol/alcoholic drinks
- Behavioral manifestations of anger, hostility, belligerence, loss of interest, or inability to concentrate
- Inability to do simple tasks, confusion, slurred speech, or retarded motor skills
- Deep preoccupation with something that can't be explained

Nursing Care of a Potential Suicide. Never assume that a suicide attempt is a means of getting the attention of the staff or family. At least 15 percent of people who try to commit suicide do it again. Keep in mind the at-risk individuals. These include:

- White males over 65 and living alone
- The very old (75 years and above)
- Persons with a recent diagnosis of a terminal illness such as AIDS
- Those suffering the sudden loss of a spouse
- The elderly with recent multiple losses

Be aware that the suicide rate is higher in acute medical wards than it is on psychiatric wards. Most of the suicides occur while the patient is under the supervision of a health provider who frequently either misses or ignores the clues of suicide. Suicide attempts may occur when the patient is either successfully recovering or getting worse. It is the responsibility of all staff members to observe their patients carefully and immediately report any signs of depression and/or suicide. You should:

- Be observant for clues of suicide attempts and report them to the appropriate person.
- Be consistent in approaches and care.
- Encourage the patient to review his life, emphasizing the positive aspects.
- Give the patient hope while being realistic.
- Work to restore the person's self-esteem, self-worth, and self-respect to preserve positive self-concept.
- Help the patient find a support network within the family, the church/synagogue, and self-help groups.
- Make the person feel acceptance as a unique, valued person.
- Never ignore the person's statements or threats about suicide.

Disorientation (Disordered Consciousness)

Disorientation is a condition in which a person exhibits a lack of reality awareness with regard to time, person, or place, Figure 28–9. In some cases, the disorientation is mild, sometimes severe, sometimes temporary but, at times, prolonged. It is important to report patient behavior, actions, and responses. The disoriented person has impaired:

- Judgment
- Memory
- Comprehension
- Orientation

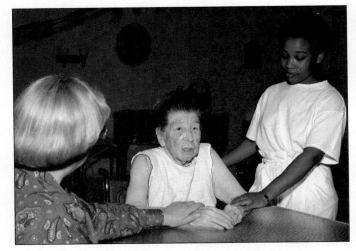

FIGURE 28–9. The disoriented person is not able to follow directions and lacks an awareness of reality.

- ■ Inability to think clearly and quickly
- ■ Bewilderment
- ■ Faulty memory
- ■ Inability to follow directions
- ■ Misinterpretation of stimuli
- ■ Confused about time
- ■ Confused about place
- ■ Confused about who he/she is

FIGURE 28–10.   Signs and symptoms of disorientation

Physical ailments and stresses that can bring about a disoriented state include:

- ■ Postsurgery
- ■ Pneumonia
- ■ Myocardial infarction
- ■ Renal infection
- ■ Head trauma
- ■ Organic brain disease
- ■ Fevers
- ■ Dehydration
- ■ Drug interaction

Figure 28–10 lists the signs and symptoms that identify the disoriented person.

Nursing Assistant Responsibilities. The nursing assistant must realize that disoriented people cannot be responsible for their actions or for protecting themselves adequately. The patient's sensory misinterpretations (delusions or hallucinations) may put others at risk. The disorientation does not allow the patient to take action for self-protection. Protection of the patient is the most important nursing responsibility. In addition, you should:

- ■ Be calm and gentle in approaching the patient since disoriented patients are startled by even minor stimuli.
- ■ Give instructions slowly, clearly, and in simple words.
- ■ Give only one instruction at a time.
- ■ Provide activities of short length that do not require strong concentration.
- ■ Build the patient's self-esteem with the reward of positive comments.
- ■ Assist patients to participate in reality-orientation activities, Figures 28–11A and B. **Reality orientation** is making the disoriented patient aware of person, place, and time by visual reminders, activities, and verbal cues.
- ■ Maintain a constant, limited routine.

- ■ Address the patient by name with each contact.
- ■ Avoid reinforcing illusions, delusions, or hallucinations.
- ■ Keep glasses, dentures, and hearing aids in place.
- ■ Speak often with the patient.
- ■ Identify yourself to the patient each time there is contact.
- ■ Be patient and repeat instructions.
- ■ Keep clock and calendar in view.
- ■ Encourage the presence of and refer to familiar objects.
- ■ Post activity board and draw attention to it.
- ■ Call attention to color coding of facility areas.

FIGURE 28–11A.   Reality-orientation activities

- ■ Use restraints only when absolutely necessary and with a physician's order, making sure all safety practices are followed. Medications that chemically restrain patient responses and the presence of a friend or family member may make physical restraints unnecessary.
- ■ Reduce disorientation by keeping rooms well lighted, cool, and quiet. Also, provide reality orientation according to the nursing care plan.

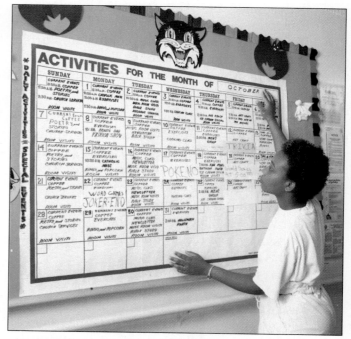

FIGURE 28–11B.   An activity board helps patients to remain reality based.

- Keep all sharps, such as knives, out of reach.
- Remove and store valuable or breakable items. If at home, make sure family knows of placement.
- Use sturdy chairs and couches.
- Put rails on windows that are close to floor.
- Provide adequate lighting.
- Protect stairways with gates.
- Do not permit poisonous plants.
- Control matches and smoking materials.
- Supervise use of stoves and appliances.
- Keep all medications out of reach.

FIGURE 28–12. Steps for maintaining a safe environment for the disoriented patient

- Noise
- Frustration at loss of control
- Feelings that their space has been invaded
- Loneliness and need for attention
- Unresolved personal difficulties in their past
- Drug interactions
- Organic brain disease
- Boredom
- Behavior of others around them
- Depression
- Dehydration
- Constipation
- Restraints
- Too much sensory stimulation

FIGURE 28–13. Factors contributing to agitation

Figure 28–12 lists guidelines for maintaining a safe environment for disoriented patients.

Agitation

Agitation is defined as inappropriate verbal, vocal, or motor activity due to causes other than disorientation or real need. It includes behavior such as:

- Aimless wandering
- Pacing
- Cursing
- Screaming
- Repeatedly asking the same question
- Spitting
- Biting
- Fighting constantly
- Demanding attention

Agitation is a significant problem for the elderly, their families, and the nursing staff. It is probably one of the foremost management problems in acute care hospitals, in home care, and in long-term care facilities.

The major factors contributing to agitation are listed in Figure 28–13. Study the list carefully because your awareness can lead to early intervention. Early intervention can often prevent serious problems.

The best way to manage the agitated patient is to:

- Not argue with or confront the person.
- Make the environment safe (secure the windows and lock the doors).
- Make sure each patient wears an identification bracelet or "patch," which is fastened securely.
- Keep a recent photo of the patient in the event the patient wanders off.
- Notify the physician, the administrator, the family, or the police department if the patient wanders away from his unit, facility, or home.
- Assign the patient brief tasks.
- Engage the patient in games, walks, swimming, and other activities if not contraindicated. These should be activities that enhance the patient's self-esteem.
- Use bean-bag seats and rocking chairs in the parlors of the nursing home or the patient's home.
- Care for the patient—watch for injuries.
- Engage the patient in conversations and in reality therapy or remotivation groups.
- Engage the patient in short-term activities. Realize that the patient's attention span is short. Thus, the patient needs rewards for short-term activities.
- Prevent the patient from becoming exhausted.
- Carefully monitor the patient's activities since the agitated patient is at risk for falls and injuries.

Hypochondriasis

The patient suffering from hypochondriasis magnifies each physical ailment. Some authorities feel that hypochondriasis is an expression of depression and is one way these individuals reduce stress. These patients need reassurance and understanding but should not be encouraged to focus or believe in their supposed illnesses. The staff must be careful not to overlook real illness when it occurs because they have become used to hearing the patient complain. Nursing assistants should report all complaints and never make a judgment that a patient is a hypochondriac.

Paranoia

Paranoia is another extreme maladaptive response to stress. It is characterized by a heightened, false sense of self-importance and delusions of being persecuted. Delusions are false beliefs about self, other people, and events. People with paranoia believe that everyone is against them. When treating the paranoid patient, you should:

- Find ways to reduce the patient's feelings of insecurity and misunderstanding.
- Keep the person as involved as possible in reality activities.

- Report and document observed responses to medication and psychotherapy.
- Monitor nutrition and fluid balance since these patients often refuse to eat or drink for fear of poisoning.
- Observe sleep patterns since the person may be fearful of being harmed while sleeping.
- Be direct and honest in all interactions.
- Not support any misconceptions or delusions that the person exhibits.
- Never argue with anyone who has delusions. It can trigger a serious confrontation.

SUMMARY

Mental and physical health are interrelated. They influence the individual's ability to cope with life within the framework of society.

Mental health is maintained through the use of different coping mechanisms such as:

- Repression
- Displacement
- Suppression
- Identification
- Projection
- Compensation
- Denial
- Conversion
- Reaction formation
- Undoing

Failure of coping mechanisms leads to maladaptive behaviors. These include:

- Excessive demands
- Disorientation
- Alcoholism
- Agitation
- Depression
- Paranoia
- Suicide attempts

The nursing assistant has specific responsibilities when caring for patients exhibiting maladaptive behaviors. These include:

- Observing and objectively reporting behaviors.
- Ensuring patient safety.
- Intervening in behaviors as directed by the care plan.

UNIT REVIEW

A. True/False. Answer the following statements true or false by circling T or F.

T F 1. Mental health refers to the adaptations made to the multiple stressors of life.

T F 2. Stressors are the physical and emotional problems that a person encounters throughout life.

T F 3. Defense mechanisms are used only by mentally unhealthy persons.

T F 4. If you know that the patient is wrong about something the patient is saying, it is proper to debate the issue with the patient.

T F 5. The best way to handle the demanding patient is by trying to determine the underlying factors for the patient's distress.

T F 6. Very few senior adults use alcohol and even fewer become alcoholics.

T F 7. The use of alcohol impairs mental alertness, judgment, reaction time, and physical coordination.

T F 8. It is dangerous for a person to drink alcohol when taking other medications.

T F 9. Alcohol is a drug.

T F 10. When intoxicated, a person could choke on food.

T F 11. Older alcoholics have a poor chance for recovery.

T F 12. Maladaptive behaviors reflect failure of usual defense mechanisms.

T F 13. Depression is the least common of the functional disorders in older people.

T F . 14. The depressed patient needs to be encouraged not to be overactive.

T F 15. Dehydration can lead the patient into a state of disorientation.

T F 16. The disoriented patient needs a stimulating environment.

T F 17. It is best to give a disoriented patient one instruction at a time.

T F 18. If a patient threatens suicide, you need not be concerned.

T F 19. The white male who is over 65 and living alone is at high risk for suicide.

T F 20. It is the responsibility of only the licensed staff to guard against suicide attempts.

T F 21. Suicides are only attempted by patients in psychiatric institutions.

T F 22. The patient who is agitated may ask the same question repeatedly.

T F 23. Agitation is a significant problem for the elderly, their families, and the staff.

T F 24. Paranoia is a maladaptive response which usually requires medication and psychotherapy.

T F 25. Paranoid individuals believe that others are out to get them.

B. Matching. Match the word in Column II with the phrase or statement in Column I.

Column I

_____ 26. conscious refusal to recognize the reality of the situation

_____ 27. excelling in one area to make up for feelings of failure in another

_____ 28. blocking out painful or anxiety-producing events or feelings

_____ 29. involuntary exclusion of the awareness of reality

_____ 30. offering socially acceptable reasons to avoid an unpleasant situation

_____ 31. substituting an object for another and behaving as if it were the original object

_____ 32. attributing one's own failing to another

_____ 33. behaving like another who is held in high regard

Column II

a. repression

b. suppression

c. projection

d. denial

e. identification

f. compensation

g. conversion

h. displacement

C. Multiple Choice. Choose the phrase that best completes each of the following sentences by circling the proper letter.

34. The patient tells you that her doctor says she has AIDS, but she knows that isn't possible. She most likely is using the defense mechanism
   a. repression.
   b. displacement.
   c. projection.
   d. denial.

35. The best way to enhance the patient's capability to cope with an unpleasant situation that has developed with another patient is to
   a. tell him to ignore it.
   b. let him know he can talk to you safely.
   c. tell him everyone has problems, his aren't so important.
   d. suggest he discuss it with his clergy.

36. The patient refuses to eat or drink because she is convinced that she is being poisoned is suffering from
    a. paranoia.
    b. depression.
    c. agitation.
    d. disorientation.

37. The patient is depressed. You can best help him by
    a. pitying him.
    b. avoiding interactions with others.
    c. agreeing that he probably deserves the way he feels.
    d. stressing his continued value to society.

38. The best way to help the patient remain oriented to reality is to
    a. keep glasses in the bedside stand so they won't be broken.
    b. isolate the patient.
    c. place a clock and calendar nearby.
    d. make explanations in a detailed way.

39. The person holding a doll and acting as if it were a baby probably is experiencing
    a. repression.
    b. denial.
    c. projection.
    d. displacement.

40. Agitation may be demonstrated by:
    a. repetitive questions.
    b. pacing.
    c. biting.
    d. all of the above.

Unit 29

Long-Term Care of the Elderly and Chronically Ill

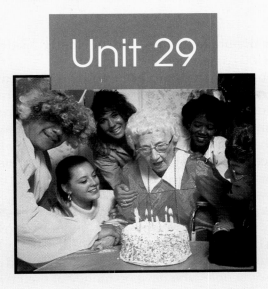

OBJECTIVES

As a result of this unit, you will be able to:

- Spell and define terms.
- List the federal requirements for nursing assistants working in long-term care facilities.
- List the rights of residents living in long-term care facilities.
- Identify the expected changes of aging.
- List the actions a nursing assistant can take to prevent infections in the long-term care facility.
- Recognize unsafe conditions in the long-term care facility.
- Demonstrate restorative techniques in the daily care of residents.
- Describe actions to use when working with residents who have dementia.
- Describe an advanced directive.

VOCABULARY

Learn the meaning and the correct spelling of the following words:

accommodation
activities of daily living (ADL)
adaptive equipment
advance directives
advocate
Alzheimer's disease
aphasia
assessment
assistive devices
care plan conference
catastrophic reaction
chronologic
debilitating
deconditioning
degeneration
dementia
dentition
diverticula
diverticulitis
diverticulosis
excoriated
flatulence
goals
hand-over-hand technique
herniations
impaction
incontinence

interdisciplinary team
legal guardian
Medicaid
Medicare
myopia
nocturia
ombudsman
organic mental syndrome
otosclerosis
pigmentation
presbycusis
presbyopia
progressive mobilization
reality orientation
reminiscing
residents
restorative care
senescent
sexuality
spasticity
sundowning
superimpose
validation therapy
verbal cues
vitality
withdrawal

Long-term Care of the Elderly and Chronically Ill

There are people with chronic health problems and permanent disability who require continuing health care, Figure 29–1. This care may be provided in the person's home or in a long-term care facility. This unit focuses on caring for persons in long-term care facilities.

Nursing assistants are valuable members of the health care team in these facilities, Figure 29–2. The skills you use in acute care facilities, such as hospitals, are also used in long-term care facilities. There are some changes in the application of these skills because of the differences between long-term and acute care.

Types of Long-term Care Facilities

There are two kinds of long-term care facilities: intermediate and skilled. Both types provide nursing care and therapies to meet the needs of residents and are usually called nursing homes. Skilled care facilities are licensed to perform more advanced procedures and techniques than intermediate facilities. Some long-term care facilities specialize in the care of people with a specific diagnosis or unusual care needs. Some are licensed to care only for children. The majority of nursing homes care for elderly residents with various diagnoses and problems.

All nursing homes are licensed by a designated state agency. These agencies survey facilities annually to ensure residents are receiving quality care.

One important issue facing our country today is the financing of long-term health care. There are few insurance policies that cover nursing home expenses. People who pay for care from private funds may find that these funds are soon exhausted.

Medicaid is a government reimbursement system whereby the federal government issues money to the states. The states determine how to distribute the money to nursing homes. These funds are used for the care of people who have no money of their own.

Medicare is another government program that partially pays for health care for persons over 65 or for those who are permanently disabled. However, Medicare covers only limited nursing home expenses.

These funds are available only to nursing homes that participate in the Medicaid and Medicare programs.

Long-term Care Population

People living in long-term care facilities are usually called residents. This is because the facility is considered their home as well as a place to receive

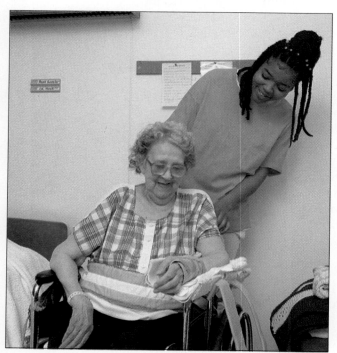

FIGURE 29–1. People with various disabilities that require assistance become part of the long-term care population.

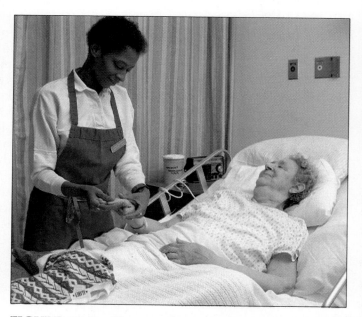

FIGURE 29–2. The nursing assistant is an important member of the health care team in a long-term care facility.

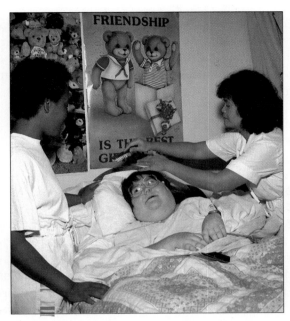

FIGURE 29–3A. This intelligent young woman with cerebral palsy needs continued supportive care.

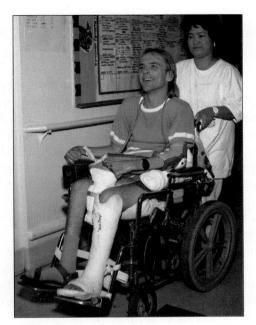

FIGURE 29–3B. This man was injured in a motorcycle accident and requires long-term rehabilitation.

health care. Many admissions are permanent, but some residents are able to go home to a less restrictive environment.

Residents are admitted to nursing homes because they have problems that require ongoing monitoring and health care. They are not admitted just because they are old. The problems of residents are a result of a disease process and are not a natural part of aging. Most nursing homes also have younger residents who are mentally or physically disabled due to chronic disease or injuries, Figure 29–3A and B. The number of people requiring long-term care is growing rapidly for several reasons:

- There are more people.
- More people are living longer, Figure 29–4.
- Modern science has enabled people to recover from illnesses or injuries that would have been fatal in the past.
- The longer a person lives, the greater the risk for acquiring a chronic, degenerative disease.
- Families are unable to provide care because of geographic distances or because everyone in the family is employed.

The percentage of persons living in nursing homes is only 1 percent for those 65 to 74 years of age. However, this increases to 22 percent for people 85 years and older. As people grow older, the

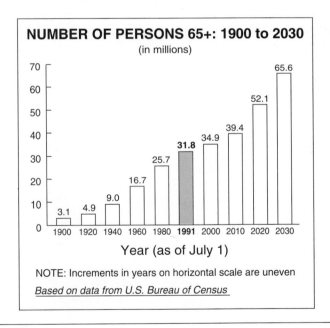

FIGURE 29–4. Number of persons 65 years of age and older: 1900-2030 *(From A Profile of Older Americans—1993, American Association of Retired Persons, 1909 K Street NW, Washington, DC 20049)*

consequences of chronic disease increase. Varying degrees of functional deficits result. Therefore, the person requires assistance in performing the activities of daily living, Figure 29–5.

Legislation Affecting Long-term Care

Recent federal legislation has brought about changes to improve the quality of care in nursing homes. This legislation is called the Nursing Home Reform Act. It is the result of the Omnibus Budget Reconciliation Act of 1987 (OBRA). Each state is responsible for implementing this legislation. It applies only to nursing homes that accept funds through Medicare and Medicaid.

Much of the OBRA content affects nursing assistants directly or indirectly:

- OBRA requires all nursing assistants working in nursing homes to complete a course of at least 75 clock hours. The course must be approved by the state agency appointed to oversee OBRA regulations. Some states require more than the minimum of 75 hours.
- After completing the course, written and manual (skills) competency tests must be passed. The tests may be taken three times.
- Nursing assistants must complete specific hours of in-service education (12 hours) per year. (Some states may require more.)

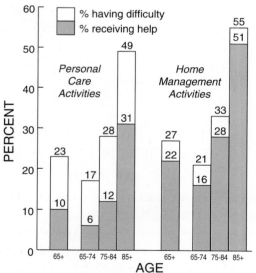

FIGURE 29–5. Percent of elderly having difficulty and receiving help with selected activities, by age: 1984 (*From* A Profile of Older Americans—1993, *American Association of Retired Persons, 1909 K Street NW, Washington, DC 20049*)

- Nursing assistants who are not employed for 24 months must repeat the course and competency tests.

Federal regulations specify the content that must be included in a nursing assistant course:

- Residents' rights
- Communication and interpersonal skills
- Infection control
- Safety/emergency procedures
- Basic nursing skills
- Personal care skills
- Mental health and social service needs
- Care of residents with Alzheimer's disease or other dementias
- Basic restorative services

Most of these topics are covered in other chapters of this textbook. This chapter provides specific information about long-term care and OBRA requirements.

Residents' Rights

Residents in nursing homes have the same rights as any citizen of the United States. The staff is responsible for assisting the resident to exercise these rights by giving the resident choices. If a resident has been legally declared incompetent, the legal guardian acts on behalf of the resident. Some rights are based on the legal and ethical foundations described in Unit 3.

These rights assure that all residents receive the care needed to reach or maintain the highest possible level of physical, mental, and psychosocial well-being. These rights are briefly described here. Those that affect the performance of the nursing assistant are described in more detail.

- Residents have the right to:
  — Free choice of physician.
  — Full information about health care status.
  — Take part in the assessment and care planning process.
- Residents have the right to
  — Refuse treatment. The laws in each state determine how this is handled.
  — Self–administer their medications if they wish to do so, and if the nurse's assessment demonstrated the resident can do this safely.
- Residents have the right to be free from abuse. Each resident has the right to be free from verbal, sexual, physical or mental abuse, corporal punishment, and involuntary seclusion. Abuse is defined as any act that is non-accidental and causes harm to the resident.

Some forms of abuse are subtle but nevertheless can cause the resident physical harm or mental anguish.

— Verbal abuse includes swearing, using inappropriate words to describe a person's race or nationality, and using obscene gestures. Embarrassing a resident by what you say is considered verbal abuse.

— Sexual abuse is the use of physical means or verbal threats to force a resident to perform sexual acts. Tormenting or teasing a resident with sexual gestures or words is a form of sexual abuse.

— Physical abuse includes hitting, slapping, pinching, kicking, or any form of physical contact that intentionally causes pain and discomfort.

— Mental abuse is a verbal threat to hurt or punish a resident. It also refers to acts of humiliation such as drawing the attention of others to a resident's behavior.

— Involuntary seclusion is the separation of a resident from other residents against the resident's will. This separation may be permitted if it is part of a therapeutic plan to reduce agitation. In such cases, there must be accurate documentation and a plan of care, and the seclusion must be effective. The decision to use seclusion must be made by the nurse.

NOTE: When a resident's behavior is described, avoid the use of words such as uncooperative, belligerent, or hostile. Instead, describe the exact actions that were observed. Often, what is called uncooperative behavior is a problem caused by faulty communication on the part of the health care provider. Residents should not be unfairly labeled.

— Physical and psychosocial neglect also are forms of abuse. This includes allowing a resident to remain soiled, not attending to the resident's personal hygiene and grooming, and actions by staff that cause the resident to withdraw or become depressed. Residents must not be subjected to abuse by anyone including staff, family members, friends, or other residents. Each health care provider must assure the safety and security of every resident. Any observed abusive behavior toward residents should be reported to the appropriate authority within the facility.

■ Residents have the right to file complaints about abuse, neglect, or misuse of property with the state agency that inspects the facility.

■ Residents have the right to be free from physical and chemical restraints. A physical restraint is any device or equipment that
— A resident cannot easily remove.
— Restricts a resident's movement.
— Does not allow normal access to one's body.

Examples of physical restraints include:
— Wrist/arm and ankle/leg restraints
— Vests
— Jackets
— Hand mitts
— Geriatric and cardiac chairs
— Wheelchair safety belts and bars
— Bed rails are considered physical restraints if they meet the definitions listed.

Psychoactive medications are considered chemical restraints because they affect the resident's mobility. The use of restraints is discussed further in the section on safety.

■ Residents have the right to privacy.
— This includes pulling privacy curtains and closing doors.
— Residents should not be unnecessarily exposed when nursing procedures are performed.
— All persons are to knock before entering the room of any resident.
— Facilities are required to provide residents with private space for telephone calls and receiving visitors.
— Facilities must also provide access to stationery, postage, and writing utensils at the resident's expense.

■ Residents have the right to confidentiality of personal and clinical records.
— Residents may inspect and purchase photocopies of the medical record upon two days' request.
— Any information learned about a resident is to be kept in confidence.

■ Residents have the right to make choices about aspects of life that are significant to them.

■ Residents have the right to voice grievances.
— Residents can take problems concerning treatment and care to someone in the facility without fear of revenge or neglect by staff.

— The appropriate staff person must promptly resolve the grievance. If residents voice complaints to a nursing assistant, it should be promptly related to the nurse.

■ The residents and family members have the right to organize resident and family councils. The facility must:
— Provide space for meetings.
— Act upon written recommendations that concern issues affecting the life of the residents.

■ Residents have the right to take part in social, religious, and community activities as long as this does not infringe on the rights of other residents. This includes the:
— Right to vote in all elections.
— Right to attend worship services and to keep religious items in the room.
— Opportunity to continue with social activities.

■ Residents have the right to know the findings of the latest survey by the state inspection agency. These results should be posted in a public area accessible to residents.

■ Residents have the right to manage personal funds.

■ Residents have the right to receive Medicare or Medicaid benefits if the resident is eligible for these benefits and if the facility participates in these programs.

■ Residents have the right to be informed about advocacy groups. These groups consist of people assigned to promote the welfare of the residents in long-term care facilities. The advocate or ombudsman supports the rights of another person or group of people with similar problems.

■ Residents have the right to visits by their families, the long-term care ombudsman, government agency representatives, and attending physician. The resident may withdraw consent to visit with any of these people.

■ Married couples have the right to share a room if they are both residing in the same facility.

■ Residents have the right to perform or not perform work for the facility if it is medically appropriate to work.

■ Residents have the right to remain in the facility unless the:
— Facility can no longer meet the resident's needs.

— Resident no longer needs the care.
— Resident's welfare requires transfer to another facility.
— Health or safety of others is endangered.
— Facility ceases to operate.
— Resident fails to pay for services.

■ The resident has the right to use personal possessions and furnishings, unless this interferes with health and safety regulations.

■ The resident, physician, family member, and legal representative must be notified within 24 hours of an accident involving a resident, a serious change in condition, major changes in treatment, and the decision to transfer or discharge.

Role of the Nursing Assistant in Long-term Care

As in the acute-care facility, the nursing assistant carries out the procedures that have been taught, assisting in the health care of elderly residents under the direct supervision of a nurse. Basic physical care, as well as special procedures, will be done to help these residents reach their maximum degree of well-being.

To be successful in this setting, you must:
■ Be patient and caring.
■ Understand the character of the older age group.
■ Be comfortable with the thought of your own aging.
■ Have the stamina to provide the assistance needed by the residents.
■ Be able to derive satisfaction from being part of a slow progress and small, if any, gains.
■ Have a sense of humor.
■ Be able to communicate effectively.

These are attributes that are important in any health setting, but in the long-term care facility they become very important.

Many of the residents will remain under your care for long periods of time, even for years. You will develop growing relationships that will become important to both care giver and care receiver. In those circumstances, communications take on greater importance. Greater significance may be attached to the attention to care or even the way thoughts are expressed in words.

Thus, the long-term care giver is a *very special person* who works in a less dramatic but important area of health care.

Characteristics of the Mature Adult

People change throughout life. These changes help identify individuals as being in specific stages of life. Some of these changes are:

- Physical changes that accompany the advancing years.
- Psychological adjustments that have been made in response to life's challenges. These are shown in attitude and behavior.

No one person moves from infancy to old age at the same rate. Each person follows her own rhythm and design. For example:

- Stature develops from small to large as growth occurs. Not everyone, however, reaches the same height at the same chronologic age.
- Some people are mature in responding to stress at age twenty. Others withdraw from stress and never learn to cope.

People are highly individual in their development and growth. It would be wrong to make assumptions based on age in years alone.

Characteristics of Adulthood

The adult:

- Has a chronologic age beyond twenty years.
- Has an adult life span defined in stages, Figure 29–6.
- Has characteristics in each stage that can only be applied generally to the group as a whole.
- Is a unique individual who may or may not conform to any or all of the group generalities.
- Has a formalized self-concept.
- Is independent and has obligations and responsibilities.
- Is a decision maker.
- May have established personal relationships.
- May be on a career track.

Admission to a nursing home represents a threat to all the adult thinks and feels. You can assist the resident's adjustment by:

- Including the resident in decisions about care.
- Giving the opportunity to make choices whenever possible.
- Recognizing that a regression to childlike behavior may be signaling frustration and fear.
- Recognizing that admission represents financial stress and a feeling that independence is lost.

Early adulthood	20–40 years
Middle adulthood	40–65 years
Late adulthood	65–75 years
Old age	75 years and over

FIGURE 29–6. Periods of adult life

Effects of Aging

The resident in the long-term facility is usually advanced in age with one or more chronic, somewhat debilitating (weakening) conditions. Some are mentally alert. Others are confused and disoriented.

There are, however, some features of aging that are characteristic for most elderly residents. Do not expect every resident to exhibit the same characteristics at the same chronologic (year) age. Remember that aging is a natural, progressive process that begins at birth and extends to death. Remember also that every resident is unique and must be treated with dignity and respect.

Physical Changes in Aging

Some investigators believe we are born with a biological time clock. This clock is programmed for a specific life span, barring accidents and disease process. As we move toward old age, changes that have been taking place gradually become more evident. For example, the elderly person:

- May lose vitality.
- May sleep less at night.
- May benefit from rest periods during the day.
- Stores less fluid in body tissue and is apt to become dehydrated. This results in a loss of elasticity and resiliency in tissues.
- Has fibrous tissue changes. These decrease the tone, mass, and strength of skeletal and smooth muscle.
- Has secretory and endocrine cells that become less functional and reduced nerve sensitivity.

Certain changes occur in every body system. They do not necessarily occur at the same rate in each system. In the nervous system:

- Response to sensory stimuli is slower and less accurate.
- Pain and awareness of injury are not always perceived with the same intensity. Because of this, serious situations may be ignored.

■ Smell and taste are less acute. Appetite tends to lag.

■ Eyes undergo changes that limit peripheral (side) vision and near vision, making additional lighting necessary.

■ Hearing diminishes, sometimes so slowly that hearing loss is significant before it is recognized. Lessening or loss of sight and hearing may make the older person feel isolated and frustrated in her ability to communicate.

The musculoskeletal system changes include:

■ Less flexible joints. Some degeneration or breakdown becomes evident.

■ Prolonged reaction time.

■ Loss of muscle strength and tone.

■ More brittle and porous bones. These changes often combine to make falls more common and serious.

■ Weakening of muscular walls, leading to herniations or pushing of organs through weakened areas of walls. One result of herniations is to make elimination more difficult.

■ Bone changes in the vertebral column resulting in loss of height, as well as postural changes, Figure 29–7.

The urinary system undergoes specific changes which include:

■ Nocturia, or getting up to void during the night. The amount of urine produced and eliminated is affected by the loss of smooth muscle tone and loss of vascular pathways. Emptying the bladder incompletely predisposes the elderly to urinary infections.

■ Enlargement of the prostate. This complicates the problem of urinary retention in elderly men.

The cardiovascular changes are reflected throughout the entire body. These are often compounded by the effects of atherosclerosis and include:

■ Narrowing of blood vessels

■ Increased blood pressure and diminished blood flow throughout the body

The digestive system, though adequate, may provide less nutrition because of:

■ Loss of sensitivity of taste buds

■ Decreased digestive enzymes

■ Poor teeth

The integumentary system shows some of the most obvious changes. These include:

■ Loss of fat and water, which leads to wrinkling and thinning of the skin.

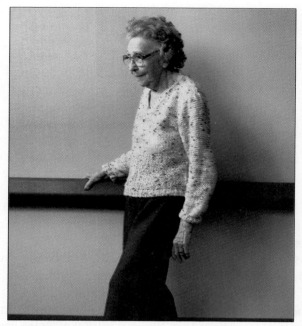

FIGURE 29–7.   Changes in the bones of the vertebral column result in postural changes.

■ A sallow skin color caused by receding capillaries.

■ Brittle and thick fingernails and toenails.

■ Pronounced areas of pigmentation, resulting in elevated patches of yellowish or brown spots, known as liver spots.

■ The development of roughened, scaly, wartlike lesions. These must be considered potentially dangerous since they may become malignant.

■ Thinner hair, which usually lightens in color.

■ A decrease in oil production, making the hair and skin dry.

The reproductive system in both females and males undergoes changes. These changes are closely related to changes in hormonal levels.

■ The older person's ability to engage in successful, satisfying intercourse is diminished but still present.

■ Some accommodation (adjustment) for slower erectile response is needed.

■ There is thinning of tissues and less lubrication of the vagina.

■ With adequate care, sexual response can continue.

Prostheses (artificial parts) are more commonly needed as age and illness take their toll. Each prosthetic device is expensive and is designed to meet the needs of a particular resident. You must learn how each prosthesis is applied, how it is cared for, and how it should be stored. Your team leader or the resident are excellent sources for this information. Some prosthetic devices include:

- Eyeglasses
- Hearing aid
- Artificial leg or eye
- Dentures

Emotional Adjustments to Aging

Emotional adjustments to aging are basically extensions of the adjustments the individual has made throughout life to the many changes in a person's circumstances. Personality characteristics and ways of reacting to stress are developed fairly early in life and tend to become a constant in the personality of the individual. In fact, as a person ages, personality traits become even more pronounced. The stress produced by the circumstances and illnesses that accompany old age do not drastically alter the individual's personality, but they do tend to enhance and, in some cases, distort the basic traits.

Old people have the same emotional needs and require the same supports for good mental health as young people, Figure 29–8. They need:

- To be loved.
- To have a sense of self-worth.
- To feel a sense of achievement and recognition.
- To have a degree of economic security.

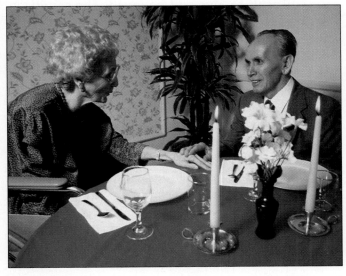

FIGURE 29–8. Older people have the same emotional needs as young people. (*Photo courtesy of Country Park Health Care Center, Long Beach, CA*)

Although these needs are common to all human beings, regardless of age, the avenues for achieving satisfaction and gratification of these needs are narrowed greatly for older people. The opportunities for social exchange and sexual expression, the two major means of gratification, are greatly reduced as the years advance.

The attitude of the Western world toward old people tends to relegate (place) them to a position of lesser and lesser significance. The older people become, the more their self-image is depreciated (devalued) both in their own eyes and in the eyes of others.

Physical ailments, far more common in the elderly because of slowed body processes, are superimposed (layered on top of) upon the changes brought about by the natural aging process. Change of body image and loss of the vigor and vitality (lively character) of former years are major losses the older person must accept—losses that further alter their self-image and self-esteem. The care giver can make an important contribution by promoting the self-esteem of those being cared for.

In old age, some accommodations must be made in the attitudes or psychological outlooks of all persons. The most healthy emotional responses are based:

- On philosophies that accept aging as a natural progressive stage.
- In life attitudes that recognize the strengths as well as the limitations of the body.
- On a form of behavior that demonstrates interest in living here and now.

Healthy psychological adjustments mean both a realistic appraisal of the present circumstance and building on the positive values while coming to terms with the negative aspects.

Some of your long-term care residents will have already made these adjustments. Some will be in the process. Your supportive caring will be important and helpful to each.

Specific Emotional Responses. The elderly or infirm resident is apt to experience some common emotional responses. Frustration is a common emotion experienced by the elderly—frustration at physical limitations and at having less control over their own lives. That is why it is important to allow the elderly the opportunity to make as many decisions as possible. Signs of frustration are often demonstrated in:

- Aggressive behavior
- Anger
- Hostility
- Demanding behavior
- Complaining
- Crying

Some residents even resort to manipulating families, staff, or other residents in an attempt to relieve their feelings of helplessness, Figure 29–9.

Anxiety and fear may be expressed in periods of depression and withdrawal. The depression experienced by the elderly is easily understood. In many instances, they:

- Are cut off from their social support systems.
- Have had to make major adjustments in their lifestyles.
- May have lost loved ones and friends.
- May have very limited finances.
- May truly feel that they no longer have any control of their destinies or even of their day-to-day activities.
- May have stretched their coping ability to the breaking point because of physical weakness and disease processes.

Withdrawal, a common frustration response, is shown by:

- Lack of communication
- Temporary confusion
- General disorientation as to time and place

You can play a major role in helping residents move successfully through these periods by:

- Reassuring them that they will not be abandoned now that they are no longer able to care for themselves.
- Treating each person with respect to reinforce self-esteem.

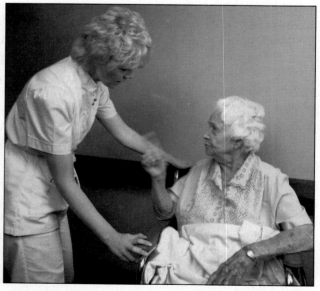

FIGURE 29–9. Aggressive behavior often signals feelings of frustration.

- Calmly helping your residents keep in touch with reality while conveying your own feelings of compassion and caring.
- Reporting changes in behavior, mood swings, and emotional responses to your supervisor so that the entire staff can form a supporting network.
- Responding to the residents' negative attitudes by being willing to listen and interact with them and emphasizing the positive.

Sexuality and the Older Adult

Sexuality is a lifelong characteristic that defines the maleness or femaleness of each person. This definition may be different for each person. All individuals are sexual whether or not they have physical sexual relations. Being old or disabled does not diminish human sexuality. However, our society tends to associate youth, beauty, and physical agility with sexuality. By using these standards, older people are not considered to be sexual beings. The person within a human being does not change. Although the hair is gray, the skin is wrinkled, and the body not so agile, the person inside still has feelings and longing for love and affection.

You learned in Unit 8 that human needs are present throughout life. You also learned that the need to love and be loved is a basic psychosocial (emotional) need. When this is not met, self-esteem decreases. With low self-esteem, human beings do not feel good about themselves. As people age, it becomes increasingly more difficult to love and be loved. The significant relationships that provided love, affection, and friendship may be lost through death or geographic distance. Some individuals living in nursing homes have spouses living elsewhere, making it difficult to maintain a loving relationship. The couple may have had an active sexual relationship as well.

As a nursing assistant, there are several actions you can take to help residents maintain their sexuality:

- Give attention to resident's grooming and appearance. This includes clothing, jewelry, hair styles, use of makeup, clean shaven face, and cologne, depending on the residents' wishes.
- Give sincere compliments on the residents' appearance.
- Use touch frequently. Touch is the only sense that does not usually diminish with aging, and yet it is the sense most likely to be deprived.

Hold a hand, give a hug, or rub a back to satisfy the resident's need to be touched.

■ Converse with residents on an adult level.

■ Support friendships among the residents. Treat all relationships with dignity and respect, Figure 29–10.

■ Married couples have the right to do in private whatever is pleasing to them unless there are medical contraindications.

■ Always knock before entering a room. If you accidentally interrupt sexual activity, leave the room and shut the door.

■ Provide privacy for residents and visiting spouses. They have a need to talk and to hold each other. Some couples may wish to continue a sexual relationship.

■ Physical sexual expression is a need for some residents that cannot be fulfilled. In these situations, the resident may choose to masturbate. This is not harmful and can bring satisfaction to the resident.

■ The health care staff is responsible for protecting vulnerable residents who are mentally incompetent or physically unable to defend themselves. Care providers or visitors cannot be allowed to sexually abuse residents. Residents who sexually abuse or harass other residents or care givers should be reported to the appropriate authority.

As a nursing assistant you can increase the residents' self-esteem. Respect and acknowledge their sexuality and treat each resident with dignity.

Nutritional Needs

Malnutrition is a problem for the aged because the older person may develop an apathy toward food that becomes progressive. Factors that contribute to lack of appetite are:

■ Decreased activity

■ Inadequate dentition (teeth)

■ Decreased saliva

■ Diminished smell and taste

■ Poor oral hygiene

■ Poor dentures

■ Eating alone

The diet for the elderly person should:

■ Be easy to chew.

■ Contain decreased amounts of refined sugars, fats, and cholesterol.

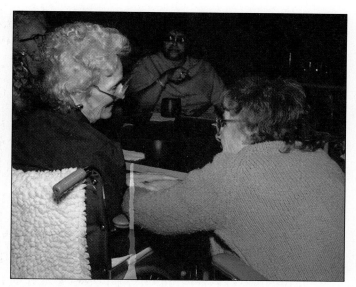

FIGURE 29–10. Heterosexual women can find validation in the loving and caring touch of another woman.

■ Have adequate proteins and vitamins to provide for optimum function and repair.

■ Have an increase of complex carbohydrates found in fruits, vegetables, and grains. These foods also provide good sources of vitamins and minerals, which tend to be deficient in the elderly diet.

■ Be monitored for weight control. Obesity is a major nutritional problem that is seen among the elderly and those who are inactive. The excess weight increases the stress of existing conditions. Calories are generally limited to about 2,000 calories for the average woman and 2,400–2,500 calories for the average man.

Because of loss of muscle tone, three intestinal problems are seen. They are:

■ Constipation—difficulty in eliminating solid waste

■ Flatulence—gas production

■ Diverticulosis—small pockets (diverticula) of weakened intestinal wall

Dietary adjustments can help reduce these problems.

■ Soft bulk foods, such as whole grain cereals and fruits and vegetables, are helpful in overcoming the constipation.

■ Skins and seeds should be avoided to prevent diverticulitis, which is an inflammation of the diverticula.

The presentation and service of the food are important in stimulating appetites. Keep in mind the following:

- Several smaller meals seem to be more easily tolerated than three large meals.
- Residents should be allowed to feed themselves as much as possible. You may assist by cutting up the food into bite-sized morsels. Even if you must do most of the feeding, allow the resident to participate as much as possible.
- Adequate liquid is absolutely essential. This is an area that is frequently neglected, leading to dehydration.
- You must encourage fluid intake and be sure that the resident actually drinks the fluids.
- Fruit and vegetable juices, eggnogs, and soups can serve the dual purpose of providing nourishment and fluids.
- Fluids must be offered at frequent intervals between meals to ensure adequate intake.

Infection Control in the Long-term Care Facility

There are no additional or special infection control techniques in long-term care facilities. Section 4 provides instructions on all infection control procedures performed in nursing homes. Effective and frequent handwashing is the most effective method for preventing the spread of disease from resident to resident, staff person to resident, or resident to staff person. Universal precautions should be implemented in the care of all persons when there is contact with blood and body fluids. Isolation techniques are used for residents with known infectious diseases.

It is important to follow these procedures because it is easy for elderly people to get infections. There are a number of reasons for this:

- Body changes due to aging make older people more susceptible to infection. The skin offers less protection because of its fragility. Any break in the skin, such as a pressure sore or skin tear, can quickly become infected.
- Changes in the urinary system cause the bladder to empty less efficiently. Urine left in the bladder contributes to urinary tract infections.
- The ability to cough and raise secretions is reduced. As a result, there is decrease ability to get rid of bacteria from the lungs.
- Elderly people do not always eat well and may be undernourished.

- Elderly people have less resistance to disease because the immune system becomes less effective as people get older.
- Resistance to disease is reduced when residents have several chronic health problems.

The elderly do not readily show signs of infection. This means they may be sick for some time before you recognize the problem. This is because:

- The elderly do not always develop a fever with an infection. The average temperature for an older person may be one or two degrees less than that of a younger person. Therefore, average temperature may represent an increase or fever.
- Some elderly persons do not feel pain as acutely as younger people. They may feel no discomfort with a bladder infection, for example.
- The elderly do not readily develop signs of inflammatory response. A skin infection usually shows redness, swelling, heat, and pain. These signs may be missing or delayed in the elderly person.
- The elderly do not necessarily have an increase in the white blood cell count. This is usually a sign of infection but is often absent in the elderly.
- Elderly people do not cough as frequently when there is a respiratory tract infection.
- Residents who are disoriented may not comprehend or be able to communicate feelings of pain or nausea.

The elderly are also more likely to develop serious complications from infections. A simple urinary tract infection can result in bacteremia (blood infection), causing the resident to be acutely ill. This can prove fatal to the person who has little ability to cope with additional health problems.

Prevention of infection in nursing home residents is an ongoing concern. There are some steps that you can take to help in this process:

- Assist residents to maintain an adequate fluid intake. This helps prevent urinary tract and respiratory tract infections and keeps the skin healthier.
- Assist residents to maintain adequate nutritional intake. Report to the nurse when residents eat less or refuse food.
- Assist residents to perform exercise programs established by the nurse or physical therapist. Follow positioning schedules and orders for range of motion exercises and ambulation. This

increases circulation, thus lowering the risk for pressure ulcers (a frequent source of infection). Exercise also improves breathing, thereby decreasing the risk of respiratory tract infections.

■ Attend to residents' personal hygiene needs. Bathing and oral care help prevent infection. Inspect the body and mouth when performing these procedures.

■ Toilet residents regularly who need assistance. This keeps the bladder empty and also assures residents that they will receive help when they need to urinate. Some residents hesitate to drink fluids for fear they will be incontinent. When caring for incontinent residents, be sure to wipe female residents using strokes from front to back. This avoids contaminating the urethra with stool or vaginal excretions.

■ Perform catheter care as directed. Avoid opening the drainage system.

■ Observe the residents carefully and report any unusual signs or changes. Urinary tract infections may be noted by changes in the urine or by incontinence. In some cases, the first sign of any infection is disorientation in people who are not usually disoriented. For persons with dementia, a change in behavior may indicate an infection. Incidents of falling often occur in residents with infections.

■ You will be asked to collect urine specimens for culture and sensitivity. The specimen should be clean catch (see Unit 24). You may need to ask for help to collect the specimen. If it is contaminated because of inadequate cleaning or improper collection, the results will be altered.

Fighting infection in the long-term care facility is everyone's responsibility. As a nursing assistant, you can do your part by performing handwashing, universal precautions, isolation techniques, and all principles of medical asepsis on a routine basis. Assist new employees to acquire these skills, and assist residents to maintain good personal hygiene practices.

Safety in the Long-term Care Facility

Each year an estimated 30–40 percent of all nursing home residents fall. There are several reasons for this:

■ Changes in vision and hearing that most older people experience cause a loss of "warning systems."

■ Problems with mobility resulting from arthritic changes, loss of flexibility, and endurance.

■ Loss of balance related to inner ear changes.

■ Frequency of urination leading to fears of incontinence, resulting in unsafe toileting habits.

■ Disorientation and faulty judgment in persons who are mentally incompetent.

■ Some elderly persons experience dizziness when coming to a standing position too quickly.

External factors can also increase the risk for falling:

■ Use of medications that affect mental status, balance, and coordination.

■ Unsafe use of assistive mobility devices.

■ Poorly planned environment.

■ Staff delay in attending to the needs of the residents.

In an effort to reduce the incidence of falls, the environment can be altered to meet the needs of elderly persons: (Also review Unit 11.)

■ Aging changes in the eye cause older people to be more sensitive to glare and to changes in lighting. They also have difficulty seeing colors at the blue-green end of the spectrum. To prevent falls due to faulty vision:
— Use nonglare wax on floors to avoid glare.
— Use blinds and curtains to prevent glare from windows.
— Place mirrors to prevent glare.
— Use nonglare glass in pictures.
— Use bright nonglare lighting with constant, even illumination.
— Use colors to mark the edges of steps and curbs that serve as caution reminders.
— Use colors in the red and yellow family that increase the ability to see changes in walls and floors.
— Encourage residents to wear sunglasses (if not contraindicated) and hats when they go outdoors.

■ Noise increases disorientation and can create anxiety even in alert persons. This increases the risk of falls. Minimizing all noises reduces this risk.

■ All tubs and showers should have chairs so residents can remain seated throughout the procedure. Lifts for tubs avoid the need for the resident to stand in the tub. Avoid using oils that can make the tub bottom slippery.

- Check residents' clothing for fit. Loose shoes and laces, slippers, long robes, and slacks increase the risk of falling.
- Observe ambulatory residents when they get out of bed and chairs, off the toilet, and when they walk.
  — Give instructions to residents who have unsafe habits.
  — Residents who self-propel their wheelchairs need instructions on how to enter and leave elevators, how to use ramps, and reminders to use the brakes.
  — Dependent residents may benefit by learning self-transfer techniques. Check with the nurse to see if this is possible.
  — When you help dependent residents transfer, always use the method indicated in the care plan.
- Side rails are a frequent cause of falls. Many nursing homes leave side rails down on one side for residents who can safely transfer without help. In some situations, half rails are more effective.

There are other actions that can be tried before using physical restraints. Some suggestions are:

- Care for the residents' personal needs promptly. This may prevent residents from attempting unsafe transfers and ambulation.
- Identify residents who are at risk for falling and make this information available to all staff. Everyone can assist in monitoring these residents.
- You may be directed by the nurse or physical therapist to instruct residents on safe mobility skills.
- Report any observations to the nurse that may increase the risk of falling, such as residents' complaints of dizziness or problems with balance and coordination.
- All staff should help in maintaining a calm, consistent environment. This can prevent anxiety and insecurity that can lead to incidents.
- Provide comfortable chairs for the residents. Special rocking chairs can be soothing for people with dementia.
- Make sure that call lights are accessible to residents.
- Cooperate with other staff in providing appropriate activities for the residents.
- Some facilities have security systems for wandering residents. A band around the ankle or wrist signals an alarm when the resident passes a sensor on the way out of an outside door, Figure 29–11.

Restraints

In the past, restraints often were used routinely as a preventive measure for falls. Research has shown that side rails and restraints do not necessarily accomplish this purpose. In fact, many falls occur with side rails up and restraints intact. This can result in serious injury or even death.

The use of restraints is the biggest cause of immobility in nursing home residents. Immobility causes other problems such as pressure sores and skin irritation, restricted circulation, loss of muscle tone, and joint stiffness. The inability to get up and go to the bathroom leads to incontinence and constipation.

Restrained residents are likely to become disoriented, depressed, hostile, and agitated. The loss of freedom imposed by restraints can lead to withdrawal and eventually the loss of the will to live.

All residents deserve to maintain their dignity and independence to the highest degree possible. This may involve taking the risks of normal, everyday life. When residents are at risk, the staff must evaluate each situation individually to determine whether the risk of potential injury outweighs the risk of complications from the use of restraints. With the OBRA

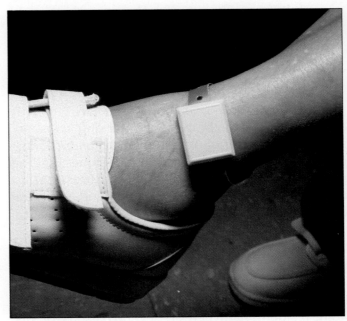

FIGURE 29–11. A special sensor may be attached to the leg or wrist of the wandering, disoriented resident. The sensor alerts the staff if the resident starts to leave the facility.

legislation, restraints are used only as the last resort after other alternatives have been tried and failed. The staff must investigate the cause of the behavior for which a restraint is needed so steps can be taken to resolve the problem without using restraints.

If restraints *must* be used, there are several actions to be followed. You can assist the nurse by reporting your observations and performing all instructions correctly:

- All resident behavior must be carefully documented.
- All alternatives that were tried must be documented.
- When the alternatives are unsuccessful, staff must consult with the resident and the resident's family or legal guardian and obtain their approval and written consent to apply a restraint or safety device.
- If approval is given, the physician must write the order. The order must include the reason for the restraint or safety device, the type of device, the length of time it can be used, and where it can be used.
- The least restrictive device is always tried first. The restraint or device should be clean, in good repair, and of the correct size.
- Always apply restraints or safety devices according to the manufacturer's directions.
- Check residents in restraints at least every 30 minutes.
- Release the restraints every 2 hours.
  — Assist residents to stand and ambulate if possible.
  — If residents cannot do this, passive range of motion exercises on all extremities should be carried out.
  — Take residents to the bathroom.
  — If residents were incontinent, change clothing, chair pads or bedding, and provide skin care.
- Check resident for any signs of skin breakdown or irritation and report these to the nurse.
- Give residents fluids and nutrition.
- Always place the call light within the resident's reach.

Unit 3 has additional information on restraints.

Other Safety Concerns

Poisonous Substances. Eating poisonous substances can cause incidents in the nursing home. Most states have regulations regarding the use and storage of dangerous chemicals. Persons with dementia may eat or drink items that other residents have in their rooms, such as shaving lotion, cologne, nail polish, and plants. Residents frequently will store food in their rooms until it spoils. Because of poor vision and reduced taste and smell, they are unaware of spoilage. To prevent accidental poisonings:

- Keep all chemicals in locked cupboards.
- Use only nonpoisonous plants in the facility.
- Provide residents with refrigerator space for perishable food items. Label containers with the residents' names.

Aspiration and Choking. Aspiration and choking occur more readily in the elderly than in young persons. The swallowing mechanism becomes less efficient as people age. Residents with dementia have an increased risk of choking. To prevent incidents of choking or aspiration:

- Be aware of residents who have problems with swallowing. Follow all instructions for giving appropriate feeding assistance to these residents.
- Position residents upright in good body alignment before meals. Have them remain in this position for at least 30 minutes after eating.
- At the end of the meal, give oral care to residents who are known to "squirrel" food in their mouths. Food can remain in the mouth for several minutes after the meal and be accidentally aspirated if the resident begins to cough.
- Monitor disoriented residents for placing nonedible items in their mouths. Remove such items from the environment.
- Know how to administer the Heimlich maneuver (see Unit 44).

Thermal Injuries. Thermal injuries (those caused by heat or cold) occur less frequently than other injuries but are still a source of concern:

- Follow procedures accurately when administering heat or cold treatments.
- Water temperatures are usually regulated but check the water before placing residents in the tub or shower.
- Check food temperatures before feeding residents. Using a microwave oven to reheat food can be dangerous because of the uneven temperatures.
- Store smoking materials in a safe place and monitor residents while smoking.

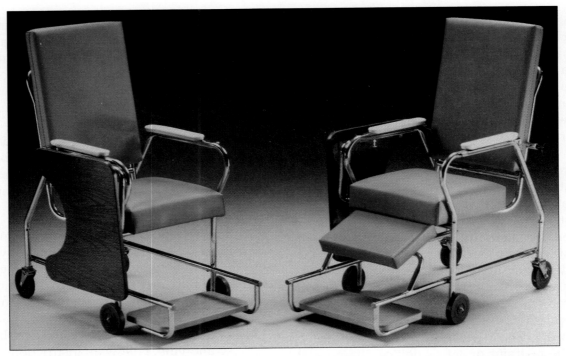

FIGURE 29–12. The geriatric wheelchair (Gerichair®) is designed to provide position changes for nonambulatory residents. The tray provides support and an area on which to eat and carry on activities. When the tray is in place, the Gerichair® is considered a form of restraint. *(Photo courtesy of Invacare Corporation)*

Safety in nursing homes is a major concern. Unlike hospitals, residents are given the freedom to move about the facility as they desire. For this reason, the entire building must be free of hazards that contribute to accidents. All employees need to be constantly aware of the residents' safety.

Exercise and Recreational Needs

Residents in long-term care facilities need the stimulation of planned recreation and exercise. The type of activity must be carefully tailored to the needs and abilities of the residents, Figure 29–12. Health workers in these facilities are often responsible for coordinating this aspect of care.

Recreation

It is important for those who do the activity planning to keep in mind:

■ The age and possible physical limitations of the participants.

■ The fact that older people have less coordination and are more apt to have hearing and vision deficiencies.

■ The fact that recreation with a purpose is considered to be the most stimulating and enjoyable form to mature people.

■ That activities that are planned by the participants are generally the most successful. Shows and skits call for many different talents. Exhibits, sales, and making gifts for others are some other examples of activities that combine recreation with purpose. These types of activities are usually enjoyed by everyone. Most care facilities have a special room where out-of-bed residents can gather.

With care, activities that even meet special rehabilitation objectives can be planned. For that reason, the occupational therapist is a valuable person to serve in a consultant capacity, both in care facilities and recreational centers. Recreational planning can thus combine physical and rehabilitative activities with enjoyment.

■ Exercising, singing, and clapping hands to music can be enjoyed to some degree by bed residents, wheelchair residents, and even those who are confused.

■ For those residents who are ambulatory, dancing can be a stimulating as well as an enjoyable activity.

■ Handicrafts and games, and even television and conversation, offer a measure of entertainment to the less active.

Restorative Care

In the past, nursing homes usually provided basic care and were concerned with meeting the physical needs of the residents. The emphasis now is on providing the care and services that a resident needs in order to reach or maintain physical, mental and psychosocial well-being. This care is called **restorative care**. A resident's condition should not deteriorate as a result of inappropriate or inadequate care.

Without meaning to, it is possible to cause residents to become helpless by not allowing them to do things that they are capable of doing. This causes residents to lose their abilities. When they can no longer care for themselves, they may feel they are less worthy people. The application of restorative care by the interdisciplinary team prevents this from happening. The **interdisciplinary team** is a group of professionals from many areas of health care who work together to solve residents' problems. The team consists of the:

- Resident
- Family or **legal guardian** (person appointed by court to manage affairs of a resident who is not competent to do so)
- Physician
- Nursing staff
- Dietician
- Social services representative
- Activities staff
- Rehabilitation staff

This staff may include the physical therapist, occupational therapist, rehabilitation nurse, and speech pathologist, depending on the needs of each resident.

There are other health care professionals who may be on the team when a resident needs their services:

- Pharmacist
- Dentist or dental hygienist
- Audiologist
- Podiatrist
- Psychiatrist or mental health consultant
- Optometrist or ophthalmologist
- Other medical and nursing specialists

The team work begins when the resident is admitted to the facility. A registered nurse coordinates an **assessment** (evaluation) with other members of the team. Nursing assistants are not directly responsible for this assessment, but your observations provide important information to other team members. After the assessment is completed, the resident, family, and team attend the **care plan conference** where the resident's needs are discussed and problems related to the resident's care are solved.

The assessment is used to identify the problems of the resident. The team plans approaches for solving the problems. The team (including the resident) sets **goals** (events to be achieved in the plan of care). This information is entered on the resident's care plan. The care plan is changed as the resident meets the goals. The team approach is successful when:

- Team members understand the philosophy, goals, and purposes of restorative care.
- Team members understand their responsibilities.
- All team members, including the resident and family, attend the care plan conference.

You can be an effective member of the interdisciplinary team by:

- Attending care plan conferences or giving the team your observations and ideas.
- Recognizing the importance of all team members.
- Appreciating each member's contribution to the team.
- Learning as much as possible about the residents and their families. This helps you understand the residents.
- Attending in-service training sessions to increase your knowledge.

Elderly people rapidly lose their self-care abilities when they have a chronic illness such as arthritis or a stroke. This causes them to be less active or mobile. Inactivity then causes other complications:

- Skin breakdown and pressure sores because of poor circulation
- Joint stiffness and contractures
- Pneumonia
- Lack of appetite, indigestion, and constipation
- Osteoporosis
- Thromboses (blood clots)
- General **deconditioning** (loss of physical and mental abilities due to inactivity)
- Mental deterioration
- Emotional changes such as apathy and depression

The major responsibilities of the nursing assistant in providing restorative care are to:

- Work with other team members in preventing complications.

■ Help residents increase their abilities to do activities of daily living.

Activities of daily living (ADLs) are the basic activities that adults carry out to sustain life. This includes mobility skills, feeding oneself, grooming and hygiene, dressing, and toileting. To help residents maintain or regain these skills:

■ Stress abilities of residents rather than their disabilities—restorative care builds on the strengths of residents.

■ Remember that activity strengthens and inactivity weakens. All residents need to participate in mental and physical activities planned for their abilities, Figure 29–13.

■ Be aware of residents' problems and why the residents cannot complete the activities of daily living. It may be from
— Paralysis from a stroke or spinal cord injury
— Inadequate range of motion due to arthritis
— Lack of endurance because of a cardiac or respiratory problem
— Lack of strength from inactivity
— Disorientation
— Loss of vision

■ Know the resident's goals.

■ Understand your responsibilities in carrying out residents' care plans. This may include:
— Giving **verbal cues** (prompting a resident through an activity by selecting words or phrases) or one-step instructions to the residents
— Utilizing hand-over-hand techniques
— Demonstrating actions for the residents to copy

■ Use these methods consistently.

■ Use assistive/adaptive equipment if it is ordered, Figure 29–14. (**Adaptive equipment** or **assistive devices** consist of items altered to make them easier to use by those with functional deficits.)

■ Be sensitive to the feelings of the residents.

■ Encourage and assist residents to do as much as possible for themselves. Be enthusiastic and believe in what you are doing.

■ Talk with the nurse if the plans cannot be carried out or if the residents are not meeting the goals.

■ Residents' progress is not always consistent. The ability to complete an activity may change

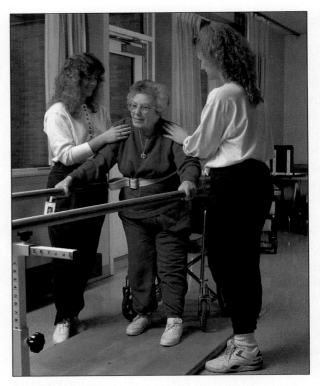

FIGURE 29–13. Exercise helps maintain muscle tone and agility. *(From Hegner and Caldwell, Assisting in Long-Term Care, copyright 1993 by Delmar Publishers Inc.)*

from day to day because of fatigue, anxiety, a change in care giver, or onset of acute illness.

Restorative Care Skills

The nurse or physical therapist evaluates each resident's potential for increasing her abilities. A process called **progressive mobilization** builds on a series of activity steps to increase the resident's abilities. Progress is different for each person. The steps of progressive mobilization begin with the following bed activities completed first with assistance and then independently by the resident:

■ Positioning
■ Passive, active, self-range of motion
■ Moving up, down, and sideways in bed
■ Rolling onto the side
■ Coming to a sitting position on the side of the bed

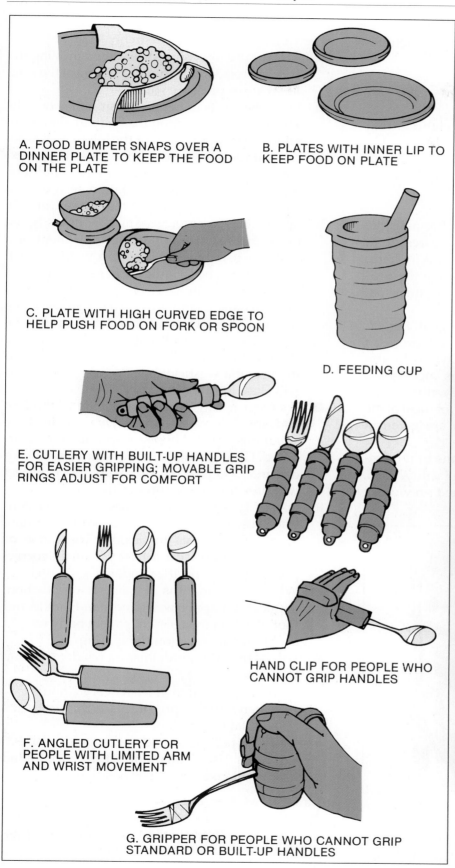

A. FOOD BUMPER SNAPS OVER A DINNER PLATE TO KEEP THE FOOD ON THE PLATE

B. PLATES WITH INNER LIP TO KEEP FOOD ON PLATE

C. PLATE WITH HIGH CURVED EDGE TO HELP PUSH FOOD ON FORK OR SPOON

D. FEEDING CUP

E. CUTLERY WITH BUILT-UP HANDLES FOR EASIER GRIPPING; MOVABLE GRIP RINGS ADJUST FOR COMFORT

HAND CLIP FOR PEOPLE WHO CANNOT GRIP HANDLES

F. ANGLED CUTLERY FOR PEOPLE WITH LIMITED ARM AND WRIST MOVEMENT

G. GRIPPER FOR PEOPLE WHO CANNOT GRIP STANDARD OR BUILT-UP HANDLES

FIGURE 29–14. Special devices can assist the elderly and handicapped to feed themselves. *(From Badasch and Chesebro, Essentials for the Nursing Assistant in Long-Term Care, 1990, Delmar Publishers Inc.)*

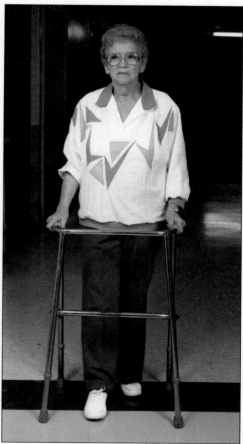

FIGURE 29–15. A walker provides support and assists stability. It allows the resident to ambulate independently with more confidence.

The next steps build on the first level and include:
- Sitting transfers
- Standing at the side of the bed
- Standing transfers with assistance of one and two persons
- Wheelchair activities including weight shifting and pushups
- Self-propelling a wheelchair

If these steps can be successfully managed, the last step is
- Ambulation

This includes learning how to walk with an assistive device (cane or walker) if one is used, Figures 29–15 and 29–16. At each step, the nurse or physical therapist may give you instructions for helping the resident perform additional exercises to strengthen specific muscles and to increase endurance.

Each of these steps has a functional goal. For example, a resident learns to transfer and propel a wheelchair in order to be able to get to the bathroom and dining room independently. This increases a resident's self-esteem and, of course, eventually decreases the work of the staff. Directions for most of the activities in progressive mobilization are given in other units.

Here are some additional instructions to remember when working in a long-term care facility. Also, review the information you have learned previously about these procedures.

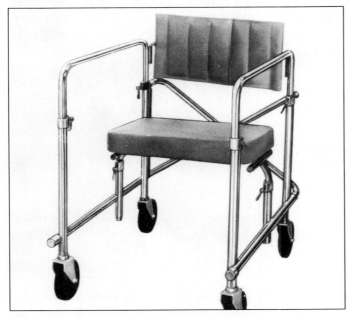

FIGURE 29–16. This type of walker has a seat that lifts for ambulation. The seat may be lowered for sitting if the resident becomes tired. *(Photo courtesy of Invacare Corporation)*

Positioning and Bed Movement.
- Always use a turning sheet when moving dependent residents to avoid shearing of the skin. This causes pressure sores.
- Place the joints in neutral position if possible. This means positioning the body in alignment with only slight flexion of the joints. It is especially important to avoid flexion or hyperextension of the neck, adduction of the shoulders, adduction and external rotation of the hips, and planter flexion of the ankles (see Unit 35).
- Spasticity is common in paralyzed limbs. **Spasticity** is resistance to passive movement of a limb due to damage to the brain or spinal cord. Contractures occur quickly in the presence of spasticity. A firm handroll may be ordered to prevent hand contractures. This is placed in the resident's hand to avoid complete flexion of the hand. Use a handroll with a smooth surface. Rough surfaces will trigger spasticity. Avoid the use of a washcloth as the resident's hand will close tightly around it.
- Footboards can increase spasticity of the foot and, for this reason, are rarely used in these situations. Special boots or splints may be ordered. Giving range of motion at least twice a day and loosening the top covers above the feet will prevent contractures of the ankle.
- Spasticity sometimes causes extension contractures. In these cases, it is more appropriate to place the joints in flexion. The nurse or physical therapist can advise you on the correct procedure for specific residents.
- When the resident is in a side-lying position, support the upper wrist and hand, ankle and foot. Position the resident so that body weight is not directly on shoulder and hip.
- Follow the same guidelines for residents sitting in chairs:
  — Change position at least every 2 hours.
  — When sitting upright, place the resident's feet flat on the floor.
  — The hips, knees, and feet should be at 90° angles. Use small pillows, towels, or folded bath blankets for chair positioning.

Range of Motion Exercises.
- Encourage residents to help with the passive exercises. Support extremities and allow residents to help with the movement.

- Passive range of motion exercises of the neck are not generally done on residents in long-term care. Arthritis is common and passive exercises can injure the neck. Instead, encourage residents to move the head independently.
- Move each joint to its full range but remember that the maximum range in an elderly person may be small.
- Do each motion slowly, smoothly, and gently to avoid causing spasticity and pain. Come to a complete stop at the end of each movement.
- Remember that many elderly persons have arthritis and osteoporosis. It is important to hold the extremities gently but firmly, using the palms of your hands and not your fingertips (see Unit 35 for complete instructions).

Transfers

- The bones of elderly persons are fragile. Grasping residents under the shoulders or around the trunk during a transfer procedure can injure residents. The use of a transfer belt is recommended for residents who cannot bear weight and who need assistance in transferring (see Unit 13).

Ambulation. The final step of progressive mobilization is ambulation. Not all residents will reach this point. Your responsibilities are to observe and assist residents with ambulation. The nurse or physical therapist selects and teaches residents how to walk and use an assistive device.

Some general rules to follow when you are ambulating residents are:

- Always use a transfer (gait) belt if the resident has problems with balance, coordination, or strength.
- If a resident has balance problems, two people should ambulate the resident so counterbalance is provided.
- If you are unsure about a resident's endurance, ask another person to follow with the resident's wheelchair.
- Always stand on the resident's weaker side. Place your hand closest to the resident in the back of the transfer belt with an underhand grasp. Place your far hand on the front of the resident's shoulder.
- A cane is held on the resident's strongest side.
- If a walker is used, all four points of the walker should strike the floor at the same time.
- A walker should never be used on stairs.

- When the resident sits down, be sure the chair is touching the back of the resident's legs. The resident's hands should be placed on the arms of the chair to lower the body into the chair.

Other Activities of Daily Living

You will be an active member of the team in assisting the resident to reach many goals. These goals may be small but represent large steps for the resident. Many residents will never reach total independence. Yet, they must be given the opportunity to do as much as possible. It is important to help residents maintain the skills they have acquired. It may take patience to wait for the resident to perform the steps of an ADL. Avoid the temptation to do it for the resident. Observe the resident for signs of frustration, fatigue or emotional upset. There will be times when a resident will not be able to perform without your help.

Some residents are inappropriate candidates for a restorative plan. It is unkind to expect persons who are dying or in the last stages of Alzheimer's disease will increase their abilities. Give them opportunities to do what they are capable of doing but at the same time be ready to provide assistance.

As you share successes with the residents in reaching their goals, you will feel a great sense of satisfaction in being a member of the interdisciplinary team.

The following procedures present basic principles of transferring the frail elderly.

Remember to perform the beginning procedure actions and procedure completion actions for each patient care procedure, Figure 29–17.

General Hygiene

Skin Characteristics

Aging skin:
- In general becomes dry and scaly with a tendency to thin. Exposure to the sun intensifies the tendency to wrinkle.
- Has less oil, so dryness from too-frequent bathing causes itching. This is sometimes referred to as bath itch. It looks like pin-point red spots.
- Is easily hurt and takes a long time to heal because circulation is less efficient.
- Has lost elasticity, adipose (fatty connective) tissue, and water. This undermines the skin foundation, causing characteristic sagging and wrinkling. Gravitational pull tends, over the

BEGINNING PROCEDURE ACTIONS	PROCEDURE COMPLETION ACTIONS
■ Wash your hands. ■ Assemble equipment needed. ■ Go to the resident's room, knock, and pause before entering. ■ Introduce yourself and identify the resident. ■ Ask visitors to leave and inform them where they can wait. ■ Provide privacy. ■ Explain what will happen and answer questions. ■ Allow resident to assist in procedure as much as possible. ■ Raise bed or table to comfortable working height.	■ Position resident comfortably. ■ Leave signal cord, telephone, and fresh water close at hand. ■ Return bed or table to lowest position. ■ Perform general safety check of resident and environment. ■ Care for equipment according to facility policy. ■ Wash your hands. ■ Report completion of task. ■ Let visitors know when they may reenter the resident's room. ■ Document action and your observations.

NOTE: Where there are open lesions, wet linen, or possible contact with resident body fluids or blood, disposable gloves are worn during the procedure. Put on gloves before contact with the resident or linen. Properly dispose of gloves after they are removed. ALWAYS APPLY UNIVERSAL PRECAUTIONS.

FIGURE 29–17. Beginning procedure actions and procedure completion actions

PROCEDURE 102 | OBRA

TRANSFERRING A RESIDENT FROM BED TO CHAIR OR CHAIR TO BED (FOR THE FRAIL ELDERLY)

1. Carry out each beginning procedure action.
2. Remember to wash your hands, identify the resident, and provide privacy.
3. To assist the resident to come to a standing position from the bed:
   - Help resident turn onto his side facing you.
   - Place your hand closest to resident's shoulders underneath the shoulders (not under the neck).
   - Place your other hand and forearm over the top and around resident's knees.
   - Tell resident to use his upper arm and hand to push off against the mattress.
   - Tell resident to use his other arm and hand to push up.
   - As resident does this, use your arm/hand under his shoulder to help him raise up and use your other arm/hand to help swing his legs (gently) off the bed.
   - This movement helps the resident's upper body automatically raise.
   - Allow resident to sit on the edge of the bed to prevent dizziness.
   - Apply transfer belt.

   NOTES:
   - The resident's hands should not be on your neck or shoulders during the transfer.
   - A confused or frightened resident may cause injury to your spinal cord.
   - The resident's hands should be used to "push off" the surface of the bed or chair.
   - Always transfer toward resident's strongest side.
   - When transferring from a chair, help resident move forward in the chair first.
4. When resident is ready to transfer from bed or chair:
   - Instruct resident to spread his knees, lean forward, and place feet slightly back. If one leg is weaker or should not bear weight, ask resident to place it out in front with the other leg slightly back.
   - Remember to maintain a broad base of support when lifting or moving residents. Your feet should be several inches apart with your knees bent.

- If resident has a weaker leg, place your knee against the resident's weak knee or use your foot to block the resident's foot on that side. This prevents the weak leg from sliding out uncontrolled.
- Tell resident that on the count of three, he should push off the bed, straighten his knees, and stand.
- If resident cannot walk, pivot around so the chair (or bed) touches the back of his legs.
- Tell resident to place his hands on the arms of the chair or the edge of the mattress and to lower self into the chair or onto the mattress.

- While resident is doing this, be sure you have a secure grasp of the transfer belt.
- Some residents want to use a walker or cane to come to a standing position before transferring or walking. These devices are used only for assistance in ambulating, not for transferring.

5. Carry out each procedure completion action. Remember to wash your hands, report completion of task, and document time, date, action (transferred resident from bed to chair or chair to bed), and resident response.

PROCEDURE 103 | OBRA | SIDE 9

ASSISTING THE RESIDENT WHO AMBULATES WITH A CANE OR WALKER

1. Carry out each beginning procedure action.
2. Wash your hands, identify resident, and provide privacy.
3. Assemble equipment needed:
   - Cane
   - Walker
   - Transfer belt
4. Check walker or cane for worn areas or loose parts. Be sure that rubber tips and rubber hand grips have adequate tread and are not cracked and worn. Place the cane or walker close by.
5. When resident's hand(s) are in place on the cane or walker, the elbow should form a 30° angle.
6. Lower bed to lowest horizontal position.
7. Instruct resident to turn on his side toward you. Provide only the assistance that is necessary.
8. Place one of your arms under resident's shoulders and the other around the top of resident's knees.
9. Instruct resident to use his arms to raise up and, at the same time, raise resident's shoulders with your arm and move his legs off the bed. The resident will come to a sitting position on the edge of the bed.
10. Assist resident to dress if necessary and put on sturdy, nonslip shoes.
11. Apply the gait (transfer) belt if necessary.
12. Instruct resident to lean slightly forward and put feet slightly back.

13. Stand in front of resident and place both your hands in the gait belt with an underhand grasp.
14. Block resident's feet with your feet to prevent them from sliding out.
15. Instruct resident to "push off" the bed with hands as you help him to stand.
16. Hand resident the cane or place the walker in front of him within reach.
17. A cane goes on the strong side. The resident should advance the cane 10 to 18 inches followed by weaker leg and then strong leg.
18. For using a walker, have resident advance the walker about 10 to 18 inches. Resident then moves weaker leg forward into the walker followed by the stronger leg.
19. If resident has a gait belt on, stand on the resident's weaker side and slightly in back with your hands in the belt.
20. After ambulation, return resident to bed or chair. Have resident walk within a step of the bed or chair. Place the cane or walker to the side and assist resident to turn around. When resident feels the bed or chair touching the back of his legs, have him reach for the arms of the chair or the mattress and lower self into the chair or bed.
21. Carry out each procedure completion action. Remember to wash your hands, report completion of task, and document time, date, action (assisted with ambulation with cane or walker), and resident reaction.

years, to make the eyelids droop. The skin in the neck often shrinks, leading to so-called age rings. Sebaceous glands in the skin are less active.

■ Has more fragile peripheral blood vessels. These are more easily seen under the thinned epidermis. Small hemorrhages can occur due to the fragility of the blood vessels. Peripheral circulation to the skin decreases so that general skin nutrition is less satisfactory.

■ Has a more sallow color and is less pink.

■ Seems drawn taut over the bony prominences of forehead, chin, and nose. This makes the eyes seem to recede in the sockets. Eyes also appear sunken due to loss of orbital fat.

■ Has areas of skin pigmentation and irregularities that seem more pronounced with advancing years.

■ Has liver spots. These are not related to the liver at all. They are elevated yellowish or brownish spots or patches that occur on exposed skin surfaces such as the backs of the hands. Their cause is unknown, but they are thought to result from environmental wear by weather and sun.

■ Has roughened, scaly, slightly elevated, wartlike lesions. They are thought to be related to sunburn damage in fair-skinned individuals.

■ Has skin tabs, moles, and warts which become more noticeable as the skin ages.

Cleanliness of the Skin

Cleanliness of the skin is essential, but a full daily bath for the older person is neither necessary nor advisable. In fact, most elderly are reluctant to bathe daily.

Sponge Baths

Although a daily bath is unnecessary, frequent sponging of specific areas is necessary. The face, groin, underarms, and other body creases need regular cleaning and care.

Skin areas that touch must be kept free from perspiration and should not be allowed to rub together. Whenever moisture, perspiration, urine, or feces are present, skin breakdown is possible. Gently wash and dry local areas.

Total Baths

Bed baths clean the skin, but they are a rather passive activity for the resident. Therefore, a tub or shower bath is desirable two or three times a week to stimulate the resident. Some points to keep in mind when bathing elderly persons are:

■ Some soaps may be drying. Superfatted soaps are less drying and less irritating.

■ The skin of an elderly resident is easily hurt and takes a long time to heal because of inefficient general circulation, so care must be taken in handling the skin.

■ The skin should be dried by patting gently rather than by rubbing. All contact with the skin must be gentle. Even pulling a sheet from under a resident too rapidly can cause trauma.

■ Lotions should be applied to dry areas to protect them. Bath oils lubricate the skin, but they are dangerous because they make the bath tub slippery. It is better to apply lotions directly to dry areas.

■ General safety factors and the resident's physical limitations should be considered before giving a tub or shower bath. Placement of hand rails, and availability of tub and shower seats, Figure 29–18, or hydraulic lifts, Figure 29–19, should be checked. Be sure you know how to use the hydraulic lift before trying to use one with the resident.

■ Warm baths may decrease cerebral circulation. This can lead to confusion. Warm baths may best be given just before the resident retires.

■ Elderly people tend to be sensitive to deodorants, so care should be used when applying them.

■ Inspect the resident's skin over bony prominences for signs of skin breakdown, including redness, warmth, and ischemic pallor.

■ The skin should be carefully observed for abnormalities and care must be taken not to disturb them. Any change in color, size, or texture should be reported immediately. Cancer of the skin, often seen in the elderly, has an excellent cure rate (93%) when treated early. This is because skin cancer tends to grow slowly and the cells tend not to spread. These lesions are usually painless. All skin lesions are suspect. You must immediately report any changes noted in the resident's skin.

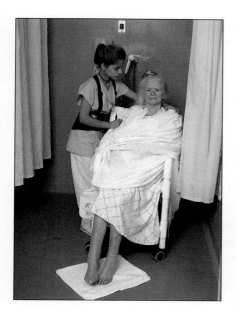

FIGURE 29–18. The shower chair allows the resident to sit safely during preparations for bathing and while bathing.

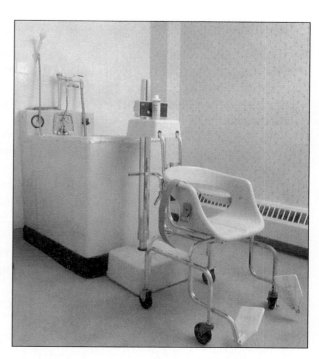

FIGURE 29–19. The bathing chair is attached to a hydraulic lift that safely lifts and swings the resident into the tub.

Hand and Foot Care

As we age, fingernails and toenails become thickened and brittle. They split frequently because of decreased peripheral circulation. Fingernails can be cleaned during the morning care period. They should not be neglected.

- A soft brush and blunt-edged orangewood stick will clean the nails without causing injury.
- The hands can be soaked in warm water and the cuticles pushed back gently with a towel.
- Softening creams and olive-oil soaks help to soften the cuticles.
- Fingernails should be cut and filed, following the contour of the fingertips (check with facility policy).
- Care should be taken not to injure the corners since improper cutting of fingernails and toenails is the biggest single cause of infections.

Foot care should also be a routine part of the morning care. This should include:

- Careful washing and drying of the feet.
- Close inspection for any abnormalities.
- Application of olive oil, lanolin, cocoa butter, hand cream, or lotion to dry, scaly skin.
- Application of a very light dusting of powder to perspiring feet.
- Cutting toenails straight across, Figure 29–20 (check with facility policy). Thickened nails, which are difficult to cut, or nails of diabetic

residents that need to be cut should always be reported to your supervisor.

- Providing slippers or shoes that fit well and are in good repair.

NOTE: Check facility policy regarding nail and foot care for diabetic residents.

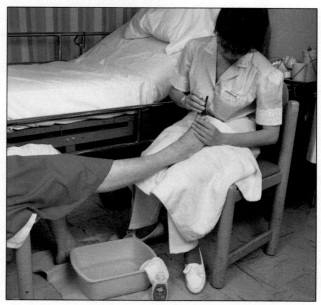

FIGURE 29–20. Foot care should be part of the daily care.

Hair Care

Hair changes in amount and color as a person ages. These changes are part of the normal aging process. Graying or loss of pigmentation (color) is usual. Some graying may be evident as early as the second or third decade.

■ Genetics probably plays an important role in the change rate. As more and more pigment is lost, the hair becomes white.

■ Decreased oil makes the hair dull and lifeless.

■ The amount of hair is reduced in some males, and the texture becomes coarser in other areas such as the eyebrows and face.

■ Balding is an aging characteristic that first appears at widely varying ages. Again, genetics has a strong influence.

Hair care is important in maintaining the resident's overall personal appearance.

■ Hair should be styled and neatly arranged.

■ An order is required for a shampoo to be given once or twice a month.

■ Dry shampoos are also available. They simplify shampoos for residents confined to bed.

■ A mild conditioning shampoo is best.

— A dryer will dry the hair quickly, decreasing the chance of chilling.

— The resident must be kept out of drafts while the hair is being washed and dried.

— Shampoos are more safely given in bed; or if the person is seated, a shampoo board can be used. Bending is difficult for older persons and their decreased sense of balance is apt to result in a fall. Shampoos may also be given in the tub or shower.

■ Hair care may be provided by a beautician or barber, if available, or by a family member or nursing assistant.

Facial Hair

Elderly women tend to have an increase in the growth and coarseness of the hair on their chins and upper lips. These can be removed:

■ With tweezers.

■ By electric needles used by a professional.

■ By shaving, with a physician's order.

Facial hair may also be lightened, by mildly bleaching it.

Elderly men need to be shaved regularly, usually daily. You may need to:

■ Only provide the equipment.

■ Use a safety razor to shave the patient yourself.

■ Assist the person to obtain barbering services.

Mouth Care

The condition of the teeth affects the aged person's total health. Hygienic routines and observations are your responsibility when an individual is no longer able to do these things for himself. See Unit 21 for specific care procedures.

Natural Teeth. Poor oral hygiene can result in loss of appetite and weight, and may be the focus of any infection. Even if teeth are missing, the remaining teeth should be cleaned regularly. Dental checkups should be given the same amount of attention as in younger years.

Dentures. False teeth, called dentures, must be cleaned daily under running water with a brush especially made for this purpose.

■ Be sure to fill the sink half full of water with a washcloth on the bottom, Figure 29–21, so that if the teeth are dropped accidentally, there is less chance of breakage.

■ Hot water and strong antiseptic solutions may injure dentures. They should not be used.

■ A place should be provided where vulcanite dentures can be stored safely in solution so

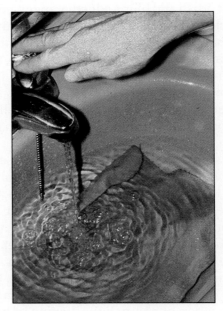

FIGURE 29–21. Before cleaning dentures under cool running water, protect the dentures by placing a washcloth in the bottom of the basin.

they will not warp while out of the mouth. Plastic dentures may be stored dry.

- Check the mouth and gums routinely for signs of irritation. Use soft brush to clean mouth and gums.
- Periodic dental examinations should be made to have the teeth checked and polished.

Mouth care is especially important for the bed resident who has lost teeth and is no longer able to keep dentures in the mouth. Check the mouth and gums for irritation. Dentures should be inspected for cracks, rough edges, and broken teeth.

- A commercial mouthwash, a warm wash of saline solution, or baking soda should be used before and after meals.
- Glycerine and lemon applied with applicators between meals are very refreshing.
- Lips should be inspected for excessive dryness or fissures.
- Creams, petroleum jelly, or glycerine applied to the lips can prevent fissures from developing into deep sores and infections.

Eyes, Ears, and Nose

Eyes, ears, and nose should also be observed daily for any signs of irritations, redness, drainage, or excess dryness of the skin that could lead to breaks and fissures. Observations of this nature by staff members should be part of routine care.

Elimination Needs

Urinary Incontinence

Urinary incontinence (loss of control) may be due to one or a combination of causes. It is not unusual to find more than one factor present at the same time. Any interruption of cerebral control such as a stroke, brain damage that destroys the control centers or pathways, confusion and decreased awareness due to general cerebral degeneration, or aphasia leading to the resident's inability to communicate to others the need for help can lead to incontinence.

- Incontinence may occur simply because the resident is unable to reach the proper facilities in time. The condition may be related to fecal impaction. Fecal impaction acts as a mechanical obstruction, causing the urine to be retained. The incontinence in this case is actually overflow. Perhaps the most common reason

for incontinence is infection. Inflammation irritates sensory nerve endings in the bladder. Mucosal and bladder contractions are increased, causing the incontinence.

- Incontinence may be temporary, lasting only a few days. For example, after a period of illness, continence may improve as the resident becomes more able to respond to the environment. Attention to the underlying causes and the temporary use of incontinence pads may be all that is needed. Every effort should be made to help the resident become continent as soon as possible with little reference to the temporary incontinence. You can do much to give emotional support and reassurance to the resident.
- Incontinence of an established nature continues even though the resident is ambulatory. This is a more difficult, but still not impossible, form of incontinence to treat. Drugs are sometimes used to achieve bladder control. Retraining may also be needed.

Retraining

Retraining usually takes from six to eight weeks of consistent effort. During these weeks, the importance of emotional support cannot be overemphasized. The entire staff must present a confident attitude, helping to assure the resident that new habits can be established. Developing new habits and achieving appropriate responses to them requires diligence, patience, and time. Successes should be praised, and lapses accepted as a natural part of the training process. The attitude and reactions of all staff members must be consistently positive.

Keep in mind that not all residents are able to cooperate to the same degree.

- The first step in retraining is to enlist the resident's cooperation.
- The second step is to make a record of the resident's incontinence times.
- The third step is to provide the resident with the opportunity to void. Nocturnal incontinence can be helped by making sure a urinal is kept at the bedside in an easily accessible spot, by taking the resident to the bathroom, or by offering the bedpan at midnight. When the record shows a specific time that incontinence occurs, the resident should be awakened routinely one hour in advance of that time.

- Fluid control may be initiated.
  — Some authorities advocate the control of fluids as an aid to continence. The fluids are increased during daytime hours and restricted at night.
  — Others believe the limitation of fluids is inadvisable because this presents a very real danger to the elderly of dehydration, increased confusion, and even uremia.
- Attention to the resident's position during elimination helps the process.
  — Sitting upright, with hips and knees flexed, and feet flat for support is the optimal position.
  — A bedside commode, Figure 29–22, may be used.
  — The height of the regular toilet seat can be raised for maximum comfort, and fitted with hand rails for safety and support, Figures 29–23A and 29–23B. A height of 20 inches is usually the most satisfactory.
  — Chairs that can be pushed over the commode are more convenient for many residents, Figure 29–23C.
  — Men find it easier to void in the standing position, but they may require support.
  — When residents must remain in bed, the bedpan should be padded and the body supported with pillows.
  — Use of an orthopedic (fracture) bedpan may provide additional comfort.

- Additional stimuli may help start the flow of urine and completely empty the bladder.
  — Offer a glass of water to drink.
  — Pour a measured amount of water over the perineum.
  — Help the resident to lean forward.
  — Run water in the sink so the resident can hear it.
  — Encourage the resident to bear down at the end of voiding to completely empty the bladder.
  — Place the resident's hand in water.
- Keeping the skin meticulously clean adds to the comfort and safety of the resident.
  — Wash the incontinent resident regularly.
  — Moisture barrier creams may be applied.

Fecal Incontinence and Constipation

Fecal incontinence is less common than urinary incontinence and is more easily controlled. Bowel retraining aims at establishing continence and preventing impaction.

- When retraining is not possible, a fecal incontinence collector may be used, Figure 29–24.
- The cause of constipation is not always evident. Certainly improper diet, lack of exercise, and inaccessibility of the lavatory are contributing factors.

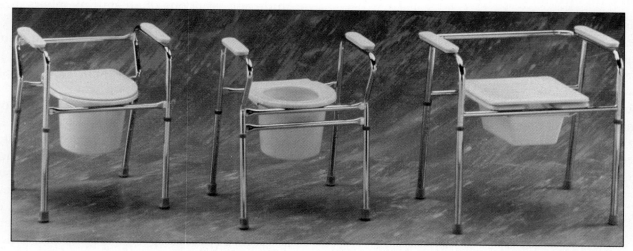

FIGURE 29–22. A bedside commode allows the resident to assume the best position during the retraining period. *(Photo courtesy of Invacare Corporation)*

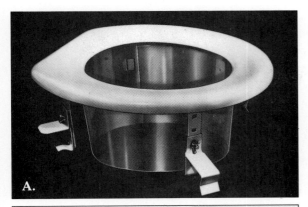

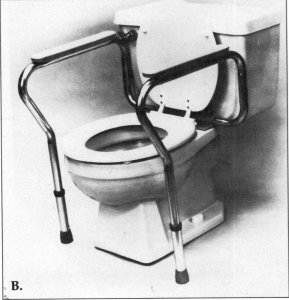

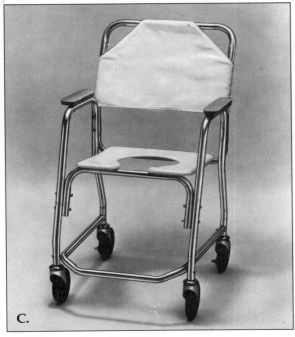

FIGURE 29–23. Equipment to assist elimination (*Photos courtesy of Invacare Corporation*)

- The most serious form of constipation results in **impaction**. The fecal mass gradually loses water if it is not eliminated from the bowel. This dehydrated mass acts as an irritant to the mucosa, and mucus production is increased. Some of the outer mass is dissolved by the mucus and there is evidence of apparent diarrhea. Any time you note diarrhea in the elderly resident, especially in one who is bedridden, you should suspect fecal impaction.

- Oil-retention enemas may be helpful when followed by a soapsuds enema. (See Unit 38 for information on administering enemas.)

- Regularity is the key to bowel retraining. Proper sitting helps considerably. The resident should be comfortably and safely positioned. Guardrails on either side of the toilet will increase the feeling of security. Privacy and an unhurried atmosphere are important.

Communication Needs and Sensory Abilities

Communication is a two-way interaction between a sender and receiver. Elderly persons may have difficulty sending messages when a stroke hampers their ability to speak or form thought properly, or when hearing or vision is impaired. They may have difficulty in receiving messages when mental deterioration clouds mental awareness.

Aphasia

The term **aphasia** means language impairment. It involves either an inability to express through speech or to understand speech. Some residents have no remaining useful language after a stroke. For them the prognosis for regaining language skills is very poor.

- For these residents, the outlook is indeed bleak. They:
  - Have no useful means of communication through reading, writing, or speaking.
  - May be unable to even gesture meaningfully.

Other residents can be retrained to some degree of useful language ability.

- The prognosis for these residents, who still have some basic skills that can be developed, is better.

A Guide to Using the Hollister®
Drainable Fecal Incontinence Collector

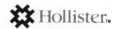 Hollister™

The Hollister® Drainable Fecal Incontinence Collector features a durable skin barrier which protects a patient's skin against contact with irritating discharge, and the same highly effective odor-barrier material used in Hollister® Ostomy Pouches.

The skin barrier comes with a 1½-inch pre-cut opening which may be enlarged. The collector also features a Convenience Drain which makes it easy to empty into a bedpan or other receptacle. If desired, the drain may be connected to a bedside container for continuous drainage.

Preparing the skin

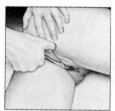

1. Carefully trim hair with a blunt-nosed scissors. **Do not** use a razor.

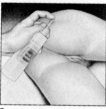

2. Wash with a mild cleanser. Rinse thoroughly and dry the skin completely.

Applying the Drainable Fecal Incontinence Collector

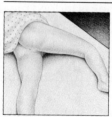

1. Have the patient assume a side-lying (Simm's) position with the upper knee up toward the chest. The patient should remain in this position for the entire procedure.

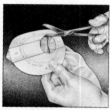

2. If necessary, enlarge the opening in the skin barrier. **Do not** cut beyond the line on the backing paper.

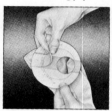

3. Remove release paper numbered 1 and 2.

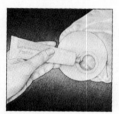

4. If desired, the remaining sections of release paper may be removed and a bead of Hollister Premium Paste (Stock No 7930) can be applied around the opening on the barrier to ensure a proper seal.

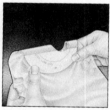

5. Fold the barrier in half and separate the patient's buttocks to expose the perianal area.

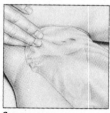

6. Press the barrier **firmly** against the skin.

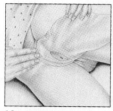

6A. For **female** patients, adhere the narrowest part of the barrier between the anus and the vagina.

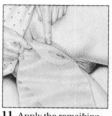

6B. For **male** patients, adhere this section of the barrier between the anus and the scrotum.

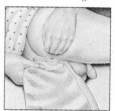

7. Apply the upper portion of the exposed skin barrier against the coccygeal area.

8. Release the buttocks.

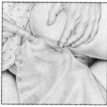

9. Remove the release paper (numbered 3 or 4, depending on the patient's position) nearest the patient's lower buttock.

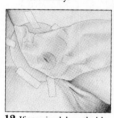

10. Press the barrier **firmly** against the skin.

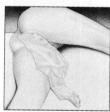

11. Apply the remaining skin barrier against the patient's upper buttock. Press **firmly.**

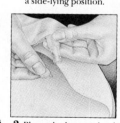

12. If required, breathable tape may be placed as shown to supplement adhesion.

Draining the Collector

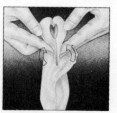

1. Have the patient assume a side-lying position.

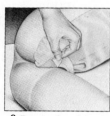

2. Place a bedpan under the drain and remove the cap.

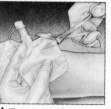

3. For continuous collection, use tubing to connect to a bedside drainage collector.

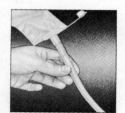

4. To accommodate more solid stool, cut off the drain.

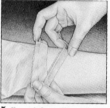

5. Reseal the collector with a Hollister® Drainable Pouch Clamp (Stock No 7765).

Removing the Fecal Incontinence Collector

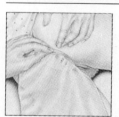

1. Gently peel the barrier away.

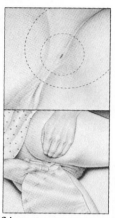

2. Fold the barrier in half and discard.

FIGURE 29–24.   The fecal incontinence collector protects the resident's skin and controls odor. Note that universal precautions must be applied: gloves must be worn for this procedure. *(Courtesy of Hollister Incorporated)*

— Their degree of aphasia means that they may make errors in reading and writing, misuse words, and show confusion over related expressions, but they can still communicate using language.

— Words that sound alike and number and time concepts might confuse them also.

— Their visual field may be imperfect, so those items in certain sections of their visual fields are disregarded when reading.

— Automatic speech, or words—frequently sprinkled with profanity—which have no real meaning or relationship to each other, is not unusual either.

Your approach to the aphasic resident is very important. It can contribute greatly to the resident's recovery. Patience is essential.

- Use short, precise sentences, speaking slowly to give the resident time to comprehend.
- Do not raise your voice. The problem is one of comprehension, not hearing.
- Use gestures to help communicate meaning.
- Talk to aphasic residents. They need examples to emulate, so you must talk to them.

Actual speech therapy requires the service of a competent speech therapist, but your cooperation is very important.

Hearing Deficits

Elderly persons who are hard of hearing:
- May have suffered ear infections or ear diseases in childhood or middle life and, as a result, have carried this socially incapacitating handicap into their later years.
- May be victims of the most common problem as a result of aging: otosclerosis. In otosclerosis, the tissues of the labyrinth and middle ear become hardened, and hearing is gradually diminished. Extreme tones are lost first, with the greatest loss in the low-pitched range. Patients with otosclerosis may also be disturbed by distressing inner sounds.

Hearing aids, which amplify sounds, can help these people. Hearing aids must be properly fitted to the individual. The resident should be carefully instructed in their use and care.

Another common cause of hearing loss in the elderly is presbycusis, known also as old-age deafness, or eighth-nerve-damage deafness. It is caused by damage to the eighth nerve. The eighth nerve is responsible for conducting sound waves. Senescent (aging) changes in this nerve, probably due to degeneration, make perception and conduction more difficult. Since hearing aids essentially increase the sound that still must be carried by the auditory nerve, they are of little value when the auditory nerve itself no longer functions.

Communication with a deaf person takes skill and practice, Figure 29–25, but it is well worth the effort. Figure 29–26 lists suggestions for making communication more effective.

Impaired Vision

Aged persons may also experience a decline in their ability to see. Many wear glasses or a prosthesis (artificial eye). Causes of vision changes include:

- Specific disease conditions such as glaucoma and cataracts. More complete explanations of these conditions are found in Unit 37.
- The aging process itself.
  — Nearsightedness is called myopia. For persons who have worn glasses for nearsightedness all their lives, the changes may make glasses no longer necessary or require a new prescription for near work.
  — Presbyopia (farsightedness) is due to a loss of elasticity in the crystalline lens of the eye.

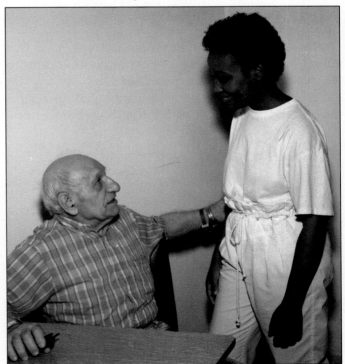

FIGURE 29–25. Face the hearing impaired resident directly and speak slowly and distinctly.

1. Speak slowly and distinctly.
2. Form words carefully; keep sentences short.
3. Rephrase words as needed.
4. Face the listener.
5. Make sure any light source is behind the listener.
6. Use facial expressions or gestures to help express meanings.
7. Encourage lip reading.
8. Diminish outside distractions.

FIGURE 29–26. Guidelines for communicating with residents who are hearing impaired

The crystalline lens of the eye changes its shape to bend light rays which are given off by objects being seen. When the lens is less functional, the object must be moved farther away to be seen clearly.

■ Drugs that the elderly person is taking for conditions unrelated to the eyes.

Any redness, burning, blurring, or excess watering may also be early indications of more serious eye conditions. These signs and symptoms must be noted and reported promptly.

Psychological Needs

Mental deterioration may stem from physical (organic) or emotional causes. A combination of both may occur in the residents in your care.

Periods of emotionally confused behavior are often temporary. They may be due to unusual stress,

such as an underlying infection or a transfer to an unfamiliar setting. At other times, the excess emotionalism signifies a progressive deterioration of mental abilities. Organic brain changes include those associated with arteriosclerosis and senile dementia of the Alzheimer's disease type.

Caring For Residents with Dementia

You will care for many residents with dementia in the long-term care facility. **Dementia** is a disorder of the brain that involves thinking, memory, and judgment. **Organic mental syndrome** is a general term that includes all dementias. Dementia is not a disease in itself but is a group of symptoms seen in a number of different diseases. **Alzheimer's disease** is the most common form of dementia. Other types of dementias are related to cardiovascular disease, Parkinson's disease, and Huntington's disease. The term dementia is used here when referring to symptoms, behavior, and nursing actions that are appropriate for people with any dementia. Alzheimer's is used when the information is specific to that dementia.

Alzheimer's Disease

Alzheimer's disease can begin during middle age but is more common in older persons. The disease affects people of all races, levels of intelligence, education, and financial status. It is progressive and cannot be cured. It has been called a "slow death of the mind." In the past the term senility was used to describe these symptoms. We know now that it is a

PROCEDURE 104 **OBRA**

SIDE 9

CARE OF EYEGLASSES

1. Carry out each beginning procedure action.
2. Remember to wash your hands, identify the patient, and provide privacy.
3. Assemble equipment needed:
   ■ Resident's eyeglasses
   ■ Cleaning solution
   ■ Clear water
   ■ Soft cleaning tissues
4. Explain what you plan to do and how the resident can help.

5. Handle glasses only by the frame.
6. Clean with cleaning solution or clear water.
7. Dry with tissues.
8. Return eyeglasses to case. Place on bedside stand or return to resident.
9. Carry out each procedure completion action. Remember to wash your hands, report completion of task, and document time, date, cleaning eyeglasses, and resident reaction.

PROCEDURE 105

CARE OF RESIDENT WITH AN ARTIFICIAL EYE

1. Carry out each beginning procedure action.
2. Remember to wash your hands, identify the resident, and provide privacy.
3. Assemble equipment needed:
   - Eyecup lined with gauze
   - Cotton balls
   - Washcloth
   - Lukewarm water
   - Cleansing solution, if ordered
4. Assist resident into bed and draw curtains.
5. Have resident close the eyes and turn head to the side of the prosthesis.
6. Wash outside eye with warm water, using one cotton ball at a time. Stroke once only with each cotton ball from medial eye to outer eye.
7. Remove eye by depressing lower eyelid with your thumb while lifting upper lid with your finger.
   - Take eye in your hand.
   - Place in eyecup.
   - Place eyecup and prosthesis in center of over-bed stand or bedside stand.
8. Clean eye socket using warm water and cotton balls. Dry area around eye gently.

9. Carry eyecup to bathroom.
   - Clean sink.
   - Half fill sink with lukewarm water.
   - Place folded washcloth in bottom of sink as added precaution against breakage.
   - Remove eye from eyecup and place in water in sink.
   - Remove all secretions from the prosthesis.
   - Use no abrasives or general solvents.
10. Empty water from eyecup.
   - Place a fresh gauze square on the bottom of the eyecup.
   - Place the wet eye on the gauze.
   - Add water if eye is to be stored in the drawer of the bedside stand.
11. Wash your hands and return to the bedside to reinsert the eye.
12. Depress lower lid and slip over prosthesis.
13. Carry out each procedure completion action. Remember to wash your hands, report completion of task, and document time, date, prosthetic eye cleaned and reinserted/stored, type of solution used, and resident reaction.

---

disease of the brain cells and is not normal aging. The cause of Alzheimer's is unknown. There is no diagnostic test. When symptoms appear, the person should have a medical workup to rule out other diseases. Nutritional problems, depression, medications, and metabolic diseases are conditions with similar symptoms. These conditions can be reversed with treatment.

Changes occur in both the structure and function of the brain. The brain shrinks and becomes smaller. If an autopsy of the brain is performed after death, changes are noted in the brain cells. These changes are called neuritic plaques and neurofibrillary tangles.

Individuals with Alzheimer's often live as long as twenty years after the onset of the disease. Their bodies can be surprisingly healthy. Families and friends have difficulty believing that the person is ill. There is much that is unknown about this disease.

Care givers can increase the quality of life for those who have the illness.

The disease generally has three stages with symptoms becoming progressively worse. The best learned skills tend to remain the longest. An English teacher, for example, may maintain verbal skills longer than usual. However, once a skill is lost, it is lost forever.

Stage I: Mild Dementia. During the first stage, most people remain at home if they have a supportive family to provide assistance. They are usually physically capable and can attend to the activities of daily living with supervision.

Characteristics of Stage I include:
- Short-term memory loss
- Personality changes with loss of spontaneity and indifference
- Decreased ability to concentrate and shortened attention span

- Disorientation to time and space
- Poor judgment
- Carelessness in actions and appearance
- Anxiety, depression, and agitation
- Delusions of persecution—the person thinks that others are conspiring to do harm

Stage II: Moderate Dementia. Symptoms of this stage are:

- Increased short-term memory loss and deterioration of memory for remote events
- Complete disorientation
- Wandering and pacing
- Sundowning. Sundowning is confusion and restlessness that occur during the late afternoon, evening, or night.
- Sensory/perceptual changes. The person is unable to recognize and use common objects, such as eating utensils, combs, and pencils. Also, the person is unable to distinguish between right and left, up and down, hot and cold.
- Perseveration phenomena. This refers to repeating an action. Examples are repeating the same word or phrase, lip licking, chewing, or fingertapping.
- Problems with walking
- Problems with speech, reading, writing
- Good eating habits continue
- Incontinent of bowel and bladder
- Catastrophic reactions, hallucinations, delusions. Catastrophic reaction is the action of a person with dementia to overwhelming stimuli.

Most people with Alzheimer's are admitted to nursing homes during the second stage. Although they may still be healthy physically, they require constant care, Figure 29–27. Most families do not have the emotional resources and physical energy to cope. Admission to the nursing home is traumatic to families. Families are vital members of the interdisciplinary team. They can provide staff with valuable information about the resident and how to deal with the problems.

Stage III: Severe Dementia. The person in Stage III:

- Is totally dependent
- Is verbally unresponsive
- May have seizures

Working with residents with Alzheimer's disease or any dementia is challenging, rewarding, and gratifying. Care givers must be compassionate, patient, calm, and have a sense of humor.

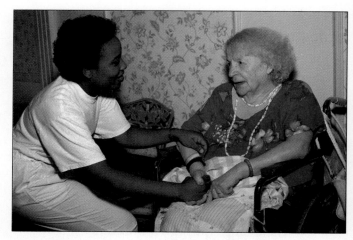

FIGURE 29–27. In stage II of Alzheimer's dementia, the resident has severe memory and concentration loss.

When you are caring for residents with dementia, remember to:

- Protect residents from physical injury.
- Allow residents to maintain independence as long as possible.
- Provide physical and mental activities within residents' abilities.
- Support residents' dignity and self-esteem.

To meet these goals, the care must be:

- Consistent.
- Provided with a structured but flexible routine.
- Given in a peaceful, quiet environment that is simple, uncluttered, and unchanged.

It is helpful to:

- Use eye contact with the residents.
- Use appropriate body language. Residents with dementia can "read" the staff. Therefore, residents' behavior will reflect the mood of the staff.
- Be able to "tune" into and accept residents without being judgmental or critical.
- Use touch appropriately. This can be soothing. But if a resident is surprised by the body contact, it can result in a catastrophic reaction.
- Avoid using logic, "reasoning," or lengthy explanations.
- Remember when the ability to use speech is lost, communication occurs through nonverbal means.
  — Biting, scratching, and kicking may be the only way the resident can express displeasure.
  — Watch for facial expressions and body language for clues to feelings and moods.

- — Learn what triggers agitation or anger. Work on preventing those situations.
- ■ Use techniques of diversion and distraction. For example, calmly take the resident by the hand and walk together or direct the resident's attention to another activity. These techniques work well because of the shortened attention span.
- ■ Realize people with dementia are not responsible for what they do or say.
  - — Their behavior is not intentional, and they cannot change.
  - — They are not aware of what they are doing.
  - — They lose the ability to control their impulses.
  - — Avoid confrontations and always allow them to "save face."
  - — No one really knows what is happening in the minds of people with dementia.

Guidelines for Activities of Daily Living

- ■ Allow the resident to do as much as possible.
  - — Use hand-over-hand technique for personal care and eating. The hand-over-hand technique means that the resident's hand is placed around an object, such as a glass. The care giver then places a hand over the resident's hand and guides the object to the resident's mouth.
  - — Give only one short, simple direction at a time.
- ■ Observe the resident's physical condition. People with dementia are usually unaware of signs of illness.
- ■ Assist residents to maintain a dignified, attractive appearance by helping them with grooming and dressing.
- ■ Monitor food and fluid intake.
  - — Too many foods at once are confusing.
  - — Place one food at a time in front of the resident.
  - — Do not use plastic utensils that can break in the resident's mouth.
  - — Provide nutritious finger foods when the resident is unable to use utensils.
  - — Avoid pureed foods as long as possible.
  - — Check food temperatures.
  - — Prepare foods for eating by buttering the bread, cutting meat, and opening cartons.
  - — Check the resident's mouth after eating for food. Squirreling food can cause aspiration.

- — Weigh residents regularly to detect patterns of weight gain or loss.
- — The dining area should be quiet and calm.
- ■ Persons with dementia eventually lose bowel and bladder continence. Taking residents to the bathroom every 2 hours keeps residents dry and prevents skin breakdown.
- ■ Residents with dementia need activities geared to their abilities.
  - — Avoid large groups or competitive activities.
  - — In later stages, use sensory stimulation with quiet music, soft touching, and calm talk.
  - — Holding puppies or kittens (pet therapy) brings pleasure to severely impaired residents.
- ■ Daily exercise needs to be planned according to residents' habits and abilities.
  - — The resident who wanders throughout the day may only need range of motion exercises.

Special Problems

Wandering and Pacing. Persons with Alzheimer's may wander or pace for hours at a time. No one knows why this occurs. Some reasons may be:

- ■ They are looking for companionship, security, or loved ones.
- ■ It is a way to handle stress.
- ■ They realize they are in a strange environment and are looking for home.

When this behavior occurs:

- ■ Allow them to wander. Using restraints only serves to increase their anxiety and frustration, resulting in other problems.
- ■ Adapt the environment to the residents, making it safe and secure. The problem may be getting lost rather than falling. When the resident walks off, walk with the resident, gradually returning to the direction of the nursing home.
- ■ Watch wandering residents for signs of fatigue. They may have forgotten how to sit down and will need reminders and demonstrations on how to get into the chair or bed.
- ■ Many companies now manufacture Alzheimer's chairs. These allow residents to rock without tipping over. A tray table top keeps residents secure and can be used for hand activities.
- ■ Nutritional needs increase with wandering so additional food intake may be necessary.

Agitation, Anxiety, and Catastrophic Reactions. Agitation and anxiety are noted by an increase in physical activity, such as pacing, or the perseveration behaviors described for Stage II. If appropriate interventions are not implemented in time, a catastrophic reaction will likely occur. This is noted by any or all of the following.

- Increased physical activity.
- Increased talking or mumbling.
- Explosive behavior with physical violence.

To avoid catastrophic reactions:

- Monitor behavior closely.
- Watch for signs of increasing agitation.
- Check to see if the resident:
  — Is hungry
  — Needs to go to the bathroom
  — Is too hot or too cold
  — Is overtired or in pain
  — Has signs of physical illness
- Check the environment for:
  — Too much noise
  — Too many people
  — Staff anxiety
  — Television programs. People with dementia cannot distinguish fiction from reality.
- People with dementia cannot make decisions. For example, the question "What do you want to wear today?" may be more than they can handle.

When agitation or catastrophic reactions occur:

- Do not use physical restraints or force in any attempt to subdue the resident. This increases agitation and can result in injury to the resident or staff.
- Avoid having several staff persons approach the resident at the same time. This is frightening to the resident.
- Use a soft, calm voice. Do not try to reason with the resident. Using touch may or may not be appropriate. Some residents respond to smooth stroking of the arms or back. Others may react violently if they are already agitated.

Sundowning. As previously mentioned, sundowning means the resident has increased confusion and restlessness during the late afternoon, evening, or night. It is sometimes prevented by avoiding too much activity before bedtime and by establishing a consistent bedtime routine.

- Overfatigue can cause sundowning. Encourage the resident to nap or rest in the early afternoon.

- Try to prevent the resident from sleeping too much during the day.
- The evening meal should be eaten at least 2 hours before bedtime. Eliminate caffeine from the resident's diet.
- Involve the resident in quiet evening activities, soft music, or interactions with a care giver or family member.
- Provide a light bedtime snack that is easily chewed and digested.
- Take the resident to the bathroom. Allow sufficient time for bladder and bowel elimination.
- Give a slow back massage.
- Check with family members and continue established habits such as wearing sox to bed, using two pillows, having a night light.
- Check the lighting of the room. Shadows and reflections are disturbing.
- If the resident awakens during the night, repeat the bedtime routine. If this is ineffective and the resident does not remain in bed, try a recliner or Alzheimer's chair.

Pillaging and Hoarding. These events do not present a major problem unless residents collect items from other resident's rooms or they hide things that are difficult to find.

- Label all residents' belongings.
- If a missing item is located, note where it was found. The resident probably will choose the same hiding place the next time.
- Check the room daily for stale food.
- Keep the resident's hands busy. Activities like folding washclothes or "fiddling" with keys on a ring may help.
- Provide a "rummaging" drawer or box for the resident.

Reality Orientation

Reality orientation (R.O.) is used for helping disoriented residents remain oriented to the environment, to time, and themselves. When it is used appropriately, it decreases anxiety in the resident. R.O. is effective in the first stage and the early part of the second stage of Alzheimer's disease. In later stages it is meaningless and increases agitation.

The basic guidelines for R.O. are:

- Always treat residents as adults, with respect and dignity, no matter how confused.

- Speak clearly and directly. Avoid the temptation to speak louder when they do not understand you.
- Give simple, brief instructions and responses.
- Establish and maintain a structured routine.
- Be polite and sincere.
- Give residents adequate time to respond.
- Allow residents to be independent as long as possible.
- Set residents' watches to correct time.
- Make sure they have clean eyeglasses and effective hearing aids if they need them.
- Place large numbered calendars in rooms and cross off the days as they pass.
- There should be large numbered clocks around the facility.
- Signs with large letters and color codes on walls, floors, or equipment help residents find their way around the facility, Figure 29–28.
- Call residents by name. Disoriented residents usually respond to their first name more quickly.
- Tell residents your name—do not expect them to remember you.
- Use R.O. in conversation with the residents, for example, "It's only March 5 today but it is warm outside."

When using R.O.:
- Do not put residents on the spot. For example, do not ask "Do you remember who I am?" or "Do you know what day this is?" If you need to verify orientation, ask them "What are your plans for today?"
- Answer questions honestly but avoid confronting the residents with information they are unable to handle. If a resident whose husband is deceased asks "Is my husband coming today?", it is cruel to answer by saying "Remember, your husband died two years ago." This response will likely trigger a catastrophic reaction. It is better to answer by asking another question such as "Tell me about your husband, Emma." She will receive pleasure from reminiscing (remembering past experiences) and will probably work up to present time on her own.
- Never argue with a resident's reality. When a resident has a delusion, arguing increases the individual's anxiety and agitation. Many delusions are based on past experiences. Because the resident is disoriented, the experience seems to be happening now.

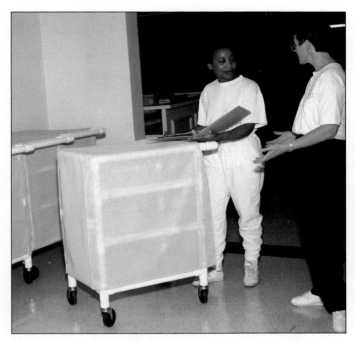

FIGURE 29–28.   Areas and equipment are color coded to help residents remain oriented to their own areas.

- Do not reinforce the resident's disorientation.
- Remember that a pleasant facial expression, relaxed body language, and a caring touch are the most important aspects of caring for confused residents.

Reminiscing

Reminiscing is a natural activity for people of all ages. We tend to reminisce when we see old friends or get together with families.
- Past experiences are remembered and enjoyed as we think of pleasant times from the past.
- As people age, the tendency to reminisce increases and is more important.
- It is an appropriate activity for residents with dementia if long-term memory is still intact.
- Reminiscing may serve as a life review. Elderly people often review the past experiences of their lives. This can bring back unpleasant memories. If these experiences are resolved, peace of mind can be found.
- Reminiscing can help people adapt to old age. It helps to maintain self-esteem. It allows them to work through personal losses.
- When we listen to residents reminisce, we understand them better.

■ Reminiscing therapy can be a group activity with a leader who is skillful and sensitive to the feelings of the members.

Validation Therapy

Validation therapy was developed by Naomi Feil. **Validation therapy** is a technique that seeks to maintain the disoriented person's dignity by acknowledging the person's memories and feelings.

It is based on these ideas:

■ Maintain the identity and dignity of the residents.

■ Help disoriented people with dementia feel good about themselves.

■ There is a reason for all behavior. What seems like confused behavior may be an acting out of memories from long ago.

■ Acknowledge feelings and memories.

■ Disoriented people have the right to express feelings when they are no longer able to be oriented to reality.

■ Living must be resolved in order to prepare for dying.

■ Sometimes, elderly persons have experienced so many losses during a lifetime that they have no coping abilities left.

■ To live in reality is not the only way to live.

■ Disoriented elderly have worth. We can give them joy by allowing them to express themselves.

■ Within each confused person is a human being who was once a child and later an adult with hopes, joys, sadness, failures, and successes. They deserve to be cared for and loved in their final years.

Death and Dying in the Long-term Care Facility

The residents you care for may live in the long-term care facility for several months or years. As you get to know them, you may develop special relationships.

Losing a friend through death is a sad experience. However, most of the residents are elderly and have significant health problems. Death is not unexpected. Death occurs in various ways. A resident may be unresponsive for a long time before dying. Some residents develop an acute illness and are unable to recover. Others quietly die in their sleep.

Most elderly people are accepting of death and may even welcome it. By the time people reach old age, they have lost much that was dear to them. However, not all people in nursing homes are old and not all of those who die are old.

Science has created the technology to extend life almost indefinitely. Many questions concerning quality of life are still unanswered. Because of the legal and ethical issues related to dying, more people are providing their families with documents called **advance directives**. These documents allow families, physicians, and nurses to follow the wishes of the individual when death occurs or is imminent (also see Unit 30). Some terms you may hear, which will also be discussed in Unit 30, are:

■ Durable Power of Attorney
   — The person who has durable power of attorney has the legal power and responsibility to make decisions or act on the behalf of another person if he/she is unable to do so for himself/herself. The person who has the durable power of attorney must be appointed by the person when that person was mentally competent.

■ Living will
   — A document that specifies exactly what a person wishes at death.
   — It generally states that no measures are to be taken to prolong life when there is little hope of recovery.
   — Living wills are legal in most states.

■ Do not resuscitate (DNR)
   — This means that in case of cardiac or respiratory arrest, the resident has directed that no cardiopulmonary resuscitation (CPR) or other lifesaving measures are to be implemented.

■ Do not hospitalize
   — There are some procedures that cannot be performed in the nursing home.
   — When residents become acutely ill, hospitalization may be necessary if lifesaving measures are to be taken.
   — Residents may choose to remain in the nursing home for supportive care.

■ Feeding restrictions
   — The resident does not wish to be fed by artificial means. This includes gastrointestinal and intravenous feedings.

■ Medication restrictions
   — The resident refuses life-sustaining medications such as chemotherapy or antibiotics.

- Other treatment restrictions
  — Blood transfusions, surgery, tracheostomy, or intubation for ventilation.
- Supportive care is not given to extend life or prolong dying but is given solely to make the last days of life as comfortable as possible. Supportive care includes:
  — Physical care for enhancing comfort such as positioning, back rubs, oral care, sponge baths, and linen changes as needed.
  —Administering food and fluids by oral means if the resident can swallow and wishes to take them.

  — Preventing and relieving pain and other physical discomforts such as nausea or shortness of breath.
  — Providing emotional support. A kind touch and listening can be very reassuring. While many residents do not fear death, they may be fearful of dying. They need to know that staff are there to help.

Residents may also have documents for organ donation, for donation of their body for medical research, or for autopsy.

You will feel sad when residents die, but you can take comfort in knowing that you made the resident comfortable.

SUMMARY

The person being cared for in the long-term health care facility is:

- Usually a mature adult
- Often elderly
- Frequently afflicted with chronic and/or debilitating conditions

Adult life spans a period of 50 years or more and is divided into:

- Early adulthood   20–40 years
- Middle adulthood   40–65 years
- Late adulthood   65–75 years
- Old age   75 years and over

Basic care will be provided using the same techniques employed in the acute setting. Adaptations will need to be made because of the greater dependency of this group of residents. Physical changes occur in each body system as the aging process progresses.

It is important for the nursing assistant to bear in mind that each person is a unique individual and must be treated with respect and dignity.

Adjustments to the aging process must be made on a physical and emotional level. The nursing assistant can be a valuable source of caring and support. Special care needs have to be met in the following areas:

- Promoting residents' rights
- Caring for personal hygiene
- Meeting dietary requirements
- Ensuring adequate exercise
- Caring for elimination
- Providing recreational needs
- Supporting emotional adjustments
- Orienting to reality
- Providing a safe environment
- Providing opportunities for social interactions
- Preventing infections

UNIT REVIEW

A. True/False. Answer the following statements true or false by circling T or F.

T F 1. Older people have the same emotional needs for good mental health as young people.

T F 2. Frustration is a common emotion experienced by the elderly.

T F 3. As people age, they become less interested in sexuality.

T F 4. Elderly people may not be aware of their need for fluids.

T F 5. Infections are not a major cause of concern in nursing homes.

T F   6. The resident's mouth should be carefully inspected and cleaned each time the dentures are cleaned.

T F   7. One of the best approaches when working with persons with dementia is to reason with them and use logic.

T F   8. Calories should be generally increased in the diet of the elderly.

T F   9. Elderly persons are generally fearful of death.

T F   10. Daily tub baths or showers are not usually necessary or recommended for elderly residents.

B. Matching. Match Column I with Column II.

Column I
_____ 11. nocturia
_____ 12. atrophy
_____ 13. reminiscing
_____ 14. debilitating
_____ 15. advocate

Column II
a. weakening
b. remembering past experiences
c. a person who supports the rights of others
d. getting up at night to urinate
e. wasting away of muscle tissue

C. Multiple Choice. Select the one best answer.

16. Characteristics of the nursing assistant that are especially important while caring for older adults include
    a. patience.
    b. kindness.
    c. sense of humor.
    d. All of the above

17. Characteristics of the elderly include
    a. increased vitality.
    b. decreased night sleep.
    c. increased appetite.
    d. increased mobility and agility.

18. Which of the following nutrients should be increased in the diet of elderly persons?
    a. Fats
    b. Vegetables, fruits and whole grains
    c. Calories
    d. Sugar

19. Restorative care emphasizes
    a. returning the individual to normal function.
    b. the limitations of the individual.
    c. the abilities and strengths of the individual.
    d. rest and inactivity.

20. Which statement is true in regard to catastrophic reactions?
    a. They are unavoidable in persons with dementia.
    b. They may be precipitated by too much sensory stimulation.
    c. Providing activity will subdue the catastrophic reaction.
    d. They are always expressions of violence.

Death and Dying

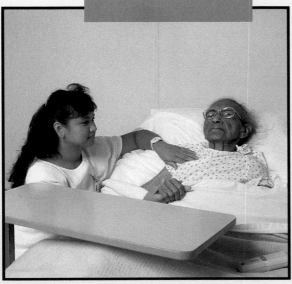

OBJECTIVES

As a result of this unit, you will be able to:

■ Spell and define terms.

■ Describe how different people handle the death/dying process.

■ Describe the signs of approaching death.

■ Describe the spiritual preparations for death practiced in the various religious denominations.

■ Demonstrate the procedure for postmortem care.

■ Describe the hospice philosophy and method of care.

VOCABULARY

Learn the meaning and the correct spelling of the following words and phrases:

acceptance	harvested
advance directive	hospice care
anger	living will
bargaining	morbid
critical list	no-code order
denial	postmortem
depression	postmortem care
directive	rigor mortis
DNR	Sacrament of the Sick
durable power of attorney	terminal

Death is the final stage of life. It may come suddenly, without warning, or it may follow a long period of illness. It sometimes strikes the young but it always awaits the old. As a nursing assistant, you will be providing care throughout the dying period and into the after-death period (postmortem). Accepting the idea that death is the natural result of the life process may help you respond to your patient's needs more generously.

The concept of death and dying is handled differently by different people, Figure 30–1. There are many reactions to the diagnosis of a terminal (life-ending) illness:

■ Some patients may have had time to prepare psychologically for their deaths. They may accept or be resigned to the inevitable.

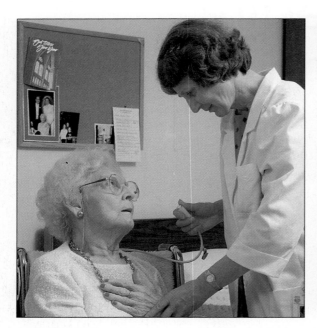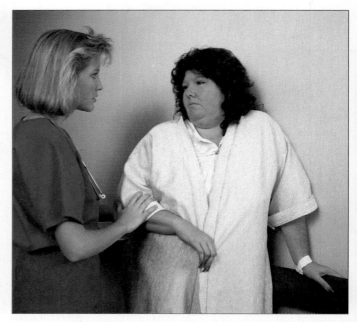

FIGURE 30–1. Reactions to a terminal diagnosis vary. Some people try to verbalize their feelings while others are reluctant to talk.

- Some may actually look forward to relief from the pain and emotional burden of a long illness and await death calmly.
- Some may be fearful or angry and demonstrate moods that swing from outright denial to depression.
- Others may reach out, trying to verbalize feelings and thoughts of an uncertain future.
- In others, despair and anxiety may give way to moments of active hostility or periods of searching, groping questions.

None of the reaction states are predictable, falling into one rigid pattern or another. You must accept the patient's behavior with understanding, interpret the patient's very real need for family support, and support the family in meeting their own needs during this adjustment period.

Five Stages of Grief

Dr. Elisabeth Kubler-Ross has identified five stages of grief that can occur in the dying patient. They are denial, anger, bargaining, depression, and acceptance, Figure 30–2. If there is adequate time and support, some patients may be able to move psychologically through each stage to a point of acceptance of their illness and death.

- **Denial** begins when the person is made aware that he is going to die. He may not accept this

information as truth, and may instead deny it. Making long-range plans that are not likely to be fulfilled may indicate that the patient is in the denial stage.
- **Anger** comes when the patient is no longer able to deny the fact that she is going to die. The patient may blame those around her, including those who are giving care, for her illness. Added stresses, however small, are likely to upset the patient who is in the anger stage, Figure 30–3. Statements such as, "It's all your fault. I should never have come to this hospital," are typical of a patient in the anger stage.
- **Bargaining** is the stage in the grief process in which the patient attempts to bargain for more time to live. He may ask to be allowed to go home to finish a task before he dies, or he may make private "deals" with God. "If you will let me live another two months, I promise I will try to be a better person." The patient in this stage is basically saying, "I know I'm going to die and I'm ready to die, but not just yet." This may be done in private and not stated verbally.
- **Depression** is the fourth stage identified in the grief process. During this stage, the patient comes to a full realization that she will die soon, Figure 30–4. She is saddened by the thought that she will no longer be with family and friends, and by the fact that she may not have accomplished some goals that she had set for

Stages of Grief	Response of the Nursing Assistant
Denial	Reflect patient's statements, but try not to confirm or deny the fact that the patient is dying. *Example:* "The lab tests can't be right—I don't have cancer." "It must have been difficult for you to learn the results of your tests."
Anger	Understand the source of the patient's anger. Provide understanding and support. Listen. Try to meet reasonable needs and demands quickly. *Example:* "This food is terrible—not fit to eat." "Let me see if I can find something that would appeal to you more."
Bargaining	If it is possible to meet the patient's requests, do so. Listen attentively. *Example:* "If only God will spare me this, I'll go to church every week." "Would you like a visit from your clergy person?"
Depression	Avoid cliches that dismiss the patient's depression ("It could be worse—you could be in more pain"). Be caring and supporting. Let the patient know that it is okay to be depressed. *Example:* "There just isn't any sense in going on." "I understand you are feeling very depressed."
Acceptance	Do not assume that, because the patient has accepted death, she/he is unafraid, or that she/he doesn't need emotional support. Listen attentively and be supportive and caring. *Example:* "I feel so alone." "I am here with you. Would you like to talk?"

FIGURE 30–2. The patient may exhibit various emotional responses to dying. The nursing assistant should be caring and supportive of the patient who is sorting out feelings.

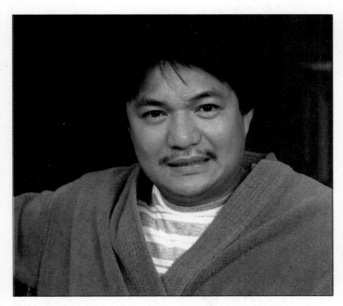

FIGURE 30–3. This patient is demonstrating feelings of frustration and anger.

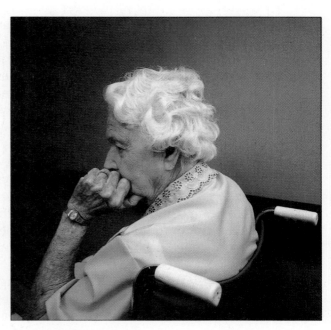

FIGURE 30–4. Depression is associated with the grieving process.

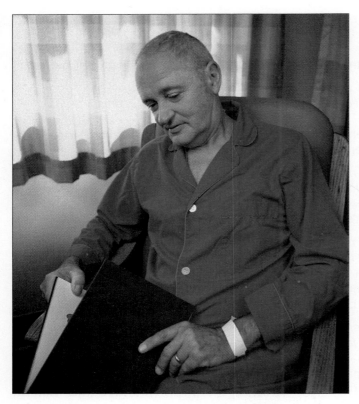

FIGURE 30–5. Do not assume that because the patient seems to be in the stage of acceptance he is unafraid.

herself. She may also express regrets about not having gone somewhere or done something. "I always promised my husband that we would go to Europe and now we'll never go."

■ Acceptance is the stage during which a patient understands and accepts the fact that he is going to die, Figure 30–5. During this stage, he may strive to complete unfinished business. Having accepted his eventual death, he may also try to help those around him to deal with it, especially family members.

Not all patients progress through these stages in sequential order. Nor does movement from one level to the next mean that the previous level will no longer be experienced. The staff must be aware of the possible psychological positions and be able to identify the patient's current reactions. For example, a patient who displays anger one day may be full of optimism and denial the next.

Denial frequently comes first, followed by anger and despair. Frustrated by feelings of helplessness, the person lashes out at those who are nearby. If each of these stages is expressed with some degree of success, the person is then able to move on to a level

of grieving, for one's self and for loved ones. When all five stages have been passed, it is believed that the patient is better able to accept the termination of life. If there is adequate time and support, Figure 30–6, many patients can be helped to reach a more accepting frame of mind.

The family and staff move through the same stages but not necessarily at the same time. It is particularly difficult when the patient is in one stage and the family is at another stage.

Preparation for Death

The knowledge of impending death comes to the patient directly from the physician or indirectly from the staff. A diagnosis of terminal illness is very difficult to conceal from the patient.

The staff, may, without realizing it, reveal the information by:

■ Exhibiting false cheerfulness
■ Being evasive
■ Making fewer visits to the patient's room
■ Spending less time with the patient

You must realize that most terminally ill patients do eventually come to realize and accept that death is part of their near future. Keep the following in mind:

■ Each patient reacts to this realization in a unique way.

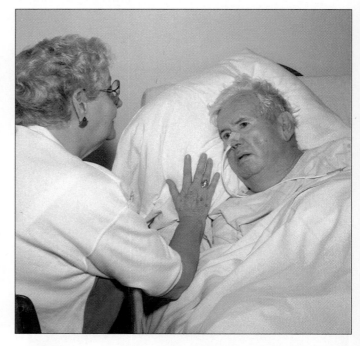

FIGURE 30–6. The support of family and friends is vital during the dying period. Liberal visiting hours are arranged.

- How many feelings the patient wishes to share and with whom are very personal decisions.
- You should be available to listen, but do not force the issue.

Upon being told of the terminal diagnosis, the patient may proceed through several stages of emotional adjustment. Initially, the:

- Patient may react to the situation by denying the truth.
- Patient may refuse all opportunities to discuss his illness with the staff or with family.
- Patient's interpersonal relationships with family and staff may become greatly strained.
- Patient may become defeated and full of despair, actively expressing a loss of hope.

Do-not-resuscitate (DNR) or No-code Order

Sometimes a no-code order or DNR (do-not-resuscitate) order is written. This means that no extraordinary means such as CPR to resuscitate the person will be used to prevent death. This allows a person to die peacefully with maximum dignity.

A no-code decision is reached after discussions by the patient, physician, and family. This is not a decision that is made by the staff. Once made, the no-code decision is entered in the patient's record. All staff members are made aware of the decision but it is kept confidential.

The nursing assistant must know which patients have DNR or no-code orders on their charts. The nursing assistant is expected to provide the same level of care for all patients, regardless of the presence or lack of a no-code order on the chart. If the nursing assistant finds it difficult to accept a no-code order, the concerns should be discussed with the supervisor. Remember that a no-code order is the patient's decision.

Many people do not want their lives to be prolonged by the use of machines. These people need to let others know of their wishes. They may put their intent in writing. Two ways in which a person can be sure their wishes are made known are the living will and the directive. The living will and the directive are not uniform legal documents throughout the United States. The requirements for each state may be different, and the procedures for making a living will and directive may also vary.

The Advance Directive

An advance directive is a document signed before the diagnosis of a terminal illness when the individual is still in good health. The physician need only consider the advance directive when circumstances change and decisions must be made with regard to patient care.

The Patient Self-Determination Act of 1990 (effective for services provided on or after December 1, 1991) requires health care providers to supply written information about state laws regarding living wills and other advance directives to patients. Health care providers must also have policies and procedures relating to these issues.

This information must be provided at the time of admission since the facility must institute life-support systems if the need arises in the absence of a clear statement of the person's wishes.

Durable Power of Attorney

At times people may feel that they will not be able to handle their own affairs or make personal decisions. In such a case, the person will sign a durable power of attorney. This is an example of an advance directive. In effect, this makes someone else responsible for handling the person's affairs and making legal and medical decisions for the person. It is to be signed by the agent (the person given the durable power of attorney) and by the principal (the person appointing the agent). It is also to be signed by an adult witness.

The durable power of attorney may or may not specifically include the authority to withhold or withdraw life-support systems. The exact authority varies from state to state. The durable power of attorney is one way to ensure that the wishes and rights of the individual will be followed and protected when the person is no longer able to make personal decisions. At other times, the court may appoint a conservator if a person has already reached a point where he/she is no longer able to make decisions or conduct personal affairs.

The Living Will

A living will is an advance directive and is a request by a person that life-sustaining procedures not be used in case of incurable injury or illness. The living will is signed before the person becomes ill and must be witnessed by two other individuals who do not stand to benefit because of the person's death. The living will must be reviewed and initialed annually.

The Role of the Nursing Assistant

As a nursing assistant, you spend much time with the patient. You have a unique opportunity to be a source of strength and comfort. You must behave in a way that instills confidence in both the patient and family. Developing the proper attitude and approach for this type of situation is not easy. It will come with experience. There are some things to keep in mind:

- Your response should be consistent. It should be guided by the patient's attitude and the care plan.
- You must be open and receptive since the terminal person's attitude may change from day to day.
- Make sure you inform the nurse of incidents related to the patient that reflect moods and needs.
- Remember, each person's idea of death and the hereafter differs. You must be open to the patient's ideas and not force your own.
- Your own feelings about death and dying influence your ability to care for the dying patient. Honestly explore your feelings by talking about them with others until you can resolve any conflicts you may have. Your acceptance of death as a natural occurrence will enable you to meet patient needs in a realistic manner.
- Give your best and most careful nursing care with special attention to comfort measures such as mouth care and fluid intake.
- You should be quietly empathetic and carry out your duties in a calm, efficient way.

When a patient's condition is critical, the physician will place his name officially on the critical list. Then the family and the chaplain will be notified.

Providing for Spiritual Needs

Many people find spiritual faith to be a source of great comfort during difficult times.

- Some religions have specific rituals that are carried out during these times. Your role is to cooperate with the patient, family, and clergyperson so that these rituals may be performed in a dignified, caring manner.
- Other religions do not have specific practices but may spend time in prayer. Allow the patient and family privacy but let them know you are close by if you are needed.
- Some patients may have no formal religious affiliation. This does not mean they do not have spiritual needs. They may request the services of a clergyperson and may not know who to call on. Relay this request to the nurse because most health care facilities will have chaplains to provide the services.
- It may be that some patients are nonbelievers in any higher spiritual being. This is their right and no one should try to change their feelings.
- Always respect the beliefs or nonbeliefs of any patient. Treat all religious items such as Bibles, medals, and rosaries with respect.
- When a Catholic patient is ill, a priest may be called for the Sacrament of the Sick, Figure 30–7. It is preferable that the family be present and leave the room only while the confession is heard. The practicing Catholic and her family consider it a privilege to have the opportunity for confession. Many patients recover completely, but this hope should not prevent the reception of this sacrament, if this is the patient's wish.
- A Bible or spiritual reading of the patient's faith, if requested, may be of some spiritual help through this crisis. Be courteous and provide privacy when the patient's clergy person visits.

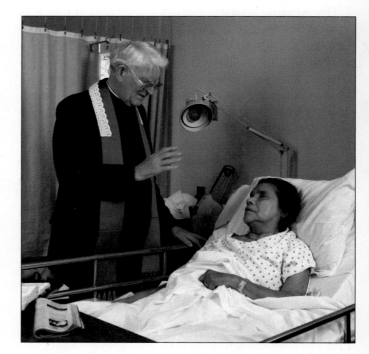

FIGURE 30–7. The Sacrament of the Sick is administered to gravely ill Roman Catholic patients.

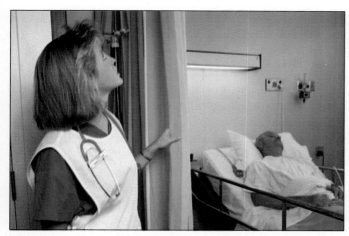

FIGURE 30–8. Provide privacy but not isolation during the dying period.

Be aware that dying is a lonely business, a journey each person must complete alone. Until the final moment comes, privacy, but not total solitude, should be the guiding rule, Figure 30–8.

It is important to remember the family and other loved ones when a patient is dying. Check the policies of your health care facility and assist in the following actions:

- Allow the family to be with the patient as they desire.
- Allow the family to assist with some of the care, if they wish to do so; for example, moistening the patient's lips or giving a backrub.
- Inform the family where they can get a cup of coffee or a meal.
- Show the family where they can use a telephone in private.
- If a family member stays during the night, offer a pillow and blanket. Some facilities provide recliners or cots for family members.
- Avoid being judgmental of family members. Remember that each person grieves in his or her own way. The emotions that others see are not necessarily an accurate indication of what the individual is feeling.

Hospice Care

Hospice care has evolved around the philosophy that death is a natural process that should neither be hastened nor delayed and that the person should be kept comfortable. Hospice care is:

- Provided to terminally ill people with a life expectancy of six months or less.
- Involved with direct physical care when needed.
- Supportive to both the family and patient.
- Provided in special hospice facilities, in other care facilities, and at home.
- Largely carried out by a home health assistant or a nursing assistant under the direction of professional health care providers.
- Follow-up bereavement counseling to help survivors accept the death of a loved one.
- A program in which volunteers play an important role, making regular personal visits to the patient and family.

Hospice care is provided by teams who work in conjunction with the terminally ill person and his family. The team usually consists of a physician, professional nurse, nursing assistant, and other professionals such as social workers and clergy as needed and desired.

The goals of hospice care include:

- Control of pain so the individual can remain an active participant in life until death
- Coordinating psychological, spiritual, and social support services for the patient and the family
- Making legal and financial counseling available to the patient and family

Since hospice care is a philosophy, it becomes part of the guide for your actions when caring for the terminally ill. This care will be provided as you give your usual care. Some things to keep in mind, however, are:

- Report pain immediately and give close attention to comfort measures.
- Encourage the person to carry out as much self-care as possible.
- Be readily available to listen. Spend as much time with the patient as possible and desired by the patient.
- Get to know the family and be supportive to them.
- Give the same care you would if a terminal diagnosis had not been made.
- Carry out all activities with dignity and respect.

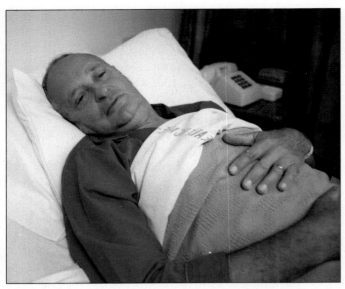

FIGURE 30–9. As death approaches, the patient becomes less responsive and bodily functions slow down.

Physical Changes as Death Approaches

As death approaches, there are notable physical changes. As changes occur, report them immediately to the charge nurse.

- The patient becomes less responsive, Figure 30–9.
- Body functions slow down.
- The patient loses general voluntary and involuntary muscle control.
- The patient may involuntarily void and defecate.
- The jaw tends to drop.
- Breathing becomes irregular and shallow.
- Circulation slows and the extremities become cold. The pulse becomes rapid and progressively weaker.
- Skin pales.
- The eyes stare and do not respond to light.
- Hearing seems to be the last sense to be lost. Do not assume that because death is approaching, the patient can no longer hear. You must be careful in what you say.

In the period before death, the patient with a terminal diagnosis needs and receives the same care as the patient who is expected to recover. Attention is paid to physical as well as emotional needs.

As it becomes clear that death will occur very soon,

you should call the nurse who will supervise the care during the final moments of life.

No-code Order

If a no-code order has been placed in the patient's record, it means that measures to maintain heart and lung activity are not to be started. Rather, the patient who has no cardiac and respiratory function is allowed to die with dignity. The no-code order is usually indicated as a DNR (do-not-resuscitate) order.

It is often difficult to carry out a no-code order when you have come to know and love the person. However, try to remember that life needs quality as well as quantity. The quality of life on mechanical support is limited. Also recognize that the no-code order reflects the patient's wishes or the wishes of those legally acting on his/her behalf.

When death has occurred:
- Do not begin postmortem care until specifically instructed to do so.
- Under no circumstances should you inform the family. This is the responsibility of the physician or the head nurse.

Moribund (Dying) Signs

After death, changes continue to take place in the body. These changes are called **moribund** (dying) changes.
- Pupils become permanently dilated.
- Heat is gradually lost from the body.
- The patient may urinate, defecate, or release flatus.
- Blood pools in dependent areas giving a purplish discoloration to those areas.
- Within 6–8 hours, body rigidity, called **rigor mortis**, develops.
- Unless embalmed within 24 hours, there is indication of progressive protein breakdown.

Postmortem Care

The patient's body should be treated with respect at all times. Before death occurs, the limbs should be straightened and the head elevated on a pillow. The body should be cleaned by gently washing it with warm water. Discharges must be washed off and wiped away.

Care of the body after death is called **postmortem care**, Figure 30–10. This may be your responsibility You may find it easier if you ask a coworker to assist.

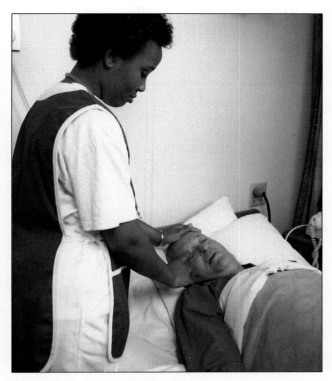

FIGURE 30–10. After death has occurred, close the person's eyes and give postmortem care.

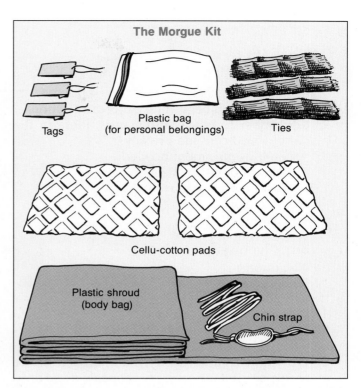

FIGURE 30–11. Supplies needed for postmortem care

■ Use gloves when giving postmortem care. The body may continue to be infectious following death.

■ Treat the body with the same dignity you would a living person.

■ Some facilities prefer to have the patient left alone until the mortuary people arrive. Your responsibility will be only to prepare the body for viewing by the family.

■ Check the hospital procedure manual before proceeding with postmortem care.

The contents of morgue kits vary, Figure 30–11, but they usually include:

■ A shroud of some kind, paper or cloth
■ A clean gown
■ Two or three tags used to identify the body
■ Gauze squares for padding
■ Safety pins

One procedure for postmortem care is described.

Organ Donations

Some people desire to share their organs with others after death. They use an organ donor card that is part of their driver's license. The card specifies if particular organs or the whole body is being donated. At times, because of a special need, the patient's family will be asked for permission so that certain body organs may be removed and saved or removed and **harvested** (reused). Such a request will be made by the physician or the nurse, never by the nursing assistant.

If the patient or family make their wishes known to you without your asking, it is important to report this to the nurse.

Postmortem Examination

In certain situations, the law requires a medical postmortem examination of the body. At other times, the family and physician may desire such an examination to understand the reasons for the patient's death. It is possible that information learned from the examination can be used to protect other family members. As in the case of organ donations, however, requesting family permission is not part of the nursing assistant's responsibilities. The nursing assistant is responsible for being supportive of the family and the decision that has been made.

PROCEDURE 106 | OBRA

GIVING POSTMORTEM CARE

1. Carry out each beginning procedure action.
2. Remember to wash your hands, identify the patient, and provide privacy.
3. Assemble equipment needed:
   - Shroud or clean sheet
   - Basin with warm water
   - Washcloth
   - Towels
   - Disposable gloves
   - Identification cards (3)
   - Cotton
   - Bandages
   - Pads as needed
4. Put on disposable gloves.
5. Remove all appliances, tubing, and used articles, if instructed to do so.
6. Work quickly and quietly; maintain an attitude of respect. If it is necessary to speak, do so only in relation to the procedure.
7. Place the body on the back, head and shoulders elevated on a pillow.
   - Close the eyes by grasping the eyelashes. Place a moistened cotton ball on each eye if the lids do not remain shut.
   - Replace dentures in the patient's mouth. Also replace artificial eye.
   - The jaw may need to be secured with light bandaging.
   - Pad beneath the bandage. Tight bandaging or undue pressure from the hands may leave marks so handle the body gently.
8. Bathe as necessary. Remove any soiled dressings and replace with clean ones. Groom hair.
9. Place a disposable pad underneath the buttocks. If the family is to view the body:
   - Put a clean hospital gown on the patient.
   - Cover the body to the shoulders with a sheet.
   - Remove disposable gloves and wash hands.
   - Make sure the room is neat and tidy.
   - Adjust the lights to a subdued level.
   - Allow the family to visit in private.
10. Put the shroud on the patient after the family leaves.
11. Collect all belongings and make a list. Wrap properly and label. Valuables remain in the hospital safe until they are signed for by a relative.
12. Fill out the identification cards and fasten:
    - One on the person's right ankle or right big toe.
    - One on the patient's clothing and valuables (securely wrapped).
    - One on the compartment in the morgue.
13. Transport the body to the morgue.
    - Call elevator to the floor and keep empty.
    - Close patient corridor doors.
    - Empty corridor.
    - With assistant, place the body on a gurney.
    - Keep patient supine with a rubber head elevator under the neck.
    - Cover with a sheet.
    - Take to the morgue.
14. Wash your hands and return to unit.
15. Report completion of the task.
16. Document date, time, placement of the body in the morgue, care of belongings, and signature.

SUMMARY

- Assisting with terminal and postmortem care is a difficult but essential part of nursing assistant duties. It requires a high degree of sensitivity, understanding, and tact.
- Both the patient and the family require support during this trying period.

- Care must be taken to provide for the individual religious preferences and practices of the patient and the family.
- The procedure for postmortem care must be carried out with efficiency and respect.

UNIT REVIEW

A. True/False. Answer the following statements true or false by circling T or F.

T F   1. All people respond to a terminal diagnosis in the same way.

T F   2. Hearing is the first sense to be lost in the dying patient.

T F   3. Death is the final stage of life.

T F   4. The nursing assistant should call the physician when the patient dies.

T F   5. Sometimes the staff, without realizing it, allows the patient to learn of a terminal diagnosis through their behavior.

T F   6. The dying patient receives the same complete care that would be given to someone expected to recover.

T F   7. The hospice philosophy has pain relief as one of its goals.

T F   8. Permanent dilation of the pupils is a moribund sign.

T F   9. Hospice-type care is only possible in the acute care facility.

T F 10. The dying person needs a great deal of understanding and realistic support.

B. Matching. Match the words in Column II with the phrase or statement in Column I.

Column I	Column II
_____ 11. refusal to accept reality	a. moribund
	b. rigor mortis
_____ 12. after death	c. denial
_____ 13. covering for the body after death	d. hospice
_____ 14. stiffening of the body after death	e. postmortem
	f. shroud
_____ 15. dying	g. anger

C. Multiple Choice. Select the one best answer.

16. Organs from a dead person may
    a. be harvested without permission.
    b. be obtained on an as needed basis.
    c. be donated with permission of the family at the time of death.
    d. never be donated.

17. Post mortem examinations
    a. are never performed.
    b. may provide valuable information.
    c. are arranged by the nursing assistant.
    d. are forbidden by law.

18. As death approaches changes include
    a. slower body responses.
    b. loss of voluntary and involuntary muscle control.
    c. slowing of circulation.
    d. all of the above.

19. Moribund changes include
    a. permanent pupil constriction.
    b. increased body heat.
    c. both a and b.
    d. neither a nor b.

20. A "no code" order on a patient's chart means
    a. Start CPR immediately.
    b. Do not resuscitate.
    c. Begin post mortem care at once.
    d. Call the family if the patient seems in danger of dying.

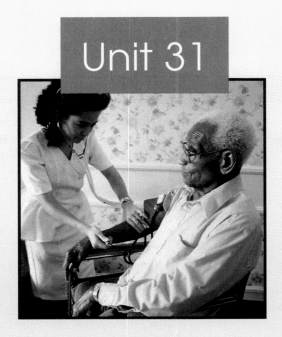

Unit 31

Nursing Assistant in Home Care

OBJECTIVES

As a result of this unit, you will be able to:

- Spell and define terms.
- List reasons why there is a trend toward more home care.
- Describe the characteristics that are especially important to the nursing assistant providing home care.
- Describe the duties of the nursing assistant working in the home setting.
- Describe the duties of the home-maker assistant.
- Carry out home care activities needed to maintain a safe and clean environment.
- Complete a time and travel report.
- Document activities for reimbursement.

VOCABULARY

Learn the meaning and the correct spelling of the following words and phrases:

client
client care records
home health assistant
home health care aide

homemaker aide
homemaker assistant
time/travel records

Trends in Health Care

The care of ill persons in their own homes is an age-old tradition. It wasn't until the middle of the twentieth century that there was a massive trend to move patient care out of the home and into the community health care facility.

The late nineteenth century saw the growth of medical schools and licensing of physicians. Schools of nursing soon followed. Hospital staffing was filled with students of these programs.

Although the permissive laws of the early 1900s gave requirements for nursing licensure, the laws did not restrict nursing practice. It wasn't until a few years later that laws to control nurse education came into being.

World War I created a tremendous demand for nurses. It resulted in increased student enrollment in hospital-based nurse training programs.

World War II brought with it a gradual increase in the:

- Need for more technical care

- Introduction of antibiotics and better techniques of infection control
- Growth of an ancillary force of workers to assist in providing nursing care
- Construction of many new health care facilities
- Hospital care of ill people

Today, the pendulum has swung back once more to treating acutely ill patients in hospitals and providing alternative care such as home care, day care, or long-term care for all others, Figure 31–1. Factors that foster this interest in home care include:

- Expensive high technology
- Introduction of diagnosis-related groups (DRGs), resulting in earlier discharge from hospitals of sicker people
- Growing population of chronically ill seniors

The duties of the home health aide include:

- Personal care and treatments
- Meal planning and preparation
- Light housekeeping

Benefits of Working in Home Health Care

You may choose to join a group that provides home health care after you have completed your training.

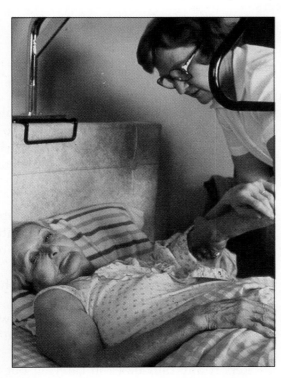

FIGURE 31–1. The trend toward home care is growing in response to increased numbers of people requiring continuing care.

There are definite advantages to working in such groups:

- Opportunities for regular employment
- Variety of nursing situations
- Part-time employment, if desired
- Satisfaction of giving complete care to one client at a time
- Opportunity to work with greater independence

The Client

The **clients** or the persons needing home care may not be as acutely ill as those you have been caring for in the hospital. They may be:

- Of various ages.
- In need of differing levels of nursing and physical care.
- Afflicted with chronic or debilitating ailments.
- Recovering from an acute illness or delivery.
- In need of assistance in carrying out the activities of daily living because of age or health status.

Home Care Provider

The nursing assistant is an important part of the health team in the acute hospital and in the long-term care facility. The nursing assistant is part of an equally important team that provides home care.

The nursing assistant may be called:

- **Home health assistant** or **home health care aide**, whose primary role is to provide assistance with nursing care.
- **Homemaker assistant** or **homemaker aide** when the primary role is to provide housekeeping chores. The homemaker assistant carries out general household tasks, prepares meals, and runs errands such as food shopping.

The nursing assistant providing health care services may be asked to carry out homemaker assistant duties in some cases.

Home Health Team

The home health team consists of the:

- Client—the person in need of care.
- Family.
  - They may act as alternate care givers.
  - They may live in the home.
  - They may or may not be supportive of the client.

■ Nursing assistant—provides for the client's safety and comfort. This care giver provides direct nursing care and is usually hired by a private agency because of past experience. The care giver is capable of working in an independent manner and is knowledgeable about disease processes and treatment. The nursing assistant has good observational skills and works with the client and the family.

■ Supervising nurse—plans the care, teaches and supervises the nursing assistant, and acts as the care coordinator.

■ Physician—writes orders and acts as a consultant and guide.

■ Other specialists as needed, such as the physical therapist, speech therapist, or nutritionist.

Source of Referral

The client may be assigned to your care through a variety of ways. You may be employed by a/an:

■ Private agency, which is paid for the services you provide.

■ Client or the family directly.

■ Health maintenance organization (HMO) of which the patient is a member.

■ Agency that receives Medicare or Medicaid reimbursement.

The Assignment Process

When a person needs home care, a referral is made to the appropriate agency. The professional nurse then makes a home visit to the client, Figure 31–2.

■ An assessment of the client's desires and needs is made.

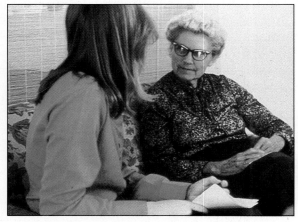

FIGURE 31–2. The professional nurse visits the home to determine the client's needs.

■ The home situation is evaluated in terms of the care to be given and safety factors to be considered.

■ A care plan is developed, Figure 31–3. It lists the goals to be achieved and the activities needed to accomplish them.

■ The amount of time of need is estimated.

The nurse discusses the plans with the client. The nurse includes the client's wishes as much as possible within the available payment plan.

The nurse then develops the assignment for the nursing assistant and/or homemaker assistant, teaching and supervising as needed.

You may be assigned to care for several clients or a particular client for a:

■ Specified number of hours daily

■ Specific period two or three days per week

■ Long-term period

■ Brief period

In some areas, the home health aide is only allowed to do certain assigned tasks when working with a third-party payer such as an insurance company or Medicare. Auditors check the tasks assigned and confirm what is actually done in the client's home.

You will need to keep appropriate records, report to the supervising nurse or physician as directed, and participate in care conferences with the other team members.

The Home Health Assistant and the Nursing Process

You are part of the nursing process. During:

■ Assessment, your observations and careful reporting can make a valuable contribution to the assembling of the objective and subjective data upon which the analysis of the client's needs is made. Make note of:

— The client's response to your care

— The interactions between family members and friends that could lead to limiting stress on the client

— Support services that may be needed

■ Planning, you contribute as you actively share in care conferences.

■ Implementation, you spend the most time with the client. You are, therefore, responsible for seeing that the plan is carried out.

— Report any difficulties in carrying out the plan.

— Work to develop ways to organize your work to make the plan more efficient.

RIVERVIEW HOME HEALTH SERVICE

8987 Walkman Ave

Parkhurst, Nebraska

Client Care Plan / Progress Notes

WT. __146__ TEMP. __98__ BP __114/80__ P __70__ R __14__ MD CONTACT __C. Boylston__

HOMEBOUND DUE TO __Spinal Cord Injury - Paraplegia.__ MEN. STATUS __Alert - Coherent__

PROBLEMS	INTERVENTIONS	TIME	PLAN	OUTCOME
① Potential altered nutrition: less than body requirements	maintain high-calorie, low-residue, high-protein diet. Reduce high calcium and gas-producing foods. Provide balanced meals morning and evening supplements		Morning Care	Tol. well
		0700	Breakfast	ate entire meal
		0815	Commode	soft formed stool
		0900	Bath, Cath Care,	
		0945	ROM	
			up in wheelchair	Tolerated well
② Potential for disuse syndrome related to effects of immobility	Exercise to tolerance, avoid fatigue. ROM. Turn and reposition q 1 hr. up in wheelchair B.I.D. Encourage self-care activities to tolerance	1030	6 z High Cal drink	
		1045	Returned to Bed	
		1130	Positioned on Rt. Side	
			Positioned on Back	
③ Alteration in bowel elimination; constipation	Stool Softener, Glycerine Suppositories, enemas, PRN. Check for BM q 3 day	1230	Lunch	½ tuna sand /tea
			up in wheelchair	
		1330	Returned to Bed	
④ Potential for infection related to indwelling Foley catheter	Routine catheter care. Change per routine schedule	1430	Positioned on left side.	
			Watching T.V.	
		1500		
⑤ Self-concept disturbance related to effects of limitations	Encourage verbalization of feelings and fears. Encourage independence. Be positive and reassuring			

DAILY SUMMARY

Diet and supplements taken fairly well. Activity tolerated. Muscles soft but some tone. Soft formed stool. Expressed frustration during transfers from bed to wheelchair. Enjoys reading and watching T.V. Seems to be gaining some confidence in transfer activities

Visit Date _____

Nursing Supervisor Report

Pt. Last Name, First Initial __Mitchell, D.__

Employee Signature __Ruthy Chek, CNA__

Joint Visit in Home _____

Conference _____

Patient's personal care and comfort measures by home aide are:

superior _____ ; good _____ ; satisfactory _____ ; need improvement _____ ;

Services provided were appropriate _____; inappropriate _____.

Comments

FIGURE 31–3. Sample client care plan/progress notes

■ Evaluation, you once more contribute to the nursing process when you share your observations about the success or lack of success of the care.

— Be accurate and concise in your reporting.

— Be honest in your appraisal of the client's progress and the point at which your services are no longer needed.

Characteristics of the Home Care Nursing Assistant and Homemaker Assistant

The home care nursing assistant and homemaker assistant must have a full measure of the characteristics you have already come to associate with a successful hospital-based assistant. There are, however, some characteristics that need to be particularly strong when an assistant works in the home.

Remember that you will be working directly with the client and her personal possessions without a supervising nurse constantly with you. This means you must demonstrate:

■ Honesty as you handle the client's possessions and shopping money. Treat the possessions with care and respect. Keep an accurate record of all money spent and receipts received.

■ Self-starter ability. This means that you must know and carry out your assigned tasks promptly and efficiently without needing someone to remind you.

■ Self-discipline so that you do not allow yourself to waste time on activities such as smoking, chatting with friends on the phone, and drinking coffee just because there isn't a supervisor to constantly check on your progress.

■ Accuracy and attention to details so that each task is performed exactly as you were taught.

■ Organization so that you plan your activities to make the best use of your in-home time. You plan your activities around the client's schedule, not your own.

■ Maturity so that judgment and assessments can be made properly.

■ Insight that gives you the ability to see the whole client as an interactive member of a family unit and community.

■ Observational skills to be able to recognize and report abnormal signs and symptoms.

■ Adaptability. Although you will need all the physical, emotional, and communication skills you learned and practiced in the clinical setting, you must be creative in adapting them to the home situation. For example, a cut plastic bag covered with a towel may be substituted for bed protectors used in the hospital. Housekeeping chores may be performed as the client rests.

■ Acceptance of clients and their home environments. Remember, your clients will be of all ethnic and religious groups and economic levels.

■ Ability to perform independently, making some decisions within the limits of your responsibilities and the scope of the assignment.

Home Health Care Duties

The duties of the home health care assistant are planned around the family routine.

These duties may include:

a. Helping with the activities of daily living

b. Special treatments such as prescribed exercises

c. Comfort measures such as positioning and special mouth care

d. Maintaining a safe environment

e. Bathing

f. Changing linen

g. Interacting with family members

Homemaker duties may include:

a. Light housekeeping

b. Shopping for meals, Figure 31–4

c. Preparing meals

You may also have to transport the client to clinic or therapy visits, Figure 31–5. You must have specific permission from your agency to perform activities

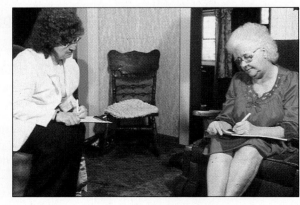

FIGURE 31–4. Sometimes, the family will make out the shopping list that you will follow.

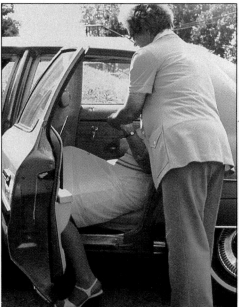

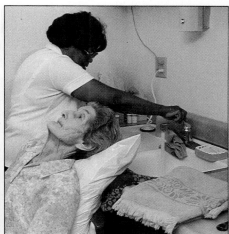

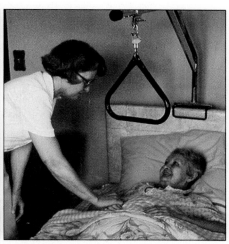

FIGURE 31–6. Procedures can be easily adapted using the client's own equipment.

FIGURE 31–7. Some equipment, such as the overhead bar, can be rented or borrowed to assist in client care.

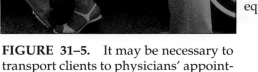

FIGURE 31–5. It may be necessary to transport clients to physicians' appointments when assigned this duty.

outside of the home. The homemaker duties *do not* include:

- Doing heavy housework such as washing windows, waxing floors, or moving heavy furniture
- Making decisions about food purchases, unless the client is unable to do so
- Becoming involved in family disputes by offering opinions or taking sides

The skills you have learned in the clinical setting can be adapted to the home environment, Figure 31–6. For example:

- Ice bags can be replaced by plastic bags sealed and wrapped in a towel.
- Reusable enema equipment can be substituted for disposable enema equipment.
- Extra pillows can be used to support position changes if the bed position cannot be changed.
- Some equipment may be rented from equipment rental companies, Figure 31–7, or borrowed from church groups or other organizations.
- The entire bed can be raised on blocks to make care giving easier if the patient is not ambulatory.
- A cotton blanket or lightweight spread can be used for a bath blanket.
- Plastic covered with a twin-size sheet can be used in place of a drawsheet.

- A cardboard box cut and taped and padded can be used as a backrest, Figure 31–8A.
- Two lightweight pieces of wood nailed at right angles can be padded and used as a footrest to hold bedding off the toes, Figure 31–8B.
- A bed tray can replace an over-bed table for eating and activities.
- A paper bag can be taped to the bed springs to dispose of soiled tissues, Figure 31–8C. The entire bag can then be closed and properly handled for disposal.
- A shoe bag tucked under the mattress and hanging by the bedside, Figure 31–8D, can be used as compartments for the patient's personal articles.
- A pillowcase hung on the back of a chair can serve as a laundry bag.

Most home health aides carry kits that contain:

- Plastic aprons
- Disposable gloves
- Observational equipment such as stethoscope, blood pressure cuff, and thermometers

The Home Environment

You are responsible for maintaining a safe and comfortable environment for the client. This means you must:

- Be alert to unsafe situations.
- Control the spread of infection.
- Care for and maintain the client's furnishings, supplies, and appliances.

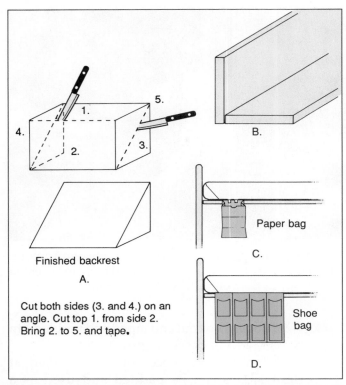

FIGURE 31–8. Making equipment using readily available materials

Avoiding Liability

You can avoid being held liable (responsible) for incidents in the home if you:

- Carry out procedures carefully as you were taught.
- Keep safety factors always in mind and be on the lookout for possible hazards.
- Seek guidance from the proper person before you take action in a questionable situation.
- Do not overstep your authority.
- Do not attempt to perform skills you have not been taught.
- Do only those tasks that are assigned to you.

Safety in the Home

Your first visit to the home provides you with an opportunity to check for safety factors. Tell the family member or supervising nurse about safety problems. For example, things to call to the attention of your supervisor include:

- Loose scatter rugs which might cause a fall as the client ambulates.

- Overloaded electrical outlets which might cause a fire when you use equipment such as an electric lift.
- Ambulatory aids that need repair, such as broken straps on braces or replacement of worn rubber tips on walkers, canes, and crutches.
- Family or client smoking when oxygen is being used in the home.

Your job is not to reorganize the client's home but to assure a safe environment.

Keep a list of emergency numbers close to the telephone. The list should include the:

- Agency
- Supervising nurse
- Physician
- Family member
- Ambulance
- Hospital
- Police department
- Fire department
- Emergency number 911 (in areas where this number is in use)

Elder Abuse

As a home health aide, you may observe clients who have possibly been abused. Unit 29 describes the various types of abuse that may be inflicted by staff members, family members, or other residents. These situations may also occur in the home:

- Some families provide loving, capable care for older, dependent relatives for many years without assistance. They may be emotionally stressed and may have also depleted their financial resources.
- In some cases there has been a long family history of one spouse abusing the other.
- Self-abuse may occur when a disabled person is unable to adequately carry out activities of daily living and is unwilling to accept help.

It is not the responsibility of the nursing assistant to determine if an individual has been abused or what type of abuse has been inflicted. It is the nursing assistant's responsibility to report to the nursing supervisor any signs or symptoms that might be the result of abuse. This includes:

- statements of the client that reflect neglect or abuse
- unexplained bruises or wounds
- signs of neglect such as poor hygiene
- a change in personality

Remember these do not necessarily indicate that the person is being abused. However, they may indicate a need for further investigation by your supervisor.

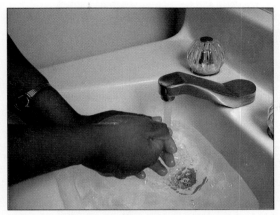

FIGURE 31–9. Wash your hands before and after each client contact and task.

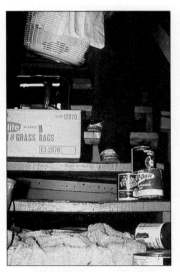

FIGURE 31–10. Do not let clutter accumulate.

Infection Control

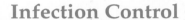

Some of the methods employed in daily cleaning help to control the spread of infection. Other requirements are:

- Washing your hands, Figure 31–9
- Keeping the kitchen and bathroom clean
- Caring for food properly
- Disposing of tissues and other wastes properly
- Cleaning up dirty dishes
- Dusting daily
- Not allowing clutter to accumulate, Figure 31–10
- Wearing a plastic apron
- Wearing latex, disposable gloves whenever there is the possibility of contacting blood and body fluids and other potentially infectious material

- Clean and put equipment away as soon as you have finished with it.
- Dust the room daily.
- Damp dust noncarpeted floors weekly or vacuum carpeted floors.
- Remove used dishes and glasses when finished and rinse right away.
- Put clean clothes away after laundering. Hang up robes when not in use.
- Line wastepaper basket with a plastic bag and empty regularly.

Housekeeping Chores

Cleaning the Client's Room

In some cases, the homemaker assistant (aide) will perform the housekeeping chores. In other cases, the home health care nursing assistant may be assigned some or all of these duties.

Keeping the client's room clean is a way to prevent infection. It also contributes positively to the client's morale. Remember that you are not to rearrange the client's things without permission.

- Pick up things so clutter will not accumulate.
- Keep cleaning equipment in one place so you do not waste time gathering it for each job as you move from room to room, Figure 31–11.

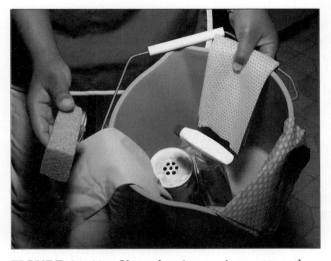

FIGURE 31–11. Keep cleaning equipment together.

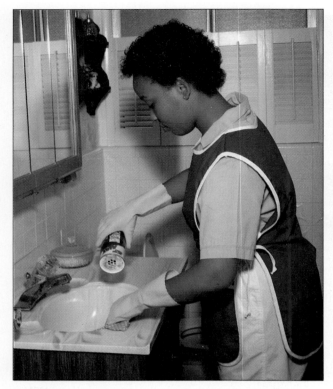

FIGURE 31–12.   Clean the bathroom daily.

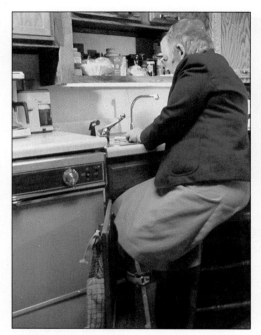

FIGURE 31–13.   Even though the client may help in the kitchen, the home health aide or homemaker assistant keeps it clean.

Cleaning the Bathroom

The bathroom can be the source of infection, so you must be careful and thorough in your daily cleaning, Figure 31–12. Use a disinfectant solution (family's choice) to clean the:

- Inside and outside of the toilet
- Shower or tub after each use
- Sink and faucets
- Countertops
- Floor; if carpeted, then vacuum daily

Be sure dirty towels are put into the laundry. Replace them with clean towels and washcloths. Use a deodorant to keep the bathroom smelling fresh and clean.

Cleaning the Kitchen

The kitchen is another area that requires special attention. An unclean kitchen can be the source of infection.

- Clean up after every meal, Figure 31–13.
- Clean up dirty dishes immediately. Do not allow them to accumulate in the sink.
  - Rinse them and wash by hand in detergent and hot water.
  - Wash glasses first, then silverware, then dishes.
  - Rinse with hot water and allow to dry in drainer.
  - Put away when dry.
- You may wash them in the dishwasher by:
  - Rinsing well.
  - Adding recommended detergent to the dishwasher.
  - Loading washer, but do not run until full.

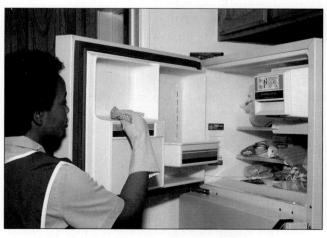

FIGURE 31–14.   Clean spills immediately.

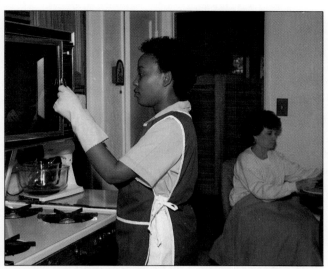

FIGURE 31–15. Clean the microwave oven after each use.

- Wash pots and pans by hand since most are not dishwasher safe.
- Clean sink, countertops, and stove.
- Dispose of garbage properly. It may be put in a disposal if one is available. Do not include bones. Wrap them tightly in newspaper and put in trash or compactor if available.
- Sweep floor after each meal.
- Place leftover foods in small covered containers and refrigerate. Use or discard within a few days.
- Keep refrigerator clean and keep food covered. Clean spills in the refrigerator immediately, Figure 31–14.
- Keep the microwave oven clean, Figure 31–15. Use a damp cloth to wipe spills immediately and to clean after each use. Make sure you heat food in microwave safe dishes only. Do not use metal of any kind in a microwave oven. For example, dishes with metallic trim are **not** used.
- Wash the kitchen floor weekly or more often if necessary.

Ask client or responsible family member for instructions on appliance use before using.

Other Duties

Two other tasks are frequently your responsibility in the home situation. They are food management and laundry.

Food Management. Plan food purchases. Food purchases are planned in conjunction with the client or family member. If consultation is not possible, keep these guidelines in mind:

- Plan menus a week in advance. Base them on good nutrition.
- Take into consideration the client's preferences, cultural background, and any religious prohibitions.
- Buy only what you need and what can be used. Large quantities are not a bargain if much of it goes unused or is wasted.
- Look for quality bargains.
- Keep track of all money spent and a list of items purchased; keep receipts.
- Make an accounting of all money handled.

Using the weekly menu, prepare foods in such a way that the client's dietary needs are met. Also:

- Wash fruits and vegetables that are to be used fresh and store in the refrigerator; store unwashed if they are not to be used right away. Remember to wash before use.
- Keep dairy products and meats refrigerated before use.
- Allow frozen meats to thaw in the refrigerator before use.
- Take into consideration the client's ordered diet, any digestive problems, and preferences.
- Keep dried and canned foods in cabinets.

Laundry. Carefully launder the client's clothes. They represent a sizable investment. This may need to be done daily. Always:

- Read labels before laundering. Some clothes must be dry cleaned or washed in special temperatures.
- Use the client's choice of detergent and read the label for instructions for amounts to use.
- Separate light and dark fabrics and wash separately.
- Wash drip-dry fabrics alone so they can be hung and dried or folded.
- Be sure clothes can be dried in a dryer and use the proper setting.
- Hang clothes after wiping off clothes lines if dryer is not available.
- After laundering, fold, iron, or hang clothes.
- Check for needed repairs and do mending before storing clothes.
- Ask client or responsible family member for operating instructions before using washer or dryer.

Record Keeping

Two types of records are compiled by the nursing assistant giving home care. They are:

1. Time/travel records, Figure 31–16. This is a record of how you spent your time in the client's home. It includes:
   a. Time of arrival
   b. Time of departure
   c. Length of time required for specific activities
   d. Travel time if working in more than one home
   e. Mileage or transportation costs

Keeping a time and travel record requires accuracy and some calculations. Fill in the record as you complete each assignment. Do not wait until the end of the day or your assigned time and then try to rely on your memory.

To compute mileage (round off to the nearest full mile):

- Record the car odometer reading before starting to your assignment.
- Record the odometer reading when you arrive at the client's home.
- Subtract the starting odometer reading from the arrival reading.
- Record this difference as the mileage.

For example, if the reading on your car odometer before starting was 45,061 and upon arrival at the client's home it is 45,068, the mileage should be recorded as 7 miles (45,068 - 45,061).

2. Client care records, Figure 31–17. This is a record of:
   a. Care given
   b. Client's response
   c. Housekeeping tasks, if assigned
   d. Observations such as:
      — Vital signs
      — Elimination
      — Intake of fluids
      — Appetite
      — Unusual conditions or behavior

RIVERVIEW HOME HEALTH SERVICE
8987 Walkman Ave
Parkhurst, Nebraska
Time and Travel Log

CARE GIVER NAME Siadto, Laura CNA   TITLE Home Health Assistant   EMPT. NO. 62718   DATE Aug. 29

PATIENT NAME/ADDRESS (Last, first)	SERVICE PROVIDED	VISIT CODE	NON BILL CODE	TIME IN	TIME OUT	CLIENT CONTACT TIME	ODOMETER READING	MILES
Volheim, Eleonore	Bedbath, Shampoo	4		8¹⁵	9⁰⁵	50 min	From: 45,061 To: 45,068	7 miles
Javonello, Sharri		1		9³⁰	9⁴⁵	15 min	From: 45,068 To: 45,083	15 miles
Doyle, Kindra	Enema, bedbath, amb	4		10¹⁰	11³⁰	1hr. 20 min	From: 45,083 To: 46,001	18 miles
Hammond, Rachel	Ass't c̄ colostomy cath care, Bath, ROM	4		11⁵⁰	1²⁰	1hr. 30 min	From: 46,001 To: 46,017	16 miles
Minzey, Aimee		2		1³⁰	1³⁵	–	From: 46,017 To: 46,025	8 miles
Galloway, Rosa		5		1⁵⁰	2⁰⁰	10	From: 46,025 To: 46,028	3 miles
							From: To:	

Total Visits 6   Total Mileage 67   Parking Fees —

Visit Code
1 IE Initial Eval & Rx   4 HC Home Care
2 FV Follow Up Visit   5 Hospital/Hospice
3 DV Discharge Visit   6 MC Maternal/Child

Nonbill Code
1. Refused Care
2. Patient Not Home
3. Non-Bill
4. Expired
5. Delivered Supplies

Supervising Nurse: Bruce Davenport R.N.

FIGURE 31–16.   Sample time and travel record

RIVERVIEW HOME HEALTH SERVICE
8987 Walkman Ave
Parkhurst, Nebraska
Client Care Plan / Progress Notes

HOME HEALTH ASSISTANT YOLANDA BROWN, CNA

CLIENT NAME NICHOLAS FRENCH   SOC. SECURITY # 728-24-8884

ADDRESS: 529 MAPLE AVE.   PARKHURST, NEBRASKA

ACTIVITY

Time	Activity
0800	arrived, Determined needs, planned activities
	client seemed fatigued "Slept poorly". On Nasal O₂ 2.5L
0830	Circumoral pallor noted. Vital Signs checked. Dyspneic on exertion.
	Put laundry into washing machine - Started breakfast.
0900	client ate 1 sl toast, 8 g oatbran cereal/milk 6 g orange juice
0930	Prepared equipment for A.M. care - Complete bath, shave and
	denture care. Asst to commode, soft brown formed stool.
1000	
1030	Made comfortable in easy chair. Reading newspaper - Nasal O₂
	Cleaned kitchen including refrigerator
1100	Linen changed - dusted and dust mopped bedroom. Vacuumed
	living room.
1130	Prepared lunch.
1200	client ate ½ chicken sandwich, 8 oz tea, chocolate pudding,
	8 oz. tomato soup.
1230	Client returned to bed for nap
1300	Cleaned lunch dishes and prepared salad, jello for evening meal
1330	Put washed laundry into dryer.
1400	Cleaned bathroom, washed kitchen floor
	Put bed linen into washer.
1430	Made out shopping list for A.M.
1500	Client awake. assisted into living room. Watching T.V.
	Ordered O₂ tank replacement.
1530	Folded and put clean laundry away. Put washed linens in dryer.
1600	client seems more rested. color improved. Resp. easier.
	Notified supervisor of clients progress.
1630	Left client's home @ 3³⁵PM.
	Y. Brown CNA

VITAL SIGNS	T	P	R	B/P
	97⁴	92	26	
INTAKE				
OUTPUT				

SUP. SIGNATURE

FIGURE 31–17. Sample client care record

SUMMARY

There is an increasing trend to provide home health care to the housebound, recuperating, and chronically ill client. The nursing assistant who provides this care may also carry out housekeeping activities.

In some situations, the duties are specifically separated into household and personal chores performed by a homemaker assistant and the nursing care activities performed by the home health care nursing assistant.

Home health care consists of:
- Maintaining a safe, comfortable environment for the client
- Managing infection control
- Carrying out proper nursing techniques under the supervision of the nurse care coordinator

The home health assistant occupies the position of:
- Member of the home health care team
- Guest in the client's home
- Provider of direct health care and household assistance

UNIT REVIEW

A. True/False. Answer the following statements true or false by circling T or F.

T F 1. World War I acted as a stimulus to the enrollment of students in hospital-based nursing programs.

T F 2. The home health care nursing assistant may be responsible for both nursing care and household tasks.

T F 3. The home health care nursing assistant makes no contribution to the nursing process since care is given at home and not in the hospital.

T F 4. Many new hospitals were built after World War II.

T F 5. Self-discipline is an important characteristic of the nursing assistant working in a home.

T F 6. The home health care nursing assistant often has both the opportunity for regular employment and flexible hours.

T F 7. The physician acts as the care coordinator for home care.

T F 8. The homemaker assistant has direct nursing care of the client as the primary responsibility.

T F 9. When washing dishes, wash the plates first, then the pots and pans, and then the glassware.

T F 10. There is much satisfaction in giving complete care to one client at a time.

B. Multiple Choice. Choose the answer that best completes each of the following sentences by circling the proper letter.

11. World War II brought about an increase in the
    a. need for more technical care.
    b. introduction of antibiotics.
    c. growth of an ancillary work force.
    d. All of the above.

12. Home care is a trend because
    a. there is little room in the hospitals.
    b. older hospitals are being torn down.
    c. people like being cared for in familiar surroundings.
    d. the cost of hospitalization has gone down in recent years.

13. The person receiving health care at home is called the
    a. patient.
    b. client.
    c. resident.
    d. recipient.

14. A special characteristic needed by a home health care nursing assistant working in a home is
    a. self-discipline.
    b. being a follower.
    c. being a fast worker.
    d. being able to take short cuts.

15. Which of the household tasks would the home health care nursing assistant not be required to do?
    a. Shop for food.
    b. Move heavy furniture.
    c. Carry out nursing procedures.
    d. Prepare food for the client.

C. Applications. Compute the following mileage traveled.

Odometer Readings

	On Departure	On Arrival	Mileage
16.	15,642	15,646	_____
17.	22,784	22,800	_____
18.	6,911	6,921	_____
19.	76,532	76,535	_____
20.	48,827	48,845	_____

SELF-EVALUATION   Section 9

A. Choose the phrase that best completes each of the following sentences by circling the proper letter.

1. When applying a hot water bag, remember
   a. to fill the bag to the top.
   b. the water should be 115°F.
   c. the bag need not be covered.
   d. None of the above.

2. The disposable coldpack
   a. provides continuous cold for 3 hours.
   b. is activated by striking or squeezing.
   c. doesn't need to be covered.
   d. needs to be checked every 30 minutes once in place.

3. If you are assigned to surgically prep the patient, remember
   a. to always use a safety razor.
   b. to shave hair opposite to the direction of growth.
   c. do not use soap because a dry shave is best.
   d. do not wash the shave area.

4. When a patient is allowed to dangle or ambulate for the first time, remember to
   a. help the patient sit up rapidly.
   b. watch closely for signs of vertigo or fatigue.
   c. stay with the patient walking a long way.
   d. take his temperature before assisting the patient up.

5. When a patient returns from surgery, you should check
   a. for drainage tubes.
   b. vital signs.
   c. the dressing.
   d. All of the above.

6. After which type of anesthesia is a patient most apt to be nauseated?
   a. Local   c. Intravenous
   b. Spinal   d. Inhalation

7. The best binder to use to hold the dressing after rectal surgery on a male patient would be a
   a. single-T binder.
   b. breast binder.
   c. double-T binder.
   d. straight abdominal binder.

8. Patients are often required to lie flat following spinal anesthesia in order to reduce the chance of
   a. nausea.   c. blood clots.
   b. headache.   d. abdominal pain.

9. The skilled nursing care facility
   a. provides care for premature babies.
   b. provides the same care as acute hospitals.
   c. cares mostly for the aged.
   d. provides only bed and board.

10. Elderly persons are characterized by
    a. loss of vitality.
    b. graying of the hair.
    c. less sensibility to pain.
    d. All of the above.

11. Foot care for the elderly should include
    a. daily washing and inspection.
    b. heavy use of powder to keep dry.
    c. cutting toenails on a curve.
    d. ignoring thick nails since they are too difficult to cut.

12. Continence retraining requires
    a. that the patient be ambulatory.
    b. that the patient consume large amounts of water.
    c. that the patient be awakened every hour during the night.
    d. the cooperation of all staff members.

13. When learning of a terminal diagnosis, the first response of the patient usually is
    a. anger.
    b. denial.
    c. depression.
    d. acceptance.

14. Signs that death is approaching include
    a. loss of general control.
    b. breathing becomes irregular and shallow.
    c. extremities become cold as circulation slows down.
    d. All of the above.

15. When a patient is in final stages of life
    a. leave patient alone.
    b. you do not have to be careful of what you say.
    c. visit frequently.
    d. mouth care is no longer needed.

16. When giving postmortem care
    a. remove dentures.
    b. leave equipment in the room.
    c. bathe as necessary.
    d. place the body in a natural sitting position.
17. The client you are caring for at home is unable to report your conduct. Therefore it is alright to
    a. talk to friends on the phone.
    b. stop for frequent coffee breaks.
    c. carry out your work in an efficient manner.
    d. help yourself to family food supplies.
    e. None of the above.
18. Which of the following would not be part of your responsibilities when caring for a client at home as a home care nursing assistant?
    a. Settling family disputes
    b. Assisting with activities of daily living
    c. Carrying out range of motion exercises
    d. Giving special mouth care if needed
    e. Shopping for meals
19. Emergency numbers you ought to keep close at hand when giving home care should include the number of the
    a. agency.
    b. supervising nurse.
    c. emergency number (911 if in use in the area).
    d. physician.
    e. All of the above.
20. When caring for the client's kitchen
    a. clean up once a day so dishes can be washed all at once.
    b. leave dirty dishes in the sink between meals.
    c. leave unused food out as long as it is in a dish.
    d. wash the floor daily.
    e. sweep the floor after each meal.

B. Name the piece of equipment pictured below.

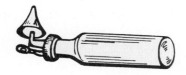

21. _____

C. Name the following examination positions.

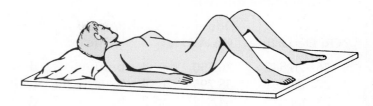

22. _____

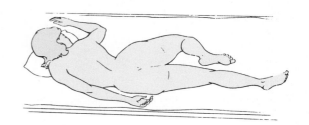

23. _____

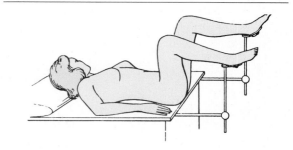

24. _____

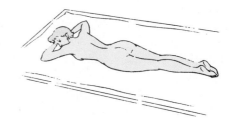

25. _____

D. Mileage Calculations. Select the correct answer for each of the following.

| | Odometer Readings | | |
On Departure	On Arrival	Mileage			
26. 26,542	26,550	a. 4	b. 10	c. 8	d. 7
27. 38,791	38,795	a. 4	b. 6	c. 12	d. 5
28. 64,839	64,842	a. 2	b. 5	c. 7	d. 3
29. 57,418	57,425	a. 7	b. 12	c. 14	d. 15
30. 52,647	52,656	a. 6	b. 7	c. 8	d. 9
31. 45,212	45,218	a. 3	b. 4	c. 6	d. 9

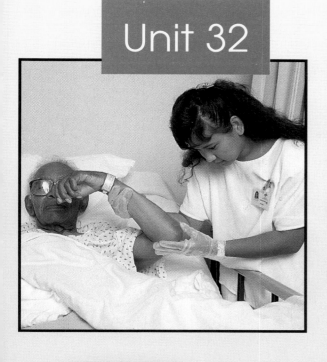

Unit 32

The Integumentary System and Related Care Procedures

OBJECTIVES

As a result of this unit, you will be able to:

- Spell and define terms.
- Review the location and function of the skin and its appendages.
- Describe some common skin lesions.
- List three diagnostic tests associated with skin conditions.
- Describe the nursing assistant actions relating to the nursing care of patients with specific skin conditions.
- Identify persons at risk for the formation of decubitus ulcers.
- Describe preventive measures for pressure sores (decubitus ulcers).
- Describe the stages of pressure sore formation and identify appropriate nursing assistant actions.
- Describe the system of classifying burns.
- List nursing assistant actions in caring for patients with burns.

VOCABULARY

Learn the meaning and the correct spelling of the following words:

allergen	excoriation
allergies	integument
anaphylactic shock	lesions
colloidal	macule
contraindicated	necrosis
crust	obese
cyanotic	pallor
debride	papule
decubitus ulcer	pressure sores
dermal ulcer	pustule
electrolytes	rubra
emollient	vesicle
eschar	wheal

Before you begin to study this unit, return to Unit 4 and review pages 47–49.

You will recall that the skin (integument):
- Covers the body.
- Protects underlying structures.
- Is an indication of overall health.
- Includes the hair, nails, and glands as appendages, Figure 32–1.

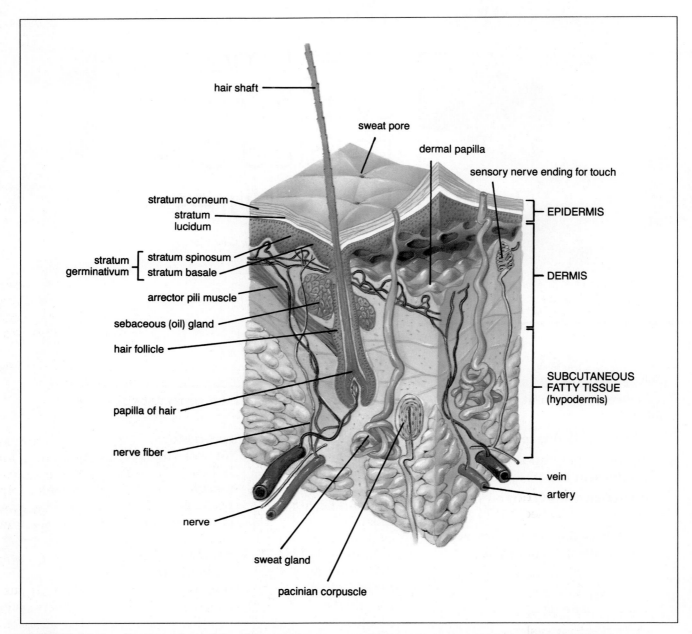

FIGURE 32–1. Cross section of the skin *(From Anatomy and Physiology Plates, copyright 1992 by Delmar Publishers Inc.)*

The skin tells us much about the general health of the body.

- A fever may be indicated by hot dry skin.
- Unusual redness—rubra, or flushing of the skin—often follows strenuous activity.
- Pallor, which is less color than normal, is a sign associated with many conditions.
- The oxygen content of the blood can be noted quickly by the color of the skin. When the oxygen content is very low, the blood is darker and the skin appears bluish or cyanotic

Common Conditions

Skin Lesions

Injury or disease causes changes in areas of the skin. These changes are called lesions. When caring for patients with skin lesions, universal precautions are followed. Some of the most common skin lesions or eruptions are:

- Macules—flat, discolored spots as in measles, Figure 32–2

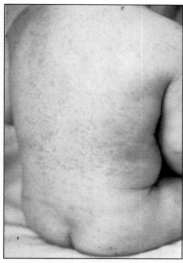

FIGURE 32–2. The macules of German measles *(Photo courtesy of the Centers for Disease Control, Atlanta, GA)*

- Papules—small, solid, raised spots as in chicken-pox
- Pustules—raised spots filled with pus as in acne
- Vesicles—raised spots filled with watery fluid such as a blister, Figure 32–3
- Wheals—large, raised, irregular areas frequently associated with itching, as in hives
- Excoriations—portions of the skin appear scraped or scratched away
- Crusts—areas of dried body secretions such as scabs

Skin lesions may be a result of systemic responses such as:

- Communicable disease—diseases that are easily transmitted, directly or indirectly, from person to person. Measles and chickenpox are two such diseases. Each has characteristic skin lesions called skin eruptions or rashes.
- People whose immune system is depressed, such as those suffering from HIV infection, may develop a specific type of cancer called *Kaposi's sarcoma*. It appears as lesions in the skin and eventually in other organs. The skin lesions begin as macules, papules, or violet lesions that gradually become bigger and darker. They are frequently seen on the trunk, neck, and head (especially on the tip of the nose). Progression of the disease may be slow or rapid.
- Allergies—also called *sensitivity reactions*, may have associated skin lesions. The vesicles of

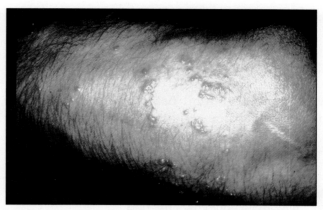

FIGURE 32–3. The fluid-filled vesicles of poison ivy *(Photo courtesy of the Centers for Disease Control, Atlanta, GA)*

poison ivy are well known. The material causing the sensitivity is called an allergen. Individuals respond to allergens in different ways.
- Anaphylactic shock—a severe, sometimes fatal, sensitivity reaction.

Observation of the skin and accurate descriptions of what you see must be carefully charted.

Diagnosing Skin Lesions

Your careful observations and accurate description of any skin lesions provide valuable information about the nature of the condition. There are several diagnostic tests that may be ordered by the physician to help establish the cause of the lesion. These tests include:

- Studying scrapings from the skin lesion under the microscope.
- Culturing the skin lesion if an infection is suspected.
- Performing skin testing if sensitivities are suspected, by introducing small quantities of substances (allergens) known to bring about an allergic (hypersensitivity) reaction in humans. Allergens include pollens, foods, dust, animal dander, and medications.

Care of Skin Lesions

When skin lesions are present, certain general nursing care is indicated. You should take the following precautions when caring for these patients.

- Closely observe the patient's skin on admission, but do not remove any dressings.
- Soap and water and rubbing lotions are often contraindicated (not permitted). Check the nursing care plan before bathing the patient or giving a back rub.

■ Do not attempt to remove any crusts from skin lesions without special instruction from your supervisor.

■ Handle the patient gently. Avoid rubbing the skin.

Emollient (colloidal) baths may be ordered to soothe and treat the condition. Emollient baths are given in tepid water to which a medication has been added, such as:

■ Baking soda   ■ Cornstarch
■ Oatmeal

Refer to Figure 32–4 for a review of the beginning procedure actions and procedure completion actions.

BEGINNING PROCEDURE ACTIONS	PROCEDURE COMPLETION ACTIONS
■ Wash your hands. ■ Assemble equipment needed. ■ Go to the patient's room, knock, and pause before entering. ■ Introduce yourself and identify the patient by checking the identification bracelet. ■ Ask visitors to leave and inform them where they can wait. ■ Care for equipment according to facility policy. ■ Provide privacy. ■ Explain what will happen and answer questions. ■ Allow patient to assist in procedure as much as possible. ■ Raise bed or table to comfortable working height.	■ Position patient comfortably. ■ Leave signal cord, telephone, and fresh water close at hand. ■ Return bed or table to lowest position. ■ Perform general safety check of patient and environment. ■ Wash your hands. ■ Report completion of task. ■ Let visitors know when they may reenter the patient's room. ■ Document action and your observations.

NOTE: Where there are open lesions, wet linen, or possible contact with patient body fluids or blood, disposable gloves are worn during the procedure. Put on gloves before contact with the patient or linen. Properly dispose of gloves after they are removed. ALWAYS APPLY UNIVERSAL PRECAUTIONS.

FIGURE 32–4 .   Beginning procedure actions and procedure completion actions

PROCEDURE 107

GIVING AN EMOLLIENT BATH

1. Carry out each beginning procedure action.
2. Remember to wash your hands, identify the patient, and provide privacy.
3. Assemble equipment needed:
   ■ Bath mat   ■ Bath thermometer
   ■ 2 bath towels   ■ Gloves
   ■ Gown   ■ Additions as
   ■ Slippers and robe   ordered
4. Be sure tub is clean and the room is warm.
5. Fill tub with tepid water (95–100°F). Check the temperature with a bath thermometer.
6. Add medication if ordered. Stir well.
7. Transfer patient safely to tub as outlined in tub bath procedure.
8. Have patient lie in the tub for 30 minutes to 1 hour as ordered.

   ■ Put on gloves. Gently sponge areas not covered with water.
   ■ Make sure patient does not become chilled.
   ■ Add warm water as needed.
9. Assist patient out of the tub. Dry the skin by patting with a soft towel. *Do not rub.* Put on clean gown.
10. Apply lotion, if ordered, by patting. Remove gloves and dispose of them according to facility policy.
11. Assist patient to bed and encourage patient to rest.
12. Put on gloves. Clean tub. Remove gloves and dispose of properly. Replace equipment according to facility policy.

13. Carry out each procedure completion action. Remember to wash your hands, report completion of task, and document date, time, emollient bath (kind of medication, temperature of water, and length of treatment), and patient reaction.

Pressure Sores (Dermal Ulcers)

Pressure sores, commonly called bedsores or **dermal ulcers** or **decubitus ulcers,** may occur in patients of any age. They are particularly common in:

- Elderly patients
- Very thin patients
- Overweight (**obese**) patients
- Persons unable to move
- Incontinent patients
- Debilitated patients
- Poorly nourished patients
- Patients confined to bed or wheelchairs
- Disoriented patients

Pressure sores are caused by extended pressure on an area of the body that interferes with circulation. The tissue first becomes reddened. As the cells die (undergo **necrosis**) from lack of nourishment, the skin breaks down and an ulcer forms. The resulting bedsore may become large and deep.

Decubiti occur most frequently over areas where bones come close to the surface. The most common sites, Figure 32–5, are the:

- Elbows
- Hips
- Heels
- Ankles
- Shoulders
- Ears
- Sacrum
- Knees (inner and outer parts)

Patients tend to develop pressure sores where body parts rub, causing friction. Common sites are:

- Between the folds of the buttocks
- Legs
- Under the breasts
- Abdominal folds
- Ankles
- Knees
- The rubbing of tubing and other equipment used in the care of patients over a long period can also cause pressure sores, Figure 32–6.

To Avoid Decubiti. Because pressure sores are far more easily prevented than cured, everyone participating in the patient's care has a responsibility to prevent skin breakdown.

When a person is admitted, the nurse will assess the patient's current status and potential for skin breakdown. This forms a baseline against which all future assessments may be measured. The assessment may be described on the patient's chart in words, pictures, diagrams, or as a score (Figures 32–7A and 32–7B). If the nursing diagnosis of actual or "potential impairment of skin integrity" is identified, every staff member must make extra effort to prevent breakdown, limit that which has already occurred, and promote the healing process.

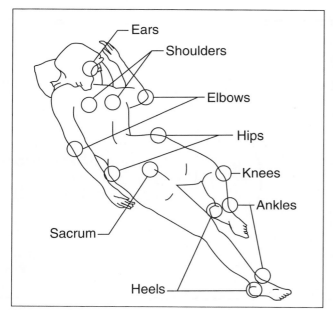

FIGURE 32–5. Common sites for pressure sores.

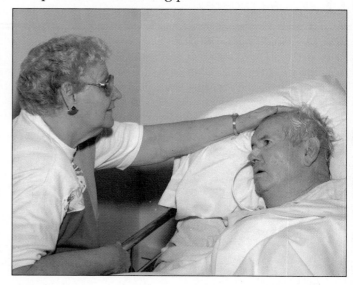

FIGURE 32–6. The rubbing of nasal catheters, nasogastric tubes, or urinary catheters can cause breakdown of skin.

PATIENTS AT RISK TO DEVELOP PRESSURE SORES: Identify any patient at risk to develop pressure sores by assessing the seven clinical condition parameters and assigning a score. Any patient with intact skin, but scoring **8 or greater** should have the nursing diagnosis *"Potential Impairment of Skin Integrity"* identified.

Clinical Condition Parameters—Risk of Pressure Sores

Clinical Condition Parameters	Score
General Physical Condition (health problem)	
Good (minor)	0
Fair (major but stable)	1
Poor (chronic/serious not stable)	2
Level of Consciousness (to commands)	
Alert (responds readily)	0
Lethargic (slow to respond)	1
Semi Comatose (responds only to verbal or painful stimuli)	2
Comatose (no response to stimuli)	3
Activity	
Ambulant without assistance	0
Ambulant with assistance	2
Chairfast	4
Bedfast	6

Clinical Condition Parameters	Score
Mobility (extremities)	
Full active range	0
Limited movement with assistance	2
Moves only with assistance	4
Immobile	6
Incontinence (bowel and/or bladder)	
None	0
Occasional (≤ 2 per 24 hours)	2
Usually (> 2 per 24 hours)	4
No control	6
Nutrition (for age and size)	
Good (eats/drinks adequately ¾ of meal)	0
Fair (eats/drinks inadequately—at least ½ of meal)	1
Poor (unable/refuses to eat/drink—less than ½)	2
Skin/Tissue Status	
Good (well nourished/skin intact)	0
Fair (poorly nourished/skin intact)	1
Poor (skin not intact)	2

Total:

FIGURE 32–7A. Assessing risk of pressure sores *(Courtesy of Artistic Press, Los Angeles, CA)*

DECUBITUS ULCER: To be assessed upon admission and every 7 days or PRN thereafter per Nursing Policy.

☐ DECUBITUS ULCER (SIZE, SITE, STAGE)

☐ PICTURE TAKEN BY:

USE DIAGRAMS TO SHOW SIZE, SITE, STAGE

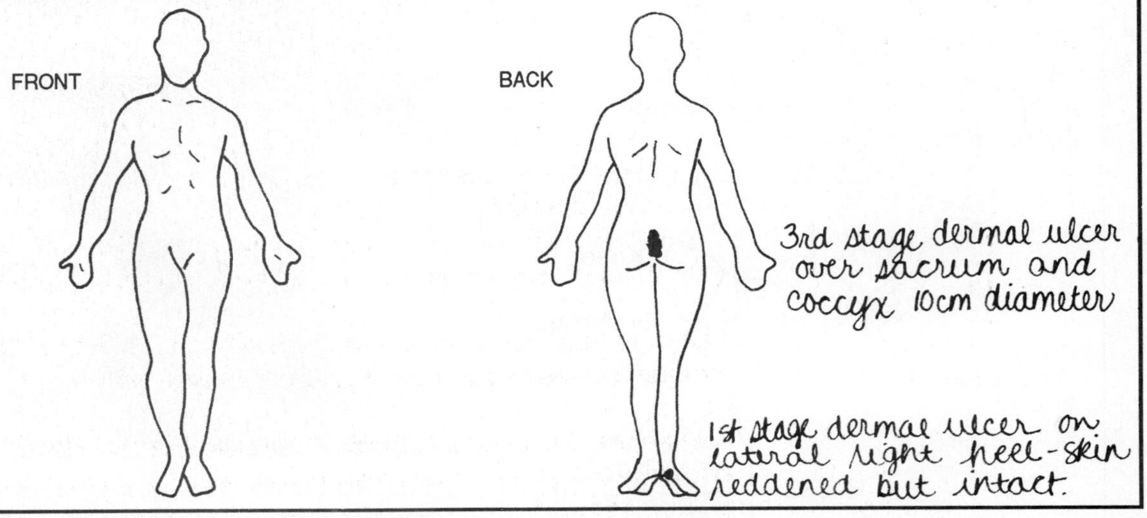

FRONT   BACK

3rd stage dermal ulcer over sacrum and coccyx 10cm diameter

1st stage dermal ulcer on lateral right heel-skin reddened but intact.

FIGURE 32–7B. Documentation of dermal ulcers is made on the patient's chart in words, pictures, and diagrams. *(From Hegner and Caldwell, Geriatrics, A Study of Maturity, 5th Edition, 1991, Delmar Publishers Inc.)*

The following care should be given:

■ Change the patient's position at least every 2 hours. A major shift in position is required. When positioning patient, be careful to avoid friction, such as sliding the patient over bedclothes or against equipment. Use lifting devices to avoid dragging.

■ Encourage patients sitting in Gerichairs® or wheelchairs to raise themselves every 10 minutes to relieve pressure, or assist patients to do so.

■ Encourage proper nutrition and adequate intake of fluids. Breakdown occurs more readily and healing is delayed when the patient is poorly nourished. Proper nutrition may require tube feedings with enriched high protein and high vitamin supplements. Patients who are able to eat should be encouraged to do so. Adequate fluids are a requirement.
Serum albumin, hematocrit, and hemoglobin levels are important laboratory values in assessing nutritional status.

■ Immediately remove feces or urine from the skin since they are very irritating to the skin. Wash and dry the area immediately.

■ Whenever giving personal care to patients, carefully inspect areas where decubiti commonly form. Report any reddened areas immediately.

■ Inspect skin daily and report the condition.

■ Keep the skin clean and dry at all times.

■ Keep linen dry and free from wrinkles and hard objects such as crumbs and hairpins.

■ Bathe patient frequently. Pay particular attention to potential pressure or friction areas. Avoid hot water and friction.

■ Massage around reddened areas frequently with rubbing solution. Do not massage directly on the site, and do not use alcohol. Use moisturizers on dry skin.

■ Use no lotion on broken skin areas.

■ Keep friction areas lightly dusted with cornstarch, but do not allow cornstarch to accumulate or cake. Overuse can cause abrasions.

■ Use a turning sheet to move dependent patients in bed.

■ Elevate the head of the bed no higher than 30 degrees to prevent a shearing effect on the tissues.

■ Carry out range of motion exercises at least twice daily to encourage circulation.

■ Check for improperly fitted or worn braces and restraints.

■ Check nasogastric tubes and catheters to be sure they are positioned in such a way as not to be a source of irritation. Keep the nasal and urinary openings clean and free of drainage. These areas must be checked frequently and carefully.

■ Use foam padding, sheepskin, or an alternating pressure mattress, Figures 32–8A, 8B, and 8C, to relieve pressure.

■ Protect areas such as heels and elbows at risk by covering with protectors, Figure 32–8D.

■ Use sheepskin and artificial sheepskin pads between patients and bottom linen, wheelchair backs or seats where excess pressure may be expected.

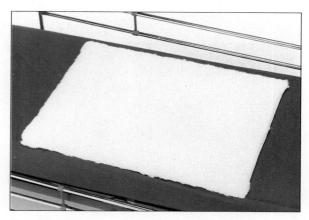

FIGURE 32–8A. Pad of synthetic sheepskin
(Photo courtesy of J.T. Posey Co., Inc.)

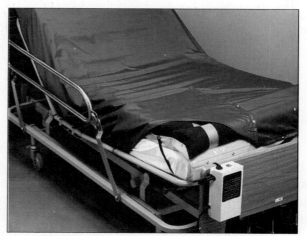

FIGURE 32–8B. Alternating low airloss mattress overlay. Alternating air pressure in mattress cells constantly changes pressure points against the patient's skin and gently massages the skin.
(Photo courtesy of National Patient Care Systems)

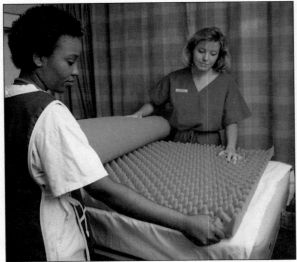

FIGURE 32–8C. An eggcrate mattress placed between patient and bed mattress adds comfort.

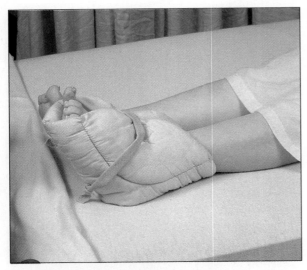

FIGURE 32–8D. Heel protector

Development of Decubitus Ulcers

Stages of Tissue Breakdown. Tissue breakdown occurs in four stages. Nursing intervention at each stage can limit the process and prevent further damage. Remember to continue with all preventive measures throughout care.

■ Stage One. In Stage One, the skin develops a redness, Figure 32–9, or blue-gray discoloration over the pressure area. In dark-skinned people, the area may appear drier. If, after peripheral massage and relief of pressure, the

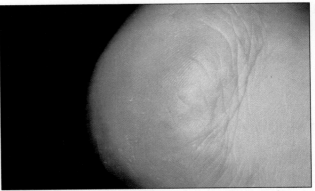

FIGURE 32–9. First indication of tissue ischemia (Stage One) is redness and heat over a pressure point such as this heel. *(Photo courtesy of Emory University Hospital, Atlanta, GA)*

blush has not subsided, it is probably the beginning of a pressure ulcer. Usually this stage of redness is reversible if effort is made to reduce or remove the pressure.

Action:

— Notify the nurse.
— Gently massage outside of the reddened area.
— Keep area around the breakdown clean and dry.
— Relieve all pressure over affected area by using mechanical aids.
— Encourage nutritious diet and adequate fluids.
— Keep any broken area covered as ordered, usually with a dry sterile dressing (DSD) or some other protective covering. The area may be covered with op-site or Bio–occlusive (clear). These are two clear, plastic-like coverings that permit air to reach the tissues but keep them moist, thus promoting healing. Holding a DSD in place without causing additional injury to the skin is not easy. The skin may be sensitive to regular tape so elastoplast, silk tape, paper tape, or cellophane may be better to use. Be careful to loosen tape with saline solution before lifting the tape when changing dressings.
— Place patient on an eggcrate mattress if ordered. The eggcrate mattress distributes the body weight over its surface and still allows for circulation of air. Make sure that the pointed side of the mattress faces the patient's body. Eggcrate-type pads also are

available to protect ankles, heels, and elbows.

— Report indications of infection such as odor or drainage, bleeding, and changes in size.

— Document the presence of potential areas for breakdown on the patient's chart using words and diagrams, Figure 32–7B.

Other measures that may be ordered include:

— Antiseptic sprays, antibiotic ointments, and dressings to control infection.

■ Stage Two. In Stage Two, the skin is reddened and there are blister-like lesions over the area, Figure 32–10. The area around the breakdown site may also be reddened. The skin may or may not be broken.

Action:

— Remove the pressure by repositioning the patient.

— Gently massage around the outside of the affected area to help prevent the development of a bedsore.

— Notify the nurse.

— Document on the patient's chart.

If this stage of involvement is neglected, further and deeper damage occurs.

■ Stage Three. In Stage Three, all the layers of the skin are destroyed, Figure 32–11. The nurse documents the size of the lesion using a commercial scale.

Action:

— Care is provided as in Stage Two and is continued faithfully if the third stage develops.

— To prevent infection, the nurse may wash the affected area with a bacteriostatic agent. Bacteriostatic agents that can be used include PhisoHex®, Caraklenz®, or Biolex® wound cleaner. The specific treatment varies with the specific physician's order.

— When there is necrotic tissue, ointments that remove the dead tissue (debride) from the area may be ordered. This treatment is performed by the physician or nurse. Elase® ointment, Biozyme® ointment, or some other tissue breakdown preparation, such as Santyl® or Travase®, may be applied for local debridement. Gelfoam sponges and gold leaf are sometimes applied directly to the lesion. These substances stimulate the development of healthy granulative tissue in the ulcer itself and decrease the toxicity of secondary infections. In some facilities, open lesions are packed loosely with gauze soaked in Carrington gel. The gel keeps the lesion moist and promotes self-debridement and healing. The pack is kept moist by being covered with hydrocolloid such as a thin sheet of Duoderm. The Duoderm must extend one inch beyond the wound edges and be held in place by a frame of either paper tape or silk tape. The dressing must be changed every 3 to 5 days, unless it is leaking.

— You may assist in daily whirlpool baths to help keep the area clean. Whirlpool baths may be given in conjunction with hyperbaric oxygenation to promote healing.

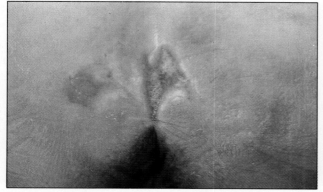

FIGURE 32–10. Stage Two is marked by destruction of the epidermis and partial destruction of the dermis. NOTE: Photo shows coccygeal (sacrum) area. *(Photo courtesy of Emory University Hospital, Atlanta, GA)*

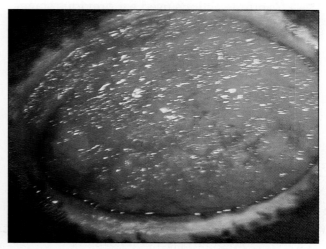

FIGURE 32–11. In Stage Three, all layers of skin have been destroyed. A deep crater has been formed. NOTE: Photo shows right hip. *(Photo courtesy of Emory University Hospital, Atlanta, GA)*

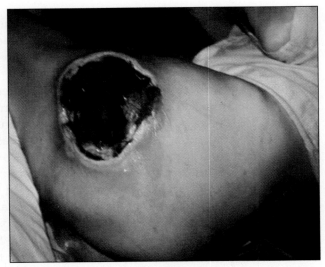

FIGURE 32–12. In Stage Four, tissue destruction can involve muscle, bone, and other vital structures. *(Photo courtesy of Emory University Hospital, Atlanta, GA)*

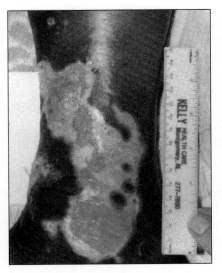

FIGURE 32–13. March 12: Right lateral ankle. Treatment with skin care products was initiated, using the following procedure:
1. The wound was cleansed.
2. Dermal wound gel was applied directly to the wound and surrounding tissue.
3. The wound was covered with vaseline gauze.
(Photo courtesy of Carrington Laboratories, Inc., Irving, TX)

— In severe cases, surgery may be needed to close the ulcerated area. You must be constantly on the alert for signs of impending skin breakdown. Remember, those patients who must remain in bed and those who are confined to Gerichairs® or wheelchairs are at the highest risk.

■ Stage Four. In Stage Four, the ulcer extends through the skin, subcutaneous tissues, and may involve bone, muscle, and other structures. Figure 32–12.

Action:
— Continue actions used for previous stages.
— A constant assessment of the breakdown includes measuring the size of the area and of observing and evaluating the extent of healing. Frequently, photos of the area are taken and are included in the chart as part of the documentation. Documentation of progress is made on a regular basis until healing is complete, Figures 32–13 and 32–14.

Burns

Any time that large sections of skin are destroyed, the body loses fluids and chemicals called **electrolytes** and is vulnerable to infection. Burns are a common cause of loss of large sections of skin.

Classification. The temperature and time exposure determine the severity of the resultant burns. Prognosis is based on the extent of the burns. Burns

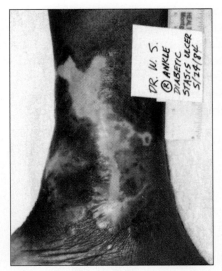

FIGURE 32–14. May 24: Right lateral ankle. Nurse's notes: "The ulcer has healed with all pink tissue present. There is no sign of infection and pigmentation has begun." *(Courtesy of Carrington Laboratories, Inc., Irving, TX)*

are commonly classified as first-, second-, and third-degree burns. Burns may also be classified according to the depth of tissue involvement.

Partial thickness burns may involve:

First degree burns

■ Epidermis. When only the epidermis is involved, the skin is pink to red. There may be some temporary swelling and pain. There is usually no permanent damage or scarring.

Second degree burns

■ Dermis. When both epidermis and dermis are involved in the burn, the color may vary from pink or red to white or tan. There is blistering and pain and some scarring.

Full thickness burns also involve differing depths of tissue:

Third degree burns

■ When the epidermis, dermis, and subcutaneous tissue are involved, the tissue is bright red to tan and brown. The area is covered with a tough, leathery coat (eschar). There is no pain initially as nerve endings have been destroyed. Later, pain and scarring will result from this injury.

■ When the epidermis, dermis, subcutaneous tissues, muscles, and bones are involved, the tissue appears blackened. Scarring will be extensive.

The Rule of Nines. This is a simple method of determining the extent of body involvement with burns. Using this method, an estimate is based on the following values:

■ The head equals 9 percent.
■ Each arm equals 9 percent.
■ The anterior trunk equals 18 percent.
■ The posterior trunk equals 18 percent.
■ Each entire leg equals 18 percent.
■ The genitalia equal 1 percent.

The diagnosis is based on the area of involvement and depth. For example, a person with burns of the right arm and upper chest that involve the epidermis and dermis might be written as partial thickness burns over 23 percent of the body.

Treatment. Initial first aid involves:

■ Ice and cold water to relieve discomfort for first degree burns only.
■ Immediate medical attention when full thickness burns or large areas are involved or burns involve face, hands, feet, or genital area.
■ Notification of the medical facility that a burned person is on the way. Give, if possible,

the extent and cause of the burn.

Once in the medical facility, the care will involve:

■ Assessment of the burn damage
■ Analgesia for pain
■ Management of fluids and electrolytes
■ Clean technique using cap, gown, mask, and gloves
■ Complete reverse isolation technique in some cases
■ Monitoring the patient for respiratory distress, shock, and anemia
■ Cleaning of the burned areas and removal of all debris
■ Application of topical antibiotics
■ Emotional support

Some hospitals have established burn centers where specially trained personnel care for burn cases. One of two approaches is in common use:

■ Open method—the burns are left uncovered. Sterile technique, also called reverse isolation technique, is used to care for the patient.
■ Closed method—the burns are covered by special ointments, wrapped in layers of gauze. The part is checked for circulation distal to the dressing and maintained in proper alignment.

New techniques such as keeping the patient submerged in a silicone solution are also being used. Each method has its advantages and disadvantages. There are four goals of treatment, whatever method is selected:

1. Replacement of lost fluids and electrolytes to combat shock.
2. Relief of pain and anxiety.
3. Prevention of contractures, deformities, and infections. Contractures are shortening of muscles, which limits motion and causes deformities. Plastic surgery may also be required.
4. Provision of emotional support and motivation.

Nursing Assistant Care. Special care emphasizes:

■ Reporting pain so that appropriate analgesics may be prescribed and given.
■ Maintaining proper alignment.
■ Gentle positioning, as ordered, to prevent contractures.
   NOTE: The burn patient may be on a Circ-o-lectric® bed, Stryker frame, or Clinitron® bed to permit frequent rotation to relieve pressure.
■ Encouraging a high-protein diet.
■ Carefully measuring intake and output.
■ Giving emotional support and encouragement.
■ Carrying out procedures that prevent infection.

SUMMARY

- The condition of the skin indicates the general health of the body. These conditions are revealed through skin:
  - Color
  - Texture
  - Lesions or eruptions
- Decubitus ulcers result from pressure on one area of the body that interferes with circulation. Decubiti:
  - Are more easily prevented than cured.
  - May occur in any patient.
  - Occur in stages which are recognizable and treatable.

- Burns:
  - Are classified according to the depth of tissue damage.
  - Require special care, often in burn centers.
- Burn therapy involves:
  - Analgesics for pain
  - Infection control
  - Replacement of lost fluids and electrolytes
  - Possible skin grafting to repair injured tissue
  - Position changes and support to prevent contractures and deformities

UNIT REVIEW

A. True/False. Answer the following statements true or false by circling T or F.

T F 1. Obesity is a predisposing cause of decubiti formation.

T F 2. The sacrum is a common site for the development of decubiti.

T F 3. To avoid decubiti, change the patient's position at least every two hours.

T F 4. If an area is reddened, massage directly over the area.

T F 5. The nails and hair are part of the integumentary system.

T F 6. When only the epidermis is damaged by burning, the patient experiences no pain.

T F 7. When using the Rule of Nines to assess burn damage, the anterior trunk is given a value of 9 percent.

T F 8. When both the dermis and epidermis are damaged by burns, blisters are apt to form.

T F 9. Reverse isolation technique is used when the closed method of burn treatment is prescribed.

T F 10. The burned patient needs great emotional support.

B. Matching. Match Column I with Column II.

Column I	Column II
_____ 11. redness	a. decubitus ulcer
_____ 12. skin	b. rubra
_____ 13. thick leathery covering that forms in severe burns	c. tactile sense
	d. emollient
	e. integument
_____ 14. bedsore	f. obese
_____ 15. feeling	g. eschar
_____ 16. flat, discolored spots, as in measles	h. crusts
	i. exoriations
_____ 17. raised spots filled with watery fluid	j. vesicles
_____ 18. large, raised area associated with itching, as in hives	k. papules
	l. macules
_____ 19. areas of dried body secretions such as scabs	m. wheals
_____ 20. portions of skin seem to be scraped or scratched away	

C. Multiple Choice. Choose the answer that best completes each of the following sentences by circling the proper letter.

21. Flat discolored spots such as those seen in measles are:
    - a. pustules.
    - b. macules.
    - c. papules.
    - d. vesicles.

22. Raised spots filled with fluid, such as blisters, are called:
    - a. pustules.
    - b. macules.
    - c. papules.
    - d. vesicles.

23. Anaphylactic shock is:
    - a. a severe sensitivity reaction.
    - b. never fatal.
    - c. a communicable disease.
    - d. associated with partial thickness burns.

24. When caring for patients with skin lesions:
    - a. rub the skin vigorously.
    - b. use soap and water when bathing.
    - c. do not attempt to remove any crusts.
    - d. use rubbing lotion.

25. You are instructed to give an emollient bath. Remember to:
    - a. have the water temperature about 105–110°F.
    - b. allow the patient to soak 2 hours.
    - c. rub the patient's skin to be sure the patient is adequately dried.
    - d. apply lotion by patting, if ordered.

D. Completion. Complete the following statements in the space provided.

26. Emollient baths are given to _____ _____

27. Three nursing assistant actions related to the care of patients with skin lesions are:
    - a. _____
    - b. _____
    - c. _____

28. Three diagnostic tests used to identify skin-related lesions are:
    - a. _____
    - b. _____
    - c. _____

29. Five patients at risk for the development of decubitus ulcers are:
    - a. _____
    - b. _____
    - c. _____
    - d. _____
    - e. _____

30. Name five common sites of decubitus formation.
    - a. _____
    - b. _____
    - c. _____
    - d. _____
    - e. _____

31. It is especially important to encourage proper nutrition and fluids in patients who have decubitus ulcers because _____ _____

32. Excessive use of cornstarch can be a problem because_____ _____

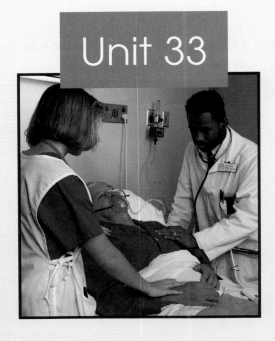

Unit 33

The Respiratory System and Common Disorders

Before beginning to study this unit, return to Unit 4 and review pages 49–52.

Remember, life cannot be maintained without oxygen, and carbon dioxide must be eliminated from the body. Diseases of the respiratory tract, Figure 33–1, that interfere with the vital exchange of oxygen and carbon dioxide bring acute distress. Nursing care is directed toward making breathing easier and preventing transmission of infection.

Patients with respiratory disease, even in pediatrics, should be taught to:

- Cover the nose and mouth when coughing or sneezing.

502

- Dispose of soiled tissues by placing them in a plastic or paper sack to be burned.
- Turn face away from others when coughing or sneezing.
- Wash hands after handling soiled tissues.

You must especially take note of and report, Figure 33–2:

- Dyspnea (difficult breathing)
- Changes in rate and rhythm of respiration
- Presence and character of respiratory secretions
- Any cough
- Changes in skin color or color of secretions

Upper Respiratory Infections (URI)

An **upper respiratory infection (URI)** follows invasion of the upper respiratory organs by microbes. The upper respiratory organs include the nose, sinuses, and throat. A common cold, which is caused by a virus, is an example of an upper respiratory infection. It is one of the most ordinary illnesses found in people. Symptoms include:

- Elevated temperature (fever)
- Runny nose
- Watery eyes

This usually self-limiting disease is best treated by:

- Use of an **antipyretic** (drug to reduce fever) such as acetaminophen
- Rest
- Increased fluid intake

URIs sometimes move down into the chest and develop into bronchitis or even pneumonia.

Pneumonia

Pneumonia is a serious inflammation of the lungs. It can be caused by a variety of infectious organisms. Three common causes of pneumonia are:

- viruses
- *Streptococcus pneumoniae* (a bacterium)
- *Pneumocystis carinii* (a protozoan)

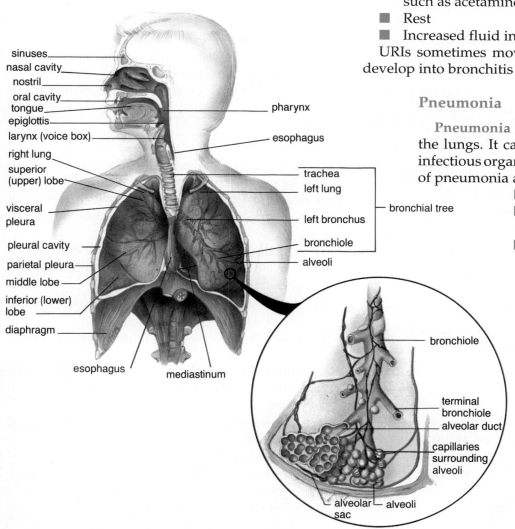

FIGURE 33–1. The respiratory system *(From Anatomy and Physiology Plates, copyright 1992 by Delmar Publishers Inc.)*

- ■ Difficulty breathing
- ■ Cough
- ■ Cyanosis
- ■ Pallor
- ■ Shortness of Breath (SOB)

FIGURE 33–2.   Reportables for the respiratory system

Pneumocystis carinii is most often seen in people who have poorly functioning immune systems. Today, most pneumonias, though serious and potentially life-threatening, respond favorably to antibiotic therapy.

Chronic Obstructive Pulmonary Disease

Chronic obstructive pulmonary disease (COPD) refers to any chronic lung disease that results in the blocking of the bronchial airways. Chronic pulmonary inflammation results in narrowing and irreversible damage to the bronchioles and alveoli and the pulmonary blood vessels. There is an increasing loss of lung elasticity.

Several conditions develop into COPD. They include asthma, bronchitis, and emphysema.

Increased levels of carbon dioxide usually stimulate respirations. People with COPD, however, adjust to high levels of carbon dioxide. Eventually they depend on special receptors that are sensitive to low levels of oxygen for respiratory stimulus (hypoxic drive).

If too much oxygen is given to the patient (flow rates are too high), the hypoxic drive is lost. For this reason, patients with COPD are usually given oxygen at 1–2 L/min.

Asthma

Asthma is the result of a sensitivity to an allergen. Other factors such as conditional stress may also cause an episode. The body responds by:

- ■ Increasing mucus production in the air passageways.
- ■ Producing spasms in the bronchial musculature.
- ■ Causing the mucous membrane lining the respiratory tract to swell.

The flow of air is obstructed on expiration. The patient experiences dyspnea and wheezing. Long-

term treatment consists of determining the allergen and eliminating it. To relieve the attack, the patient is given medication to decrease the swelling and **dilate** (enlarge) the bronchioles. Low levels of oxygen are also generally administered in the hospital. Chronic asthma leads to COPD.

Bronchitis

Chronic **bronchitis** develops from frequent infections or chronic irritations of the respiratory tract such as occur with smokers. It, too, can ultimately result in COPD.

Chronic bronchitis is characterized by:

- ■ Excessive mucus secretions in the bronchi
- ■ Thickened, reddened bronchial walls
- ■ Chronic, recurrent, productive cough

Treatment, in general, includes:

- ■ Antibiotics to combat infection
- ■ Drugs to loosen the **phlegm** (secretions from deep in the respiratory tract)
- ■ Techniques to improve ventilation and drainage

Emphysema

Almost 20,000 Americans die of emphysema every year. The number of cases is increasing. This condition develops gradually, usually over a period of years. Characteristics of **emphysema** include the following:

- ■ The tiny alveoli lose some of their elasticity.
- ■ The alveoli cannot become smaller as they should during expiration.
- ■ A portion of carbon dioxide remains trapped in the alveoli.
- ■ There is less possibility of good gas exchange.

As a result:

- ■ Interference with the exchange in the lungs puts additional strain on the blood vessels and heart.
- ■ The heart may enlarge under the strain and then fail.
- ■ These patients are susceptible to infections.
- ■ Expiration is difficult so that patients with emphysema characteristically lean forward with shoulders raised as they try to force the carbon dioxide out of their lungs, Figure 33–3.

General Care. The care of the emphysema patient includes all the care required of any patient with COPD:

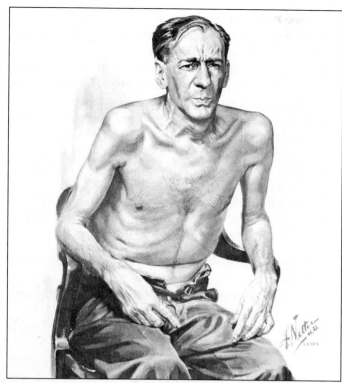

FIGURE 33–3. Characteristic posture of patient with emphysema. The patient leans forward on his arms and purses his lips. *(©Copyright 1968, CIBA-GEIGY Corporation. Reproduced with permission, from the Clinical Symposia, illustrated by Frank H. Netter, M.D. All rights reserved.)*

- Assisting with the proper breathing techniques such as pursed lip breathing
- Encouraging breathing exercises
- Positioning to improve ventilation
- Assisting with use of incentive spirometer
- Assisting with postural drainage
- Providing care during low flow oxygen therapy
- Paying attention to nutrition and fluid intake
- Treating infections with antibiotics and drugs to loosen and thin respiratory secretions
- Encouraging patients to avoid crowds, especially during the flu season
- Encouraging patients not to go out of doors when the temperature is 35°F–40°F or lower since the cold can trigger spasms
- Encouraging patients not to smoke
- Maintaining humidity with a room humidifier if ordered

Tuberculosis

In recent years, there has been an increase in the number of people diagnosed with tuberculosis.

Many people were infected with the tuberculosis organism in their younger years. Now that they are elderly, the disease has reactivated. Many patients with HIV infection are diagnosed with tuberculosis. For those with compromised immune systems, tuberculosis is an opportunistic infection.

Tuberculosis is one of the oldest known diseases. It still ranks highly as a cause of death. It is caused by microorganisms that are transmitted to others by droplets from sneezing and coughing. The organisms usually attack the lungs, but other parts of the body may also be invaded.

Tuberculosis Infection. When the organisms first enter the body, the body responds by walling off the germs with special protective white blood cells. A walled-off area is called a tubercle. The organisms are not necessarily destroyed but may remain alive within the tubercle. The person is said to have a tuberculosis infection. As long as the organisms remain walled off, they are not transmitted to others and the condition is arrested (contained).

Tuberculosis Disease. If there are many organisms or if the resistance of the person being infected is low, then not all of the organisms are walled off. In this case, the organisms spread, resulting in damage to the lungs or other body organs. The person is said to have tuberculosis disease.

Tuberculosis may also develop later in a person with an arrested case. Malnutrition, debilitation, aging, or HIV infection lower the resistance of the person and the organisms are no longer contained but spread, causing further damage to the body.

Not all cases of tuberculosis make people feel ill. A tubercle may be formed without the person knowing it. Therefore, it is important to:
- Perform a skin test to learn if infection is present.
- Health care workers are skin tested before employment and yearly thereafter to be sure they are infection free. Residents in long-term care are also skin tested yearly.
- Improve the overall health of the patient.
- Treat the patient with drugs until the disease process is arrested. Drugs must be taken regularly for many months.
- Prevent transmission to others.

Signs of tuberculosis disease include:
- Fatigue
- Hemoptysis (spitting of blood)
- Fever
- Night sweats
- Weight loss
- Coughing

Respiratory precautions are carried out when patients have a diagnosis of tuberculosis disease.

Diagnostic Techniques

Some techniques used to diagnose problems of the respiratory system include:
- Tissue biopsy (microscopic examination of specimen of tissue removed from patient)
- Cultures of secretions
- Volume studies that measure the amount of air entering or leaving the lungs during different respiratory movements
- Radiographic techniques such as X-rays, CAT scans, and MRIs
- Direct visualization procedures such as bronchoscopy

Special Therapies Related to Respiratory Illness

Oxygen Therapy

Oxygen is often ordered by the physician. Remember that when oxygen is in use, special precautions are required to prevent fires and to administer the oxygen safely. Information about general fire control is presented in Unit 11.

Fire Safety. The following safety measures must be emphasized in areas where oxygen is being used:
- Be certain that there are no open flames and that no one smokes or has matches.
- Provide a hand call bell.
- Post no smoking or oxygen-in-use signs.
- Remove unneeded electrical equipment.
- Use cotton bedspread, blanket, bed linens, and gown or pajamas.
- Before using electrically operated equipment discontinue the flow of oxygen (only after obtaining approval of the charge nurse).

In Case of Fire. If a fire breaks out, the safety of the patient is most important.
- Sound the alarm by using the call board that connects to the switchboard.
- Manual alarms close by may also be activated, but do not leave the unit to find one.
- If you have been trained in the use of a fire extinguisher, you may use it on small fires.
- Move the patients out of the area as quickly as possible. Bed patients are moved in their beds.

Ambulatory patients need to be escorted and directed to safety. Patients closest to the fire are moved to safety first.
- Be prepared to follow instructions when someone in authority assumes control. In the meantime, carry out the policies of your facility.
- Once the patients are safe, go back to the unit and check to be sure the oxygen is shut off and electrical equipment is disconnected.
- Shut doors and fire doors if they are part of the safety equipment.
- Be sure to keep all exits accessible.
- In all situations, get patients to safety, follow facility policy, and keep calm.

Giving Oxygen. Patients may receive oxygen by one of several methods:
- Nasal cannulas: small tubes placed at the entrance to the nose, Figure 33–4.
- Nasal catheter: a small plastic or rubber tube that is inserted into the nose, Figure 33–5.
- Mask: cuplike mask held in place over the nose and mouth by hand or by straps around the head, Figure 33–6.
- Tent method, Figure 33–7.
- Intermittent positive pressure breathing (IPPB): Oxygen is administered intermittently under pressure by professional personnel such as respiratory therapists, Figure 33–8. This technique helps to expand the lungs.

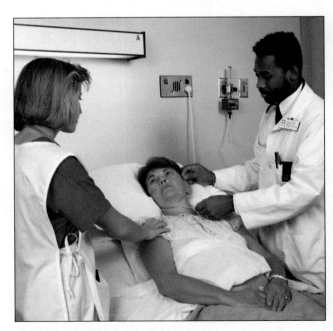

FIGURE 33–4. Oxygen administered by nasal cannula

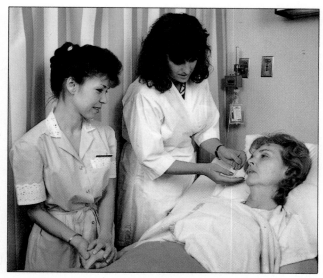

FIGURE 33–5. Oxygen administration by nasal catheter

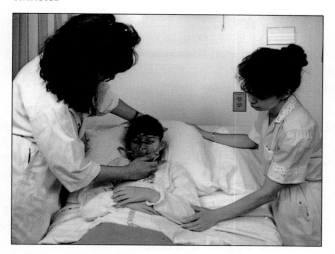

FIGURE 33–6. Oxygen administration by mask

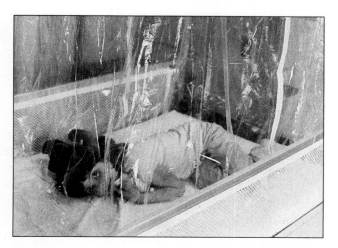

FIGURE 33–7. Oxygen may be administered by means of a tent.

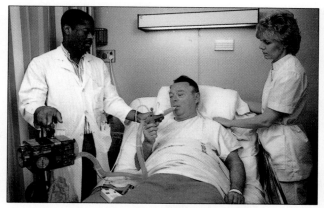

FIGURE 33–8. Oxygen administration by intermittent positive pressure breathing (IPPB)

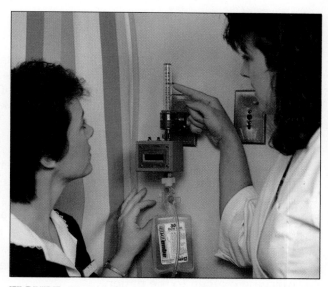

FIGURE 33–9. Oxygen generally is piped directly into each patient's unit.

Maintaining an Oxygen Source. Some hospitals have oxygen piped from wall units directly into the patient's room, Figure 33–9. In others, the oxygen source is a tank that is brought to the patient's room when therapy is ordered, Figure 33–10. The amount of oxygen (rate of flow measured in liters) is ordered by the physician. You should:

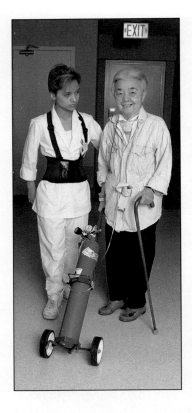

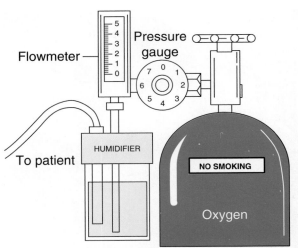

FIGURE 33–11. Note attachment of flowmeter gauge to oxygen tank. Check flowmeter and gauge whenever the patient is receiving oxygen. Note that the tank is green. Tanks of gas are color coded for safety.

FIGURE 33–10. Patients can be ambulatory by using small portable tanks of oxygen attached to a mask or nasal cannula.

- Know the rate that has been ordered and set for your patient if instructed to do so by the nurse.
- Notify the nurse immediately if you find a change in the rate.
- Be able to read the flow rate meter.
- Be sure there are no obstructions in the tube carrying oxygen to the patient.

If a tank is used as an oxygen source, be sure that:

- There is sufficient oxygen. Check the gauge, Figure 33–11, each time you go to the bedside.
- An additional oxygen tank is readily available for the exchange.
- Empty tanks are marked and returned promptly to the proper area for refilling.
- The tank is secure and cannot fall. Straps may hold it to the bed or it may be held in a tank holder.

Maintaining Moisture. Pure oxygen is very drying and thus is damaging to tissues. Therefore, oxygen should be moisturized by passing it through water before reaching the patient. Water is used for this purpose. Be sure the level of water is maintained in accord with your facility policy. Since many patients with respiratory difficulty breathe through their mouths, special attention to mouth care is essential.

Methods of Oxygen Delivery. As previously mentioned, oxygen may be delivered to the patient by several different methods. The same basic care is required for each method, with modifications.

Nasal Cannula. Delivery of oxygen by nasal cannula is the most common method used today. The oxygen is delivered through a tube that has two small plastic prongs or nipples. The prongs are placed at the entrance to the patient's nose. A strap around the patient's head holds the prongs in place.

- Make sure the strap is secure but not too tight.
- Check for signs of irritation where the prongs touch the patient's nose.
- Check that mucus has not blocked the prong openings. Clean if necessary.

The Mask.

- Place mask over nose and mouth.
- Be sure the straps are secure but not too tight.
- Periodically remove the mask. Wash area under it. Dry carefully.

The Nasal Catheter.

- Keep patient's face free of any nasal discharge.
- Make sure that there are no kinks or undue pressure on the tubing. Tape is used to secure the catheter at the nose and temple. A linen tunnel around the tube allows for patient mobility.

Mistogen® Units (Croupettes). A croupette is a small, portable unit similar to the oxygen tent. The croupette:

- Is used to provide oxygen and a high degree of humidity at a cool temperature for children and babies.
- May cover the entire baby or just the head and shoulders of an older child.
- Requires the same precautions as other methods.
- May or may not have a canopy across the top.

Babies and children in Mistogen® units may suffer sensory deprivation. They need additional attention and care. In selecting toys for them, be sure to consider toys that will not soak up moisture, are not mechanical, and are not made of wool.

NOTE: Oxygen, being heavier than air, accumulates in the bottom of the unit. Ice is kept in the back of some units to maintain a lowered temperature.

The Oxygen Tent.

- Place a rubber cover over the mattress to prevent loss of oxygen and moisture through it.
- Check plastic canopy for leaks.
- Be sure oxygen is turned on before patient is covered with the canopy and patient is out of the tent before turning oxygen off.
- Tuck in the canopy under the mattress to prevent leakage.
- Secure the canopy across the front of the bed:
  — Place an additional sheet folded lengthwise over bed with the opening of the fold toward the patient.
  — Place the open end of the canopy between the folds.
  — Tuck the edges of the sheet under the sides of the mattress.
- Work quickly through zippered openings.

NOTE: The oxygen tent is usually used today only when cooling, in addition to oxygen, is needed.

Respiratory Positions

Positioning of the patient to permit expansion of the lungs and a straightened airway is helpful to patients with respiratory distress.

High Fowler's Position. In the high Fowler's position, the patient is in a sitting position with the backrest elevated, Figure 33–12.

- Position three pillows behind the patient's head and shoulders. Adjust knee rest.
- Keep feet in proper position.
- Check for signs of skin breakdown over coccyx due to shearing forces.

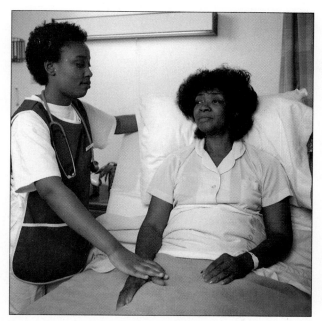

FIGURE 33–12. Note the patient is in a high Fowler's position.

Orthopneic Position. The orthopneic position may be used as an alternative to the high Fowler's position, Figure 33–13.

- The position of the bed remains the same.
- The bedside table is brought across the bed and a pillow or two are placed on top.
- The patient leans forward across the table with arms on or beside the pillows.
- Another pillow is placed low behind the patient's back for support.

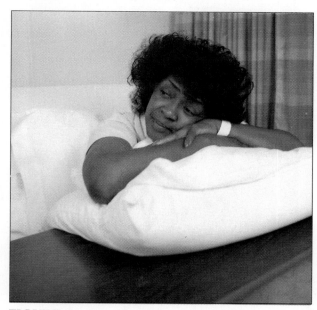

FIGURE 33–13. The orthopneic position

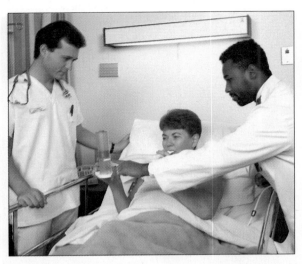

FIGURE 33–14. Breathing exercises using an incentive spirometer

Breathing Exercises

The nurse or respiratory therapist teaches the breathing exercises. You may be asked to assist with them. In each of the following exercises, the patient blows with pursed lips to increase the expiratory phase. The exercises ordered may be:

- Blowing against water resistance.
- Blowing a feather or ping pong ball across the table.

- Incentive spirometry, Figure 33–14. For a complete description of this therapy, see Unit 27.

Other Techniques

Aerosol Therapy

Nebulizers deliver moisture or medication deep into the lungs. Drugs that thin the mucus (mucolytics) or dilate the bronchi are often prescribed. The stream of moisture or medication may be delivered by a hand-held nebulizer or driven by oxygen, compressed air, or compressor pump, Figure 33–15. The medication may be given in conjunction with an intermittent positive pressure breathing (IPPB) machine. If oxygen is used, the rate of administration and the depth of the patient's respirations must be carefully monitored. The treatment must be stopped if the respiratory rate and rhythm decrease by 25 percent.

Concentrations of 100 percent oxygen delivered continuously for 5 to 10 minutes can have a depressing effect on respirations. This is particularly hazardous to patients suffering from COPD.

After administering the mucolytics, nurses and therapists use various techniques to loosen the mucus and clear the air passageways.

- Chest tapping (also called percussion)—a technique of striking the chest with the tips of the fingers with hands cupped to loosen secretions, Figure 33–16.

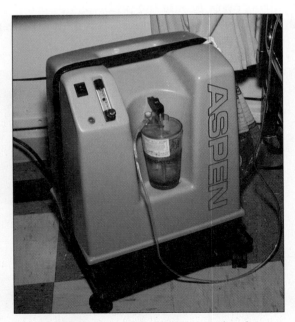

FIGURE 33–15. Nebulizers may be driven by compressed air instead of oxygen.

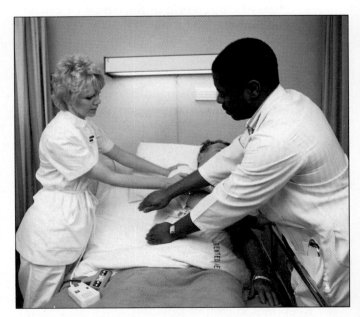

FIGURE 33–16. The nursing assistant helps position the patient as the therapist performs chest tapping to loosen secretions.

The patient may perform chest tapping on himself/herself, but you will have to be sure that the patient is safe as position is changed and maintained.

■ Postural drainage—positioning the patient either on the bed or on a tilt table to encourage drainage from the respiratory tree, Figure 33–17.

Postural drainage requires close supervision to avoid injury to the patient as different positions are assumed.

■ Suctioning to remove loose secretions. If suctioning is used, it must be performed gently. You can help by providing comfort to the patient as a nurse or respiratory therapist carries out the procedure. Suctioning is considered to be an advanced procedure (see Unit 43) and is performed only by those specially trained to do so.

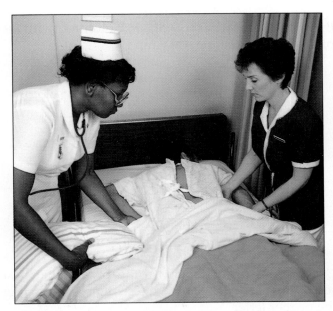

FIGURE 33–17. A pillow placed under the patient's abdomen helps drain the chest.

SUMMARY

The organs of respiration function to take in and exchange oxygen and output carbon dioxide. Diseases that affect the respiratory tract make breathing difficult. These conditions include:

■ Upper respiratory infections
■ Chronic obstructive pulmonary diseases (COPD)

Special techniques which can make breathing easier include:

■ Oxygen therapy
■ Incentive spirometry
■ Chest tapping
■ Postural drainage
■ Suctioning
■ Positioning
■ Mouth care

Special precautions must be taken to avoid transmission of disease. These precautions include handwashing, disposing of soiled tissues, and avoiding coughing and sneezing in the direction of others. Observations that need to be reported and documented include:

■ Rate and rhythm of respiration
■ Changes in skin color
■ Character and presence of respiratory secretions
■ Cough, including character. For example, amount, color, and odor of sputum, if present

UNIT REVIEW

A. True/False. Answer the following statements true or false by circling T or F.

T F 1. In asthma, there is increased production of mucus which blocks the respiratory tract.

T F 2. Antipyretic drugs fight infection.

T F 3. An allergen causes a sensitivity reaction.

T F 4. URI stands for underrated respiratory injections.

T F 5. Patients with tuberculosis always show signs and symptoms such as cough and weight loss.

T F 6. Always post a sign when oxygen is in use.

T F 7. The oxygen flow rate is ordered by the physician.

T F 8. Oxygen should always be moisturized before reaching the patient.

T F 9. When oxygen is administered by mask, make sure the straps are very tight.

T F 10. In the high Fowler's position, the patient leans forward across the over-bed table.

B. Matching. Match the word in Column II with the phrase or statement in Column I.

Column I   Column II

_____ 11. inflammation of   a. emphysema
           the lungs
                                    b. hemoptysis
_____ 12. an example of
           COPD   c. pneumonia

_____ 13. difficult breathing   d. dyspnea

_____ 14. controlled   e. spirometer

_____ 15. spitting up blood   f. arrested

                                    g. tubercle

C. Multiple Choice. Choose the phrase that best completes each of the following sentences by circling the proper letter.

16. Patients with respiratory disease should
    a. cover the nose and mouth when coughing.
    b. turn face toward others when sneezing.
    c. wash hands only after toileting.
    d. dispose of soiled tissues by dropping them in the nearest trash can.

17. When oxygen is in use
    a. allow smoking near an oxygen tent.
    b. provide electric signal cords.
    c. use cotton blankets.
    d. discontinue the flow of oxygen before using a safety razor.

18. You should know that
    a. patients receiving oxygen do not require special mouth care.
    b. oxygen need not be humidified when a mask is used.
    c. oxygen need not be moisturized when administered with a nasal catheter.
    d. oxygen is very drying to tissues.

19. When your patient is receiving oxygen, you should
    a. monitor intake and output.
    b. know the ordered rate.
    c. check the flow rate once each shift.
    d. check the flow rate every three hours.

20. When administering oxygen by mask, in addition to routine care and precautions, you should
    a. make sure straps are not too tight.
    b. periodically remove the mask to wash and dry under it.
    c. make sure mask covers nose and mouth.
    d. All of the above.

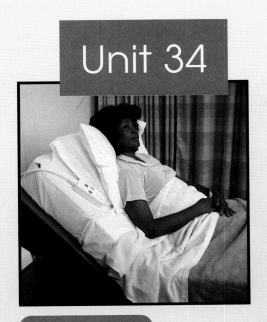

Unit 34

The Circulatory (Cardiovascular) System and Common Disorders

The circulatory or cardiovascular system may be thought of as a transportation system. It takes nourishment and oxygen to the cells and carries away carbon dioxide and other waste products. The system is kept in motion by the force of the heartbeat. Diseases that attack any part of this system interfere with the overall function. Before studying this unit, you may wish to review Unit 4.

Remember, the circulatory system is a continuous network made up of the:

■ Heart—central pumping station, Figure 34–1

■ Blood vessels, Figures 34–2A, 2B, and 34–3

■ Lymphatic vessels   ■ Spleen

■ Lymph nodes   ■ Blood

Diseases of this system are very common. Longstanding diseases of the cardiovascular system are eventually reflected in the pulmonary and renal systems as well.

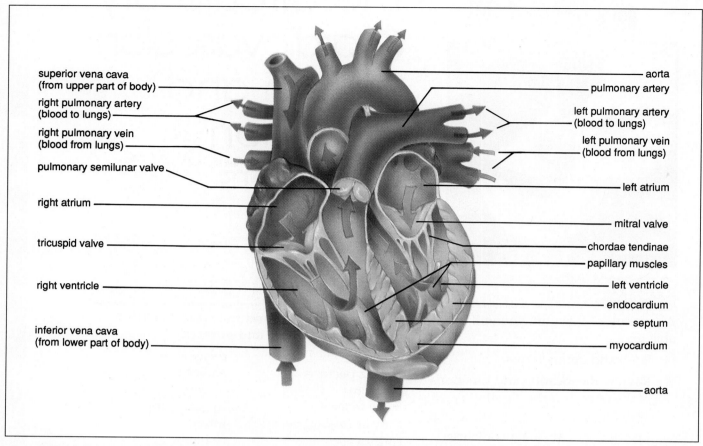

FIGURE 34–1. In this schematic representation of the heart, the red arrows show the circulation of oxygen-rich blood from the lungs. The blue arrows show the circulation of oxygen-poor blood returning from the body.

Diagnostic Tests

Some techniques used to diagnose problems of the cardiovascular system include:

- Blood chemistry tests, such as electrolyte panels
- Complete blood cell counts (CBC)
- Electrocardiograms (ECG or EKG)
- Cardiac catheterization and angiogram—introduction of catheter and dyes into the vascular system under fluoroscopy
- Ultrasound—sound waves are bounced against tissues to reflect variations in tissue density

Common Conditions

Diseases of this system include:

- Diseases relating to the blood vessels.
- Diseases of the heart.
- Blood **dyscrasias** (abnormalities). These diseases can involve the bone/bone marrow, liver, or spleen.

Refer to Figure 34–4 for the observations the nursing assistant is to report in patients with disorders of the circulatory system.

Peripheral Vascular Diseases

The blood vessels that serve the outer parts of the body, particularly those of the hands and feet, are referred to as **peripheral** (toward the outer part) blood vessels. Diseases of these vessels affect parts of the body through which they pass. The health of these vessels also influences the heart function.

Peripheral vascular diseases that affect the arteries diminish the flow of blood to the extremities. Tissues, through which the narrowed arteries pass, may not be getting the nourishment they need. Areas affected are the extremities: namely the arms, legs, and brain. The signs and symptoms associated with decreased peripheral circulation are:

- Coldness
- Tingling sensation
- Loss of sensitivity

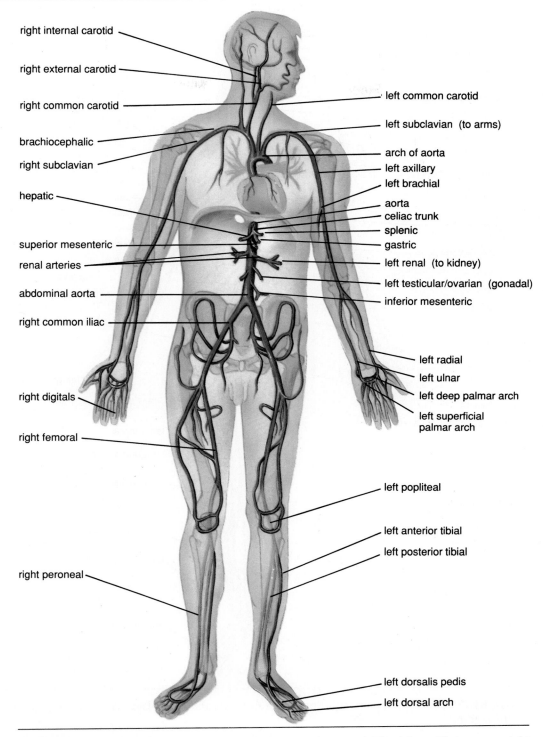

right internal carotid

right external carotid

right common carotid

brachiocephalic

right subclavian

hepatic

superior mesenteric

renal arteries

abdominal aorta

right common iliac

right digitals

right femoral

right peroneal

left common carotid

left subclavian (to arms)

arch of aorta

left axillary

left brachial

aorta

celiac trunk

splenic

gastric

left renal (to kidney)

left testicular/ovarian (gonadal)

inferior mesenteric

left radial

left ulnar

left deep palmar arch

left superficial palmar arch

left popliteal

left anterior tibial

left posterior tibial

left dorsalis pedis

left dorsal arch

FIGURE 34–2A. Arterial circulation (*From Anatomy and Physiology Plates, copyright 1992 by Delmar Publishers Inc.*)

Treatment is aimed at:

■ Increasing local circulation

— Positioning and specific prescribed exercises can promote arterial flow and venous return.

— Sometimes an oscillating (rocking) bed is employed to improve the circulatory flow.

The oscillating bed rocks up and down in cycles, raising the patient's feet 6 inches above his head and then lowering them 12–15 inches. The steady rhythm provides both passive exercise for the patient and some circulatory stimulation.

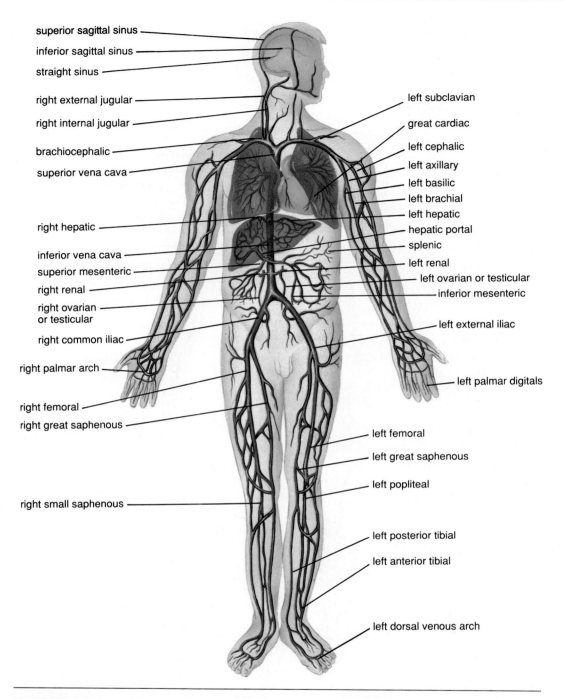

FIGURE 34–2B. Venous circulation *(From Anatomy and Physiology Plates, copyright 1992 by Delmar Publishers Inc.)*

— Permit nothing that would hamper the patient's circulation. Promptly report any new tissue breakdown.
— Discourage circular garters, crossing the legs, and exposure to cold.
— Forbid smoking.
— Discourage use of knee gatch on bed or pillows under the knees.

■ Preventing injuries that heal poorly
— Give special attention to preventing injury to the arms and legs and to preventing pressure areas, since such injuries heal poorly when circulation is limited.
— Supply warmth by increasing the room temperature and using lightweight blankets and well-fitting, warm socks.

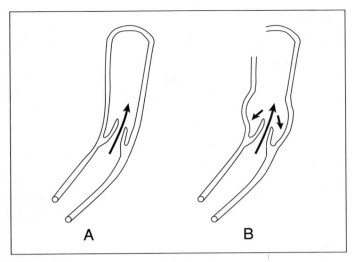

FIGURE 34–3. Vein with normal valve (A) and vein with weakened valve and varicosity (B)

— Avoid the use of hot water bottles because these patients may not realize they are being burned.

Atherosclerosis

Atherosclerosis is a common form of vascular disease.

■ Roughened areas known as atheromas, which are growths developed over deposits of fatty materials, form on the vascular walls and narrow the vessels.

■ The vessels of the heart and brain, and those leading to the legs from the body are often affected.

■ The atheromas gradually grow larger until they eventually block blood flow to the parts and organs served by the affected vessels.

■ Sometimes clots that have formed over the

■ Color change, pallor or cyanosis, redness

■ Cool to touch

■ Hot to touch

■ Changes in pulse rate or rhythm

■ Changes in blood pressure

■ Edema

■ Disorientation

FIGURE 34–4. The nursing assistant is expected to report these observations in patients with disorders of the circulatory system.

---

irregular areas in the vessel walls break off and travel as emboli to block distant vessels.

■ The narrowing of vessels can lead to serious complications such as:
— Formation of blood clots
— Angina pectoris
— Myocardial infarct (MI)
— Strokes (CVA)
— Gangrene

The exact cause of this vascular disease is unknown, but several factors seem to predispose to its development. These factors include:

■ Hypertension
■ Diabetes mellitus
■ Overweight
■ Heredity
■ Smoking
■ Stress
■ Lack of exercise
■ Diets high in cholesterol and fats

Treatment includes:

■ Exercise
■ Proper diet
■ Reduction of stress
■ Control of smoking and obesity *fat*

Hypertension

Hypertension is another name for high blood pressure. It may have no known origin or it may follow illnesses that affect such organs as the:

■ Blood vessels
■ Kidneys
■ Liver

High blood pressure:

■ Promotes the development of atherosclerosis, which further narrows the vessels. This increases the blood pressure even more.
■ Increases the stress on the heart.
■ Increases the damage to the blood vessel walls so they are more apt to rupture.
■ Further limits the blood flow to the organs of the body.

Treatment may consist of:

■ Drugs that lower the blood pressure
■ Diets low in sodium and that promote weight loss
■ Discouraging smoking
■ Surgical sympathectomy (a procedure in which the nerves that cause blood vessels to constrict are cut. When the nerves are cut, the blood vessels dilate.)

■ Teaching the patient to practice moderation in lifestyle
■ Biofeedback techniques to lower the blood pressure

Angina Pectoris

Angina pectoris is known as cardiac "pain of effort." You will recall that the blood vessels nourishing the heart are the coronary arteries. These vessels often are the site of atherosclerotic changes. In an angina attack, the vessels are unable to carry enough blood to meet the demand of the heart for oxygen. This may develop:

■ Gradually over a period of time as atheromas develop.
■ Suddenly, as the vessels constrict.

Factors that precipitate (bring on) an attack include:
■ Exertion
■ Heavy eating
■ Emotional stress

Treatment consists of:
■ Diagnosing hidden causes. A treadmill stress test is one method for doing this.
■ Teaching the patient to avoid stress and sudden exertions.
■ Drugs that relax the coronary arteries.
■ Coronary artery bypass surgery.
■ Angioplasty, a surgical procedure to open the vessels.

Heart Conditions

Myocardial Infarction (Coronary Heart Attack)

The term myocardial infarction (MI), or heart attack, refers to a period in which the heart suddenly cannot function properly. There are different kinds of heart attacks. They differ in their severity and prognosis (expected outcome). Remember that the heart is muscle tissue and may become tired just as any muscle may tire. The cells of the heart require nourishment and oxygen just as do all other cells.

A heart attack occurs when the coronary arteries, which nourish the heart, are blocked. Part of the heart muscle supplied by these vessels becomes ischemic (loses its blood supply). Unless circulation is restored quickly, the cells die (infarction). If too much tissue dies, the person cannot survive. Coronary heart attack is also called:

■ Coronary occlusion—blockage of coronary arteries

■ Coronary thrombosis when a thrombus (stationary blood clot) forms at the site, blocking the blood flow
■ Coronary embolism—when a moving clot or insoluble particle, an embolus, which has originated elsewhere and moved, becomes lodged in the artery

Signs and Symptoms. The signs and symptoms of a heart attack include:
■ Pain—may resemble severe indigestion. It is more often described as "crushing" chest pain which radiates to jaw and left arm, Figure 34–5.
■ Nausea.
■ Irregular pulse and respiration.
■ Perspiration.
■ Feelings of anxiety.
■ Indications of shock, which include drop in blood pressure and pallor.

Immediate treatment has saved many people. The treatment is directed toward:
■ Relieving the pain
■ Reducing heart activity
■ Altering the clotting ability of the blood
■ Administering drugs to dissolve the clot

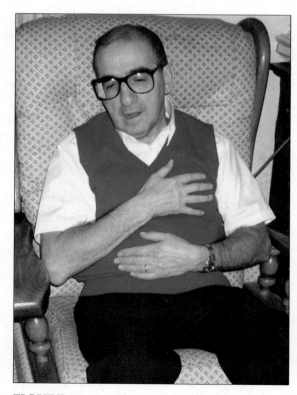

FIGURE 34–5. The patient suffering a heart attack experiences crushing chest pain that radiates.

Nursing Care. During the acute stage, heart attack patients require professional care. Many hospitals have provided intensive cardiac care units for these patients. Nursing care supports the therapy ordered. Special attention must be given to:

- Noting signs of a recurrence and reporting immediately to the nurse
- Watching for bleeding and reporting immediately
- Providing support of the activities of daily living
- Monitoring vital signs

Congestive Heart Failure (CHF)

The heart, like any other muscle, will enlarge and tire if it has to work against increasing pressure. When narrowed blood vessels due to atherosclerosis increase the resistance to blood flow and when there is severe damage to major organs like the liver and spleen, it is more difficult to maintain the circulation. The heart muscle may also have been damaged and weakened from myocardial infarction. The heart must pump harder to maintain the internal flow of blood.

- At first, the heart enlarges (hypertrophies) and makes up for (compensates) the additional workload.
- Eventually, however, it reaches a point where it can no longer compensate.
- Heart failure follows.

This form of heart disease is also known as congestive heart failure or cardiac decompensation.

Signs and Symptoms. The signs and symptoms are the result of the heart being unable to pump the blood with sufficient force.

- Edema (swelling) develops in dependent tissues and blood flow slows, congesting the vessels and allowing more fluid to enter the body spaces and tissues.
- Fluid accumulates in the lungs.
- Cyanosis occurs since fluid in the lungs makes gas exchange less efficient.
- Pulse becomes irregular and rapid.

Treatment. Treatment involves:

- Drugs to help the heart beat more strongly and regularly and to increase the output of fluids (diuresis) by the kidneys
- Low-sodium diet
- Restriction of fluids, if ordered

- Careful monitoring of I & O
- Daily weighing to monitor level of fluid retention
- Monitoring apical pulse—observing for pulse deficit, Figure 34–6
- Oxygen therapy
- Positioning patient in orthopneic position or high Fowler's to improve ventilation
- Assistance as needed with activities of daily living

Cerebrovascular accidents (CVA) is another name for strokes. This condition is dealt with in Unit 37.

Blood Abnormalities

Blood abnormalities are often called blood dyscrasias, as previously mentioned.

Anemia

Anemia is a condition that results from a decrease in the quantity or quality of red blood cells. There are several causes, such as:

- Poor diet
- Low production of new red blood cells
- Blood loss as in hemorrhage

Types of anemia include:

- Pernicious—inability to absorb vitamin B_{12} most often seen in the elderly. Vitamin B_{12} is required by the body to produce red blood cells.

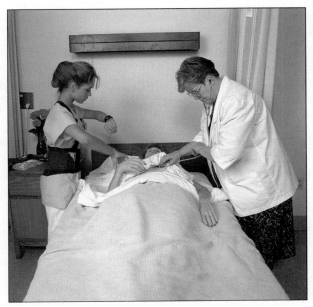

FIGURE 34–6. A pulse deficit may result from ineffective myocardial contractions.

- Sickle cell—inability to form normal hemoglobin. Sickle cell anemia is transmitted genetically. It is seen most often in blacks.
- Deficiency—inadequate intake of iron, inability to absorb iron, or excessive loss of iron.
- Dietary—inadequate intake of iron or vitamins in diet.

Signs and Symptoms. The anemic person:
- Has little energy.
- Appears pale.
- May have dyspnea.
- May experience digestive problems.
- May have a rapid pulse.

Treatment. Treatment is aimed at:
- Improving the quantity and quality of the blood by giving iron supplements
- Eliminating the basic cause of the disease
- Giving blood transfusions as needed

Nursing Care. Nursing care includes providing for:
- Rest
- Adequate diet
- Special mouth care (see Unit 21)
- Monitoring vital signs
- Prompt reporting of any signs of bleeding
- Emotional support

Leukemia

Leukemia is sometimes called cancer of the blood. The cause of the many forms of leukemia is not known. This disease may strike young or old. The number of white blood cells increases, but the white blood cells may be of poor quality. The number of erythrocytes and platelets decreases. Patients with leukemia are highly susceptible to infection. During the course of the disease, minor trauma causes bleeding.

Treatment. Treatment is aimed at:
- Easing symptoms and keeping the patient comfortable.
- Maintaining normal blood levels. Transfusions may be needed to combat the anemia that accompanies the condition.
- Combating infection by using antibiotics.
- Slowing the production of abnormal white cells through chemotherapy and/or radiation therapy.

Nursing Care. The nursing care of patients with leukemia is similar to that given to anemic patients.
- Patients are allowed to be up and care for themselves as long as possible.

- Handling must be gentle to avoid injury and bleeding.
- Special care is given to the mouth.
- When respiratory difficulties develop, special positioning and oxygen may be required.
- The nursing team provides emotional support.

SUMMARY

The cardiovascular system is the transportation system of the body.
- The heart and blood vessels make up a closed network. This network carries the blood and the products of and for metabolism.
- Diseases can affect the heart or blood vessels with a related effect on many parts of the body, especially the respiratory tract.
- Because heart disease is so prevalent, the nursing assistant will likely provide care for many cardiovascular patients.

UNIT REVIEW

A. True/False. Answer the following statements true or false by circling T or F.

T F   1. The person with atherosclerosis is encouraged to smoke.

T F   2. The treadmill test is done to detect hidden cardiac stress.

T F   3. When warmth is needed by someone with peripheral vascular disease, a hot water bottle should not be used.

T F   4. Another name for a heart attack is coronary infarction.

T F   5. In leukemia, there is an increase in white cells.

T F   6. The heart muscle shrinks as it undergoes hypertrophy.

T F   7. An embolus is a moving blood clot.

T F   8. Anemia is an example of a blood dyscrasia.

T F   9. Hypertension is best treated with a high-sodium diet.

T F   10. The person with CHF should be monitored for pulse deficit.

B. Matching. Match the words in Column II with the statement or phrase in Column I.

Column I	Column II
_____ 11. largest artery in the body	a. hypertension
	b. edema
_____ 12. death of the heart muscle	c. myocardial infarction
_____ 13. another term for stroke	d. plasma
	e. aorta
_____ 14. high blood pressure	f. CVA
_____ 15. blocking of the blood supply to the heart	g. hypotension
	h. coronary occlusion

C. Multiple Choice. Choose the phrase that best completes each of the following sentences by circling the proper letter.

16. Which of the following is not a predisposing cause of atherosclerosis?
    a. Emboli
    b. Diabetes mellitus
    c. Heredity
    d. Stress

17. You suspect the patient needs immediate attention for a possible heart attack because the person
    a. has chest pain.
    b. is perspiring profusely.
    c. feels anxious.
    d. All of the above.

18. Nursing care of the anemic person might include
    a. blood letting.
    b. transfusions.
    c. frequent checking of vital signs.
    d. Both b and c are correct.

19. The patient suffering from anemia has a
    a. high energy level.
    b. pink, rosy skin.
    c. low energy level.
    d. slower than normal respiratory rate.

20. An attack of angina pectoris could be brought about by
    a. heavy meals.
    b. physical exertion.
    c. emotional stress.
    d. All of the above.

D. Completion. Complete the following statements in the space provided.

21 Five specific tests used to diagnose cardiac, vascular or blood abnormalities are:
    a. _____
    b. _____
    c. _____
    d. _____
    e. _____

22. Six predisposing factors to atherosclerosis are:
    a. _____
    b. _____
    c. _____
    d. _____
    e. _____
    f. _____

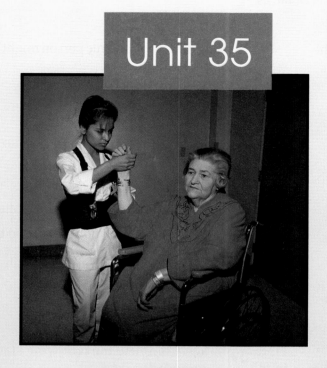

Unit 35

The Musculoskeletal System and Common Disorders

OBJECTIVES

As a result of this unit, you will be able to:

- ■ Spell and define terms.
- ■ Review the location and functions of the musculoskeletal system.
- ■ Demonstrate nursing assistant actions in performing passive range of motion (ROM) exercises.
- ■ List seven specific diagnostic tests for musculoskeletal conditions.
- ■ Describe some common diseases of the musculoskeletal system.
- ■ Describe the nursing assistant actions related to the care of patients with conditions and diseases of the musculoskeletal system.

VOCABULARY

Learn the meaning and the correct spelling of the following words:

abduction
adduction
amputation
arthritis
balanced suspension
 skeletal traction
bursitis
cartilage
cervical traction
chymopapain
closed (oblique)
 fracture
comminuted fracture
compression fracture
countertraction
degenerative joint
 disease (DJD)
dorsiflexion
eversion
flexion
fracture
fusion
greenstick fracture
hyperextension

inversion
laminectomy
open (compound)
 fracture
open reduction/
 internal fixation
osteoarthritic joint
 disease (OJD)
osteoarthritis
pelvic belt traction
phantom pain
plantar flexion
pronation
prosthesis
radial deviation
range of motion
 (ROM)
rheumatoid arthritis
rotation
spica cast
supination
trapeze
ulnar deviation
vertebrae

Before beginning to study this unit, you may wish to go back to Unit 4 and review pages 56–64. Also study Figures 35–1, 35–2, and 35–3.

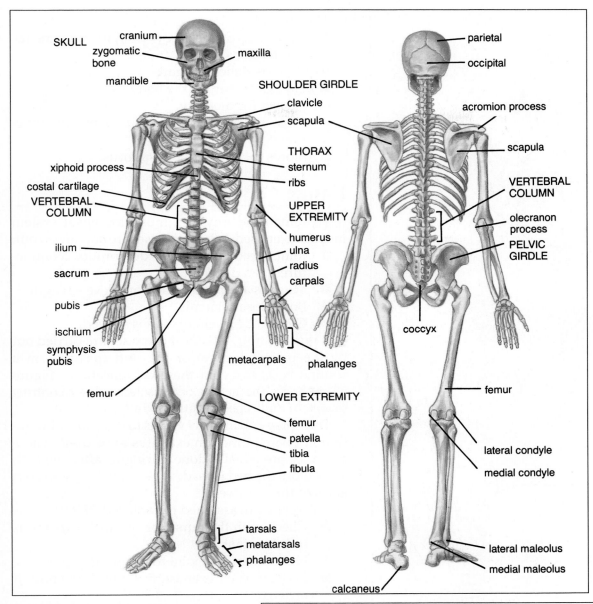

FIGURE 35–1. The human skeleton *(From Anatomy and Physiology Plates, copyright 1992 by Delmar Publishers Inc.)*

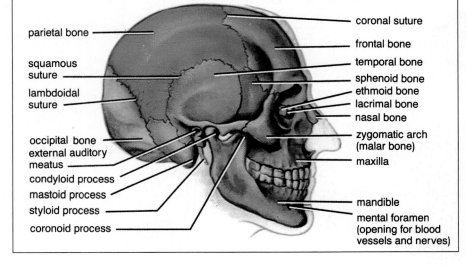

FIGURE 35–2. Bones of the skull *(From Anatomy and Physiology Plates, copyright 1992 by Delmar Publishers Inc.)*

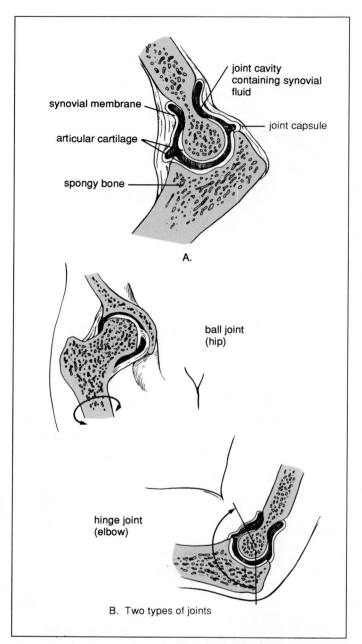

FIGURE 35–3. Parts and types of joints

The musculoskeletal system:

■ Is made up of muscles, bones, joints, ligaments, and tendons.
■ Protects delicate organs.
■ Gives structure to the body.
■ Allows for mobility.
■ Must be properly stressed to remain functional.
■ Stores calcium and phosphorus.

Range of Motion

To remain healthy, the musculoskeletal system must be exercised. When exercises are not carried out:

■ Joints become stiff and deformities (contractures) can develop.
■ Muscles atrophy (shrink) and lose strength.
■ Bones lose minerals.
■ General body circulation is slowed.

Range of motion (ROM) exercises are carried out by the patient (active) or the staff (passive) on a routine basis to avoid these complications. Figure 35–4 shows the action of muscles as they contract (shorten) and relax (lengthen) due to exercise.

The nurse will instruct you as to the type or limitation of range of motion exercises to be done. These exercises are usually done during or after the bath and before the bed is made. They may be carried out at other times as well.

When you are assigned to carry out ROM:

■ Check with the nurse for specific instructions or limitations.
■ Never exercise a joint to the point of pain.
■ Perform each exercise five times, or more if ordered.

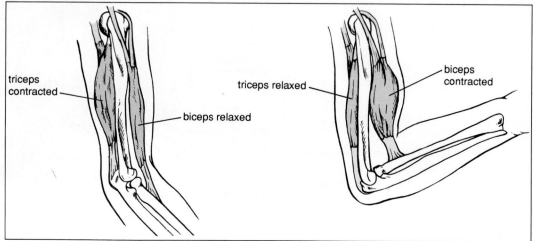

FIGURE 35–4. Coordination of muscles

BEGINNING PROCEDURE ACTIONS	PROCEDURE COMPLETION ACTIONS
■ Wash your hands. ■ Assemble equipment needed. ■ Go to the patient's room, knock, and pause before entering. ■ Introduce yourself and identify the patient by checking the identification bracelet. ■ Ask visitors to leave and inform them where they can wait. ■ Care for equipment according to facility policy. ■ Provide privacy. ■ Explain what will happen and answer questions. ■ Allow patient to assist in procedure as much as possible. ■ Raise bed or table to comfortable working height.	■ Position patient comfortably. ■ Leave signal cord, telephone, and fresh water close at hand. ■ Return bed or table to lowest position. ■ Perform general safety check of patient and environment. ■ Wash your hands. ■ Report completion of task. ■ Let visitors know when they may reenter the patient's room. ■ Document action and your observations.

NOTE: Where there are open lesions, wet linen, or possible contact with patient body fluids or blood, disposable gloves are worn during the procedure. Put on gloves before contact with the patient or linen. Properly dispose of gloves after they are removed. ALWAYS APPLY UNIVERSAL PRECAUTIONS.

FIGURE 35–5. Beginning procedure actions and procedure completion actions

■ Stop the exercise if pain or discomfort develops, and report to the nurse.

■ Support each joint above and below the joint being exercised. Provide support *at* the joints to prevent pressure on the muscles.

■ Note that special corrective exercises are performed by the physical therapist.

Refer to Figure 35–5 to review the beginning procedure actions and the procedure completion actions to be carried out for each personal care procedure.

PROCEDURE 108 | OBRA

SIDE 9

PERFORMING RANGE OF MOTION EXERCISES (PASSIVE)

NOTE: This procedure may be carried out as an independent procedure or as part of the bath. Repeat each action five times. It will be described here as an independent procedure.

CAUTION: Passive range of motion that involves the neck is usually carried out by a physical therapist or a registered nurse. Patients, who can, are encouraged to exercise this area themselves. Check your facility policy regarding ROM neck exercises.

1. Carry out each beginning procedure action.
2. Remember to wash your hands, identify the patient, and provide privacy.
3. Assemble equipment needed:
    Bath blanket

■

4. Position patient on back close to you.
5. Adjust the bath blanket to keep the patient covered as much as possible.
6. Supporting the elbow and wrist, exercise shoulder joint nearest you as follows:
    a. Bring the entire arm out at right angle to the body (horizontal abduction), Figures 35–6A and B.
    b. Return the arm to a position parallel to the body (horizontal adduction).
7. a. With arm parallel to the body, roll entire arm toward body (internal rotation of shoulder).
    b. Maintaining the parallel position, roll entire arm away from body (external rotation of shoulder).

continues

FIGURE 35–6. Shoulder abduction and adduction. Supporting the elbow and wrist, bring the entire arm out at right angle from the body.

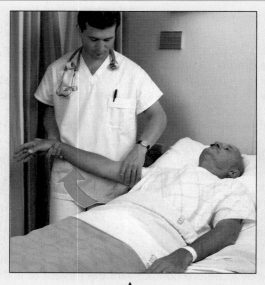

A.

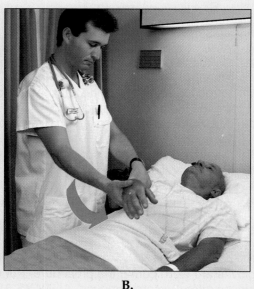

B.

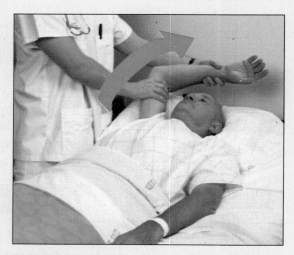

FIGURE 35–7. Shoulder flexion. With shoulder in abduction, flex elbow and raise entire arm over head.

8. With shoulder in abduction, flex elbow and raise entire arm over head (shoulder flexion), Figure 35–7.
9. With arm parallel to body (palm up—**suppination**), flex and extend elbow, Figures 35–8A and B.
10. Flex and extend wrist, Figures 35–9A and B. Flex and extend each finger joint, Figures 35–10A and B.
11. Move each finger, in turn, away from the middle finger (abduction), Figure 35–11A, and toward the middle finger (adduction), Figure 35–11B.
12. Abduct the thumb by moving it toward the extended fingers, Figure 35–12.
13. Touch the thumb to the base of the little finger, then to each fingertip (opposition), Figure 35–13.

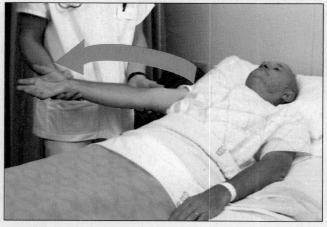

FIGURE 35–8A. Elbow extension and flexion. Supporting the upper arm and wrist, straighten elbow.

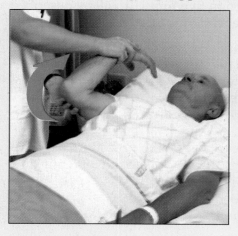

FIGURE 35–8B. Then bring lower arm toward upper arm.

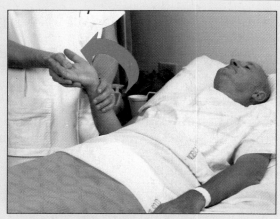

FIGURE 35–9A. Wrist extension and flexion. Supporting arm above wrist and hand, straighten wrist.

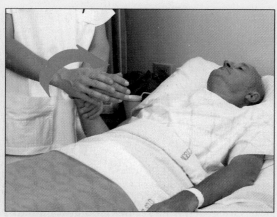

FIGURE 35–9B. Place hand over patient's hand while supporting wrist and bend wrist.

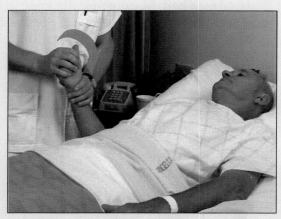

FIGURE 35–10A. Finger flexion. Supporting wrist with one hand, cover patient's fingers and curl them to make a fist.

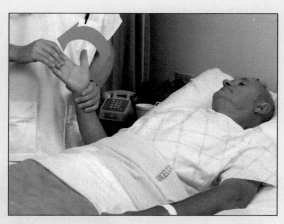

FIGURE 35–10B. Finger extension. Slip fingers over flexed fingers and straighten fingers.

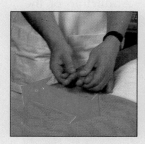

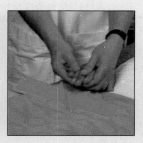

FIGURE 35–11A. Abduction of the fingers

FIGURE 35–11B. Adduction of the fingers

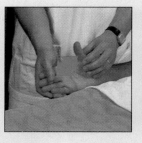

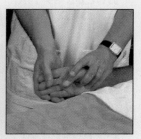

FIGURE 35–12. Abduction and adduction of thumb and fingers. Supporting the hand, draw the thumb toward and away from the extended fingers.

FIGURE 35–13. Thumb opposition. Supporting the hand, touch each finger with the thumb.

continues

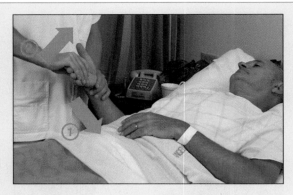

FIGURE 35–14. Wrist inversion and eversion. Grasp wrist with one hand and patient's hand with the other and bring wrist toward body and then away from body.

14. Turn hand palm down (pronation), then palm up (supination).
15. Grasp patient's wrist with one hand and the patient's hand with the other. Bring wrist toward body (inversion) and then away from the body (eversion), Figure 35–14.
16. Point hand in supination toward thumb side (radial deviation), then toward little finger side (ulnar deviation).
17. Cover the patient's upper extremities and body. Expose only the leg being exercised. Face the foot of the bed.
18. Supporting the knee and ankle, move the entire leg away from body center (abduction) and toward the body (adduction), Figures 35–15A and B.
19. Turn to face bed. Supporting the knee in bent position (flexion), raise the knee toward the pelvis (hip flexion), Figure 35–16. Straighten the knee (extension), Figure 35–17, as you lower the leg to the bed.

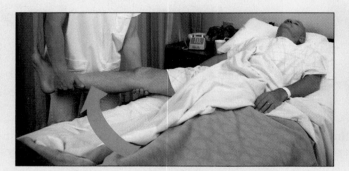

FIGURE 35–15A. Abduction of the hip. Supporting patient's knee and ankle, move entire leg away from body center.

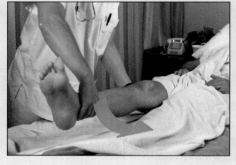

FIGURE 35–15B. Adduction of the hip. Supporting leg, return toward center of body.

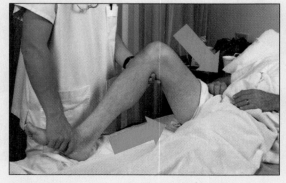

FIGURE 35–16. Hip and knee flexion. Supporting patient's knee and ankle, flex knee and hip.

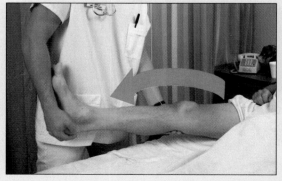

FIGURE 35–17. Knee extension. Supporting knee and ankle, straighten knee.

20. a. Supporting leg at knee and ankle, roll leg in a circular fashion away from body (lateral hip rotation).
    b. Continuing to support leg, roll leg in the same fashion toward the body (medial hip rotation).
21. Grasp patient's toes and support ankle. Bring toes toward the knee (**dorsiflexion**), Figure 35–18A. Then point toes toward the foot of the bed (**plantar flexion**), Figure 35–18B.
    NOTE: The patient may be more comfortable if the knee is slightly flexed during this motion.
22. Gently turn patient's foot inward (inversion),

Figure 35–19, and outward (eversion), Figure 35–20.
23. Place your fingers over patient's toes. Bend toes (flexion) and straighten toes (extension).
24. Move each toe away from the second toe (abduction), Figure 35–21A, and then toward the second toe (adduction), Figure 35–21B.
25. Cover the leg with the bath blanket. Raise the side rail and move to the opposite side of the bed.
26. Move the patient close to you and repeat Steps 6–24.

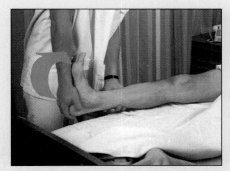

FIGURE 35–18A. Ankle flexion. Grasp the patient's heel with one hand using your upper arm to support the foot. Dorsiflex the ankle by bringing the toes and foot toward the knee.

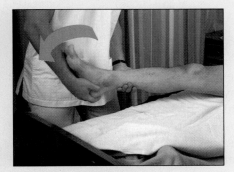

FIGURE 35–18B. Plantar flex the ankle by drawing the foot in a downward position.

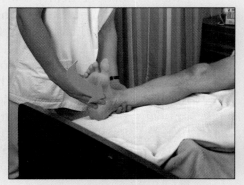

FIGURE 35–19. Foot inversion. Grasp patient's foot and gently turn it inward.

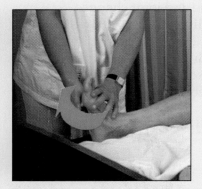

FIGURE 35–20. Foot eversion. Grasp patient's foot and gently turn it outward.

continues

27. If the procedure is part of the bath, complete the procedure for making an occupied bed (Unit 19).
28. Carry out each procedure completion action. Remember to wash your hands, report completion of task, and document date, time, range of motion exercises, and patient reaction.

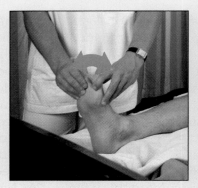

FIGURE 35–21A. Toe abduction. Move each toe away from the second toe one at a time.

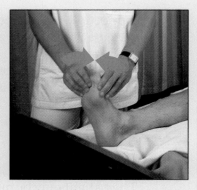

FIGURE 35–21B. Toe adduction. Move each toe toward the second toe one at a time.

Diagnostic Techniques

Some techniques used to diagnose problems of the musculoskeletal system include:
- Radiographic techniques such as X-ray.
- Electromyography (EMG)—test to measure the effectiveness of muscle/nerve interaction.
- Measurements of alkaline and acid phosphatases.
- Bone marrow examination—sample of the bone marrow is removed and evaluated.
- CAT scan to check for bone, muscle, and joint conditions.
- Radioisotope scanning—technique often can detect early bone and joint changes.
- Arthroscopy—direct visualization of a joint.
- MRI—examination of musculoskeletal tissues that shows conditions of tissues around bones to help diagnose tumors, ruptured disc between two vertebrae, and other conditions.

Common Conditions

Bursitis

Bursae are small sacs of fluid found around joints. They help to reduce friction when muscles move. At times, the bursae can become inflamed, and the tissues around a joint become painful. This condition is known as bursitis. Treatment of bursitis includes:
- Applications of heat to promote healing
- Immobilization so that the joint cannot move to relieve pain around the joint

- Removal of excess fluid from the joint by aspiration with a needle
- Administration of steroids

Arthritis

The term arthritis means inflammation of the joints. It may develop following an acute injury or it may be chronic and progressive. There are two forms of chronic arthritis:

1. Rheumatoid arthritis—this form affects the joint tissues, the joint lining, and can affect any other body system. It is a serious form of arthritis that can affect persons of any age. The cause is not specifically known. It is believed to be an autoimmune response.
2. Osteoarthritic joint disease (OJD) or degenerative joint disease (DJD)—this form affects the cartilage covering the ends of the bones as they form the joint. Cartilage breaks down and the ends of the bones rub together, causing pain and deformity. The joints most often affected are the weight-bearing joints. Several factors seem to contribute to the disease process. These factors include:
   - Aging
   - Trauma
   - Obesity

Treatment of arthritis includes:
- Balance of rest and exercise
- Joint immobilization where there is pain
- Weight control to relieve pressure on the joints
- Medicating to relieve pain and reduce the in-

flammation
- Providing physical therapy when inflammation subsides to maintain joint mobility
- Replacing badly damaged joints by surgery
- Use of adaptive equipment to enable the patient to get most range of motion from injured joints
- Exercising arthritic joints in warm water (with or without whirlpool action)

Fractures

A fracture is any break in the continuity of a bone. Falls are the common cause of fractures. If the bone breaks through the skin, the situation is identified as an open compound fracture. If the bones do not break through the skin, the fracture is known as closed. There are several kinds of fractures, Figure 35–22:
- Closed or oblique fractures—those in which the bones remain in proper position (alignment).
- Greenstick fractures—The bone is not broken completely through. This is typical of fractures in young children. Children's bones are flexible since growing is incomplete. Their bones tend to bend like young tree limbs, breaking on one side only. This gives rise to the name "greenstick."

- Compression fractures—seen in spongy bone such as the vertebral bodies. The bone is compressed or crushed.
- Comminuted fractures—result in a bone that is fragmented or splintered into more than two pieces.
- Open (compound) fractures—bone is broken and skin is open. The bone may break through the open skin.

Treatment. Fractures of any kind are treated by keeping the part that is injured immobilized in proper position until healing takes place. Injured bones take from several weeks to several months to heal. Immobilization is achieved through the use of:
- Pins, Figure 35–23
- Screws
- Bone plates
- Casting
- Traction

Special beds and attachments are used to make nursing care easier. The patient may be placed on a Stryker frame or the Circ O lectric® bed.

Be sure you know how to operate each bed and attachment before attempting care. In many facilities, an RN must be present when the bed is turned. Know and follow the policy of your facility.

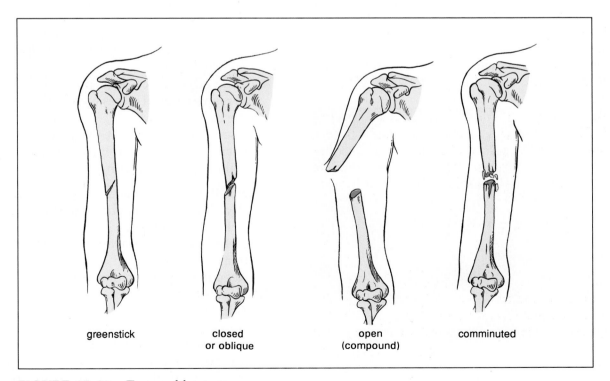

greenstick   closed   open   comminuted
                  or oblique   (compound)

FIGURE 35–22. Types of fractures

Care of Patients with Casts. Two types of cast materials are commonly used:

1. Plaster of Paris, which can take up to 48 hours to dry completely
2. Fiberglass, which dries very rapidly

Cast material is wet when it is applied. During the drying period, the cast gives off heat. Special care for the newly casted patient includes:

■ Supporting the cast and body in good alignment with pillows covered by a cloth pillow slip, and keeping the cast uncovered.
■ Turning the patient frequently to permit air circulation to all parts of the cast. Maintain support. Use palm of hand, not fingers, to support the wet cast.
■ Close observation of the uncasted areas of the extremities, such as the fingers and toes, for signs of decreased circulation. Report coldness, cyanosis, swelling, increased pain, or numbness immediately.
■ Close observation of skin areas around the cast edges for signs of irritation, Figure 35–24. Rough edges should be covered with adhesive strips to prevent skin irritation.
■ Recall the following key of reportables when checking the patient:
  — C = color
  — M = motion
  — E = edema
  — T = temperature

Special Care After Cast Is Dry. After the cast has completely dried:

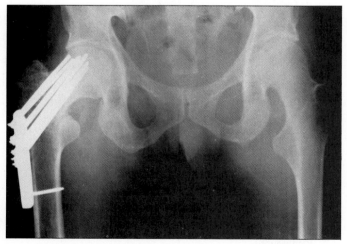

FIGURE 35–23. Fractured bones are held in place with plates, pins, and screws.

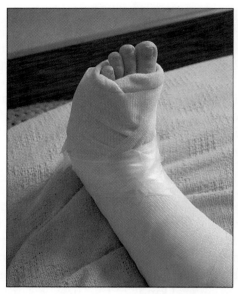

FIGURE 35–24. Carefully and frequently check skin areas around the edges of the cast for signs of irritation.

■ Turn the patient to the noncasted area. This is particularly important in moving a patient with a body cast (spica cast) because turning to the casted side may result in cracking the cast.
■ Always support the cast when turning or moving a patient.
■ Encourage use of an overhead bar, known as a trapeze, to assist the patient in helping herself, Figure 35–25.
■ Tape edges of casts to prevent pressure and abrasive areas, if edges were not covered when the cast was applied.
■ Use plastic to protect the cast edges that are near the genitals and buttocks to help prevent soiling during toileting.

Care of Patients in Traction. Traction is designed to pull two body areas slightly apart to:

■ Relieve pressure.
■ Help tightly contracted (spasmodic) muscles relax.
■ Keep in proper position as healing takes place.

Traction is of two types:

■ Skin traction where traction is applied to the skin.
■ Skeletal traction where traction is applied through the skin to the bone.

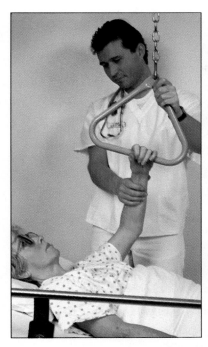

FIGURE 35–25. The overhead trapeze greatly assists in patient care.

Traction is applied by attaching weights to a part of the body above or below the area to be treated. The patient's body weight serves as countertraction by pulling in the opposite direction to the traction. Belts, head halters, or tapes may be applied to the patient's skin to hold the traction. Traction may be applied continuously or intermittently.

Skeletal traction uses tongs or pins placed into bones with weights applied to the tongs or pins. Skeletal traction is always continuous once applied. The weights for skeletal traction must not be lifted or removed until the traction is to be discontinued.

When patients are in traction:
- Do not disturb the weights or permit them to swing, drop, or rest on any surface.
- Keep the patient in good alignment. Make sure that the body is acting properly as countertraction by keeping the head of the bed low.
- Check under head halter or pelvic belt for areas of pressure or irritation.
- Make sure straps of halters and belts are smooth, straight, and properly secured.
- Keep covers off ropes and pulleys.

Not all patients remain in traction continually. If pelvic belt traction, Figure 35–26, or cervical traction with a head halter, Figure 35–27, is to be discontinued, the following steps should be taken:

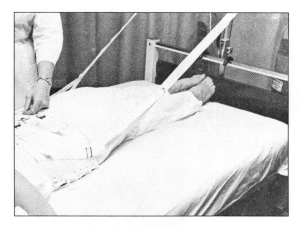

FIGURE 35–26. Pelvic belt traction

- Slowly raise the weights to the bed. Avoid abrupt or jerking movements as this may cause the patient pain. If two sets of weights are being used, raise them at the same time and rate.
- Remove the weight holder and weights from the connection with the halter or belt and place them on the floor. Remove the head halter or pelvic belt.
- To reapply traction, reverse the procedure.
- Remember never to jerk or drop the weights quickly or lower them unevenly. Always apply weights smoothly to avoid causing the patient pain.

Balanced Suspension Skeletal Traction. Patients in balanced suspension skeletal traction have more serious injuries as compared to injuries requiring skin traction. Patients also tend to remain in this type of traction for a longer period compared with skin trac-

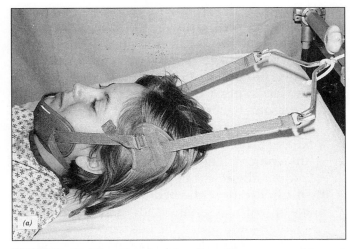

FIGURE 35–27. Cervical traction (*Photo courtesy of Leona A. Mourad*)

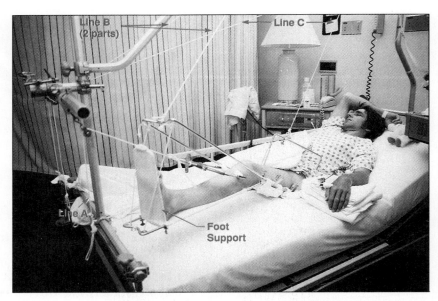

FIGURE 35–28. Balanced suspension skeletal traction *(Photo courtesy of Leona A. Mourad)*

- Line A is the primary or traction line through the tibia.
- Line B suspends the Harris splint, which supports the thigh, and the Pearson attachment. This holds the legs so they move as one as they are tied together to one line or rope.
- Line C is tied to the top of the Harris splint, then goes to the head of the bed for countertraction.
- A trapeze over the bed allows the patient to raise with assistance for back care, linen changes, and toileting.

tion. However, the same basic principles of traction apply. Usually there is one primary line of traction. The extra ropes and weights provide suspension and countertraction.

Study Figure 35–28. It will help you understand how balanced suspension skeletal traction is maintained.

- First locate the primary pull. Line A extends from a pin inserted in the tibia to the weights and provides the primary traction for the fractured femur.
- A Harris splint supporting the thigh is tied to a Pearson attachment. The Pearson attachment supports the patient's leg.
- Clamps hold a foot plate onto the Pearson attachment. The foot plate holds the foot in proper alignment to prevent footdrop.
- A trapeze over the bed allows the patient to raise with assistance for back care, linen changes, and use of the bedpan.

NOTE: The continuous passive motion machine (CPM) is used after hip and knee surgery to provide

slow, continual movement. The physical therapist instructs the patient in its use and supervises the patient to be sure the limb is properly positioned in the appliance.

Bedmaking. Bedmaking for orthopedic patients varies according to the type of traction.

- Two half sheets are often used in place of a large sheet for the bottom.
- Bottom linens may be changed from top to bottom rather than side to side.
- The top linen is arranged according to the patient's special needs. Half sheets and folded bath blankets can be worked around the traction to keep the patient covered and comfortable.

Fractured Hip

It is common to have patients in your care who have fractured hips. Elderly people are especially at risk for falling and breaking their hips. The fracture may be repaired through a surgical procedure called open reduction/internal fixation. This means the surgeon makes an incision, manipulates the fractured bone into alignment, and then inserts a device such as a nail, pin, or rod to hold the ends of the fractured bone in place. If you are assigned to a patient who has had this surgery you must:

- Know how to position the patient in bed. It is important to avoid adduction and internal and external rotation of the affected hip.
- Know the correct procedure if the patient is allowed to ambulate. The patient is usually not allowed to bear weight on the affected side for a few weeks after surgery.

Ruptured or Slipped Disc

There are 31 bones in the spinal column. These bones are called vertebrae. Between most of these bones, small discs or pads of cartilage with soft, gel-like centers are found. These discs help to cushion the back bones. The anterior of the vertebrae support the head and body. The posterior portions form a tunnel that surrounds the delicate spinal cord and nerves. It is possible for a disc to bulge (slip) out of place or for the soft center to rupture. In either case, pressure is placed on the spinal nerves, Figure 35–29A and 35–29B.

Depending on which disc is injured, the patient may experience, in different parts of the body:

- Pain
- Numbness
- Tingling
- Weakness of one or more muscles

Treatment. Treatment is directed toward relieving pressure on the nerve roots. Three techniques are employed:

1. Traction.
2. Surgery to remove the protruding portion of the disc (laminectomy). The surgery sometimes includes a fixation (fusion) of the vertebral bones.
3. Injections of an enzyme called chymopapain. The enzyme, which dissolves the herniated material, is injected into the ruptured disc area while the patient is in the operating room. When the patient returns from surgery, he is given routine postoperative follow-up. The major side effect is the possibility of an anaphylactic reaction (severe hypersensitivity reaction). Since this occurs rather rapidly upon

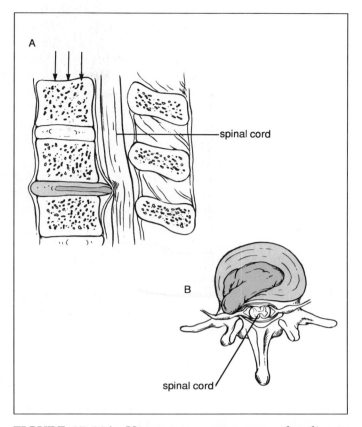

FIGURE 35–29A. Uneven pressure causes the disc to bulge, putting pressure on the nerve root (slipped disc). B. A herniated (ruptured) disc puts pressure on the nerve root as its gel-like center oozes backward.

injection, you would probably not witness it, as the patient would still be in surgery or recovery. However, the reaction can occur several weeks later. Some patients still require further surgery to remove disc pieces to relieve pain.

Lower Extremity Amputation

You may care for patients who have had one or both legs surgically removed (amputated). A leg may need to undergo amputation because of circulatory problems, a malignancy, or because of an accident in which the leg is severely damaged.

It is common for people to experience phantom pain after the removal of a limb. Patients with phantom pain may feel pain or tingling where the limb used to be. These feelings may persist for months. The pain is real, although it is difficult to explain.

When you are positioning a patient who has had an amputation of the lower extremities, remember:

- Avoid abduction and flexion of the patient's hip—because the weight of the lower leg is not there, the hip on the affected side will quickly become contracted if flexion is allowed.
- If the patient has a below the knee amputation (BKA), avoid flexion of the knee so that a contracture does not form.

After the surgery, the patient will either have the stump wrapped with elastic bandage or will wear a stump shrinker. It is important that these be on at all times except during the bath. It is the nurse's responsibility to apply either of these items. If you notice that the bandage or shrinker is loose or needs to be reapplied, notify the nurse. The purpose of these items is to make sure that the stump will heal in the appropriate shape.

If you bathe a patient, follow these directions:

- Gently wash the stump with soap and warm water, rinse well and pat dry.

- Observe the stump for:
  - redness
  - swelling
  - drainage from the incision
  - open areas in the incision or anywhere else on the stump.

After an amputation, some people are fitted with an artificial leg (**prosthesis**). They have to learn how to walk and sit when the prosthesis is worn. A prosthesis is custom made for the person who will be wearing it. A special health care professional measures the patient and makes the prosthesis. The physical therapist teaches the patient how to apply the prosthesis and how to walk with it. If you are responsible for helping a patient put on a prosthesis, be sure you know how to attach and secure it because each device is different.

Various types of materials are used to make prostheses. They need to be cleaned regularly, and the method of cleaning depends on what materials were used to make the prosthesis.

SUMMARY

- Orthopedic injuries often require long periods of immobilization.
- Routine range of motion exercises must be carried out for all uninjured joints to:
  — Prevent deformities and joint stiffening.
  — Promote general circulation.
  — Prevent mineral loss from the bones.

- Special nursing care to patients in casts and traction:
  — Ensures proper alignment.
  — Prevents pressure areas.
  — Avoids skin breakdown.

UNIT REVIEW

A. True/False. Answer the following statements true or false by circling T or F.

T   F   1. Chymopapain is used to treat arthritis.

T   F   2. If ROM is not carried out faithfully, the patient's future mobility is threatened.

T   F   3. When carrying out ROM, always support the parts being exercised at the joint.

T   F   4. The nursing assistant will carry out special corrective exercises.

T   F   5. Aging is a contributory factor to osteoarthritis.

T   F   6. When the patient has a painful arthritic joint, it should be exercised vigorously.

T   F   7. An over-bed bar (trapeze) will assist orthopedic patients to move more easily and to help themselves.

T   F   8. A fracture is any break in a bone.

T   F   9. Before operating beds or attachments used with orthopedic patients, the nursing assistant must be sure of his/her competency to operate this equipment.

T   F   10. It only takes a few moments for a cast to completely dry.

T F 11. Patients recovering from fractured hips are generally not allowed to bear weight on the affected side for several weeks.

T F 12. If a patient has an open reduction/internal fixation for a fractured hip, it means a cast will have been applied.

T F 13. Phantom pain after an amputation is imaginary and of no concern to caregivers.

T F 14. The nursing assistant is responsible for teaching patients with prostheses how to use them.

T F 15. It is important to prevent contractures after an amputation.

B. Matching. Match the phrases or statements in Column I with the words in Column II.

Column I

_____ 16. correct position

_____ 17. small fluid-filled sacs found around joints

_____ 18. name given to a cast covering hips and one or both legs

_____ 19. fracture where bone breaks through skin

_____ 20. inflammation of joints

Column II

a. arthritis

b. spica

c. closed

d. bursae

e. simple

f. alignment

g. open

C. Multiple Choice. Choose the phrase that best completes each of the following sentences by circling the proper letter.

21. When assigned to perform ROM, you should
    a. exercise every joint.
    b. exercise joints to the point of pain.
    c. check with the nurse for any limitations before starting.
    d. perform each exercise four times.

22. A greenstick fracture
    a. occurs mainly in children.
    b. fragments the bone.
    c. occurs mainly in the elderly.
    d. None of the above.

23. While a leg cast is drying
    a. cover it tightly so moisture won't be lost.
    b. maintaining general alignment is not important.
    c. carefully observe the extremities for circulation.
    d. use only fingertips to handle the cast.

24. When caring for the patient in traction
    a. maintain proper alignment.
    b. lift the weights rapidly.
    c. allow weights to rest on the floor.
    d. allow the patient's feet to press against the footboard.

25. Your patient has a ruptured disc. You should note and report
    a. tingling.
    b. paralysis.
    c. numbness.
    d. All of the above.

D. Completion. Complete the following statements in the space provided.

26. Seven tests used to diagnose problems of the musculoskeletal system are:
    a. _____
    b. _____
    c. _____
    d. _____
    e. _____
    f. _____
    g. _____

27. Three factors contributing to the process of osteoarthritis are:
    a. _____
    b. _____
    c. _____

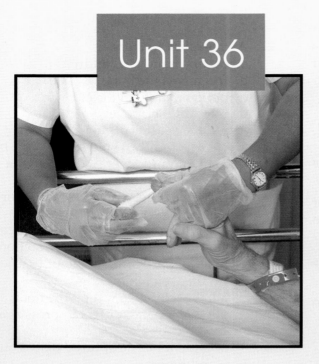

Unit 36

The Endocrine System and Common Disorders

As a result of this unit, you will be able to:

■ Spell and define terms.

■ Review the location and functions of the endocrine system.

■ List five specific diagnostic tests associated with conditions of the endocrine system.

■ Describe some common diseases of the endocrine system.

■ Recognize the signs and symptoms of hypoglycemia and hyperglycemia.

■ Describe nursing assistant actions related to the care of patients with disorders of the endocrine system.

■ Perform blood tests for glucose levels if facility policy permits.

■ Perform the Ketostix test for the presence of ketones in the urine.

Learn the meaning and the correct spelling of the following words and abbreviations:

Addison's disease
assimilated
basal metabolism rate (BMR)
Cushing's syndrome
diabetes mellitus
endocrine glands
glucometer
glucose
glycogen
glycosuria
hypercalcemia
hyperglycemia
hypersecretion
hyperthyroidism
hypertrophy
hypoglycemia
hyposecretion
hypothyroidism
insulin

insulin dependent diabetes mellitus (IDDM)
iodine
ketosis
morbidity
mortality
noninsulin dependent diabetes mellitus (NIDDM)
parathormone
polydipsia
polyphagia
polyuria
protein bound iodine (PBI) test
simple goiter
tetany
thyroxine

Before beginning to study this unit, you may wish to review Unit 4, pages 64–68.

The endocrine glands, Figure 36–1:

■ Secrete hormones.

■ Control body activities and growth.

■ Are found as distinct glands or clusters of cells.

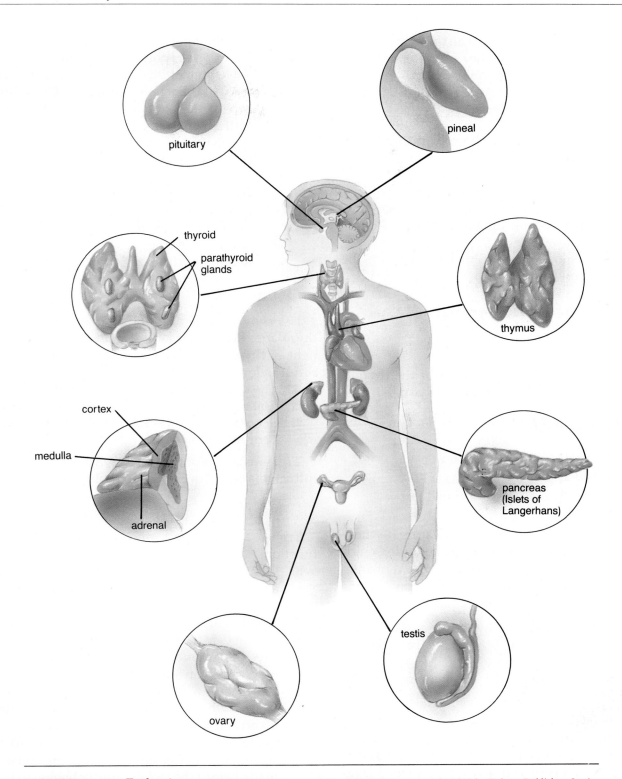

FIGURE 36–1. Endocrine system *(From Anatomy and Physiology Plates, copyright 1992 by Delmar Publishers Inc.)*

■ Are subject to disease that can result in hyposecretion (underproduction) or hypersecretion (overproduction) of hormones.

Diagnostic Techniques

Techniques used to diagnose problems of the endocrine system include:
■ Blood assays for hormone levels.
■ Urine assays for hormone levels.
■ Radioisotope scanning for thyroid disease.
■ Radioactive iodine uptake for thyroid function.
■ Basal metabolic rate (BMR) to measure the speed of oxygen uptake.

Disorders of the Thyroid Gland

Hyperthyroidism

Hyperthyroidism, or overactivity of the thyroid gland, results in hypersecretion of thyroxine. The person shows:
■ Irritability and restlessness
■ Nervousness
■ Rapid pulse
■ Increased appetite
■ Weight loss
■ Sensitivity

Nursing Assistant Actions. When caring for these patients, the nursing assistant must be understanding and have patience. The room should be kept quiet and cool. The patient's increased nutritional needs should be met with foods that are liked.

Treatment. Treatment of hyperthyroidism is designed to reduce the level of thyroxine through:
■ Surgical thyroidectomy
■ Radiation to reduce the number of functional cells

Thyroidectomy. It may be necessary to treat hyperthyroidism with surgery. You may be assigned to assist in the postoperative care. Following surgery:
■ The patient is placed in a semi-Fowler's position, with neck and shoulders well supported. Remember at all times to support the back of the neck. Hyperextension of the neck may damage the operative site.
■ Assist with oxygen, if ordered, using all oxygen precautions.

■ Give routine postoperative care.
■ Check for and report the following:
— Any signs of bleeding (this may drain toward the back of the neck). The pillows behind the patient should be checked, as well as the dressings.
— Signs of respiratory distress.
— Inability of the patient to speak. Initial hoarseness is common, but any increase should be reported.
— Greatly elevated temperature and pulse, pronounced apprehension, or irritability.
— Numbness, tingling, or muscular spasm (tetany) of the extremities.

Hypothyroidism

Hypothyroidism results in an undersecretion of thyroxine. Recall that iodine is an essential component of thyroxine. A lack of iodine in the diet can result in low thyroxine production.
■ The condition is called simple goiter.
■ The thyroid gland enlarges (hypertrophies).
■ Secretions produced have low thyroxine content.

Treatment. Hypothyroidism has been successfully managed with thyroxine replacement.

Thyroid Tests

Tests are usually performed to determine thyroid function.
■ One such test, a blood test, is the protein bound iodine (PBI) test. It requires little advance preparation.
■ Another thyroid test, the basal metabolism rate, or (BMR), may be ordered. This test measures the amount of oxygen used by the cells when a person is at complete rest. It also determines levels of the thyrostimulating hormone (TSH), which is produced by the pituitary gland and stimulates thyroid activity. It is done in the morning before breakfast and after a restful night. Certain preparations must be made before the test. If your patient is to have a BMR:
— Do not awaken for AM care.
— Withhold breakfast and fluids.
— If necessary, provide a bedpan rather than allow patient to get up.
— It is most important to maintain a quiet, restful environment.

Disorders of the Parathyroid Glands

Parathormone is secreted by the parathyroids and regulates the levels of electrolytes, calcium and phosphates. Hypersecretion of this hormone results in:

- Excessively high levels of blood calcium (**hypercalcemia**)
- Development of renal calculi
- Loss of bone calcium

Hypersecretion is usually caused by tumors. Tumors can be treated through surgical excision.

Hyposecretion can lead to:

- Abnormal muscle-nerve interaction
- Severe muscle spasm (tetany)

This can be an emergency situation, requiring management of the muscle spasms and administration of calcium. In the chronic state, calcium replacements and increased dietary calcium are prescribed.

Disorders of the Adrenal Cortex

The adrenal cortical secretions regulate:

- Development and maintenance of sexual characteristics
- Carbohydrate, fat, and protein metabolism
- Fluid balance
- Electrolyte levels of sodium and potassium

Hypersecretion results in **Cushing's syndrome**, which is characterized by:

- Weakness due to loss of body protein
- Increased blood sugar levels (hyperglycemia)
- Edema
- Hypertension
- Loss of potassium and retention of sodium
- Masculinization of a female

Therapy is primarily surgical and supportive.

Hyposecretion results in **Addison's disease**, which is characterized by:

- Loss of sodium and retention of potassium
- Abnormally low blood sugar (hypoglycemia)
- Dehydration
- Low stress tolerance

Addison's disease is treated by hormone replacement therapy and techniques to combat dehydration.

Diabetes Mellitus

The United States has the highest rate of diabetic **morbidity** (illness) and **mortality** (death) in the world. Each year 250,000 new cases of **diabetes mel-**litus are added to the over four million known cases. Many new cases are discovered during routine physical examinations. In addition, it is estimated that millions more people are unaware that they are diabetics.

Although forms of the condition can appear at any age, it is more common in the middle and later years. About 80% of all diabetics are over 40 years of age. As many as 5% of those over 65 require treatment.

The incidence of diabetes mellitus increases as people age. In the elderly, the disease:

- Is much more stable and predictable than in the young.
- Has fewer incidents of **ketosis** (diabetic coma) or insulin shock. When insulin shock or diabetic coma does occur in the elderly, either can be severe, resulting in heart attacks or strokes.
- May not require insulin for management. Less than half the elderly patients with diabetes require insulin.

These statistics tell us that many of our patients will have this condition.

The reason why diabetes develops is not fully understood. Factors that seem to play a role in the incidence of diabetes are:

- Heredity
- Obesity
- Age
- Infectious agents
- Autoimmune reactions

All diabetics should wear or carry a Medic Alert identification so that proper and immediate care can be provided in an emergency. It is also recommended that the diabetic carry food that provides a quick source of carbohydrates.

Disease Mechanism

In diabetes, the normal metabolism of fats, carbohydrates, and proteins is unbalanced. Normally, when carbohydrates are absorbed into the bloodstream, the blood sugar (glucose) level rises. The pancreas responds to an increase of **glucose** by secreting more insulin. **Insulin** is the hormone that is primarily responsible for:

- Lowering the blood sugar level by allowing glucose to cross the cell membrane.
- Increasing the oxidation of glucose by the tissues.
- Stimulating the conversion of glucose to glycogen by the liver. **Glycogen** is a storage form of energy.
- Decreasing glucose production from amino acids.
- Stimulating glucose formation into fat for storage.

In diabetes, there is insufficient insulin for these metabolic functions.

■ Glucose cannot be properly utilized for energy.
■ Fats and proteins are incompletely broken down. This leads to an accumulation of ketone bodies in the forms of acetone and other acids.
■ The excess glucose is eliminated along with water and salts through the kidneys. This causes dehydration and electrolyte imbalance.
■ The characteristic symptoms of excessive thirst, hunger, and increased urination are directly related to the loss of fluids, electrolytes and sugar.

Types of Diabetes Mellitus

Diabetes mellitus is typed and named according to the need for insulin. Examples are insulin dependent diabetes mellitus and noninsulin dependent diabetes. Either form of diabetes may occur at any age. However, IDDM appears more commonly in younger years and NIDDM is more common in older people.

1. **Insulin dependent diabetes mellitus (IDDM)** (Type I). This first appears in youth and in those under 40 years of age. The disease tends to be severe and unpredictable. It usually requires insulin. Typical signs and symptoms are:
   ■ **Polyuria** (excessive urination)
   ■ **Polydipsia** (thirst)
   ■ **Polyphagia** (hunger)
   ■ **Glycosuria** (sugar in the urine)
2. **Noninsulin Dependent Diabetes Mellitus (NIDDM)** (Type II). This is sometimes known as old-age diabetes or ketosis-resistant diabetes. It usually begins in later years. It is ten times more common than the juvenile form. About half of the patients show obvious signs (as listed above). The rest show less well-defined symptoms. These may include:
   ■ Easy fatigue   ■ Burning on urination
   ■ Skin infections   ■ Pain in fingers and
   ■ Slow healing   toes
   ■ Itching   ■ Vision changes
   ■ Pruritus vulvae (itching of the vulva)

Obesity is a common problem. Often only one or two symptoms are apparent in the elderly person. The older person may:
■ Complain of constant fatigue.
■ Have a skin lesion that takes an unusually long time to heal.

■ Experience vision changes that may be mistakenly attributed to general aging.

Complications

Long-standing diabetes mellitus is often complicated by:
■ Diabetic retinopathy such as retinitis proliferans
■ Renal disease — kidney
■ Circulatory impairments, which often result in gangrene, Figure 36–2, and amputation
■ Poor healing
■ Diabetic coma
■ Insulin shock

Care of the diabetic is largely directed toward preventing and managing complications. It also involves managing the following three areas of the diabetic's life:
■ Diet
■ Exercise
■ Use of insulin or oral antidiabetic agents

Diet

Diet is an important part of diabetic treatment. Physicians are not in full agreement as to the degree of rigidity with which a diet must be followed by all patients.
■ Weight reduction is favored.
■ Weight reduction alone may be sufficient to bring the condition under control in NIDDM.

The Exchange Systems. The diabetic exchange system of foods was formulated by a committee with representatives from the American Diabetic Associa-

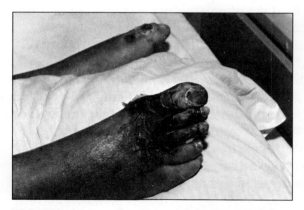

FIGURE 36–2. Gangrene of the toes and foot often means eventual amputation. *(From Hegner and Caldwell, Geriatrics: A Study of Maturity, copyright 1991, Delmar Publishers Inc.)*

tion and the diabetic branch of the U.S. Public Health Service. The use of food lists based on the exchange system has simplified the task of measuring food by weight. Measurements can now be made using a standard 8-ounce measuring cup, teaspoon, and tablespoon.

Exercise

Exercise is an important part of the overall treatment. The amount and type of exercise that is routinely engaged in is balanced by the food intake and insulin or hypoglycemic drug requirements.

Antidiabetic Drugs

Diabetes mellitus is treated by one of two main drug groups. One is administered subcutaneously. The other is given orally.

At the present time, there are several types of insulin. They vary in their:
- Speed of action
- Duration
- Potency or strength

Insulin is:
- Administered by the nurse. The nurse rotates the administration sites.
- Given by injection.
- Increasingly given through use of an insulin pump. The insulin pump delivers a prescribed amount of insulin on a regular basis into the patient's body.
- Used to treat IDDM.
- Persons living at home are taught to administer their own insulin.

NOTE: When insulin is self-administered, it is important to report any missed injections or signs of infection around the administration site.

Hypoglycemic drugs are:
- Administered by the nurse.
- Given by mouth.
- Used to treat NIDDM.

Two serious complications related to diabetes mellitus are the conditions of hypoglycemia and hyperglycemia.

Hypoglycemia (Low Blood Sugar)

Hypoglycemia occurs when the blood glucose level is below normal. It:
- May occur rapidly.
- Occurs far less commonly when oral antidiabetic agents are given.

- Is referred to as insulin reaction or insulin shock when due to an overdose of insulin.

Hypoglycemia can be brought on by:
- Skipping meals
- Diarrhea
- Unusual activity
- Omission of planned snack
- Stress
- Vomiting
- Interaction of drugs

Signs and Symptoms. The signs and symptoms of hypoglycemia include:
- Shallow, rapid respiration
- Rapid pulse
- Hunger
- Pale, moist skin
- Excitement and nervousness

If the patient is awake and alert, treatment includes:
- Orange juice or
- Milk or
- Another easily absorbed carbohydrate such as hard candy

If the patient is unconscious, the physician or nurse may give glucagon that causes a rapid elevation of blood sugar.

Hyperglycemia (High Blood Sugar)

Hyperglycemia (diabetic coma) or ketosis:
- Occurs when there is insufficient insulin for metabolic needs.
- Is less apt to occur in NIDDM.
- Usually develops slowly, sometimes over a 24-hour period.
- May be seen as confusion or drowsiness or a slow slippage into coma in the patient who is confined to bed.

Hyperglycemia may be brought on by:
- Stress
- Illness such as infection
- Dehydration
- Injury
- Forgotten medication

Treatment includes:
- Administration of insulin
- Fluids and electrolytes

Signs and Symptoms. The signs and symptoms of diabetic coma include:
- Early headache, drowsiness, or confusion
- Sweet, fruity odor to the breath
- Deep breathing
- Full, bounding pulse

- Low blood pressure
- Nausea or vomiting
- Flushed, dry, hot skin

Nursing Assistant Responsibilities

You must:

- Know the signs of insulin shock and diabetic coma.
- Be alert for the signs of diabetic coma or insulin shock and report them immediately to the nurse.
- Know the storage location of orange juice or other easily assimilated (absorbed) sources of carbohydrates.
- Keep easily assimilated carbohydrates such as orange juice, crackers, hard candy, or Karo syrup available if caring for the diabetic at home.
- Make sure you serve the patient proper trays of food.
- Not give extra nourishments without special permission.
- Keep a record of the food consumed, on the patient's chart.
- Report uneaten meals to the nurse.
- Give special attention to the care of the diabetic patient's feet.
  - Wash daily, carefully drying between toes.
  - Inspect feet closely for any breaks or signs of irritation.
  - Report any abnormalities to the nurse.
  - Do not allow moisture to collect between toes.

- The toenails of a diabetic should be cut only by a podiatrist, a specialist who is trained in foot care.
- Shoes and stockings should be clean, free of holes, and fit well. Anything that might injure the feet or interfere with the circulation must be avoided.
- Do not allow the patient to go barefoot.
- Test blood for presence of sugar, if permitted.
- Test urine (if ordered) for presence of ketones.
  - All urine to be tested should be freshly voided. It is well to have patients empty their bladders about an hour before the test is to be done. Collect the specimen for testing immediately before the test is to be done.
  - As a precaution, test the initial sample of urine just in case a second, fresh specimen cannot be obtained. The second specimen is preferred since this urine has recently accumulated while the first sample may have been in the bladder for an unknown period of time.
  - If the patient cannot void, be sure to report this to the nurse.
  - When the test is completed, record the results on the appropriate record. Report results to the nurse.

Refer to Figure 36–3 to review the beginning procedure actions and the procedure completion actions to be followed.

BEGINNING PROCEDURE ACTIONS	PROCEDURE COMPLETION ACTIONS
■ Wash your hands. ■ Assemble equipment needed. ■ Go to the patient's room, knock, and pause before entering. ■ Introduce yourself and identify the patient by checking the identification bracelet. ■ Ask visitors to leave and inform them where they can wait. ■ Care for equipment according to facility policy. ■ Provide privacy. ■ Explain what will happen and answer questions. ■ Allow patient to assist in procedure as much as possible. ■ Raise bed to comfortable working height.	■ Position patient comfortably. ■ Leave signal cord, telephone, and fresh water close at hand. ■ Return bed to lowest position. ■ Perform general safety check of patient and environment. ■ Wash your hands. ■ Report completion of task. ■ Let visitors know when they may reenter the patient's room. ■ Document action and your observations.

NOTE: Where there are open lesions, wet linen, or possible contact with patient body fluids or blood, disposable gloves are worn during the procedure. Put on gloves before contact with the patient or linen. Properly dispose of gloves after they are removed. ALWAYS APPLY UNIVERSAL PRECAUTIONS.

FIGURE 36–3.   Beginning procedure actions and procedure completion actions

Blood Glucose Monitoring

Procedures to test blood for the presence of glucose and urine for the presence of sugar and acetone vary according to equipment. It is important that instructions be followed exactly to avoid an incorrect reading because insulin may be administered according to the results. Currently, most testing for glucose levels uses some type of electronic device. The device uses a sample of blood rather than urine for testing.

The following procedure gives a general list of steps to follow. Remember to follow the manufacturer's instructions for the use of a specific device. Check with your supervisor to be sure the facility policy permits nursing assistants to perform this procedure.

PROCEDURE 109

USING A GLUCOMETER 3®

1. Carry out each beginning procedure action.
2. Remember to wash your hands, identify the patient, and provide privacy.
3. Assemble equipment needed:
   - Blood glucose monitoring device
   - Antiseptic wipes
   - Disposable gloves
   - Glucolet II lancet
   - Band-Aid®
   - Test strips

NOTE: Calibrate meter according to manufacturer's instructions every time a new bottle of test strips is opened.

4. Put on disposable gloves.
5. Clean patient's finger with antiseptic wipe and let dry.
6. Use the lancet to prick the side of the distal part of the patient's finger to obtain a drop of blood. Apply drop to test strip without smearing the drop.
7. Prepare the specimen of blood according to the manufacturer's instructions.
8. Carefully time and read the scale.
9. Wipe patient's finger with antiseptic wipe.
10. Put Band-Aid® on patient's finger.
11. Remove and discard disposable gloves according to facility policy.
12. Carry out each procedure completion action. Remember to wash your hands, report completion of task, and document. Documentation may include reporting test results to the nurse or recording results on the diabetic flow sheet according to facility policy.

PROCEDURE 110

USING ACCU-CHEK III®

1. Carry out each beginning procedure action.
2. Remember to wash your hands, identify the patient, and provide privacy.
3. Assemble equipment needed, Figure 36–4:
   - Accu-chek III®
   - Soft touch lancing device
   - Chemstrip bG® test strip
   - Dry cotton balls or rayon balls
   - Antiseptic wipe
   - Disposable gloves

NOTE: Calibrate meter according to manufacturer's instructions if display window number and code number on Chemstrip vial do not match.

Device needs to be recalibrated after battery is replaced.

NOTE: The series of photos shows self-testing of blood glucose. The procedure is the same when performed on a patient. Put on disposable gloves if taking a blood sample from a patient.

4. Wash the patient's hand with soap and water and dry.
5. Select finger to be pricked. Use an antiseptic wipe to clean area, Figure 36–5, and let dry.
6. Remove a test strip from the container. Recap container immediately, Figure 36–6.
7. Use an autolet to obtain specimen, Figure 36–

continues

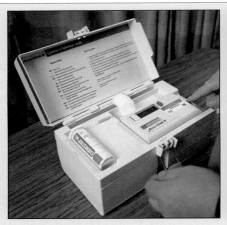

FIGURE 36–4. Assemble equipment needed.

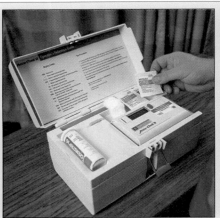

A.

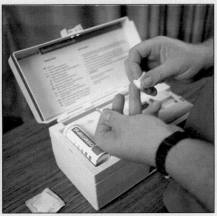

B.

FIGURE 36–5. Select an alcohol wipe **(A)** and clean the area to be used to draw blood **(B). NOTE:** The nursing assistant who is demonstrating this procedure is a diabetic and was performing his own routine blood glucose test. Whenever such a test is performed on another person, protective gloves must be worn.

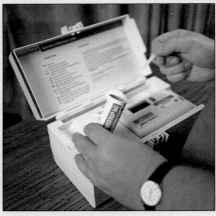

A.

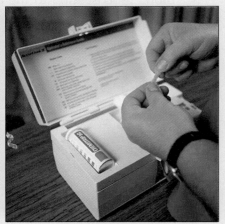

B.

FIGURE 36–6. Select a Chemstrip bG® from container. Touch only the end of the strip **(A).** Close cover on container right away **(B).**

FIGURE 36–7A. Remove the cover of the lancet.

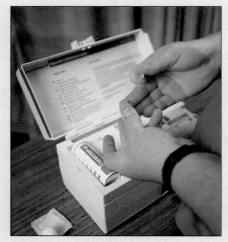

FIGURE 36–7B. Puncture the finger to obtain a sample.

7A. Use the side of the fingertip because it is less sensitive, Figure 36–7B. Put a Band-Aid® over the area.

8. Put drop of blood on test strip, Figure 36–8

9. Insert test strip into meter, Figure 36–9.

10. Follow the manufacturer's instructions for obtaining a reading on the meter, Figure 36–10.

11. Remove and properly discard Chemstrip® from meter.

12. Dispose of lancet properly, Figure 36–11.

13. If blood sample was obtained from patient, remove and dispose of gloves according to facility policy.

14. Carry out each procedure completion action. Remember to wash your hands, report completion of task, and document. Documentation may include reporting the test reading on the diabetic flow sheet.

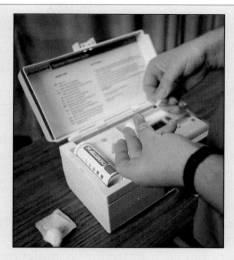

FIGURE 36–8. Put drop of blood on test strip.

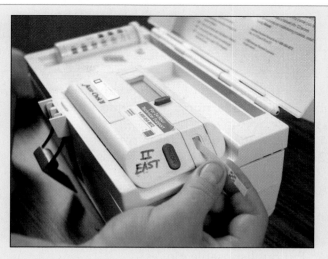

FIGURE 36–9. Insert test strip into machine.

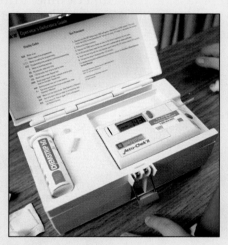

FIGURE 36–10. Wait for reading to register.

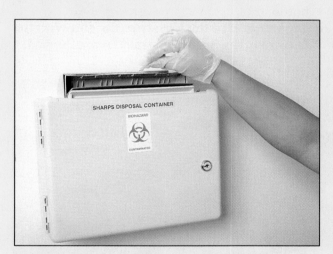

FIGURE 36–11. Dispose of lancet properly.

PROCEDURE 111

TESTING URINE FOR ACETONE: KETOSTIX® STRIP TEST

NOTE: If the results of the blood glucose tests are above normal, the nurse may request the urine be tested for acetone.

1. Carry out each beginning procedure action.
2. Remember to wash your hands, identify the patient, and provide privacy.
3. Assemble equipment needed:
   - Disposable gloves
   - Ketostix reagent strips
   - Sample of freshly voided urine in container
4. Put on disposable gloves.
5. Remove one test strip from bottle and recap bottle.
6. Dip one end of the test strip (the end with the reagent areas) into the urine, Figure 36–12A.

7. Remove and hold strip horizontally.
8. Fifteen seconds later, compare the strip with the color chart on the bottle label, Figure 36–12B. Match it as closely as possible to one of the colors on the chart. Do not touch wet strip to bottle label.
9. Dispose of strip and urine specimen unless orders have been given to save it.
10. Remove and properly dispose of gloves according to facility policy.
11. Carry out each procedure completion action. Remember to wash your hands, report completion of task, and document time, urine tested for acetone using Ketostix strip, and patient reaction.

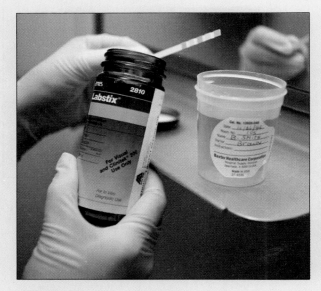

FIGURE 36–12A. Remove a test strip from bottle. Recap bottle. Dip strip into fresh urine sample. Do not touch wet strip to label of bottle.

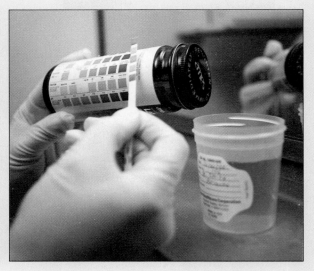

FIGURE 36–12B. Compare strip with color chart to determine results.

SUMMARY

Endocrine glands:
- Secrete hormones that influence body activities.
- Are subject to disease and malfunction.

Common conditions of the endocrine system are those involving:
- The thyroid gland. These are hyperthyroidism or hypothyroidism.
- The pancreas. A major condition is diabetes mellitus.

Diabetes mellitus:
- Affects many people.
- May be treated with a balance of:
  — Diet
  — Exercise
  — Hypoglycemic drugs or insulin
- Requires conscientious nursing care to avoid serious complications.
- Requires understanding by the patient of the need to follow the therapeutic program.

UNIT REVIEW

A. True/False. Answer the following statements true or false by circling T or F.

T F 1. The person with polyphagia has a high urine output.

T F 2. The morbidity rate for diabetes mellitus is very high.

T F 3. Glucose is another name for blood sugar.

T F 4. The person with hyperthyroidism is slow moving and lethargic.

T F 5. Hyperthyroidism causes people to lose weight.

T F 6. You should keep the room of a patient with hyperthyroidism quite warm.

T F 7. Obesity may play a role in the incidence of diabetes mellitus.

T F 8. If the patient with NIDDM appears drowsy and confused, you should suspect the possibility of ketosis.

T F 9. Foot care is especially important for the diabetic patient.

T F 10. Disposable gloves should be used when testing blood for sugar using the ACCU-CHEK II® glucometer.

B. Match. Match the phrases or statements in Column I with the words in Column II.

Column I	Column II
_____ 11. internal secretion produced by glands	a. polydipsia
	b. polyphagia
_____ 12. diabetic coma	c. polyuria
_____ 13. illness rate	d. glycosuria
_____ 14. excess thirst	e. endocrine gland
_____ 15. sugar in the urine	f. hormone
_____ 16. produces hormones	g. ketosis
_____ 17. excess hunger	h. mortality rate
_____ 18. death rate	i. morbidity rate
_____ 19. blood sugar	j. obesity
_____ 20. overweight	k. glycogen
	l. NIDDM
	m. insulin shock
	n. glucose

C. Multiple Choice. Choose the phrase that best completes each of the following sentences by circling the proper letter.

21. Your patient has had a thyroidectomy. You should
    a. keep patient flat in bed.
    b. watch for and report signs of respiratory distress.
    c. carry out ROM exercises immediately.
    d. position patient in a left Sims' position.

22. Lack of iodine in the diet can result in
    a. hypothyroidism.
    b. hyperthyroidism.
    c. diabetes mellitus.
    d. ketosis.

23. Your patient is scheduled for a BMR. You know
    a. this test is performed in the late afternoon.
    b. breakfast will be withheld.
    c. the patient should be given bathroom privileges.
    d. a stimulating environment is important.

24. Your patient is an insulin dependent diabetic. You know this
    a. is a stable form of the disease.
    b. affects older persons.
    c. requires hypoglycemic drugs.
    d. is a less stable form of the disease.

25. Insulin is an important hormone since it
    a. lowers blood sugar.
    b. raises blood sugar.
    c. stimulates the conversion of glycogen to glucose.
    d. breaks fat down to form glucose.

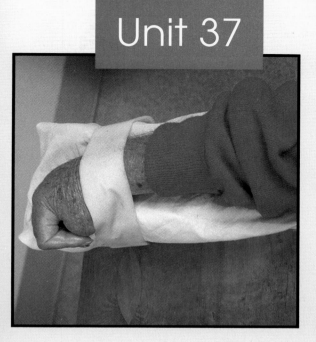

The Nervous System and Common Disorders

OBJECTIVES

As a result of this unit, you will be able to:

- Spell and define terms.
- Review the location and functions of the organs of the nervous system.
- List nine diagnostic tests used to determine conditions of the nervous system.
- Describe some common diseases of the nervous system.
- Describe nursing assistant actions related to the care of patients with conditions and diseases of the nervous system.
- State ways of assisting a person who is blind become oriented to new surroundings.
- Explain the proper care, handling, and application of a hearing aid.

VOCABULARY

Learn the meaning and the correct spelling of the following words:

akinesia
aphasia
apoplexy
aura
cataracts
cerebrospinal fluid (CSF)
cerebrovascular accident (CVA)
convulsion
epilepsy
expressive aphasia
global aphasia
grand mal seizure
hemiplegia
intracranial pressure
Jacksonian seizure
meninges
meningitis
multiple sclerosis
otitis media
otosclerosis
paralysis
paraplegia
petit mal seizure
quadriplegia
receptive aphasia
retinal degeneration
senile macular degeneration
status epilepticus
stroke
transient ischemic attack (TIA)
tremors

Before studying this unit, you may wish to review Unit 4, pages 68–75.

The nervous system is a highly complex network of nerve tissue and chemical secretions that controls all body activities. Damage to this system through injury or disease requires the most specialized nursing care. Remember that the nervous system includes the organs of special senses. Study Figures 37–1 through 37–7 to refresh your memory of the parts of the nervous system.

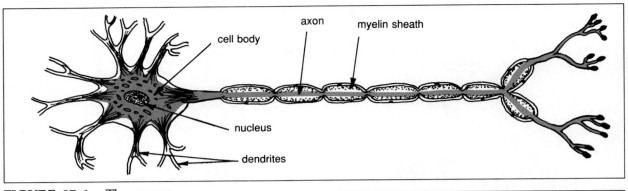

FIGURE 37–1. The neuron

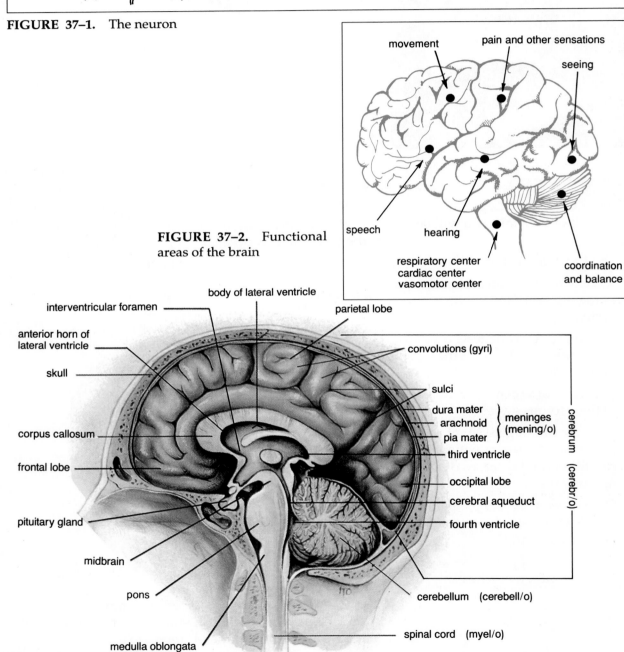

FIGURE 37–2. Functional areas of the brain

FIGURE 37–3. Cross section of the brain *(From Anatomy and Physiology Plates, copyright 1992 by Delmar Publishers Inc.)*

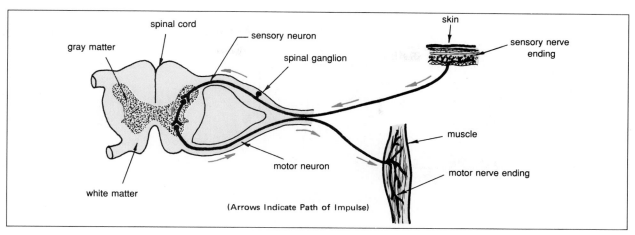

FIGURE 37–4. The reflex arc

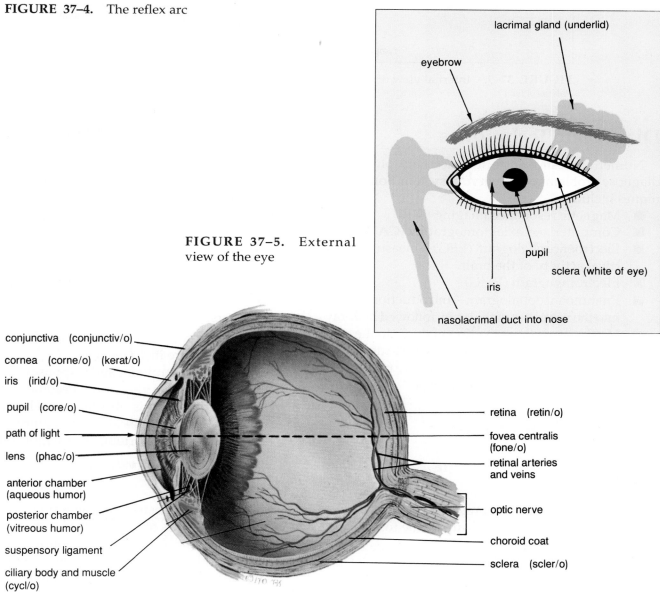

FIGURE 37–5. External view of the eye

FIGURE 37–6. Internal view of the eye *(From Anatomy and Physiology Plates, copyright 1992 by Delmar Publishers Inc.)*

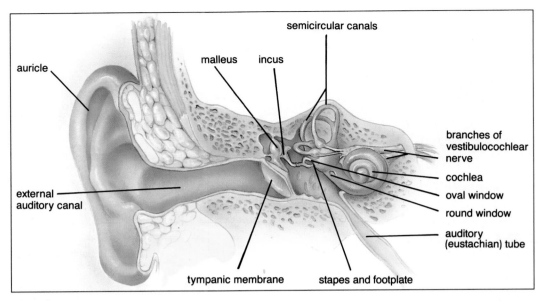

FIGURE 37–7. Internal view of the ear *(From Anatomy and Physiology Plates, copyright 1992 by Delmar Publishers Inc.)*

Diagnostic Techniques

Numerous tests and techniques help physicians diagnose problems of the nervous system. Some techniques include:

- Magnetic resonance imaging (MRI)
- Computerized axial tomography (CAT) scan
- Electroencephalogram (EEG)—measures electrical activity of the brain
- Electromyogram (EMG)
- Pneumoencephalogram—introduction of air into the ventricles of the brain, followed by X-ray
- Myelogram—introduction of dye into the central nervous system, followed by X-ray
- Tonometry—measures intraocular pressure
- Audiometry—measures hearing

Common Conditions

Increased Intracranial Pressure

The structures within the skull exert a normal amount of pressure. This pressure is called the intracranial pressure. The pressure is due to:

- Nervous tissue
- Cerebrospinal fluid
- Blood flowing through cerebral vessels

Any change in the size or amount of these components changes the pressure. Increased intracranial pressure can result from:

- Head injury. Bleeding from damaged blood vessels and edema puts pressure on the delicate nervous tissue.
- Inflammation or infection with edema.
- Intracranial bleeding due to ruptured blood vessels. This is called a cerebrovascular accident (CVA).
- Toxins.
- High temperature.
- Blockage of the normal flow of cerebrospinal fluid.
- Tumors.

Signs and Symptoms. Indications of increased intracranial pressure include:

- Alteration in pupil size and response to light. In the normal eye, the pupil becomes smaller when a flashlight is directed at each eye. The equality of the pupils and their ability to react to light is an important observation when a head injury occurs.
- Headache.
- Vomiting.
- Loss of consciousness and sensation.
- Paralysis—loss of voluntary motor control.
- Convulsions (seizures)—uncontrolled muscular contractions that are often violent.

How long all or part of the symptoms remain depends upon the extent and cause of damage to the brain cells. Remember also that paralysis is not always accompanied by sensory loss.

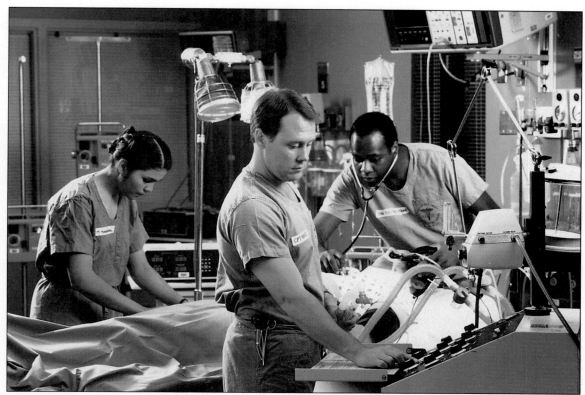

FIGURE 37–8. Critical nursing care *("Be All You Can Be" Courtesy U.S. Government, as represented by the Secretary of the Army)*

Specific Nursing Care. Patients who are acutely ill with head injuries or increased intracranial pressure require skilled nursing care, Figure 37–8. The nurse will handle certain responsibilities. These include monitoring the patient's:

■ Level of consciousness
■ Degree of orientation to time and place
■ Reaction to pain and stimuli
■ Vital signs

If, as you are assisting in the care, you note any change in the patient's response or behavior, it must immediately be brought to the nurse's attention. Changes that might be very significant include:

■ Incontinence
■ Uncontrolled body movements
■ Disorientation
■ Deepening or lessening in the level of consciousness
■ Dizziness
■ Vomiting
■ Alterations in speech

Once improved, the patient may be moved from a critical to an intermediate unit. From there, the patient may go to a long-term care facility for a possibly long period of convalescence. The nursing measures first established in the critical care unit must be maintained throughout this extended period.

Loss of sensation and decreased mobility make these patients more prone to pressure sores, infection, and contractures. You must continue to:

■ Give special skin care.
■ Carry out range of motion exercises, Figure 37–9.

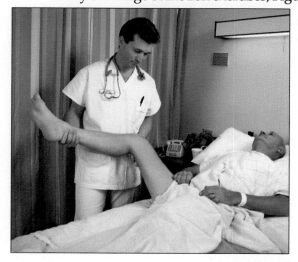

FIGURE 37–9. It is particularly important to carry out range of motion exercises when patients are paralyzed.

■ Check skin over pressure points frequently.

■ Change the patient's position regularly, Figure 37–10.

■ Report early signs of infection.

■ Monitor elimination. Loss of muscle tone and inactivity may lead to constipation and impaction.

■ Check drainage tubes such as indwelling catheters. They must receive careful attention.

■ Provide reality orientation as needed.

■ Be alert to any signs of mood changes and plan extra time to provide essential support.

Patients recovering from these illnesses often experience anxiety and depression.

■ Keep a careful check on vital signs of any patient with a head injury. A special record (neurosurgical watch) may be kept for recording all observations, Figure 37–11.

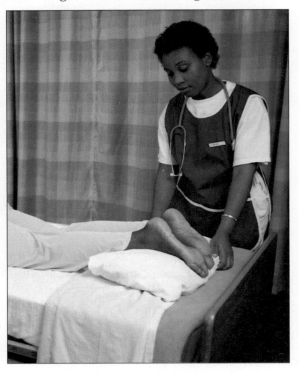

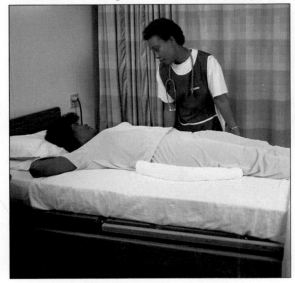

A. The patient's weak hand is tucked under the pillow with fingers open. Rolled sheet or bath blanket is used to maintain position of leg.

B. When it is not possible for the patient's legs to hang over the end of the mattress, a large pillow can be used to support the feet so that the toes do not touch the mattress.

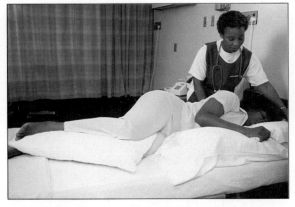

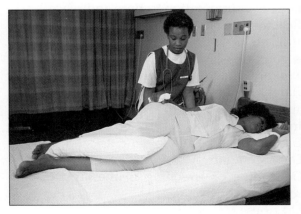

C. In this side-lying position, a pillow is used to support the weak arm. Another pillow is used to support the weak leg and foot.

D. Here is one more side-lying position. The weak arm is placed on a pillow right behind the patient. Notice the roll under the hand.

FIGURE 37–10. Four positions of the patient following a CVA. **NOTE:** The protective side rails, which would normally be up and locked in position, have been omitted in each of the photos for clarity.

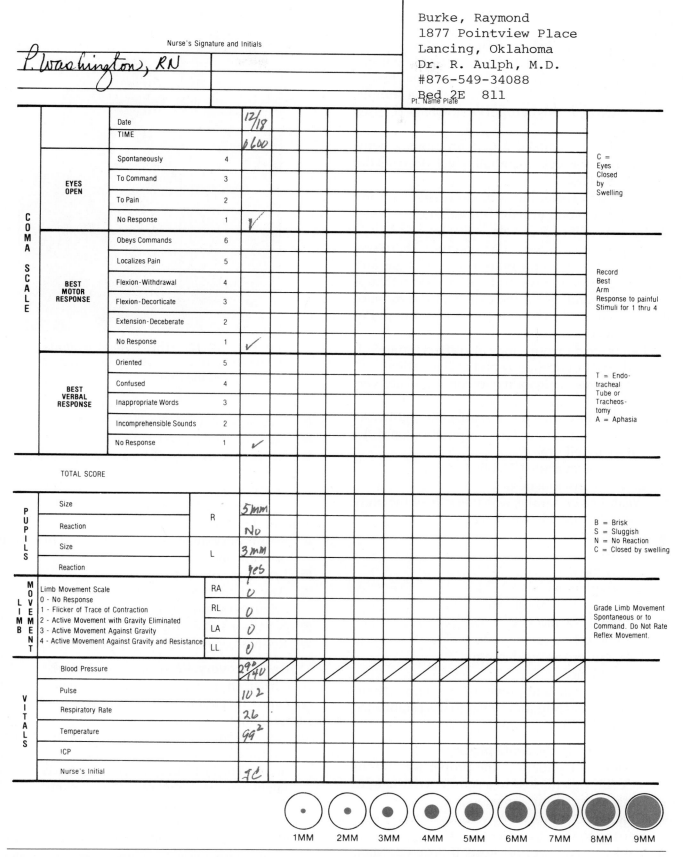

				12/18										
		Date		12/18										
		TIME		0600										
C O M A S C A L E	**EYES OPEN**	Spontaneously	4											C = Eyes Closed by Swelling
		To Command	3											
		To Pain	2											
		No Response	1	✓										
	BEST MOTOR RESPONSE	Obeys Commands	6											Record Best Arm Response to painful Stimuli for 1 thru 4
		Localizes Pain	5											
		Flexion-Withdrawal	4											
		Flexion-Decorticate	3											
		Extension-Deceberate	2											
		No Response	1	✓										
	BEST VERBAL RESPONSE	Oriented	5											T = Endo-tracheal Tube or Tracheos-tomy A = Aphasia
		Confused	4											
		Inappropriate Words	3											
		Incomprehensible Sounds	2											
		No Response	1	✓										
	TOTAL SCORE													

P U P I L S	Size	R	5 mm											B = Brisk S = Sluggish N = No Reaction C = Closed by swelling
	Reaction		No											
	Size	L	3 mm											
	Reaction		yes											

L I M B M O V E M E N T	Limb Movement Scale 0 - No Response 1 - Flicker of Trace of Contraction 2 - Active Movement with Gravity Eliminated 3 - Active Movement Against Gravity 4 - Active Movement Against Gravity and Resistance	RA	0											Grade Limb Movement Spontaneous or to Command. Do Not Rate Reflex Movement.
		RL	0											
		LA	0											
		LL	0											

V I T A L S	Blood Pressure	290/140											
	Pulse	102											
	Respiratory Rate	26											
	Temperature	99²											
	ICP												
	Nurse's Initial	PC											

Nurse's Signature and Initials

P. Washington, RN

Burke, Raymond
1877 Pointview Place
Lancing, Oklahoma
Dr. R. Aulph, M.D.
#876-549-34088
Bed 2E   811
Pt. Name Plate

1MM 2MM 3MM 4MM 5MM 6MM 7MM 8MM 9MM

FIGURE 37–11. This type of documentation is made on patients with neurological trauma. Note the guide for eye pupil size.

Stroke

A **stroke** is also called a **cerebrovascular accident (CVA)** or **apoplexy**. It affects the vascular system and the nervous system. The complete or partial loss of blood flow to the brain tissue is frequently a complication of atherosclerosis or brain hemorrhage. Causes of CVA include:

- Vascular occlusion due to a thrombus, atherosclerotic plaques, or emboli which obstruct the flow of blood
- Intracranial bleeding as blood vessels rupture, releasing blood into the brain tissue
- Spasms of blood vessels

Remember, most nerve pathways cross. Therefore, damage on one side of the brain results in signs and symptoms on the opposite side of the body. Symptoms vary depending on the extent of interference with the circulation and on the area and amount of tissue damaged.

- Left brain damage—may also affect the speech and communication centers. The patient will have **aphasia** (inability to communicate verbally).
- Right brain damage—may affect thought processes, memory, written computation, and the ability to tell time.

Symptoms of an acute CVA include:

- Loss of consciousness
- Weakness or paralysis on one side of the body (**hemiplegia**), Figure 37–12.
- Dizziness
- Nausea
- Headache
- Disorientation
- Inability to communicate
- Difficulty swallowing
- Loss of feeling on one side
- Thought processes deranged
- Incontinence

The nursing goal is to prevent any complications that will delay rehabilitation. This goal is established on admission and is a continuing goal.

Nursing Care. In the acute phase:

- Position the patient in the proper way on the side. Elevate the bed to a semi-Fowler height.
- Keep side rails up for safety.
- Change position every two hours, always supporting to maintain alignment.
- Apply elastic support hose, if ordered. Make sure they are kept smooth.

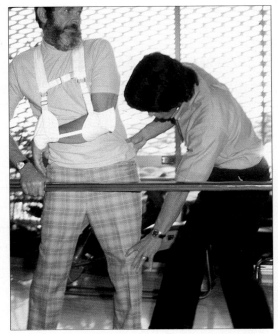

FIGURE 37–12. This patient exhibits left hemiplegia due to a stroke centered in the right side of the brain.

- Check drainage if a catheter has been inserted.
- Monitor vital signs frequently.
- Keep airway clear, frequently wiping the mouth. Inform the nurse if suctioning is needed.
- Carry out ROM exercises as ordered.

Note and report:

- Respiratory distress such as labored breathing or cyanosis
- Levels of consciousness
- Any uncontrolled muscular activity such as seizures or muscle spasms
- Need for suctioning
- Redness of skin over bony prominences

During Recovery. Recovery from a stroke is often a very frustrating experience for the patient. Care givers must be patient. In your approach to the patient, remember two things:

1. The patient has more than enough frustration for the two of you so be careful not to let yours show. The last thing the patient needs is your silent reinforcement of his helplessness.
2. It is well known that the degree and speed of recovery are directly related, in most cases, to the patience and encouragement of the care givers with whom the patient has close contact.

When patients are able to eat, allow them to assist themselves as much as possible. Until this happens, feeding the stroke patient requires time and a lot of patience. Be sure to place food on the unaffected side of the mouth. Continue with the same basic care. Allow patients to do as much as they can for themselves. Rehabilitation efforts include:

- Assisting in bowel and bladder training as directed
- Giving careful attention to the skin to prevent breakdown
- Encouraging the stroke victim to communicate
- Assisting with ambulation to prevent falls
- Maintaining a positive and supportive attitude at all times

Convalescence is often long. The nursing care is demanding, requiring much patience and understanding.

Aphasia

Stroke victims often suffer from aphasia or language impairment, Figure 37–13. They have difficulty forming thoughts or expressing them in coherent ways. This is extremely frustrating and frightening for the patient and family.

- **Receptive aphasia** means the person cannot comprehend communication.
- **Expressive aphasia** means the person cannot properly form thoughts or express them in a coherent way.
- **Global aphasia** means the person has lost all language abilities.

Aphasic patients make errors in the choice of words and expressions. They misuse words. They may also say profane words automatically and unintentionally. A speech therapist works with the aphasic person. The nursing assistant can help by:

- Speaking in short concise sentences.
- Using gestures to explain the meaning.
- Speaking often with the patient to provide practice.
- Being very patient and supportive of the person's attempts to communicate.
- Using a picture board to which the patient can point.

In the convalescent/rehabilitation phase, continue care started in the acute phase, such as:

- Changing position
- Carrying out ROM
- Applying elastic support hose if ordered
- Providing catheter care if a catheter is in place

Transient Ischemic Attack (TIA)

A **transient ischemic attack** (**TIA**) or ministroke is a temporary period of diminished blood flow to the cerebrum. The more often the TIAs occur, the more damage is done to the nerve cells. This situation may lead to dementia or loss of mental functioning. Muscle weakness and loss of coordination may also result, Figure 37–14. One or a series of TIAs is often a warning signal of impending stroke.

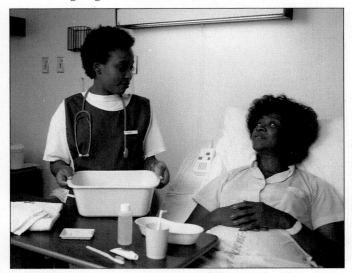

FIGURE 37–13. The receptive aphasic patient understands only part of a sentence and may answer incorrectly. *(From Hegner and Caldwell, Geriatrics, A Study of Maturity, 5th Edition, 1991, Delmar Publishers Inc.)*

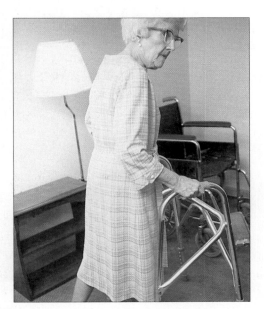

FIGURE 37–14. Transient ischemic attacks (TIA) have left this patient weakened so that a walker is needed for safe ambulation.

Roygan

Parkinson's Syndrome

Parkinson's syndrome is believed to be caused by not having enough neurotransmitters (dopamine) in the brain stem and cerebellum. The symptoms are progressive over many years. Some people will show minor changes. Others will have much more pronounced symptoms.

Signs and Symptoms. Signs and symptoms of Parkinson's syndrome include:

- **Tremors** (uncontrolled trembling). Tremors of the hands commonly affect the fingers and thumb in such a way that an affected person will appear to be rolling a small object such as a pill between them. These tremors occur frequently. They usually begin in the fingers, then involve the entire hand and arm, and finally affect an entire side of the body. Starting on one side, the tremors eventually involve both sides of the body. Tremors are more evident when the person is inactive. A typical posture of a patient suffering from Parkinson's syndrome is shown in Figures 37–15A and B.
- Muscular rigidity (loss of flexibility). The muscular rigidity is more evident when the patient is inactive. It seems to be lessened when the person sleeps or is engaged in activities such as walking or other exercises that require large muscle involvement. The rigidity makes the person with Parkinson's syndrome more prone to falls and injury.
- **Akinesia** (difficulty and slowness in carrying out voluntary muscular activities). Persons with advanced Parkinson's typically have:
  - A shuffling manner of walking
  - Difficulty starting the process of walking
  - Difficulty stopping smoothly once walking has started
  - Affected speech, causing words to be slurred and poorly spoken
  - Facial muscles that lose expressiveness and emotional response
- Loss of autonomic nervous control. Because of loss of autonomic nervous control, persons with Parkinson's:
  - May drool.
  - Become incontinent.
  - Become constipated.
  - Retain urine.
- Mood swings and gradual behavioral changes. You may notice that the person experiences mood swings. A patient may appear up and positive one moment, and then be depressed the next. The depression tends to be progressive. Personality and behavioral changes may occur that cause psychotic breakdowns and dementia in later stages.

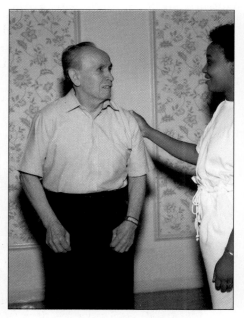

A. Ventral view

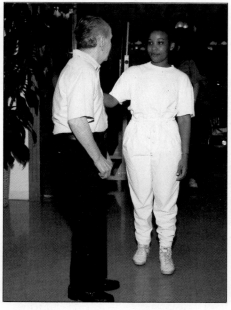

B. Lateral view

FIGURE 37–15. Note the typical posture from a ventral and lateral view of the patient suffering from Parkinson's disease.

Treatment. The treatment consists of:
- Surgery for some younger persons
- Drug therapy
- Therapy to limit the muscular rigidity and to meet the basic physical and emotional needs

Nursing Care. Nursing care of the person with Parkinson's syndrome includes:
- Maintaining a calm environment since patient symptoms are more intense when the patient is under stress.
- Assisting and supervising the activities of daily living. For example, directing food into the mouth and then keeping it there to be chewed and swallowed is very difficult for many persons with Parkinson's syndrome.
- Providing emotional support and encouragement.
- Carrying out a program of general and specific exercises.
- Providing protection for patients with dementia.

Multiple Sclerosis

Multiple sclerosis generally occurs in young adults. It is the result of the loss of insulation (myelin) around central nervous system nerve fibers. This interferes with the ability of the nerve fibers to function.

Multiple sclerosis is a progressive, gradually disabling condition. It progresses at varying rates. Early in the disease process there may be:
- Visual disturbances
- Weakness
- Unusual fatigue

As the disease progresses:
- Speech becomes slowed.
- There is gradual loss of bowel and bladder control.
- Paralysis often occurs, Figure 37–16.

Treatment. There is no known way to stop the progression of the disease. Treatment consists of maintaining functional ability as long as possible through general health practices and physical therapy.

Seizure Disorder (Epilepsy)

Seizure disorder (**convulsions, epilepsy**) involves recurrent, transient attacks of disturbed brain function. It is characterized by various forms of convulsions called seizures. Not all seizures are alike. A seizure occurs when one or more of the following is present:

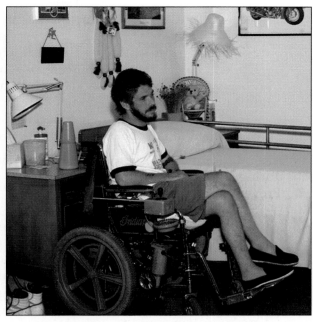

FIGURE 37–16. In multiple sclerosis, there is a gradual loss of motor control and sensory interpretation.

- An altered state of consciousness, which may be momentary or prolonged
- Convulsive uncontrolled movements
- Disturbances of feeling or behavior

Seizures may develop:
- Congenitally, associated with a difficult birth.
- Following a head injury.
- As a result of increased intracranial pressure.
- As a result of lesions of the brain such as tumors.
- As a result of cerebrovascular accidents.
- As a result of high fever, especially in infants and children.

Seizure activity may be classified as follows:
- **Partial seizures**
  — There may or may not be loss of consciousness.
  — Seizures generally begin in one part of the body and involve only one side of the body.
- **Generalized seizures**
  — These include grand mal seizures. There is bilateral generalized motor movement and muscular rigidity. Consciousness is lost and special awareness may or may not precede convulsive movements. The sensory awareness or aura may be in the form of lights, sounds, or aromas and is part of the seizure.
  — Petit mal seizures are characterized by momentary loss of muscle tone. They may involve temporary erratic behavior without awareness. For example, the individual

stops his present activity and carries out an unrelated repetitive activity for a few moments. Then he returns to the original activity with no awareness of the interruption.

■ **Status epilepticus** is a condition in which one convulsive seizure follows another so rapidly that the person does not gain consciousness between them. It is a very serious condition.

Nursing Care During Seizures. The main nursing focus during a seizure is to:

■ Prevent injury by:
— Staying with the person
— Assisting the person to lie down if there is time.
— Making no attempt to restrain the person's movements or put anything in the mouth.
— Moving away any object the person might hit to protect the person from injuring self.
— Placing a pillow under the person's head.
■ Maintain an airway by:
— Loosening clothing, particularly around the neck.
— Turning the person's head to one side so that saliva or vomitus drains out.
— Opening an airway, if necessary, by lifting the person's shoulders and allowing the head to tilt back.

If you find a person who is convulsing:

■ Do not leave the person.
■ Do not move the person.
■ Maintain an airway.
■ Ring or call for assistance.
■ Protect the person from self-inflicted injury.
■ Watch the person carefully.

Observation of the patient should be made during and following the convulsion. Breathing should be carefully monitored. Ring for assistance, if possible, but do not leave the patient alone. As much as possible, protect the patient from injuring self during the convulsion.

Spinal Cord Injuries

Injuries to the spinal cord result in loss of function and sensation below the level of the injury. These patients are particularly prone to contractures and pressure areas. Special terms have been given to the conditions resulting from such injury:

■ **Quadriplegia**—both arms and legs are paralyzed (paralyzed from the neck area down)
■ **Paraplegia**—lower part of the body is paralyzed

Responsibilities of the Nursing Assistant. Spinal cord injury patients need long-term nursing care which includes:

■ Listening—many persons with spinal cord injury are taught to give directions to caregivers who are doing for the person what the individual cannot do for self.
■ A consistently calm and patient approach, because the loss of sensory and motor functions often makes self-care difficult.
■ Acceptance of the patient's expressions of anger, fear, and depression, as well as clumsy attempts at self-care. Remember that the patient's ability to think is not necessarily impaired. Frustration is even greater because these patients can no longer will their actions.
■ Giving careful skin care since:
— Incontinence not only causes the patient embarrassment and discomfort but makes the skin prone to breakdown.
— The lack of nervous stimulation decreases circulation to the skin.
— Pain and pressure cannot be felt.
■ Attention to elimination needs. For example, suppositories may be given daily. A catheter may be inserted into the bladder, so catheter and drainage care will be needed. Special pads within plastic incontinence pants may also be used, Figure 37–17. Success has been achieved in bladder and bowel retraining, but it requires consistent professional supervision.
■ Constant care to prevent contractures. This care involves:
— Regular turning
— Proper positioning
— ROM exercises

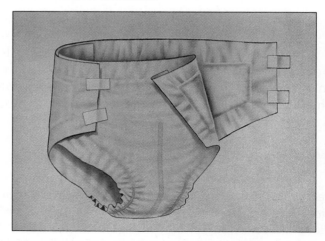

FIGURE 37–17. Wings® contoured incontinence briefs
(Wings® is a registered trademark of Professional Medical Products, Inc.)

- Proper attention and care to prevent:
  — Respiratory infections
  — Urinary tract infections
  — Pressure ulcers

Meningitis

Meningitis is an inflammation of the meninges. It is usually caused by microorganisms.

Signs and Symptoms. The signs and symptoms of meningitis are:
- Headache
- Nausea
- Stiffness of the neck
- Convulsions
- Chills
- Elevated temperature

Treatment. This condition is treated with antibiotics. If it is communicable, strict isolation precautions are taken.

Spinal Punctures

Spinal lumbar punctures (L.P.) are done to withdraw cerebrospinal fluid (CSF) for examination or to introduce medications such as during anesthesia before surgery.

The physician inserts a long, sterile needle between the lumbar vertebrae into the fluid-filled space between the arachnoid mater and pia mater. The pressure of the cerebrospinal fluid is measured. A sample is withdrawn and placed in a sterile test tube.

There are special positions in which the patient can be placed in preparation for the spinal puncture.
- The patient is placed on the side facing away from the doctor. The knees are drawn up to the abdomen. The head is bent down on the chest with the arms comfortably flexed, Figures 37–18A and B.
- An alternative position is one in which the patient is seated on the edge of the bed with the shoulders hunched forward, Figure 37–19. The patient may lean on an over-bed table.
- It is important that the patient not move during the procedure so be sure to offer ample support.

Tests on the cerebrospinal fluid give information about pressure within the system. Other tests measure the presence of blood, proteins, and infectious materials. Each abnormal finding or value provides clues to the condition of the central nervous tissues.

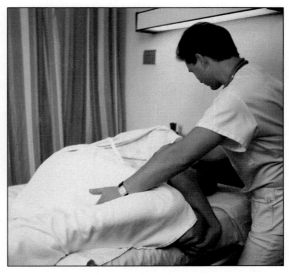

A.

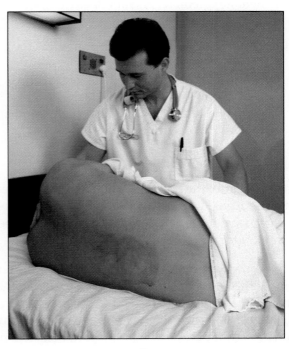

B.

FIGURE 37–18. One position of the patient for a cerebrospinal puncture. Draw the patient's knees up to his abdomen and his head toward his chest.

For example:
- Blood in the cerebrospinal fluid indicates bleeding into the system. This occurs in hemorrhagic stroke patients.
- Lowered sugar or increased white blood cells are indicative of bacterial infections.

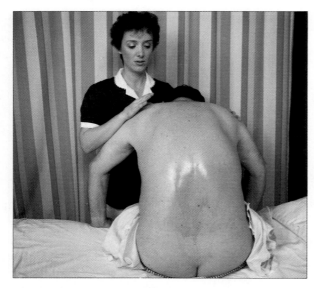

FIGURE 37–19. An alternative position of the patient for a cerebrospinal puncture.

Following Care. After a spinal puncture, the patient:

- Is usually kept flat in bed for eight hours to reduce the possibility of headache.
- Does not have the head of the bed elevated and is not provided with a pillow.

Cataracts

Cataracts cause the normally clear lens of the eye to become cloudy. The cloudy (opaque) lens will not allow light rays to pass through. Therefore, the person is no longer able to see.

Treatment. Removal or replacement of the lens permits light rays to enter the eye. Sight is then restored. The lens is needed to adjust vision to different distances. When the lens is removed, glasses must be worn to compensate for the loss. In selected patients, it may be possible to insert an intraocular lens at the time of surgery.

The cataract surgery is usually performed under local anesthesia unless the patient is frightened. In that case, a general anesthesia may be used.

The surgery is usually performed either as an outpatient procedure or in a day surgery center. The patient is admitted to the center in the morning and remains one to two hours after surgery or until vital signs are stable.

Nursing Care. Nursing care of the cataract patient includes:

- Routine postoperative care related to the specific anesthesia used.
- Relief of pain. Be sure to report discomfort and *especially* any sharp pain in the involved eye.
- Positioning the patient on the noninvolved side or back with the head of the bed slightly elevated.
- Being sure all needed items, such as signal cords, are within easy reach.
- Assisting with all activities so as to minimize strain.
- Encouraging the patient not to move rapidly, bend over, or cough. This might cause strain.
- Checking dressing and reporting drainage to the nurse.
- Taking extra precautions if the patient is confused or restless.
- Checking vital signs until stable.

Orders regarding postoperative activity usually include:

- Protecting the eye for the first four weeks.
- Avoid straining activities such as bending over, lifting objects over 20 pounds, or strenuous coughing.
- No water in the eye for the first three weeks.
- Removing crusts around eyelashes with antibiotic ointment and/or Q-Tip.
- Using eyedrops as directed.
- Not sleeping on the operative side.
- Informing the physician if there is an increase in pain or loss of vision.

Retinal Degeneration

Breakdown of the retina, known as **retinal degeneration** or **senile macular degeneration**, occurs over a period of months or years. The incidence increases with age. Central vision is progressively lost as the macula (area of acute central vision) is damaged. Subretinal hemorrhages lead to scarring of this important area.

Treatment. Early treatment with laser therapy can seal the tiny capillaries to prevent further damage to the macula.

Blindness

Cataracts, glaucoma, eye infections, and other eye conditions, such as an ocular tumor, can cause blindness. People who are legally blind may still have partial vision. The degree of visual limitation must be considered when giving care. It is also important to consider the patient's attitude to the limitations. Adjustment to blindness is both a physical and an emotional process.

Allow the blind or nearly blind person the opportunity to do as much as possible in personal care and other activities. Many blind people are capable and independent. In fact, most blind people do well with minimal help and support once they are fully oriented to their surroundings.

You should:

- Orient the blind person to anything new that is introduced into the environment.
- Place furniture in simple arrangements. Do not move furniture.
- Provide support until the person is familiar with the physical arrangement of the living space.
- Return all personal belongings to their proper places.
- When serving food, describe the food and its placement on the plate as if the plate were the face of a clock.

Otitis Media

Otitis media is an infection of the middle ear. Infections of the nose and throat can move along the eustachian tube to the middle ear, causing inflammation of the middle ear. Fluid and pus form within the middle ear. This may result in fusion (locking) of the middle ear bones. Increased pressure may cause the eardrum to rupture. Both conditions decrease the ability to transmit sound waves. This condition, which is rare in adults, is common in children.

Treatment. Antibiotics are usually given. A surgical opening (myringotomy) is sometimes made in the eardrum to drain the pus. Small tubes (PE/Sheperd's) may be inserted.

Otosclerosis

Otosclerosis is a progressive form of deafness of unknown cause. The process involves the growth of new, abnormal bone in the bony labyrinth. This growth prevents the stapes from vibrating properly.

Hearing is improved by the use of a hearing aid. Surgery (stapedectomy) removes the excess bone and replaces it with a prostheses.

Deafness

Some of your patients will be hard of hearing or completely deaf. A hearing aid will sometimes improve the patient's level of hearing and comprehension. Lip reading or sign language may be needed to communicate. In general, when communicating with someone who is hard of hearing:

- Be sure the hearing aid is in place, if used, and functioning.
- Keep voice pitch low.
- Speak slowly and distinctly.

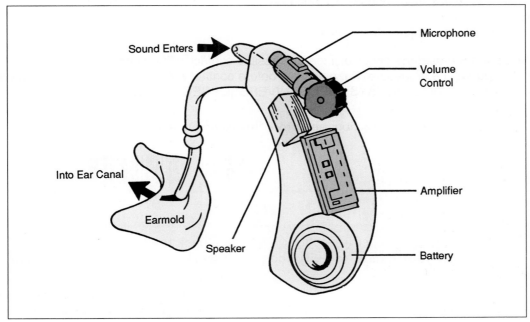

FIGURE 37–20. Parts of the hearing aid *(From Hegner and Caldwell,* Assisting in Long-Term Care, *copyright 1993 by Delmar Publishers Inc.)*

- Form words carefully. Keep sentences short.
- Rephrase words as needed.
- Face the listener.
- Have the light behind the listener.
- Use facial expression or gestures to help express meanings.
- Encourage lip reading.
- Reduce outside distractions.

Care of the Hearing Aid

The hearing aid is an instrument that must be handled carefully. There are several parts, Figure 37–20:

- Ear mold—should be washed with soap and water daily. Make sure it is dry before attaching it to the receiver.
  NOTE: If the unit is one piece, do not use water. Give unit to the nurse if it needs cleaning.

- Cannula—may be cleaned with a small applicator or pipe cleaner.
- Transmitter—usually attached to the glasses or placed behind the ear.

If the appliance is not working properly, check to be sure that the:

- On-off switch is in the "On" position.
- Batteries are in the proper position. Replace batteries if necessary.
- Cord is intact with no cracks or breaks.
- Ear mold is clean.
- Ear canal is not blocked by wax.

Review Figure 37–21 showing the beginning procedure actions and procedure completion actions for all patient care procedures before studying the following procedures.

BEGINNING PROCEDURE ACTIONS	PROCEDURE COMPLETION ACTIONS
■ Wash your hands.	■ Position patient comfortably.
■ Assemble equipment needed.	■ Leave signal cord, telephone, and fresh water close at hand.
■ Go to the patient's room, knock, and pause before entering.	■ Return bed or table to lowest position.
■ Introduce yourself and identify the patient by checking the identification bracelet.	■ Perform general safety check of patient and environment.
■ Ask visitors to leave and inform them where they can wait.	■ Wash your hands.
■ Care for equipment according to facility policy.	■ Report completion of task.
■ Provide privacy.	■ Let visitors know when they may reenter the patient's room.
■ Explain what will happen and answer questions.	■ Document action and your observations.
■ Allow patient to assist in procedure as much as possible.	
■ Raise bed or table to comfortable working height.	

NOTE: Where there are open lesions, wet linen, or possible contact with patient body fluids or blood, disposable gloves are worn during the procedure. Put on gloves before contact with the patient or linen. Properly dispose of gloves after they are removed. ALWAYS APPLY UNIVERSAL PRECAUTIONS.

FIGURE 37–21. Beginning procedure actions and procedure completion actions

---

PROCEDURE 112 **OBRA**   SIDE **9**

APPLYING A BEHIND-THE-EAR HEARING AID

1. Carry out each beginning procedure action.
2. Remember to wash your hands, identify the patient, and provide privacy.
3. Assemble equipment needed:
   - Hearing aid

4. Check the appliance to be sure batteries are working and tubing is not cracked, Figure 37–22.
5. Check to make sure the hearing aid is off or the volume is turned to its lowest level.

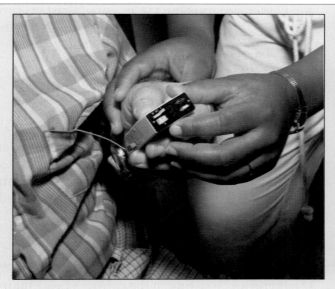
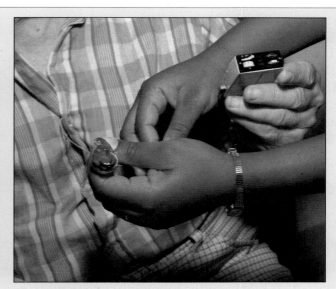

FIGURE 37–22. Check the appliance to be sure batteries are working and tubing is not cracked.

6. Check the patient's ear for wax buildup or any abnormalities.
   NOTE: If the patient complains that the hearing aid hurts or doesn't fit properly, it may need to be refitted as ear structure changes with age. Report this to the nurse.
7. Handle the aid carefully.
   - Do not drop it.
   - Do not allow it to get wet.
   - Store it carefully with the switch in the off position when it is not in use. Some aids should have batteries removed when being stored.
8. Hand the aid to the patient so that you support the appliance as the patient inserts the earmold into the ear canal.

Alternate Actions:

9. Place the hearing aid over the patient's ear, allowing the ear mold to hang free.
10. Adjust the hearing aid behind the patient's ear.
11. Grasp the ear mold and gently insert the tapered end into the ear canal.
12. Gently twist the ear mold into the curve of the ear, pushing upward and inward on the bottom of the ear mold, while pulling on the ear lobe with the other hand.
13. Turn on control switch and adjust volume to a comfortable level.
14. Carry out each procedure completion action. Remember to wash your hands, report completion of the task, and document time, date, hearing aid applied, and patient reaction.

PROCEDURE 113 | OBRA

REMOVING A BEHIND-THE-EAR HEARING AID

1. Carry out each beginning procedure action.
2. Remember to wash your hands, identify the patient, and provide privacy.
3. Explain to the patient what you plan to do.
4. Turn off the hearing aid.
5. Loosen the outer portion of the ear mold by gently pulling on the upper part of the ear.
6. Lift the ear mold upward and outward.
7. Make sure on-off switch is in off position. Store hearing aid in a safe area.
8. Carry out each procedure completion action. Remember to wash your hands, report completion of the task, and document time, date, hearing aid removed, and patient reaction.

SUMMARY

The nursing assistant assists the registered nurse in the care of patients with neurological conditions. Although the registered nurse is responsible for neurological assessment and intervention, the alert nursing assistant can be valuable.

- Observations of changes in levels of consciousness, response, and behavior must be accurately and promptly reported.
- The nursing assistant supplies comfort and support during the critical care period.

- Under supervision, the nursing assistant provides specific care for patients who have the following conditions:
  — CVAs.
  — Seizures.
  — Head injuries.
  — Spinal cord injuries.
  — Diseases of or trauma to eyes and ears.

Diseases and injuries of the nervous system often require a long recovery period. During the convalescent period, the nursing assistant plays an important role. Patience, empathy, and skill are needed in full measure to assist these patients in their recovery.

UNIT REVIEW

A. True/False. Answer the following statements true or false by circling T or F.

T F 1. The patient with right brain damage will not be able to speak.

T F 2. The patient has aphasia so it is not necessary to speak to him since he can't understand anyway.

T F 3. The patient suffering from CVA will need assistance in carrying out ROM.

T F 4. Paralysis means loss of voluntary muscle control.

T F 5. The patient with Parkinson's syndrome characteristically has a "pill-rolling" tremor to the hands.

T F 6. Status epilepticus is a serious condition.

T F 7. The Parkinson's syndrome patient often has mood swings.

T F 8. The quadriplegic person is paralyzed on the left side only.

T F 9. Fluid may be withdrawn from the spinal canal for examination.

B. Multiple Choice. Choose the answer that best completes each of the following sentences by circling the proper letter.

10. Increased intracranial pressure can develop from
    a. head injuries.
    b. infections.
    c. CVAs.
    d. All of the above.

11. If you are assisting in the care of a head-injury patient, you should note and report
    a. disorientation.
    b. alterations in speech.
    c. changes in levels of consciousness.
    d. All of the above.

12. You come into a room and find a patient having a seizure. You should
    a. leave and find help.
    b. restrain the patient's movements.
    c. raise the foot of the bed.
    d. remove any object the patient might hit.

13. The person with Parkinson's syndrome
    a. needs much emotional support.
    b. needs a hearing aid.
    c. suffers from blindness.
    d. None of the above.

C. Matching. Match the phrases or statements in Column I with the words in Column II.

Column I	Column II
_____ 14. uncontrolled trembling	a. akinesia
	b. aphasia
_____ 15. CVA	c. tremors
_____ 16. difficulty and slowness in carrying out voluntary muscular activities	d. seizure
	e. sclera
	f. stroke
_____ 17. language impairment	
_____ 18. convulsion	

D. Completion. Complete the following statements in the space provided.

19. Four actions the nursing assistant can take to help orient a person who is blind are:

    a. _____

    b. _____

    c. _____

    d. _____

20. Four actions a nursing assistant can take to check a hearing aid that is not working properly are:

    a. _____

    b. _____

    c. _____

    d. _____

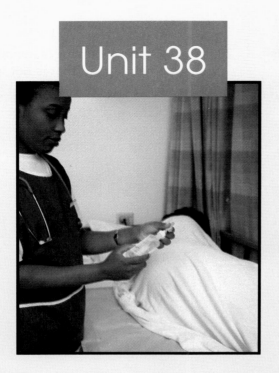

Unit 38

The Gastrointestinal System and Common Disorders

OBJECTIVES

As a result of this unit, you will be able to:

- Spell and define terms.
- Review the location and functions of the organs of the gastrointestinal system.
- List specific diagnostic tests associated with disorders of the gastrointestinal system.
- Describe some common disorders of the gastrointestinal system.
- Describe nursing assistant actions related to the care of patients with disorders of the gastrointestinal system.
- Identify different types of enemas and state their purpose.

VOCABULARY

Learn the meaning and the correct spelling of the following words:

bile
cholecystectomy
cholecystitis
cholelithiasis
colon
colostomy
duodenal resection
duodenal ulcer
flatus
gastrectomy
gastric resection
gastric ulcer
gastroscopy
hernia
herniorrhaphy
hydrochloric acid (HCl)

impaction
incarcerated
  (strangulated)
  hernia
nasogastric tube
  (NG tube)
peristalsis
proctoscopy
sigmoidoscopy
stoma
stool
suppository
ulcer
ulcerative colitis
urgency

Before beginning this unit of study, you may wish to go back to Unit 4 and review pages 75–78.

You learned that the digestive tract extends from the mouth to the anus. It receives the help of the teeth, tongue, salivary glands, liver, gallbladder, and pancreas in breaking food into simple substances. These substances are used by the body cells to carry on their work of supplying nutrition and eliminating wastes. Study the diagrams in Figures 38–1, 38–2, and 38–3.

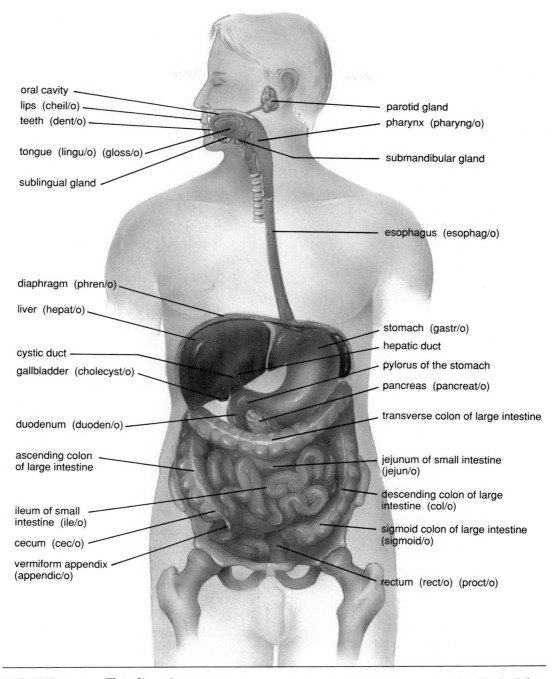

FIGURE 38–1. The digestive system *(From Anatomy and Physiology Plates, copyright 1992 by Delmar Publishers Inc.)*

Common Conditions

Malignancy

Malignancies (cancers) of the gastrointestinal tract are very common. The symptoms they cause depend on their location.

Among the symptoms are:

- Obstruction. The blocking of the passageway is sometimes the first major indication of a long-growing tumor.
- Indigestion.
- Vomiting.
- Constipation.

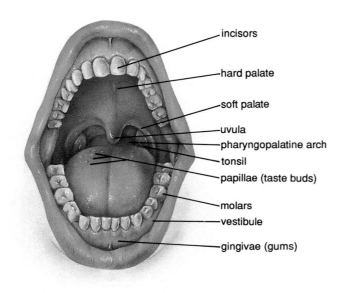

incisors

hard palate

soft palate

uvula

pharyngopalatine arch

tonsil

papillae (taste buds)

molars

vestibule

gingivae (gums)

FIGURE 38–2.   The mouth

■ Changes in the shape of the stool (bowel movement).

■ Flatus (gas).

■ Blood in the stool.

Treatment. Malignancies of the intestinal tract are usually treated surgically by removing the affected part. For example:

■ Esophagectomy—removal of the esophagus

ORGAN	IMPORTANT ENZYMES	FOOD ACTED UPON
Salivary glands	Salivary amylase	Starches
Stomach	Pepsin Lipase Renin (infants)	Proteins Fats Milk protein
Pancreas	Lipase Amylase Trypsin	Fats Starches Proteins
Small intestine	Lactase Sucrase Maltase Peptidase	Lactose (sugar) Sucrose (sugar) Maltose (sugar) Protein

FIGURE 38–3.   Enzymes and digestion

■ Subtotal gastrectomy—removal of part of the stomach

■ Colectomy (bowel resection)—removal of a part of the colon (large intestine).

■ Colostomy—creation of an artificial opening in the abdominal wall and bringing a section of the colon to it for the elimination of feces

■ Ileostomy—creation of an artificial opening in the abdominal wall and bringing a section of ileum through it for the elimination of waste

Ulcerations

An ulcer (sore or tissue breakdown) can occur anywhere along the digestive tract. Common places are the:

■ Colon—ulcerative colitis. In colitis, malnutrition and dehydration are brought about by loss of fluids in frequent, watery, offensive stools with mucus and pus.

■ Stomach—gastric ulcer.

■ Duodenum—duodenal ulcer.

Treatment. Treatment of ulcerative colitis includes:

■ Medications to slow peristalsis (wave-like contractions of the intestines) and reduce patient anxiety.

■ Modification of diet to include high protein, high calories, and low residue. The low-residue diet is one in which the foods are almost completely digested. There is little waste with this type of diet.

■ Medications (steroids) to reduce inflammation.

Patients with gastric or duodenal ulcers have periodic burning pain about two hours after eating. Most patients improve when they are placed on a diet in which foods that cause distress are not served. Medications are given to neutralize the hydrochloric acid (HCl), to coat the stomach, and to decrease anxiety. It is sometimes necessary to remove part of the stomach (gastrectomy or gastric resection) or duodenum (duodenal resection). Following such surgery, the patient is:

■ Placed on NPO. Special mouth care is therefore needed.

■ Placed on gastrointestinal drainage. A nasogastric tube (NG tube), Figure 38–4, is inserted through the patient's nose and extends into the stomach. The tube is attached to a drainage bottle. Miller-Abbott and Canter tubes are inserted into the intestinal tract. Be careful not to disturb the tubes. Check frequently to ensure that the drainage is not blocked. If drainage becomes blocked, report it to your supervisor at once. The type and amount of drainage are noted and recorded.

Hernias

A hernia results when a structure such as the intestine pushes through a weakened area in a normally restraining wall. The danger of such abnormal protrusions is that some of the protruding tissue can become trapped in the weakened area. Circulation then becomes limited so that the tissue is in danger of dying. This is called an incarcerated (strangulated) hernia

Frequent sites of herniation are:
- Groin area (inguinal hernia)
- Near the umbilicus (umbilical hernia)
- Through a poorly healed incision (incisional hernia)
- Through the diaphragm (hiatal hernia)

Treatment. Hernias are usually repaired surgically with a herniorrhaphy

Gallbladder Conditions

Two common conditions affecting the gallbladder are:
- Cholecystitis—an inflammation of the gallbladder.
- Cholelithiasis—the formation of stones in the gallbladder. The stones may obstruct the flow

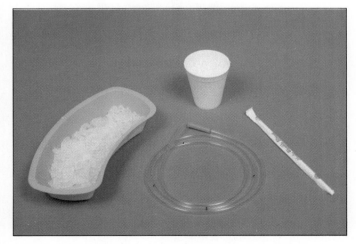

FIGURE 38–4. Preparing for nasogastric tube insertion

of bile (fluid that aids digestion), giving rise to signs and symptoms such as:
- Indigestion
- Pain
- Jaundice—yellow discoloration of the skin and whites of the eyes

Treatment. Cholecystitis and cholelithiasis may be treated by:
- Low-fat diet.
- Surgery to remove the gallbladder and stones. This surgical procedure is called a cholecystectomy
- Laser therapy to break up the stones.

Drains are often placed in the operative areas. Large amounts of yellowish-green drainage may be expected.

In addition to the routine postoperative care:
- Position the patient in a semi-Fowler's position.
- Do not disturb drains.
- If you notice fresh blood on the dressing, increased jaundice, or dark urine, report it immediately to your team leader.

Special Diagnostic Tests

Some techniques used to diagnose problems of the gastrointestinal system include:
- Gastrointestinal (GI) series—for this test a liquid called barium is either swallowed (upper GI series) or given as an enema (lower GI series). X-rays are then taken.
- Direct visualization procedures:
  - **Proctoscopy**—visualization of the rectum
  - **Sigmoidoscopy**—visualization of the sigmoid colon
  - **Gastroscopy**—visualization of the stomach

In preparation for the tests, the entire GI tract must be emptied before the X-rays.
- No food is permitted for eight hours or longer.
- Enemas are given before the series until only the clear liquid returns.
- Laxatives are given the night before the test.

Cholecystogram (Gallbladder Series)

A gallbladder (GB) series is an X-ray examination similar to the GI series except that the dye tablets are swallowed. Orders for preparing patients for this test vary. Cleansing enemas are frequently ordered. A special diet may also be required beforehand.

Enemas

A cleansing enema is the technique of introducing fluid into the rectum in order to remove feces and flatus (gas) from the colon and rectum. Enemas are given:

- To aid illumination during X-rays.
- Before surgery.
- Before testing.
- During bowel retraining programs.
- To relieve constipation.
- To instill drugs.

The fluids often ordered for the enemas are:

- Soap suds solution (SSE)
- Salt solution (saline)
- Tap water (TWE)
- Phosphosoda

These solutions create a feeling of urgency in the patient's bowel. Solutions are expelled a short time after they are given. Urgency is a term used to describe the need to empty the bowel. When enemas are given in preparation for diagnostic X-rays or to instill drugs, the fluid is retained as long as possible.

Position

The best position for the patient to receive an enema is in the left Sims' position. Fluid flows into the bowel more easily when the patient is in this position. The left Sims' position and several alternative positions are shown in Figure 38–5.

At times, the enema may need to be administered with the patient on the bedpan in the supine position. The supine position can be used if the patient is unable to hold the fluid or to assume the Sims' position.

- The patient's knees are flexed and separated.
- An orthopedic (fracture) bedpan is more comfortable than a regular bedpan. It may need to be padded when the patient is very thin.

Some patients may not be able to hold the enema fluid. For this reason, disposable gloves are worn when administering an enema.

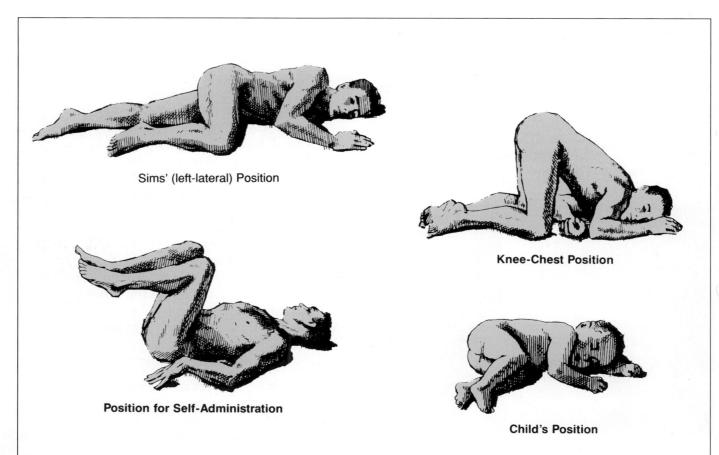

Sims' (left-lateral) Position

Knee-Chest Position

Position for Self-Administration

Child's Position

FIGURE 38–5. Alternative positions for enema administration *(Courtesy of C.B. Fleet Co., Inc.)*

BEGINNING PROCEDURE ACTIONS	PROCEDURE COMPLETION ACTIONS
■ Wash your hands. ■ Assemble equipment needed. ■ Go to the patient's room, knock, and pause before entering. ■ Introduce yourself and identify the patient by checking the identification bracelet. ■ Ask visitors to leave and inform them where they can wait. ■ Care for equipment according to facility policy. ■ Provide privacy. ■ Explain what will happen and answer questions. ■ Allow patient to assist in procedure as much as possible. ■ Raise bed or table to comfortable working height.	■ Position patient comfortably. ■ Leave signal cord, telephone, and fresh water close at hand. ■ Return bed or table to lowest position. ■ Perform general safety check of patient and environment. ■ Wash your hands. ■ Report completion of task. ■ Let visitors know when they may reenter the patient's room. ■ Document action and your observations.

NOTE: Where there are open lesions, wet linen, or possible contact with patient body fluids or blood, disposable gloves are worn during the procedure. Put on gloves before contact with the patient or linen. Properly dispose of gloves after they are removed. ALWAYS APPLY UNIVERSAL PRECAUTIONS.

FIGURE 38–6. Beginning procedure actions and procedure completion actions

General Considerations

Some general considerations to keep in mind are:
■ If the patient is to get up following the enema and use the bathroom, make sure the bathroom is available and not in use before giving the enema.
■ When possible, the enema should be given before the patient's bath or before breakfast.
■ Do not give an enema within an hour following a meal.

Before studying the following procedures, review the beginning procedure actions and the procedure completion actions in Figure 38–6.

■ Remember that you must have a physician's order for any enema.

Disposable Units

Disposable units are available to give:
■ Oil-retention enemas
■ Soapsuds enemas
■ Commercially prepared enemas

Administration of disposable enemas is simple. Time is saved in preparing and cleaning the equipment. The techniques for using reusable equipment for oil-retention or soapsuds enemas are the same. The procedures when using a prepackaged prepared solution follow.

PROCEDURE 114

SIDE
9

GIVING AN OIL-RETENTION ENEMA   20 MIN

1. Carry out each beginning procedure action.
2. Remember to wash your hands, identify the patient, and provide privacy.
3. Assemble equipment needed:
    ■ Bedpan and cover, commode, or toilet
    ■ Toilet tissue
    ■ Towel, soap, basin with water
    ■ Prepackaged oil for retention enema

■ Bed protector
■ Bath blanket
■ Disposable gloves

4. Instruct the patient that it will be necessary to hold the solution at least 20 minutes, Figure 38–7.
5. Place chair at foot of bed and cover with towel. Place bedpan on it.

continues

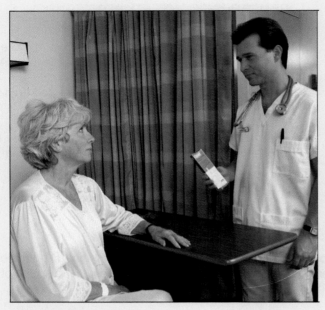

FIGURE 38–7. Explain to the patient the purposes of the enema and answer any questions.

6. Cover patient with bath blanket and fanfold linen to foot of bed.
7. Place bed protector under buttocks.
8. Help patient assume the Sims' position.
9. Open the prepackaged oil-retention enema.
10. Put on gloves.
11. Expose the patient's anus. Remove cap from enema and insert the prelubricated tip into anus as the patient takes a deep breath, Figure 38–8.
12. Squeeze container until all the solution has entered the rectum.
13. Remove container and place in package box to be discarded.
14. Encourage patient to remain on the side.
15. Remove and dispose of gloves according to facility policy.
16. Check patient every five minutes until fluid has been retained for 20 minutes.
17. Wash your hands and put on gloves.
18. Position patient on bedpan or commode or assist to bathroom.
19. If patient is on the bedpan, raise head of bed to comfortable height.
20. Place toilet tissue and signal cord within easy reach of patient. If patient is in bathroom, stay nearby. Caution patient not to flush toilet.

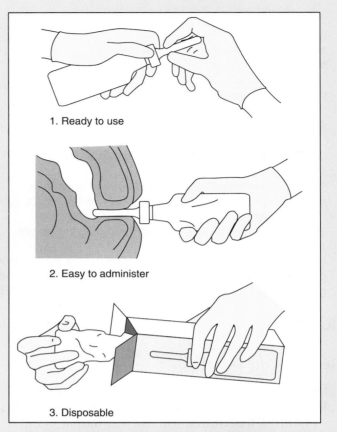

1. Ready to use

2. Easy to administer

3. Disposable

FIGURE 38–8. Administering an oil-retention enema *(Courtesy of C.B. Fleet Co., Inc.)*

21. Dispose of disposable material per facility policy.
22. Remove bedpan or assist patient to return to bed.
    - Observe contents of bedpan or toilet.
    - Cover pan and dispose of or flush toilet.
23. Cleanse the anal area of the patient, if required.
24. Remove gloves and dispose of properly.
25. Give patient soap, water, and towel to wash and dry hands.
26. Replace top bedding and remove bath blanket and bed protector. Dispose of according to facility policy.
27. Carry out each procedure completion action. Remember to wash your hands, report completion of task, and document time, oil retention enema, and patient reaction.
    NOTE: An oil-retention enema is usually followed by a soapsuds enema. The oil softens the feces and the soapsuds stimulates evacuation of the bowel.

PROCEDURE 115

GIVING A SOAPSUDS ENEMA

1. Carry out each beginning procedure action.
2. Remember to wash your hands, identify the patient, and provide privacy.
3. Assemble equipment needed:
   - Disposable enema equipment, which is commercially available, consisting of a plastic container, tubing, clamp, and lubricant
   - Disposable gloves
   - Bedpan and cover, commode, or toilet
   - Bed protector (Chux)
   - Toilet tissue
   - Bath blanket
   - Towel, soap, basin with water

   NOTE: If disposable equipment is not available, you will also need:
   - Funnel
   - Tubing, clamp, and rectal tube
   - Connecting tube
   - Graduated pitcher with warm, soapy water, 105°F
   - Lubricant
4. In the utility room:
   a. Connect tubing to solution container, Figure 38–9A.
   b. Adjust clamp on tubing and snap shut, Figure 38–9B.

c. Fill container with warm water (105°F) to the 1000 ml line (500 ml for children), Figures 38–9C and D.
d. Open packet of liquid soap and put the soap in the water, Figure 38–9E.
e. Using the tip of the tubing, mix the solution (mix gently so that no suds form) or rotate the bag to mix. Do not shake.
f. Run small amount of solution through tube to get rid of air and warm the tube. Clamp the tubing, Figures 38–9F and G.
5. Place chair at foot of bed and cover with towel. Place the bedpan on it.
6. Cover the patient with a bath blanket and fanfold linen to foot of bed.
7. Place bed protector under buttocks.
8. Help patient to turn on left side and flex knees (Sims' position).
9. Place container of solution on chair so tubing will reach patient.
10. Adjust bath blanket to expose anal area.
11. Put gloves on.
12. Expose anus by raising upper buttock.
13. Lubricate tip of tube. Insert tube 2–4 inches into the anus. Have the patient take a deep breath and bear down to relax the anal sphincter.

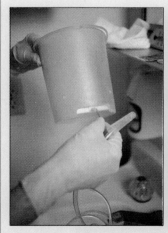

FIGURE 38–9A. Attach tubing to container.

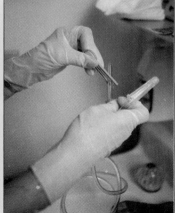

FIGURE 38–9B. Slip clamp over tubing.

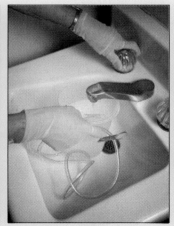

FIGURE 38–9C. Fill container with warm water.

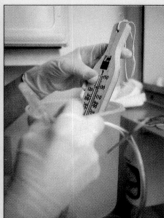

FIGURE 38–9D. Use a bath thermometer to be sure temperature of water is about 105°F.

continues

14. Never force the tube. If tube cannot be inserted easily, get help. There may be a tumor or a mass of feces blocking the bowel. Such a mass of feces is known as impaction.
15. Open the clamp and raise the container 12 inches above the level of the anus so that the fluid flows in slowly.
    ■ Ask the patient to take deep breaths to relax the abdomen.
    ■ If the patient complains of cramping, clamp tube and wait until cramping stops.
    ■ Then open the tubing to continue fluid flow.
16. When enough solution has been given, clamp the tubing.
17. Tell the patient to hold breath while upper buttock is raised and tube is gently withdrawn.
18. Wrap tubing in paper towel. Put it in the disposable container.
19. Place patient on bedpan or commode or assist to bathroom. Remove gloves and discard according to facility policy.
20. Raise head of bed to comfortable height if patient is on bedpan.
21. Place toilet tissue and signal cord within reach of patient. If patient is in bathroom, stay nearby. Caution patient not to flush toilet.
22. Take tray into utility room. Put on gloves.
    a. Rinse enema equipment thoroughly in cool water.
    b. Wash in warm soapy water. Dry equipment.
    c. Return it to bedside or discard according to facility policy.
    d. Remove gloves and discard according to facility policy. Wash your hands.
23. When patient is ready, wash your hands. Put on gloves to remove bedpan or assist patient to return to bed. Observe contents of bedpan. Cover bedpan. Dispose of contents according to facility policy or flush toilet.
24. Cleanse anal area of patient, if necessary. Remove bed protector.
25. Remove gloves and dispose of properly.
26. Give the patient soap, water, and a towel to wash hands.
27. Replace top bedding.
    a. Remove bath blanket.
    b. Air the room.
    c. Leave room in order.
    d. Unscreen unit.
28. Clean and replace all other equipment used according to facility policy.
29. Carry out each procedure completion action. Remember to wash your hands, report completion of task, and document time, date, enema (type, amount, and temperature of solution), returns (color, consistency, unusual materials, flatus), and patient reaction.

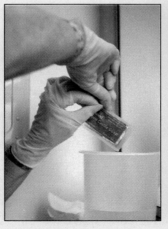

FIGURE 38–9E. Add soap from packet.

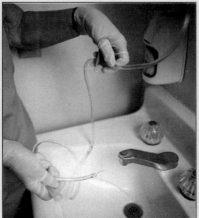

FIGURE 38–9F. Let a small amount of water flow through the tube to expel air.

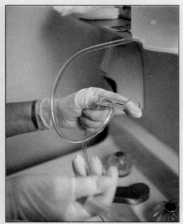

FIGURE 38–9G. Clamp tubing.

Giving An Enema with a Preprepared Chemical Enema Solution

The preprepared enema solution is an easy-to-use enema. It is frequently ordered for patients in the hospital, as well as in the home. These units have proved most successful for patients who are unable to hold the large amount of fluid that is necessary when a soap or saline solution is being used.

■ The chemical solution is already measured, prepared, and ready to use.

■ It is a special solution that draws fluid from the body to stimulate peristalsis.

■ The amount of solution administered is about four ounces.

■ The tip of the container is prelubricated.

■ The enema solution is in an easy-to-handle plastic container.

■ The solution is sometimes used at room temperature.

■ You may be asked to warm it by placing it in warm water before administration. Check with the nurse regarding your facility's policy.

PROCEDURE 116

SIDE **9**

GIVING A COMMERCIALLY PREPARED ENEMA

1. Carry out each beginning procedure action.
2. Remember to wash your hands, identify the patient, and provide privacy.
3. Assemble equipment needed:
   - Disposable prepackaged enema
   - Bedpan and cover, commode, or toilet
   - Bed protector
   - Disposable gloves
   - Pan of warm water (if enema solution is to be warmed)
4. Open package and remove plastic container with enema solution. Place solution container in warm water (if it is to be warmed).
5. Place bedpan and cover on the chair close at hand. Explain to the patient what you will be doing, Figure 38–10.
6. Lower head of bed to horizontal position. Raise side rail on opposite side of bed.
7. Assist patient to assume the left Sims' position. Refer to Figure 38–11.
8. Place bed protector under the patient.
9. Put gloves on.
10. Expose only the patient's buttocks by drawing the bedding upward in one hand.
11. Remove the cover from the enema tip. Gently squeeze to make sure tip is patent.
12. Separate buttocks, exposing anus, and ask patient to bear down slightly.
13. Insert lubricated enema tip 2 inches into the rectum.

14. Squeeze the plastic container slowly from the bottom of the container until all fluid has entered the patient's body.
15. Remove the tip from the patient and place the container in the box. Encourage the patient to hold the solution as long as possible.
16. Remove and dispose of gloves according to facility policy.
17. When the patient feels the urge to defecate (usually 5–15 minutes), assist patient to the bathroom/commode or position on the bedpan.

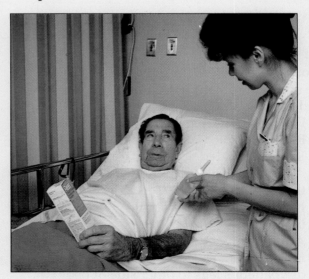

FIGURE 38–10. The nursing assistant explains to the patient that he must hold only the contents of the container.

continues

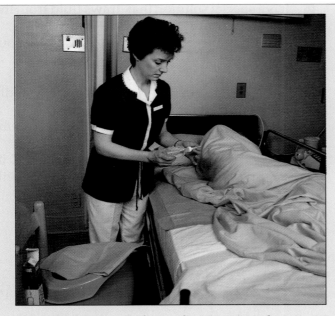

FIGURE 38–11. Before administering the enema, assist the patient into the left Sims' position and place a bed protector over the bed linens.

18. Raise the head of the bed to a comfortable height if the patient is on the bedpan.
19. Place toilet tissue and signal cord within reach of the patient. If patient is in bathroom, stay nearby. Caution patient not to flush toilet.
20. Return to the patient when signaled. Put on gloves.
21. Remove bedpan or assist patient to return to bed. Observe contents of bedpan or commode. Cover bedpan and remove bed protector.
22. Dispose of contents according to facility policy.
23. Remove and dispose of gloves properly. Wash your hands.
24. Give the patient soap, water, and a towel to wash hands.
25. Put on gloves. Take equipment to the dirty utility room and dispose of it according to facility policy.
26. Carry out each procedure completion action. Remember to wash your hands, report completion of task, and document time, date, enema (type, amount, and temperature of solution), if warmed, character and amount of returns, flatus, and patient reaction.

PROCEDURE 117

GIVING A ROTATING ENEMA

NOTE: The procedure for the rotating enema varies only slightly from the regular soapsuds enema. The same equipment is used, and about 1000 ml of fluid is allowed to flow into the rectum.

1. Follow steps 1–8 for the soapsuds enema.
2. Raise foot of bed about 30 degrees, Figure 38–12.
3. Insert lubricated tip 2–4 inches into the rectum.
4. Allow about 300 ml of fluid to flow slowly into the rectum.
5. Help patient to turn on back while holding tube in place.
6. Administer about 300 ml more of the solution.
7. Holding tube in place, move solution can under patient's legs to other side of bed.
8. Assist patient to turn on right side and administer the remaining solution.
9. Follow steps 16–29 for the soapsuds enema.

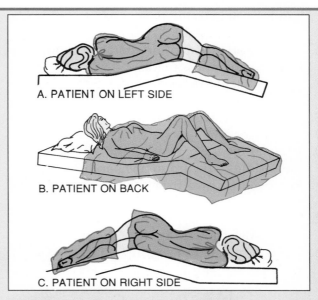

FIGURE 38–12. Positions for rotating enema

The Harris Flush

The Harris flush is used to relieve abdominal distention caused by gas. In this procedure, a small amount of fluid is injected into the rectum. It is then allowed to return by lowering the irrigation can. The Harris flush is also called a return-flow enema.

Other Gas-expelling Methods

The rectal tube is used to reduce the amount of flatus (gas) that is in the bowel. Flatus distends the intestines, causing pain and stress on incisions.

- The disposable tube is used once in a 24-hour period for no more than 20 minutes each time.
- Relief is sometimes dramatic as soon as the tube is inserted.
- Be sure to check the amount of abdominal distention.
- Question patient about degree of relief.

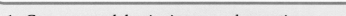

PROCEDURE 118

GIVING A HARRIS FLUSH (RETURN-FLOW ENEMA)

1. Carry out each beginning procedure action.
2. Remember to wash your hands, identify the patient, and provide privacy.
3. Assemble equipment needed:
   - Plastic container
   - Enema tubing and clamp
   - Lubricant
   - Covering for tray
   - Bed protector
   - Toilet tissue
   - Solution: 500 ml tap water at 105°F
   - Disposable gloves
4. Pour the solution into the plastic container and cover. Carry tray to bedside.
5. Place a bed protector under the patient.
6. Put lubricant on a square of tissue. Lubricate the end of the enema tubing.
7. Allow a small amount of fluid to run through the tubing to remove air.
8. Put gloves on.
9. Insert tube into rectum about 4 inches.

10. Handle the Harris flush in the following way to bring about peristalsis:
    a. Open clamp, raise irrigating can to a height of 12–18 inches above the patient's hips, and allow about 200 ml of fluid to run into the rectum.
    b. Lower irrigating can about 12 inches below the level of the bed and allow fluid to flow out of rectum into can.
11. Continue procedure until some gas is expelled. When all fluid has been returned, clamp tube and remove.
12. Remove bed protector.
13. Return tray to utility room. Dispose of contents of can. Clean equipment as for regular enema. Remove gloves and dispose of properly.
14. Carry out each procedure completion action. Remember to wash your hands, report completion of task, and document date, time, Harris flush (temperature of solution and flatus expelled), and patient reaction.

PROCEDURE 119

INSERTING A RECTAL TUBE AND FLATUS BAG

1. Carry out each beginning procedure action.
2. Remember to wash your hands, identify the patient, and provide privacy.
3. Assemble equipment needed:
   - Disposable rectal tube and flatus bag
   - Lubricant
   - Tissue
   - Tape
   - Paper towel
   - Disposable gloves
4. Lower the head of the bed to horizontal position.

continues

5. Assist the patient to assume the left Sims' position.
6. Put gloves on.
7. Expose only the patient's buttocks by drawing the bedding upward in one hand.
8. Lubricate tip of rectal tube.
9. Separate buttocks, exposing anus, and ask patient to bear down gently.
10. Insert lubricated tip of rectal tube 2–4 inches.
11. Secure rectal tube in place with small piece of adhesive.
12. Remove gloves and dispose of properly.
13. Adjust bedding and make patient comfortable. Leave unit neat and tidy and signal cord close at hand.
14. Wash your hands.
15. Return to unit in 20 minutes. Wash your hands.
16. Identify patient and screen unit. Explain what you plan to do.
17. Put on gloves.
18. Gently remove rectal tube and place on paper towel.
19. Dispose of wrapped rectal tube and bag according to facility policy.
20. Remove and dispose of gloves according to facility policy.
21. Carry out each procedure completion action. Remember to wash your hands, report completion of task, and document date, time, rectal tube inserted (time), removed (time), degree of relief, and patient reaction.

Rectal Suppositories

A suppository is given to stimulate bowel evacuation or to instill medications. Medicinal suppositories must be inserted by the nurse. You may be asked to insert suppositories that soften the stool and promote elimination, if you have been trained in this advanced procedure and if your facility allows it. Instructions are detailed in Unit 43.

Care of the Patient with a Colostomy

Sometimes disease of the bowel makes it necessary to remove or rest part of the bowel. To make this possible, a section of the bowel is brought to the surface of the abdomen and an opening is made. The procedure is called a colostomy and the new opening is called a stoma. Care of the patient with a colostomy is an advanced procedure and is covered in Unit 43.

The following advanced procedures are included in Unit 43:
- Inserting Rectal Suppositories
- Giving Routine Stoma Care (Colostomy)
- Routine Care of an Ileostomy (Patient in Bed)
- Routine Care of an Ileostomy (Patient in Bathroom)

These procedures are to be carried out only after adequate practice and supervision and only in accord with specific facility policy.

SUMMARY

- The organs in the digestive system are very complex. Because of their complexity, disease of these organs is fairly common. Common conditions include:
  — Cancer
  — Ulcerations
  — Hernias
  — Inflammation such as cholecystitis
- Procedures performed on this system include:
  — Enemas. Enemas are also performed before surgery on other parts of the body.
  — Insertion of rectal tubes to relieve flatus.
  — Irrigations such as colostomy irrigations.
- Great care must be exercised when performing the procedures. Remember that the comfort and privacy of the patient should be protected at all times.

UNIT REVIEW

A. True/False. Answer the following statements true or false by circling T or F.

T F 1. A herniorrhaphy is the surgery performed when there is bowel malignancy.

T F 2. The drainage from a new cholecystectomy patient would be expected to be yellowish-green.

T F 3. The patient is placed preferably in the left Sims' position for the administration of an enema.

T F 4. When administering an enema using a preprepared chemical solution, approximately 4 ounces are given.

T F 5. It is a wise idea to be sure that the bathroom is free before giving an enema.

T F 6. A flatus tube is used to reduce abdominal distention from gas.

T F 7. A physician's order is needed before an enema can be given.

T F 8. When giving a soapsuds enema, approximately 2000 ml are used.

T F 9. Gastric ulcers are located in the esophagus.

T F 10. Irrigating a new colostomy is a nursing assistant task.

B. Matching. Match the word or phrase Column I with the word in Column II.

Column I	Column II
_____ 11. gas	a. stool
_____ 12. yellow discoloration of skin	b. flatus
	c. cholelithiasis
_____ 13. large bowel	d. cyanosis
_____ 14. feces	e. cholecystectomy
_____ 15. gallstones	f. colon
	g. jaundice

C. Multiple Choice. Choose the answer that best completes each of the following sentences by circling the proper letter.

16. Signs of possible gastrointestinal malignancy might be
    a. good appetite.   c. weight gain.
    b. change in stool color. d. pallor.

17. Your patient has just returned from surgery for gallstones. She will be most comfortable in the
    a. dorsal recumbent position.
    b. lithotomy position.
    c. semi-Fowler's position.
    d. left Sims' position.

18. Enemas are given before
    a. surgery.   c. testing.
    b. delivery.   d. All of the above.

19. The oil-retention enema is usually
    a. preceded by a soapsuds enema.
    b. retained one hour.
    c. followed by a soapsuds enema.
    d. given in the semi-Fowler's position.

20. Urgency is a term that means
    a. need to urinate.
    b. need to empty the bowel.
    c. pain from flatus.
    d. need to vomit.

D. Completion. Complete the following statements in the space provided.

21. The enema given to soften feces is known as

_____.

22. The purpose of a soapsuds enema is to _____

_____.

Unit 39

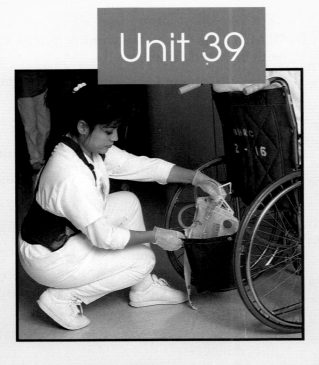

The Urinary System and Common Disorders

OBJECTIVES

As a result of this unit, you will be able to:

- Spell and define terms.
- Review the location and function of the urinary system.
- List five diagnostic tests associated with conditions of the urinary system.
- Describe some common diseases of the urinary system.
- Describe nursing assistant actions related to the care of patients with urinary system diseases and conditions.

VOCABULARY

Learn the meaning and the correct spelling of the following words:

catheter	intravenous
cystitis	pyelogram (IVP)
cystoscopy	lithotripsy
dialysis	nephritis
dysuria	pyelogram
Foley catheter	renal calculi
hematuria	renal colic
hydronephrosis	retrograde pyelogram
indwelling catheter	urinalysis

Before beginning to study this unit, review Unit 4, pages 78–80. Refer also to Figures 39–1 and 39–2 to review the components of the urinary system.

You will recall that the urinary system consists of the kidneys, ureters, bladder, and urethra. The functions that this system performs are vital. It:

- Excretes liquid wastes.
- Manages blood chemistry.
- Manages fluid balance.

Because the chemistry of the blood and urine reflect the chemistry of the cells, many tests are performed on urine specimens. It is important that the urine sample be obtained and preserved properly (refer to Unit 24).

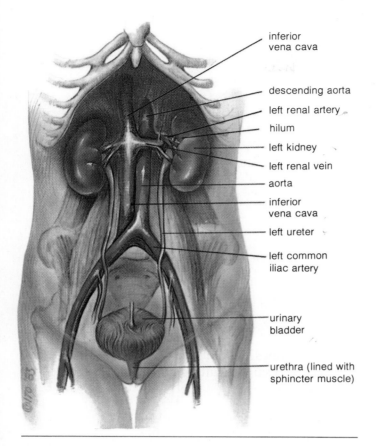

FIGURE 39–1. The urinary system *(From Fong, Ferris, and Skelley, Body Structures and Functions, 7th Edition, 1989, Delmar Publishers Inc.)*

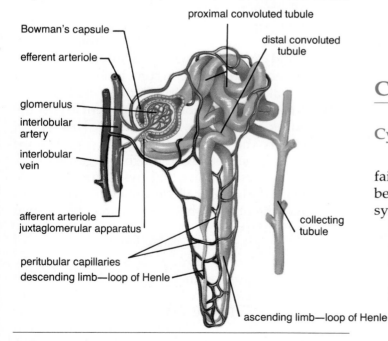

FIGURE 39–2. The nephron is the functional unit of the kidney that produces urine. One million of these units are found in the cortex of each kidney. *(From Anatomy and Physiology Plates, copyright 1992 by Delmar Publishers Inc.)*

Diagnostic Tests

Techniques used to diagnose problems of the urinary tract include:

- Magnetic resonance imaging (MRI)
- CAT scan
- Urinalysis

  One common method for learning about the condition of the kidneys is to examine the urine (**urinalysis**). You learned how to collect a specimen for routine urinalysis in Unit 24.

- **Cystoscopy**—is a test usually performed during surgery. It enables the physician to look inside the bladder. An instrument called a cystoscope is inserted through the urethra. Following this examination, frequency of urination is to be expected but heavy bleeding or a complaint of sharp, intense pain should be reported at once.

- **Pyelogram**—an X-ray examination of the urinary tract, similar to the GB and GI series. The dye may be given intravenously (**intravenous pyelogram or IVP**) or inserted during cystoscopy (**retrograde pyelogram**) through the urethra. Preparation of the patient usually includes cleansing enemas. Satisfactory results of the X-ray examination are largely based on proper patient preparation.

- Blood chemistries
  - Blood urea nitrogen (BUN)
  - Creatinine

Common Conditions

Cystitis

Cystitis, or inflammation of the urinary bladder, is fairly common. It is particularly common in women because of the shortness of the urethra. Signs and symptoms of cystitis include:

- Frequent urination
- **Hematuria** (blood in the urine)
- **Dysuria** (painful urination and/or burning upon urination)
- Bladder spasm

Treatment. Treatment is aimed at relieving the symptoms and eliminating the cause. Treatment includes:

- Sitz baths
- Rest
- Bacteriostatic agents
- Increased fluid intake
- Antibiotics

Nephritis

Nephritis means inflammation of the kidney. Nephritis:

- May follow an attack of infectious disease or may result from general arteriosclerosis. In either case, kidney cells are destroyed. This results in decreased urine production.
- May follow a disease course that is acute (rapid) or chronic (slow).
- Causes hypertension and edema.

Treatment. Treatment includes:

- Absolute bedrest
- Low-sodium diet
- Restricted fluid intake, at times
- Frequent checks on vital signs
- Accurate I & O

If both kidneys are involved, the patient will require regular dialysis until the diseased kidneys are replaced with a healthy kidney (kidney transplant). **Dialysis** is the process of removing the waste products from the blood by a hemodialysis machine—commonly called an artificial kidney.

Many patients on dialysis receive treatment in a hospital dialysis unit or in special outpatient dialysis centers. Other patients receive dialysis at home using portable dialysis machines. The patient's overall physical condition is an important factor in determining if home dialysis is an option.

Renal Calculi

Renal calculi are kidney stones. They can cause obstruction when they become lodged in the urinary passageways.

Signs and Symptoms. There may be no sign of the development of renal calculi until some obstruction develops. Then:

- The pain is sudden and intense. It is called **renal colic**.
- Calculi may be passed in the urine.

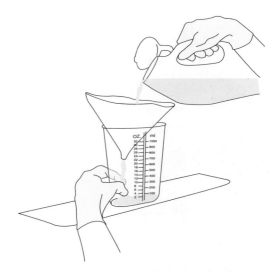

FIGURE 39–3. The urine can be strained through filter paper to retrieve kidney stones that are excreted through the bladder.

- As stones pass along the tract, tissue damage may occur, resulting in hematuria (blood in urine)

Treatment. The goal of treatment is to relieve the blockage and eliminate the stones.

- Encouraging fluids increases urine output. This helps to move the stones along the tract.
- All urine must be strained through gauze or filter paper, which is inspected for stones before it is discarded, Figure 39–3. Stones that are found can be analyzed. With information from the stones, the diet can sometimes be changed to make the formation of stones less likely.
- When it is impossible for the patient to pass the stones, surgery may be necessary. This type of surgery can be done by passing a cystoscope through the urethra or through a surgical incision. With the cystoscope, the physician is able to see inside the bladder and locate stones. The stones may then be crushed so they may be flushed out in the urine.
- At other times, the stones may be reached and removed only through a surgical incision. When a surgical incision is made, the patient usually returns from surgery with two drainage tubes in place. One tube is inserted in the urinary bladder. The other tube is inserted in the ureter or kidney.
  - The nurse will see that proper drainage is established.

— In addition to routine postoperative care, you must check frequently to be sure the drainage is not blocked by kinks in the tubes or by the patient's body lying on the tubes.
— The amount and type of drainage from each area should be carefully noted.

■ **Lithotripsy** is a relatively new technique. It uses carefully directed sound waves to crush the stones without making any surgical incision. The patient receiving this form of treatment is usually in the hospital less than 24 hours.

Hydronephrosis

Hydronephrosis results from accumulation of fluid within the kidney. The increasing pressure of urine causes pressure on the kidney cells. As a result, kidney cells are destroyed. The fluid accumulates in the kidney because something is blocking its flow. The flow may be blocked by:

■ Renal calculi
■ Kinking or twisting of the ureters
■ Tumors, especially benign prostatic hypertrophy
■ Distended bladder

Symptoms. Symptoms may be acute and similar to those of renal calculi or occur so gradually as to go unnoticed until much damage has been done.

Treatment. The condition is treated by draining the urine above the blockage to relieve pressure and then correcting the cause.

Renal Dialysis

As a result of disease or trauma, the kidneys may not be able to carry out their life-sustaining function of filtering impurities from the blood. In this case, mechanical dialysis is substituted to remove impurities from the blood.

Patients requiring this treatment usually have tubing permanently placed in the arm to make it easier to connect to the dialysis machine. The graft attaches to an artery and a vein to provide ready access to the blood circulatory system. When not in use, the tubing from the artery and the tubing from the vein are joined.

NOTE: The nursing assistant should never use the arm with a graft to measure blood pressure.

When dialysis is performed, the two sections of tubing are separated and attached to the dialysis machine. Blood passes from the artery to the machine where impurities are separated. The blood is then returned to the patient's vein by way of the graft. The process takes six to eight hours. It is usually performed two to three times per week. Patients with chronic renal failure may be maintained in this manner for some time, often for more than one year.

Sometimes a compatible kidney can be obtained from a donor and transplanted into the person suffering from renal failure. If the kidney is not rejected, it will take on the life-sustaining role of the original kidneys.

Responsibilities of the Nursing Assistant

Be sure you understand the orders for each individual patient before you assist in their nursing care. Orders regarding positioning, drainage, and activity for urological (urinary) patients vary.

There are some important measures that will apply to most urinary patients in your care:

■ Accurately measure intake and output, Figure 39–4.
■ Promptly report signs and symptoms of:
— Bleeding
— Chilling
— Elevated temperature
— Reduced output
— Increased edema
— Pain

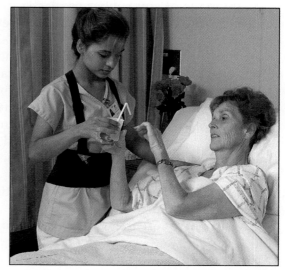

FIGURE 39–4. Once the patient is finished, carefully measure the amount of fluid consumed and mark the amount on the I & O chart.

- ■ Explain the purpose
- ■ Post force fluids sign
- ■ Offer fluids each time there is patient contact
- ■ Make sure fresh water is close at hand
- ■ Offer a variety of fluids
- ■ Keep accurate I & O

FIGURE 39–5.   Guidelines for encouraging fluids

- ■ Explain the purpose
- ■ Post fluids restricted sign
- ■ Provide frequent mouth care
- ■ Keep water pitcher out of sight
- ■ Serve fluids in small container
- ■ Serve small amount of fluid at a time
- ■ Keep accurate I & O

FIGURE 39–6.   Guidelines for limiting fluids

- ■ Properly care for urinary drainage.
- ■ Know the proper steps to take for forcing fluids, Figure 39–5, and for limiting fluids, Figure 39–6.

Urinary Drainage

Many patients with urinary problems will be on urinary drainage.

- ■ Urine is drained from the bladder through a tube called a catheter, Figure 39–7.
- ■ French catheters are hollow tubes. They are usually made of soft rubber or plastic. These catheters are used to drain the bladder. They do not remain in the bladder.
- ■ Foley catheters have a balloon surrounding the neck. The balloon is inflated after the catheter is introduced into the bladder. This is known as an indwelling or retention catheter.

The insertion of a catheter is a sterile procedure. It is performed by the nurse or physician. Closed urinary drainage systems, Figure 39–8, protect the patient from the possibility of infection.

You have definite responsibilities when patients have urinary drainage:

- ■ Make sure tubes are in good position and unblocked.
- ■ Measure output carefully. Note color and anything else unusual.

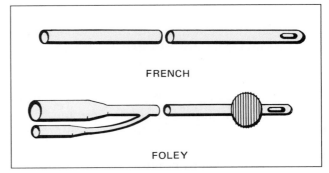

FRENCH

FOLEY

FIGURE 39–7.   Two types of catheters used to drain urine

- ■ Keep the end of the drainage tubing above the urine in the bag.
- ■ Do not permit the drainage bag to touch the floor; it may be connected to the bed frame. Drainage bags must never be attached to the side rails. Always keep the bag below the patient's bladder level.
- ■ Keep the drainage tubes smoothly coiled in the bed so that there is a direct drop to the drainage bag.
- ■ Do not disconnect from catheter.

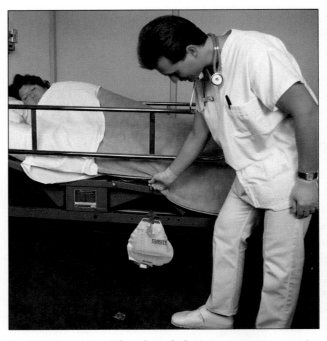

FIGURE 39–8.   The closed drainage system carries the urine directly from the patient to the container. There is less danger of infection to the patient using this type of closed system.

BEGINNING PROCEDURE ACTIONS	PROCEDURE COMPLETION ACTIONS
■ Wash your hands. ■ Assemble equipment needed. ■ Go to the patient's room, knock, and pause before entering. ■ Introduce yourself and identify the patient by checking the identification bracelet. ■ Ask visitors to leave and inform them where they can wait. ■ Care for equipment according to facility policy. ■ Provide privacy. ■ Explain what will happen and answer questions. ■ Allow patient to assist in procedure as much as possible. ■ Raise bed or table to comfortable working height.	■ Position patient comfortably. ■ Leave signal cord, telephone, and fresh water close at hand. ■ Return bed or table to lowest position. ■ Perform general safety check of patient and environment. ■ Wash your hands. ■ Report completion of task. ■ Let visitors know when they may reenter the patient's room. ■ Document action and your observations.

NOTE: Where there are open lesions, wet linen, or possible contact with patient body fluids or blood, disposable gloves are worn during the procedure. Put on gloves before contact with the patient or linen. Properly dispose of gloves after they are removed. ALWAYS APPLY UNIVERSAL PRECAUTIONS.

FIGURE 39–9. Beginning procedure actions and procedure completion actions

Catheter Care

Once the Foley catheter is inserted, the urinary meatus must be kept clean and free of secretions. The area around the meatus is washed daily with a solution approved by your facility or with soap and water. In some facilities, this procedure may be performed on each shift. This care is called indwelling catheter care.

Indwelling catheter care may be performed:
■ During the routine morning care.
■ As part of perineal care.
■ As a separate procedure.
Report signs of irritation or complaints of discomfort, and changes in the character or quantity of drainage.

Refer to Figure 39–9 to review the beginning procedure actions and procedure completion actions for all patient care procedures.

PROCEDURE 120 | **OBRA**   SIDE **10**

GIVING INDWELLING CATHETER CARE

1. Carry out each beginning procedure action.
2. Remember to wash your hands, identify the patient, and provide privacy.
3. Assemble equipment needed:
   ■ Disposable gloves
   ■ Bed protector
   ■ Bath blanket
   ■ Plastic bag for disposables
   ■ Daily catheter care kit
   ■ Antiseptic solution
   ■ Sterile applicators
   ■ Tape

4. Be sure opposite side rail is up and secure. Position patient on back, legs separated and knees bent, if permitted.
5. Cover patient with bath blanket and fanfold bedding to foot of bed.
6. Ask patient to raise hips. Place bed protector underneath patient.
7. Position bath blanket so that only genitals will be exposed.
8. Arrange catheter care kit and plastic bag on side of bed toward foot. Open kit.

continues

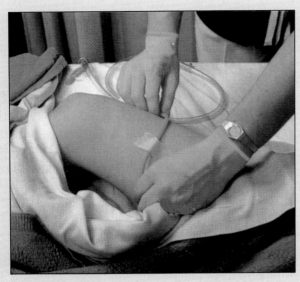

FIGURE 39–10. Check the catheter tubing to be sure it is taped properly and securely and that there is sufficient slack.

9. Put on gloves and draw drape back.
10. For the male patient:
    ■ Gently grasp penis and draw foreskin back, if not circumcised.*
    ■ Using an applicator dipped in antiseptic solution, for each stroke, cleanse the glans from meatus toward shaft for approximately 4 inches.
    ■ Dispose of each used applicator in plastic bag after one stroke.
    ■ Use a new, freshly dipped applicator for each stroke.
      Alternate Action: Going around the catheter on each side, wash with soap and water. Dry in the same manner. Make sure to return the foreskin (if not circumcised) to its proper position.

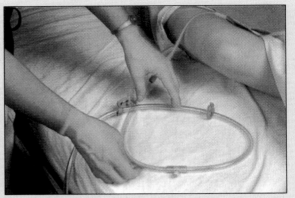

FIGURE 39–11. Check that the tubing is coiled on the bed.

For the female patient:
■ Separate the labia.
■ Using an applicator freshly dipped in antiseptic, stroke from front to back.
■ Dispose of each used applicator in plastic bag after one stroke.
  Alternate Action: Wash catheter down about four inches from meatus with soap and water and dry.
11. Check catheter to be sure it is taped properly, Figure 39–10. Retape and adjust for slack, if needed.
12. Check to be sure tubing is coiled on bed, Figure 39–11, and hangs straight down into drainage container. Check level of urine in container. End of tubing should not be below urine level. Empty bag and measure, if necessary. Do not raise bag above level of tubing.
13. Remove gloves and discard in plastic bag.
14. Replace bedding and remove bath blanket.
15. Fold bath blanket and leave in bedside stand for reuse.
16. Carry out procedure completion actions. Remember to wash your hands, report completion of task, and document time, date, catheter care, antiseptic solution used, and patient reaction.

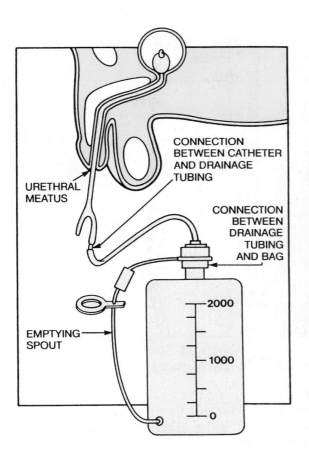

Refer to Figure 39–12. Note the possible sites of contamination, which could lead to infection, in the closed urinary drainage system.

External Drainage Systems (Male)

External urinary drainage systems are preferred for male patients who require long periods of urinary drainage. In external drainage, a catheter is not inserted in the urethra. Thus, there is less danger of infection. A condom (sheath) is connected or some other type of external drainage appliance is applied to the penis. Procedure 122 explains how to replace condom drainage. The nursing assistant checks the security of the appliance frequently and will change and reapply it daily during morning care. There are different types of drainage systems available. Urine may be collected in a bag that hangs from the bed or wheelchair or in a bag attached to the patient's leg.

FIGURE 39–12. Special care must be taken to protect the possible sites of contamination in the closed urinary drainage system.

PROCEDURE 121 OBRA

SIDE 10

DISCONNECTING THE CATHETER

NOTE: It is preferable never to disconnect the drainage setup, but at times it is necessary. If sterile caps and plugs are available, they should be used. If not, the disconnected ends must be protected with sterile gauze sponges.

1. Carry out each beginning procedure action.
2. Remember to wash your hands, identify the patient, and provide privacy.
3. Assemble equipment needed:
   - Alcohol
   - Disposable gloves
   - Gauze sponges
   - Sterile caps/plugs
   - Clamps

4. Clamp the catheter.
5. Disinfect the area to be disconnected with alcohol. Put on gloves.
6. Disconnect the catheter and drainage tubing. Do not put them down or allow them to touch anything.
7. Insert a sterile plug in the end of the catheter. Place a sterile cap over the exposed end of the drainage tube, Figure 39–13.
8. Secure the drainage tube to the bed in such a way that it will not touch the floor.
9. Remove and dispose of gloves according to facility policy.

continues

10. Carry out each procedure completion action. Remember to wash your hands, report completion of task, and document date, time, catheter disconnected, ends protected (how), and patient reaction.

NOTE: Reverse the procedure to reconnect the catheter. If you find an unprotected, disconnected tube in the bed or on the floor, *do not reconnect it. Report it at once.*

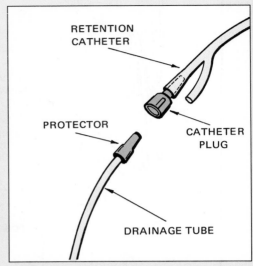

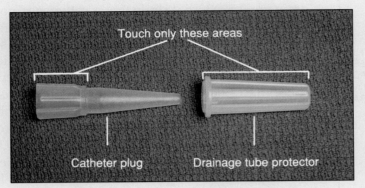

FIGURE 39–13. (A) sterile catheter plug and protective cap.

FIGURE 39–13. (B) plug and protective cap in place

PROCEDURE 122

SIDE
10

REPLACING A URINARY CONDOM

1. Carry out each beginning procedure action.
2. Remember to wash your hands, identify the patient, and provide privacy.
3. Assemble equipment needed:
   - Basin of warm water
   - Washcloth
   - Condom with drainage tip
   - Disposable gloves
   - Bed protector/bath blanket
   - Plastic bag
   - Tincture of benzoin
   - Towel
   - Paper towels
4. Arrange equipment on overbed table.
5. Lower side rail on the side on which you are working.
6. Cover patient with bath blanket and fanfold bedding to foot of bed. Place bed protector under patient's hips.
7. Adjust bath blanket to expose genitals only.
8. Put on gloves.
9. Remove condom (sheath) by rolling toward tip of penis. Place in plastic bag, if disposable.

Place on paper towels to be washed and dried, if reusable.
10. Carefully wash and dry penis. Observe for signs of irritation. Check to see if condom has "ready stick" surface.
    - If not, a thin spray coat of tincture of benzoin may be applied to the penis.
    - Do not spray on head of penis.
    - Let dry.
11. Apply fresh condom and drainage tip to penis by rolling it toward base of penis. If the patient is uncircumcised, be sure that the foreskin remains in good position.
12. Reconnect drainage system.
13. Remove gloves. Dispose of according to facility policy.
14. Adjust bedding and remove bath blanket. Fold bath blanket and leave in bedside stand.
15. Carry out each procedure completion action. Remember to wash your hands, report completion of task, and document date, time, urinary condom drainage replaced, and patient reaction.

PROCEDURE 123 | OBRA

COLLECTING URINARY DRAINAGE IN A LEG BAG

1. Carry out each beginning procedure action.
2. Remember to wash your hands, identify the patient, and provide privacy.
3. Assemble the following equipment:
   - Equipment for applying external drainage using a condom (see Procedure 122)
   - Alcohol wipes
   - Gloves
   - Drainage tubing
   - Clean leg bag with straps.
4. Follow procedure for replacing a urinary condom (Steps 3–11 of Procedure 122).
5. Attach leg drainage bag, Figure 39–14.

   If leg bag is to be reused:
   a. Place emesis basin under connection of drainage tubing.
   b. Open alcohol wipe.
   c. Cover end of newly applied condom with alcohol wipe.
   d. Disconnect soiled condom sheath tubing from drainage bag tubing. Put into emesis basin.
   e. Using a second alcohol wipe clean the connector of the leg bag tubing.
   f. Connect the two ends and check for security.

   If leg bag is not to be reused:
   a. Place entire apparatus in emesis basin.
   b. Open alcohol wipe.
   c. Wipe end of condom sheath tubing and end of the connecting tubing of the fresh leg bag.
   d. Connect the two ends and check for security.
   e. Disconnect used condom sheath and drainage bag.
   f. Follow facility policy regarding disposal of used condom and care and cleaning reuseable leg bag.
6. Remove gloves and dispose of according to facility policy.
7. Adjust bedding and remove bath blanket. Fold bath blanket and leave in bedside stand.
8. Carry out each procedure completion action. Remember to wash your hands, report completion of task. and document date, time, urinary condom drainage replaced, attached to leg bag drainage and patient reaction.

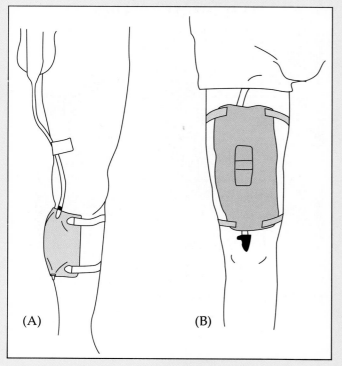

(A)   (B)

FIGURE 39–14. Leg bag attached to condom urinary drainage. (A) shows the leg bag attached to the calf of the leg. (B) shows the leg bag attached to the thigh.

PROCEDURE 124 | OBRA

EMPTYING A URINARY DRAINAGE UNIT

1. Carry out each beginning procedure action.
2. Remember to wash your hands, identify the patient, and provide privacy.
3. Assemble equipment needed:
   - Graduated container
   - Disposable gloves
   - Sterile cap or sterile 4 × 4 (needed if container has no bottom drain tube)
   - Alcohol swab
4. Put on gloves.
5. If drainage bag has a drain in the bottom, place a graduate under it.
6. Open drain and allow the urine to drain into the graduate, Figure 39–15. Do not allow the tip of the tubing to touch the sides of the graduate, Figure 39–16.
7. Close the drain and wipe it with the alcohol swab. Replace it in the holder.

8. If there is no opening, the tube must be removed before emptying. Protect the end of the drainage tube with a sterile cap or a sterile sponge.
9. Empty urine into the graduate.
10. Remove protective cover from the end of the tube. Reinsert the tube into the bag. Be careful not to touch the sides of the bag with the tip of the tube.
11. Note the amount and character of urine.
12. Check position of drainage tube.
13. Take graduate to utility room and empty it.
14. Wash and dry graduate and store it according to facility policy.
15. Remove gloves and dispose of according to facility policy.
16. Carry out each procedure completion action. Remember to wash your hands, report completion of task, and document date, time, urinary drainage emptied (amount and character of drainage), and patient reaction.

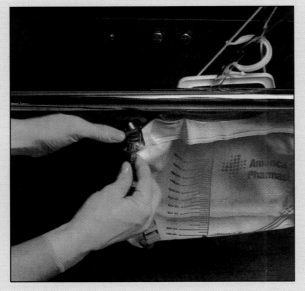

FIGURE 39–15. Open the drain on the bottom of the collection bag.

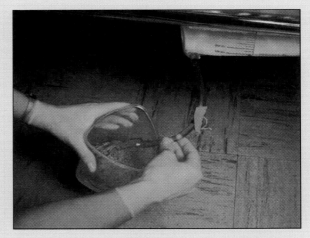

FIGURE 39–16. Allow the urine to drain into the graduate. Note that the end of the tubing is not touching the sides of the container.

SUMMARY

Two vital nursing measures necessary in the care of patients with urinary dysfunction are:
- Maintaining adequate urinary drainage
- Keeping drainage equipment contamination free

The urinary tract is considered a sterile area. Special sterile techniques must be used when the physician or nurse introduces a catheter into this area. The nursing assistant must know how to safely:
- Disconnect the catheter from the drainage setup.
- Empty and measure the drainage.
- Ambulate the patient with constant urinary drainage.

UNIT REVIEW

A. True/False. Answer the following statements true or false by circling T or F.

T F   1. Insertion of a sterile catheter into the urinary bladder is a routine nursing assistant task.

T F   2. Gloves should be worn when emptying a urine collection bag.

T F   3. It is preferable never to disconnect a urinary drainage setup.

T F   4. The pain associated with kidney stones is referred to as renal colic.

T F   5. If you find an unprotected, disconnected catheter on the floor, you should reconnect it immediately.

T F   6. The hemodialysis machine takes the place of nonfunctioning kidneys.

T F   7. Forcing fluids encourages increased output, which is important in treating kidney stones.

T F   8. A catheter with an inflatable balloon is called a French catheter.

T F   9. French catheters are indwelling catheters.

T F 10. Cystitis is a fairly common problem for women.

B. Matching. Match the phrase in Column I with the words in Column II.

Column I	Column II
_____ 11. indwelling catheter	a. micturate
_____ 12. inability to expel formed urine	b. hematuria
	c. cystitis
_____ 13. urinate	d. retention
_____ 14. inflammation of the bladder	e. dysuria
	f. Foley catheter
_____ 15. blood in the urine	g. suppression

C. Multiple Choice. Choose the phrase that best completes each of the following sentences by circling the proper letter.

16. Your patient has a diagnosis of nephritis. Your care will include
    a. keeping the patient very active.
    b. serving a high-sodium diet.
    c. measuring I & O accurately.
    d. eliminating vital sign measurements so the patient can rest more.

17. Your patient has renal calculi. Included in your care will be
    a. saving all urine.
    b. straining urine.
    c. limiting fluids.
    d. inserting a catheter.

18. A common cause of hydronephrosis is
    a. renal calculi.
    b. twisting of the ureter.
    c. tumors.
    d. All of the above.

19. Important signs and symptoms to note when there is a diagnosis involving the urinary system include
    a. chilling.
    b. pain.
    c. temperature evaluation.
    d. All of the above.

20. Indwelling catheter care is:
    a. performed once each week.
    b. performed during AM care.
    c. omitted safely as long as patient is in bed.
    d. None of the above.

D. Completion. Complete the following statements in the space provided.

21. The nursing assistant who finds a disconnected catheter in the bed should: _____
    _____
    _____

22. A routine check of a patient on urinary drainage should include: _____
    _____
    _____
    _____
    _____
    _____

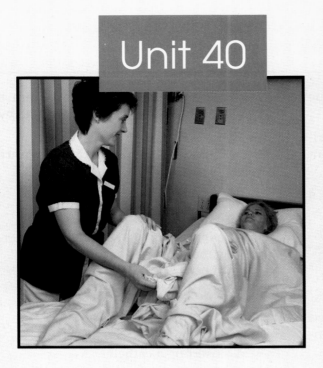

Unit 40

The Reproductive System and Common Disorders

OBJECTIVES

As a result of this unit, you will be able to:

- Spell and define terms.
- Review the location and functions of the organs of the male and female reproductive systems.
- List six diagnostic tests associated with conditions of the male and female reproductive systems.
- Describe some common disorders and conditions of the male reproductive system.
- Describe some common disorders and conditions of the female reproductive system.
- Describe nursing assistant actions related to the care of patients with conditions and diseases of the reproductive system.
- State the nursing precautions required for patients who have sexually transmitted diseases.

VOCABULARY

Learn the meaning and the correct spelling of the following words and phrases:

AIDS (acquired immune deficiency syndrome)
amenorrhea
benign prostatic hypertrophy
biopsy
chancre
colporrhaphy
cystocele
dilatation and curettage (D & C)
dysmenorrhea
gonorrhea
hemorrhoids
herpes simplex II
hysterectomy
irrigate
leukorrhea
lumpectomy
mammogram
mammography

mastectomy
menorrhagia
metrorrhagia
oophorectomy
orchidectomy
panhysterectomy
Pap smear
pelvic inflammatory disease (PID)
prostatectomy
radical mastectomy
rectocele
salpingectomy
sexually transmitted disease (STD)
simple mastectomy
sterility
syphilis
trichomonas vaginitis
venereal warts
vulvovaginitis

Before beginning your study of this unit, you may wish to review Unit 4, pages 80–83. Also review Figures 40–1 and 40–2A and B to refresh your memory of the components of the male and female reproductive systems.

You will recall that:

■ There are similarities and differences between the male and female reproductive tracts.

■ The purposes of both male and female organs are:
— Reproduction
— Sexual expression
— Hormone production

Diagnostic Tests

Techniques used to diagnose problems of the reproductive system include:

■ Cultures for microorganisms
■ Urinalysis for hormone levels
■ Biopsy of tissue samples
■ Pap smear—test using cells from the cervix to detect possible cancer of the cervix. The test:
— Is painless.
— Can be performed in the physician's office during the routine pelvic examination.
— Should be done regularly.

■ Dilatation and curettage (D & C)—a surgical procedure used to help diagnose conditions of the uterus, including tumors. The D & C is an operation in which the opening of the cervix is made larger and the uterus is scraped with a surgical instrument known as a curette.

■ Cystoscopy—used to evaluate prostate conditions.

Conditions of the Male Reproductive Organs

The male organs are subject to the same kinds of disease processes that affect other body parts. Examples of these conditions are tumors and infections. A very common problem experienced by many men involves the prostate gland.

Prostate Conditions

Benign prostatic (of the prostate gland) hypertrophy:

■ Is an enlargement of the prostate gland without tumor development.

■ Causes narrowing of the urethra, which passes through the center of the prostate gland.

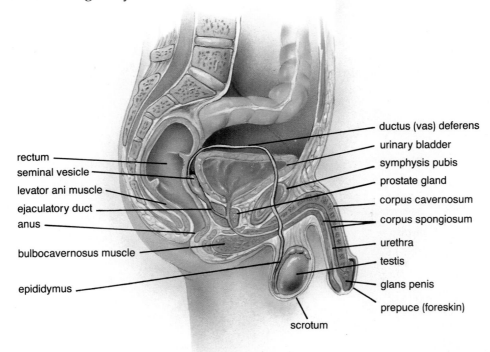

rectum
seminal vesicle
levator ani muscle
ejaculatory duct
anus
bulbocavernosus muscle
epididymus

ductus (vas) deferens
urinary bladder
symphysis pubis
prostate gland
corpus cavernosum
corpus spongiosum
urethra
testis
glans penis
prepuce (foreskin)
scrotum

FIGURE 40–1.   Lateral view of the male reproductive organs *(From Anatomy and Physiology Plates, copyright 1992 by Delmar Publishers Inc.)*

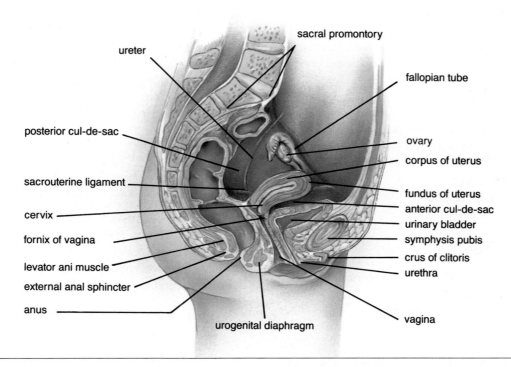

FIGURE 40–2A. Lateral view of the internal female reproductive organs *(From Anatomy and Physiology Plates, copyright 1992 by Delmar Publishers Inc.)*

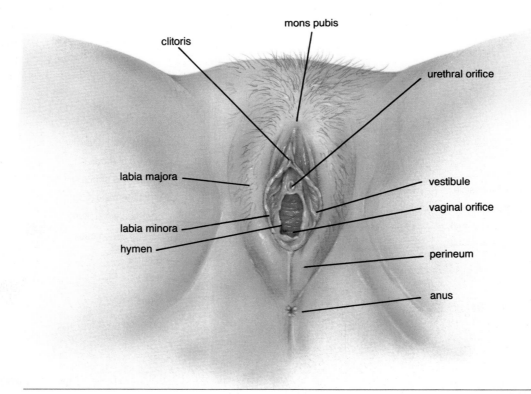

FIGURE 40–2B. External female reproductive organs *(From Anatomy and Physiology Plates, copyright 1992 by Delmar Publishers Inc.)*

- Can cause sufficient enlargement to cause urinary retention.
- Is noncancerous.

Signs and Symptoms. Signs and symptoms of prostate conditions involve difficulty in:
- Starting the stream of urine
- Emptying the bladder completely

Treatment. Various surgical approaches are used to remove all or part of the prostate gland (prostatectomy) to relieve urinary retention.
- Transurethral prostatectomy (TURP)—only enough of the gland is removed, working from inside the urethra, to permit urine to pass.
- Perineal prostatectomy—the entire gland is removed through surgical incisions in the perineum.
- Suprapubic prostatectomy—an incision is made just above the pubis and part of the gland is removed.

Male patients are likely to be disturbed by the necessity of prostate surgery. Men often fear that they will not be able to have sexual intercourse after a prostatectomy. They feel that their manhood is threatened.

Postsurgical Care. In addition to routine postoperative care, the prostatectomy patient:
- Will have a Foley catheter in place following the surgery.
- May have a suprapubic drain through the suprapubic incision.
- May have a perineal drain in the perineal incision.

As a nursing assistant:
- Be careful the tubes do not become twisted, stressed, or dislodged when positioning the patient.
- Carefully note the amount and color of drainage from all areas.
- Report at once any sudden increase in bright redness or the appearance of clots that seem to block the tube.
- Report to the nurse if dressings become wet with urinary drainage.
- Be patient and understanding of the patient's emotional stress.
- Refer questions of possible sexual limitations to the nurse so that the patient may be provided with accurate information and support.

At times, it will be necessary to irrigate (wash out) the drainage tubes. This is a sterile procedure that will be carried out by the nurse or physician.

Cancer of the Testes

Cancer of the testes is seen commonly today. It may require the removal of the testicles (orchidectomy). This procedure is performed when there is testicular malignancy. When an early diagnosis is made, treatment can be started early. Orchidectomy can then be avoided.

Testicular self-examination is an important way to locate lumps or changes in the testes. This procedure should be performed by all adult males:
- At least once each month
- During a warm shower so the scrotum will be relaxed
- With soapy fingers
- By palpating each testis between the fingers and thumb

Conditions of the Female Reproductive Organs

Rectocele and Cystocele

Rectoceles and cystoceles are hernias. They usually occur at the same time.
- **Rectoceles** are a weakening of the wall shared between the vagina and rectum. These hernias frequently cause constipation and hemorrhoids (varicose veins of the rectum).
- **Cystoceles** are a weakening of the muscles between the bladder and vagina. Cystoceles cause urinary incontinence.

Treatment. A surgical procedure called colporrhaphy tightens the vaginal walls.

Nursing Care. In addition to routine postsurgical care, you may assist in:
- Ice packs
- Heat lamps
- Sitz baths
- Sterile vaginal douches (irrigations)
- Checking carefully for signs of excessive bleeding or foul discharge

Infections

Vulvovaginitis. Vulvovaginitis is often caused by a fungus infection caused by *Candida albicans*.
- There is a thick, white, cheesy vaginal discharge.

- Inflammation and itching are intense.
- Douches are not given for this condition.
- Special drugs and creams are prescribed to fight the infection.

Tumors

Benign and malignant tumors of the uterus and ovaries are frequent. Malignancies of the cervix are very common. The cure rate is very high if treated in time.

Signs and Symptoms. The most common indications of tumors of the uterus and ovaries are changes in the menstrual flow such as:
- Menorrhagia (excessive flow)
- Amenorrhea (lack of menstrual flow)
- Dysmenorrhea (difficult or painful menstrual flow)
- Metrorrhagia (bleeding at completely irregular intervals)

Treatment. Several different types of procedures may be performed to treat tumors of the female reproductive tract, including chemotherapy, radiation, and surgery. Some surgical procedures are:
- Total hysterectomy—removal of the entire uterus, including the cervix.
- Oophorectomy—removal of an ovary. In younger women, at least a portion of the ovary is left to continue hormone production whenever possible.
- Salpingectomy—removal of a Fallopian tube.
- Panhysterectomy—removal of the uterus and both ovaries and tubes. The surgical approach may be abdominal or vaginal. If a panhysterectomy is performed, the patient experiences surgically induced menopause. The more uncomfortable symptoms are usually relieved with hormone supplements.

Postoperative Care. In addition to the usual postoperative care, the care following a hysterectomy will include:
- Caring for Foley drainage.
- Possibly caring for a nasogastric tube, which may be in place to relieve abdominal distention and nausea.
- Giving special attention to maintaining good circulation because slowing of the blood supply to the pelvis may result in clot formation.
- Introducing fluids and foods gradually after the initial nausea subsides.

- Carefully observing the patient for low back pain.
- Monitoring urine output and bleeding.
- Checking both the abdominal incisional area and the vagina for presence and type of drainage.

Breast Surgery

Tumors, both benign and malignant, are commonly found in the breasts.

Diagnosis. Breast tumors are often first found during self-examination or through mammography (X-ray examination). Most of these masses turn out to be benign tumors. The self-examination procedure should be:
- Performed by all adult females.
- Carried out each month on the last day of the menstrual flow.
- Carried out on one selected day of the month, after menopause.
- Carried out faithfully in a routine manner.

Mammography. Mammograms are X-rays of the breasts. A mammogram:
- Can identify the presence of tumors up to two years before the tumor can be felt during self-examination.
- Should be performed between the ages of 35 and 40 years to provide a baseline evaluation.
- Thereafter, should be performed every one to two years until age 50.
- Should be performed yearly after age 50.

Biopsy. Biopsy (examining a sample of living tissue) is used to make a diagnosis. The biopsy sample is obtained through a needle. The procedure may be performed in the physician's office or in the hospital. Biopsy tissue may also be obtained during a D & C.

Mastectomy means removing the breast. All or part of the breast tissue may be removed in a mastectomy.
- A simple mastectomy includes removal of the breast tissue only.
- A radical mastectomy includes the breast tissue, underlying muscles, and the glands in the axillary area. This procedure is not performed as often as it was previously.
- A lumpectomy removes the abnormal tissue and only a small amount of the breast tissue.

Any form of mastectomy requires a great deal of psychological adjustment for the patient. There is the fear of disfigurement and the fear of loss of femininity. To restore the outward physical appearance of the

BEGINNING PROCEDURE ACTIONS	PROCEDURE COMPLETION ACTIONS
■ Wash your hands. ■ Assemble equipment needed. ■ Go to the patient's room, knock, and pause before entering. ■ Introduce yourself and identify the patient by checking the identification bracelet. ■ Ask visitors to leave and inform them where they can wait. ■ Care for equipment according to facility policy. ■ Provide privacy. ■ Explain what will happen and answer questions. ■ Allow patient to assist in procedure as much as possible. ■ Raise bed or table to comfortable working height.	■ Position patient comfortably. ■ Leave signal cord, telephone, and fresh water close at hand. ■ Return bed or table to lowest position. ■ Perform general safety check of patient and environment. ■ Wash your hands. ■ Report completion of task. ■ Let visitors know when they may reenter the patient's room. ■ Document action and your observations.

NOTE: Where there are open lesions, wet linen, or possible contact with patient body fluids or blood, disposable gloves are worn during the procedure. Put on gloves before contact with the patient or linen. Properly dispose of gloves after they are removed. ALWAYS APPLY UNIVERSAL PRECAUTIONS.

FIGURE 40–3. Beginning procedure actions and procedure completion actions

mastectomy patient, there are many excellent breast forms now available. Breast implants are an alternative way of restoring the physical form of the breast. There are also support groups to aid in the psychological adjustment.

Postoperative Care. In addition to the routine postoperative care, you will:

■ Realize that since a large amount of blood can be lost during a mastectomy, transfusions are likely to be ordered. You will monitor a blood transfusion as you would monitor an intravenous infusion.

■ Check pressure dressings frequently for signs of excess bleeding.

■ Check the bed linen since blood may drain to the back of the dressing.

■ Report immediately numbness or swelling in the arm of the operative side.

■ Be ready to offer support since walking may be difficult for the patient who may feel unbalanced.

■ Be ready to offer your fullest emotional support.

■ Assist patient in rehabilitative exercises.

■ Refer questions about fears of disfigurement and loss of femininity to the nurse, who will see that the patient is provided with accurate information and support.

Refer to Figure 40–3 to refresh your memory of the beginning procedure actions and the procedure completion actions to be carried out for each patient care procedure.

Sexually Transmitted Diseases (STD)

Sexually transmitted diseases (STDs) affect both men and women. Although most sexually transmitted diseases can be treated and cured, patients do not develop immunity to repeated infections. It is often possible to transmit the organisms causing STDs from:

■ Mucous membrane to mucous membrane such as from genitals to mouth or genitals

■ Mucous membrane to skin, such as genitals to hands

■ Skin to mucous membrane, such as hands to genitals

Any disease that is transmitted mainly in this way is a STD. There are many sexually transmitted diseases. Some are seen more commonly than others. It is important to realize that patients may:

■ Not always be aware that they have been infected.

■ Be too embarrassed to tell you about the problem.

■ Not realize the serious damage these infectious diseases can do to the body.

PROCEDURE 125

BREAST SELF-EXAMINATION

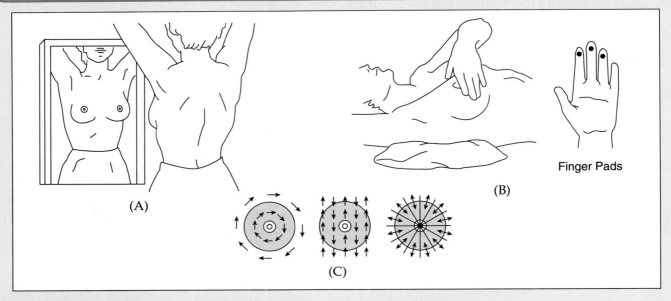

FIGURE 40–4. Breast self-examination. *(Courtesy of the American Cancer Society)*

1. Disrobe above waist and stand or sit in front of a mirror. Observe breasts for changes in shape or size.
   NOTE: Some women prefer to perform breast self-examination standing in the shower.
2. Raise arms above your head, Figure 40–4A. Note any "dimpling" of the breast tissue, redness or swelling, or changes in the nipples.
3. Lie down and put a pillow under your right shoulder, Figure 40–4B. Place your right arm behind your head.
4. Use the finger pads of your three middle fingers on your left hand to feel for lumps or thickening. Your finger pads are the top third of each finger.
5. Press firmly enough to know how your breast feels. If you're not sure how hard to press, ask your health care provider, or copy the way your health care provider uses the finger pads during a breast examination. Learn what your breast feels like most of the time. A firm ridge in the lower curve of each breast is normal.
6. Move around the breast in a set way, Figure 40–4C. You can choose the circle (A), the up and down line (B), or the wedge (C). It will help you to make sure that you've gone over the entire breast area, and to remember how your breast feels.
7. Now examine your left breast using right hand finger pads.
8. If you find any changes, see your doctor right away.

The most common sexually transmitted diseases are gonorrhea, herpes simplex II, and syphilis. Other sexually transmitted diseases are caused by Chlamydia, human papilloma virus, HIV, and the Trichomonas parasite.

Trichomonas Vaginitis

Trichomonas vaginitis is caused by a parasite, the *Trichomonas vaginalis*. This condition:
■ Is sexually transmitted.
■ May affect the male reproductive tract with no signs and symptoms.

- In females, causes a large amount of white, foul-smelling vaginal discharge called leukorrhea.
- Can be controlled with medication.
- Requires that both sex partners receive treatment.

Gonorrhea

Gonorrhea is a serious STD caused by the bacterium *Neisseria gonorrheae*. The disease causes an acute inflammation.

- In the male:
  — Greenish-yellow discharge appears from the penis within 2–5 days after contact.
  — There is burning on urination.
  — The disease can spread throughout the reproductive tract, causing sterility (inability to reproduce).
- In the female:
  — Eighty percent may have no signs or symptoms until after the disease is spread.
  — Pelvic inflammatory disease (PID) can lead to formation of abscesses and sterility.
  — It is possible to spread the disease before being aware of being infected.
- It is important for all sex partners to be treated with antibiotics.
- When a pregnant woman has gonorrhea, her baby's eyes may be permanently damaged if they are contaminated by the disease during birth. As a preventative measure, all babies' eyes are routinely treated with silver nitrate drops or antibiotics shortly after birth.

Syphilis

Syphilis also is caused by the microorganism *Treponema pallidum*. Both sexes show the same effects of the disease. If untreated, this disease passes through three stages.

1. First stage—a sore (chancre) develops within 90 days of exposure. The chancre heals without treatment. Since it is not painful, it may go entirely unnoticed.
2. Second stage—may be accompanied by a rash, sore throat, or other mild symptoms suggestive of a viral infection. Again, the signs and symptoms disappear without treatment. The disease is infectious during the first and second stages and may be transmitted to a sexual partner. By this time, the microorganisms have gained entrance into vital organs such as the heart, liver, brain, and spinal cord.

3. Third stage—the stage in which permanent damage is done to vital organs. It may not appear for many years.

An additional danger of syphilis in pregnancy is that the microorganism can attack the fetus, causing it to die or be seriously deformed.

Herpes

Herpes simplex II (genital herpes) is an infectious disease caused by the herpes simplex virus. It is transmitted primarily through direct sexual contact. The person who has herpes:

- May develop red, blister-like sores on the reproductive organs.
- Has sores that are associated with a burning sensation.
- Usually has sores that heal in about two weeks.
- Must remember that the fluid in the blisters is infectious.
- May shed organisms even when an outbreak is not present.

People with the herpes infection may have only one episode or may have repeated attacks. In many cases, repeated attacks are milder. In addition to the local discomfort:

- There seems to be a greater incidence of cancer of the cervix and miscarriages among female sufferers than among women who do not have this condition.
- Newborn children can be infected when the pregnant mother gives birth.
- The mother with an active case of herpes simplex II is usually delivered by cesarean section.

Treatment reduces the discomfort and degree of communicability. There is no cure at the present time.

Venereal Warts

Venereal warts are caused by a virus.

- Lesions develop on the genitals on both skin and mucous membranes.
- The warts are cauliflower-shaped, raised, and darkened.
- They may be removed by ointments or surgery but often recur.
- They may cause discomfort during intercourse and may cause bleeding when dislodged.
- Predispose to development of cancerous changes.
- One of the most rapidly growing forms of STD.

Chlamydia Infection

Chlamydia are small infectious organisms that can invade mucous membranes of the body. These organisms can be:

■ Introduced into the eyes infecting the conjunctiva. This causes inflammation (conjunctivitis) and a more serious condition called trachoma. Trachoma can lead to blindness.

■ Sexually transmitted and commonly cause infections of the reproductive tract.

■ The cause of serious pelvic inflammatory disease (PID) with scarring and even systemic infections. The scarring can result in sterility.

■ Responsible for signs and symptoms similar to those of gonorrhea, except that the discharge is usually yellow to whitish in color.

■ Treated with antibiotics.

Patients with pelvic infections are usually checked for gonorrhea. If they are found negative for gonorrhea, they are frequently diagnosed as having nongonorrheal urethritis (NGU) or nonspecified urethritis (NSU) because many different organisms may cause the infection. However, chlamydia organisms are the most common cause.

Acquired Immune Deficiency Syndrome (AIDS)

AIDS is a viral disease. It is transmitted primarily through direct contact with the bodily secretions of an infected person. There is a greater incidence of the disease among:

■ Intravenous drug users
■ Female prostitutes
■ Homosexual males and bisexual males
■ Hemophiliacs
■ Babies of mothers who are infected
■ Sexual partners of AIDS victims
■ Heterosexuals with multiple sexual partners

The incidence of AIDS among hospital workers not otherwise exposed is very low. It is, however, a disease that can be transmitted to anyone who has direct blood-to-secretion contact with infected bodily fluids such as blood or semen.

There are three ways the AIDS virus (HIV) is transmitted:

1. Blood to blood through:
   a. Transfusion of infected blood (rarely occurring now)
   b. Treatment of hemophilia with clotting factor (rarely occurring now)
   c. Needle sharing among drug abusers

   d. Accidental needle prick with contaminated needle
   e. Unsterile instruments used for procedures such as ear piercing or tatooing
2. Unprotected vaginal or anal intercourse when one partner is infected:
   a. Male to female
   b. Female to male
   c. Male to male
3. Infected mother to infant during:
   a. Pregnancy
   b. The birth process
   c. Nursing

The AIDS Virus

The AIDS virus (HIV):

■ Has more than one variant
■ Does not live for long outside the body.
■ Is affected by common chemicals such as bleach.
■ Depresses the body's immune system.
■ Makes the infected person more susceptible to infections.
■ Makes the infected person more likely to experience complications such as:
   — *Pneumocystis carinii* pneumonia—a serious lung infection
   — Kaposi's sarcoma—a serious malignancy that affects many body organs. Figure 40–5 shows typical skin lesions of Kaposi's sarcoma
   — Brain involvement leading to dementia
   — Other opportunistic infections

The presence of *Pneumocystis carinii* pneumonia or Kaposi's sarcoma is diagnostic for AIDS.

Disease Progression. Not everyone who comes in contact with the HIV virus becomes infected. In 1993 several other opportunistic infections in the presence of HIV infection were added to broaden the diagnostic base.

Incubation Period. There is always a period between contact with the organism and the start of the signs and symptoms.

■ The incubation period may be as long as many years.
■ Most people become seropositive (show antibodies to HIV in the bloodstream) within three to six months after infection.
■ No signs or symptoms of the disease are usually seen during the first six months to one year following exposure.

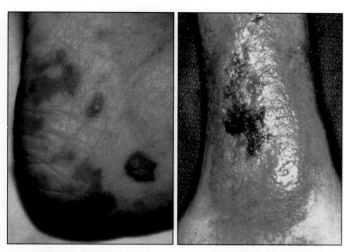

FIGURE 40–5. Typical skin lesions of Kaposi's sarcoma *(Photos courtesy of The Centers for Disease Control and Prevention, Atlanta, GA)*

- This asymptomatic period may last seven to ten years or longer.
- One-fourth to one-half of people exposed to the virus show evidence of disease within five to ten years of antibody development (becoming seropositive).
- Two tests used to diagnose HIV infection are:
  — ELISA (positive is presumptive for AIDS)
  — Western blot (positive is confirming for AIDS)

Signs of Disease Progression

A series of infections is the next step in the progression of the disease. The person is seropositive and experiences:
- Increasingly suppressed immune response
- Chronic illness
- Signs and symptoms which include:
  — Fatigue or listlessness
  — Weight loss of 10% of body weight
  — Recurrent fever of 100°F
  — Drenching night sweats
  — Swollen lymph nodes
  — Diarrhea
  — Variety of opportunistic infections

One-fourth to one-third of the people develop AIDS within five years of the start of signs and symptoms.

Treatment. There is no specific cure for AIDS at the present time.
- No vaccine has been developed to prevent the infection from developing, but much effort is being applied to the search for a vaccine.
- A blood test has been developed. It detects antibodies in the blood (chemicals produced by the infected person to the virus). This test permits the blood supply to be checked before blood is given to people needing transfusions.
- The same test detects the presence of antibodies to HIV in a person's own blood.
- Presence of the antibodies indicates exposure to HIV. It does not indicate the specific course the disease will take.
- AZT (azidothymidine) is sometimes prescribed for the treatment of AIDS for individuals who have had a confirmed case of *Pneumocystis carinii* pneumonia or a low lymphocyte count. Blood transfusions may be needed because this medication can cause a low red blood cell count. AZT needs to be taken every four hours around the clock and it is important that all doses be taken on time.
- Therapy is directed toward treating each infection vigorously as it arises.

Drugs such as AZT and DDI are given to slow disease progression.

At the present time, there is *no evidence* that AIDS is transmitted:
- Through kissing, touching or hugging
- By eating at the same table with an infected person
- By toilet seats
- Through insect bites

Nursing Precautions. Any infection can be transmitted directly into the bloodstream through open cuts or small breaks in the skin or mucous membranes. Universal precautions and, where appropriate, isolation techniques are required when caring for patients with infections such as STDs, hepatitis B, or AIDS, which are easily transmitted.

Personal Precautions. There are some personal activities that an individual can carry out to lessen the risk of contracting hepatitis B, AIDS, or sexually transmitted diseases.
- Abstain from casual sexual encounters.
- Know your sexual partner well before engaging in sexual activity.
- Limit the number of sexual partners.
- Always use a latex condom throughout sexual contact.
- Wash well following sexual intercourse.
- Use approved germicides that can be applied to vagina, penis, and condom.
- Provide to your partner and be provided with a negative ELISA test result covering the three-month period before sexual activity.

PROCEDURE 126

GIVING A NONSTERILE VAGINAL DOUCHE

1. Carry out each beginning procedure action.
2. Remember to wash your hands, identify the patient, and provide privacy.
3. Assemble equipment needed:
   - Disposable douche
   - Bed protector (Chux)
   - Toilet tissue
   - Bath blanket
   - Cotton balls
   - Disinfectant
   - Cup
   - Irrigating standard
   - Gloves
   - Bedpan and cover
   - Paper bag
4. Pour a small amount of the specified disinfecting solution over the cotton balls in the cup.
5. Measure water in douche container. Temperature should be about 105°F. Add powder or solution as ordered.
6. Hang douche bag on standard. Close clamp on tubing. Leave protector on sterile tip.
7. Assemble the remaining equipment at bedside where it can be easily reached. Screen unit.
8. Wash your hands. Put on gloves.
9. Assist the patient into the dorsal recumbent position.
10. Place bed protector beneath the patient's buttocks.
11. Remove the perineal pad from front to back and discard in paper bag.
12. Drape patient with bath blanket, Figure 40–6. Fanfold top bedding to foot of bed.
13. Place bedpan under patient and ask her to void, Figure 40–7.
14. Cleanse perineum.
    - Use one cotton ball with disinfectant for each stroke.
    - Cleanse from vulva toward anus.
    - Cleanse labia majora first.
    - Expose labia minora with thumb and forefinger and cleanse.
    - Give special attention to folds.
    - Discard cotton balls in emesis basin.

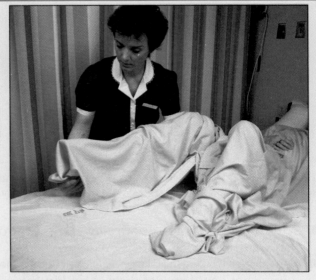

FIGURE 40–6.   Drape the patient.

15. Open clamp to expel air. Remove protector from sterile tip of disposable douche, Figure 40–8.
16. Allow small amount of solution to flow over inner thigh and then over vulva. Do not touch vulva with nozzle.

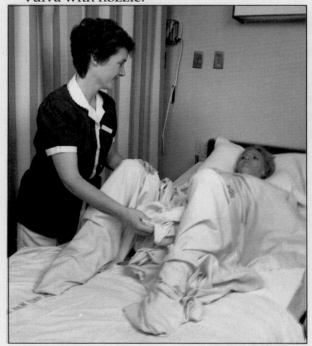

FIGURE 40–7.   Lift the center flap after positioning the patient on the bedpan.

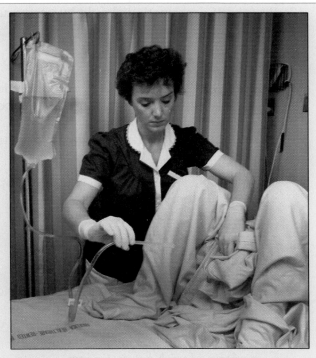

FIGURE 40–8. Insert the nozzle slowly and gently.

17. Allow solution to continue to flow and insert nozzle slowly and gently into the vagina with an upward and backward movement for about 3 inches.

18. Rotate nozzle from side to side as solution flows.
19. When all solution has been given, remove nozzle slowly and clamp tubing.
20. Have patient sit up on bedpan to allow all solution to return.
21. Remove douche bag from standard and place on paper towels.
22. Dry perineum with tissue. Discard tissue in bedpan.
23. Cover bedpan and place on chair.
24. Have patient turn on side. Dry buttocks with tissue.
25. Place clean pad over vulva from front to back.
26. Remove bed protector and bath blanket. Replace with top bedding.
27. Observe contents of bedpan. Note character and amount of discharge, if any. Discard contents of bedpan according to facility policy. Remove gloves and dispose of them according to facility policy.
28. Carry out each procedure completion action. Remember to wash your hands, report completion of task, and document time, date, vaginal irrigation (type, amount, temperature of solution), character of returns, and patient reaction.

Perineal Care

Perineal care is a simple procedure that greatly adds to the comfort of many patients. The technique reduces odor and provides an opportunity to closely inspect the patient for abnormalities. Daily attention to the perineum is also given in conjunction with indwelling catheter care.

Perineal care can be given with soap and water during the bath and after each incontinent episode. The procedures for giving routine perineal care (male and female) can be found in Unit 20.

SUMMARY

- A knowledge of the normal male and female reproductive structures is important for the nursing assistant who wishes to understand the related nursing care.
- Disposable equipment available in many hospitals makes nursing care more convenient and safer for the patient.
- The nursing assistant must be understanding and patient when providing care for patients with reproductive problems, because any surgery on the reproductive organs may have a strong psychological effect on the patient.

UNIT REVIEW

A. True/False. Answer the following statements true or false by circling T or F.

T F 1. D & C is a surgical procedure that can help establish a diagnosis related to the female reproductive system.

T F 2. Following a panhysterectomy, you should check the patient for increased bleeding.

T F 3. Salpingectomy means removal of the ovaries.

T F   4. Foul-smelling leukorrhea is associated with the condition called trichomonas vaginitis.

T F   5. The female with gonorrhea may not know she has been infected with the disease.

T F   6. Untreated gonorrhea passes through three stages.

T F   7. Syphilis presents an additional danger that is caused by a bacterium.

T F   8. AIDS is a sexually transmitted disease that is caused by a bacterium.

T F   9. The discharge in gonorrhea is white in color and very irritating.

T F 10. There is a cure for AIDS at the present time.

B. Matching. Match the phrases in Column I with the words in Column II.

Column I	Column II
_____ 11. inability to repro-duce	a. dysmenorrhea
_____ 12. inflammation of the vagina	b. mastectomy
	c. circumcision
_____ 13. painful menstrua-tion	d. leukorrhea
	e. sterility
_____ 14. removal of a breast	f. vaginitis
_____ 15. whitish discharge	

C. Multiple Choice. Choose the phrase that best completes each of the following sentences by circling the proper letter.

16. You are to give a nonsterile douche. You will remember to
    a. place the patient in a high Fowler's position.
    b. use a solution with a temperature of about 115°F.
    c. insert the nozzle about 3 inches into the vagina.
    d. allow the nozzle to touch the vulva.

17. Breast self-examination should be performed
    a. daily.   c. monthly.
    b. weekly.   d. yearly.

18. When giving routine perineal care
    a. drape the patient in the left Sims' position.
    b. use a solution with a temperature of about 110°F.
    c. perform the procedure in the bathroom.
    d. use cotton balls to wipe the area dry.

19. Your patient has just returned from a suprapubic prostatectomy. You know that
    a. there will be no incision.
    b. there will be a Foley catheter drain.
    c. there will be a suprapubic drain.
    d. Both b and c.

20. When carrying out testicular self-examination, you know the procedure should be
    a. done once each month.
    b. performed in a warm shower.
    c. performed with soapy fingers.
    d. All of the above.

D. Completion. Complete the following statements in the space provided.

21. Precautions to be followed in caring for patients with STD include:
    a. _____
    b. _____
    c. _____
    d. _____
    e. _____

22. Women over fifty should have a mammogram _____

23. Breast self-examination should be performed _____
    _____

SELF-EVALUATION   Section 10

A. Match Column I with Column II.

Column I

_____ 1. break in a bone

_____ 2. ovaries and testes

_____ 3. simple sugar

_____ 4. bringing the arm toward the midline

_____ 5. chemical messengers

_____ 6. scabs

_____ 7. color less than normal

_____ 8. cerebrovascular accident

_____ 9. carry blood toward the heart

Column II

a. flexion

b. abduction

c. pallor

d. adduction

e. crusts

f. fracture

g. hormones

h. stroke

i. gonads

j. veins

k. glucose

l. cyanosis

B. Choose the phrase that best completes each of the following sentences by circling the proper letter.

10. Patients in pelvic traction require special care. Remember to
    a. allow weights to rest on the floor.
    b. allow the patient's feet to rest on the foot of the bed.
    c. adjust the belt and straps smoothly and snugly.
    d. All of the above.

11. The best position for the patient with respiratory problems is
    a. lithotomy.
    b. high Fowler's.
    c. prone.
    d. Sims'.

12. You may be asked to weigh the cardiac patient daily because
    a. decreased appetite may cause weight loss.
    b. increased appetite may cause weight gain.
    c. fluid tends to collect in the tissues, increasing weight.
    d. urine output is increased causing weight loss.

13. Remember in caring for patients with arteriosclerosis that
    a. hot water bottles may cause serious burns.
    b. injuries heal well.
    c. circulation is very adequate.
    d. a cool room is most comfortable.

14. The patient who has suffered a CVA usually
    a. is paralyzed.
    b. speaks clearly.
    c. is able to assist in his care.
    d. has a short convalescence.

15. Fractures of children's bones are frequently incomplete. These fractures are called
    a. compound.
    b. simple.
    c. comminuted.
    d. greenstick.

16. A patient with skin lesions must
    a. be washed off with soap and water.
    b. have crusts removed daily.
    c. have frequent back rubs with alcohol.
    d. be handled gently.

17. A bed patient may develop pressure areas if
    a. position is not changed at least every 2 hours.
    b. bed is kept dry and clean.
    c. the patient is bathed frequently.
    d. pressure areas are frequently massaged.

18. When assigned to give an emollient bath, remember to
    a. gently sponge areas not submerged in water.
    b. have temperature of water 100°F.
    c. allow the patient to soak only 5 minutes.
    d. help the patient remain active after the bath.

19. The patient with emphysema has respiratory problems because
    a. he cannot inspire completely.
    b. he cannot expire completely.
    c. he inspires more deeply than usual.
    d. he expires more deeply than usual.

20. In caring for patients receiving oxygen, remember
    a. no smoking is permitted in the area.
    b. electric call bells may be used.
    c. woolen blankets are used for warmth.
    d. electrical equipment may be used without discontinuing the oxygen.

21. Following a thyroidectomy, check your patient carefully for
    a. signs of respiratory distress.
    b. inability to speak.
    c. bleeding.
    d. All of the above.

22. During a convulsion, remember to
    a. force the mouth open and insert a mouth gag.
    b. restrain the patient.
    c. move objects away that the patient may hit.
    d. not turn the head to one side.

23. Your patient has anemia. You should carry out which of the following nursing procedures?
    a. Oxygen by cannula
    b. Special mouth care
    c. Vital signs
    d. Urine measurement

24. You are assigned to care for a convalescing patient who has suffered a stroke. You will pay particular attention to
    a. skin care.
    b. development of contractures.
    c. evidence of infection.
    d. All of the above.

25. When a patient is aphasic, you can communicate with him best if you
    a. raise your voice.
    b. leave the patient alone much of the time.
    c. ask lengthy questions.
    d. speak in short, concise sentences.

26. Patients at risk for decubiti are those who are
    a. well nourished.
    b. young.
    c. incontinent.
    d. up and about.

27. The nursing assistant helping to care for the burn patient should
    a. carefully measure I & O.
    b. provide emotional support.
    c. assist in preventing infection.
    d. All of the above.

28. The nursing assistant caring for the diabetic patient
    a. may give nourishments freely.
    b. knows the signs of diabetic coma and insulin shock.
    c. cuts the patient's toenails.
    d. need not monitor how much food is eaten.

29. The nursing assistant must remember that when the patient has arterial–venous shunt for renal dialysis,
    a. use the arm with the shunt to measure an accurate blood pressure.
    b. do not use the shunted arm to determine pulse rate.
    c. do not use shunted arm to measure blood pressure.
    d. it is not necessary to measure ordered intake and output.

30. During which of the following procedures should the nursing assistant wear disposable gloves?
    a. Giving enemas.
    b. Giving perineal care.
    c. Giving indwelling catheter care.
    d. All of the above.

31. During a seizure, the nursing assistant should
    a. secure clothing around the neck for support.
    b. keep the head flat, facing forward.
    c. run quickly and get help.
    d. None of the above.

32. When caring for a spinal cord injured patient, the nursing assistant should
    a. recognize that pain and pressure will be felt more acutely.
    b. realize the patient requires extra care to prevent contractures.
    c. know the patient will not need skin care since voluntary movement will not be impaired.
    d. use a hurried approach to care to stimulate the patient into action.

33. The nursing assistant preparing a patient for an 8 AM gastrointestinal series might expect to find as part of the instructions
    a. high-calorie breakfast.
    b. enemas until clear in the morning of test.
    c. surgical prep of abdomen.
    d. no visitors the night before the test.

34. To make insertion of a rectal tube easier, the nursing assistant might suggest the patient
    a. take a breath and bear down.
    b. exhale as the tube is inserted.
    c. lie with legs extended.
    d. cross legs.

35. When preparing to give a preprepared chemical enema, the nursing assistant knows
    a. water will need to be added.
    b. approximately 500 ml of solution will be used.
    c. special care will have to be taken of the glass container holding the fluid.
    d. the tip of the container is prelubricated.

36. The nursing assistant assigned to give a Harris flush recognizes that
    a. all the fluid will be retained.
    b. the purpose is to evacuate feces from the bowel.
    c. all the fluid is usually returned.
    d. gloves need not be worn during the procedure.

37. The nursing assistant is 52 years old and should have a mammogram
    a. yearly.
    b. every other year.
    c. every three years.
    d. every five years.

38. The nursing assistant has frequent herpes simplex II outbreaks and recognizes that such circumstances
    a. puts females at less risk of cancer of the cervix.
    b. puts females at greater risk of miscarriage.
    c. makes vaginal delivery the preferred route.
    d. cannot affect a newborn in any way.

39. The nursing assistant caring for the patient with AIDS must bear in mind that
    a. AIDS is caused by a bacteria.
    b. the organism is transmitted primarily through the exchange of respiratory secretions.
    c. ELISA and Western blot are tests done to identify the presence of AIDS antibodies.
    d. HIV infection never progresses to full AIDS.

40. Syphilis and gonorrhea are diseases that are commonly sexually transmitted. Other sexually transmitted diseases include:
    a. chlamydia infections.
    b. papilloma viral infections.
    c. HIV infection.
    d. All of the above.

The Obstetrical Patient and Neonate

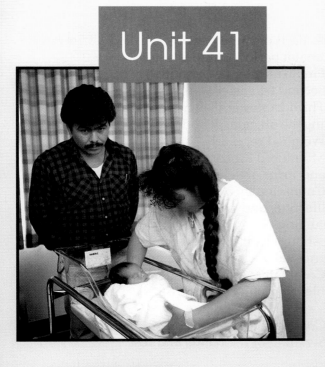

NOTICE TO THE READER

By state law, you may not be permitted to perform some of the advanced procedures given in this section. Consult with your instructor/supervisor to be sure you know your legal responsibilities. Do not perform or assist in any procedure you are not permitted by law to do.

OBJECTIVES

As a result of this unit, you will be able to:

- Spell and define terms.
- Assist in the prenatal care of the normal pregnant woman.
- List reportable observations of the woman in the prenatal period.
- List the presumptive, probable, and positive signs of pregnancy.
- Assist in the care of the normal postpartum patient.
- Properly change a perineal pad.
- Recognize reportable observations of patients in the postpartum period.
- Recognize reportable signs and symptoms of urine retention in the postpartum patient.
- Assist in the care of the normal newborn.
- Demonstrate three methods of safely holding a baby.
- Assist in carrying out the discharge procedures for mother and infant.

VOCABULARY

Learn the meaning and the correct spelling of the following words:

afterbirth
amniocentesis
amniotic fluid
amniotic sac
Apgar score
birthing centers
cesarean
circumcision
colostrum
dilation stage
efface
endoscope
episiotomy
expulsion stage
fetal monitor
fetoscopy
fetus
foreskin
fundus
gestational age
involution
isolette
labor

lactation
lochia
meconium
neonate
obstetrical
placenta
placental stage
positive signs of pregnancy
postpartum
prenatal
presumptive sign of pregnancy
probable signs of pregnancy
rooming in
status
trimester
ultrasound
umbilical cord
vaginal examination
vernix caseosa

When a baby is ready to be born, it is normally upside down in the mother's uterus with its head toward the birth canal, Figure 41–1. Before the baby is born, it is known as a fetus. It is surrounded by a membranous bag called an amniotic sac. The fetus floats in a liquid called amniotic fluid.

The fetus gets nourishment from the mother through the umbilical cord. The umbilical cord is attached to the fetus and the placenta (afterbirth). The placenta is attached to the wall of the mother's uterus.

After the baby is born and separated from the umbilical cord, the placenta, amniotic sac, and remaining cord are expelled as the afterbirth. After a period of time, the mother's uterus, or womb, which had greatly stretched to accommodate the pregnancy, will return to its normal size and shape.

There are three phases of pregnancy. They are:
- Prenatal (before birth)
- Labor and delivery
- Postpartum (after birth)

The nursing assistant, who is especially trained, helps provide care and support throughout each phase.

Prenatal Care

The care of the mother begins in the prenatal period when she first learns she is pregnant. You may meet her as you work in a doctor's office or in an obstetrical (pregnancy) clinic.

The prenatal period is divided into three-month periods. Each of these periods is called a trimester The prenatal period includes:
- First trimester (1–3 months)
- Second trimester (4–6 months)
- Third trimester (7–9 months)

During the prenatal period, the pregnant woman is:
- Weighed regularly.
- Monitored for complications—blood pressure and urine are checked.
- Counseled by a nurse or physician about diet, lifestyle, and any problems that might be occurring.

You should call to the attention of the nurse anything unusual. Examples of items to report are:
- Complaints of persistent headache
- Elevated blood pressure
- Vaginal bleeding
- Complaints of dizziness
- Swelling of the hands and feet

Signs of Pregnancy

A woman usually first suspects that she is pregnant when she stops her menstrual flow. Many factors can cause an interruption of the normal monthly menstrual cycle. Therefore, this is only a presumptive sign of pregnancy, Figure 41–2. Other presumptive signs include:
- Morning sickness
- Frequent voiding
- Fatigue

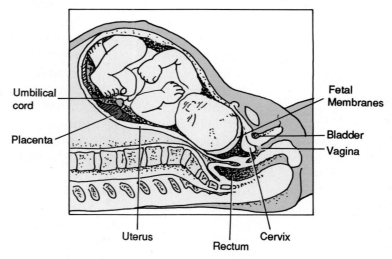

FIGURE 41–1.   The usual position of the fetus at term. This is known as a head (vertex) presentation. *(From Sloane,* Biology of Women, *copyright 1993 by Delmar Publishers Inc.)*

PRESUMPTIVE SIGNS
■ Cessation of menses (amenorrhea)
■ Breast enlargement
■ Darkening of areola
■ Fatigue
■ Morning sickness
■ Linea nigra (line of pigmentation along midline of abdomen)
POSITIVE SIGNS
■ Hearing the fetal heartbeat
■ Feeling fetal movement
■ Visualization by X-ray or ultrasound

FIGURE 41–2. Some signs of pregnancy

■ Tenderness and fullness of breasts
■ Darkened areas of pigmentation around nipples (areola)

As the pregnancy progresses, she will notice other changes. These are the **probable signs of pregnancy**. They include:

■ Enlargement of the abdomen
■ Positive pregnancy tests

The physician will be able to detect changes in the uterus and may even feel the fetal outline. The **positive signs of pregnancy** include:

■ Hearing the fetus
■ Feeling the fetus
■ Seeing the fetus through X-ray or ultrasound procedures

Preparation for Birth

Parents are encouraged to participate fully in the birth of their baby. Special training for the birth begins in the prenatal period. It prepares the parents to participate in the birthing process. Many parents choose to participate in natural childbirth. This technique of birthing:

■ Allows the mother to be awake and fully participate in the birth.
■ Encourages the father or an alternative support person to act as coach for the mother.
■ Necessitates little, if any, pain-controlling medication. One of the most popular of these methods is called the Lamaze method. Further advances have combined the Lamaze method with a refinement developed by Frederick Leboyer.

The Leboyer Method

The Leboyer method of natural childbirth is based on the principle of "birth without violence." With this technique:

■ All unnecessary stimuli are limited.
■ Lighting is lowered as much as possible without making the birth area unsafe.
■ No noise is permitted or only soft music is allowed in the delivery room.
■ The cord is not cut or tied until the pulsations cease.
■ The baby is placed on the mother's abdomen for approximately 3–6 minutes following delivery.
■ The mother traces the outline of the baby's eyes with her fingers while gently stroking its back. Shortly thereafter the baby is:
— Placed, with its head carefully supported, in a tub of warm water for another 3–6 minutes.
— Carefully dried and wrapped.
— Returned to the mother for an extended period.

This technique is believed to encourage parental interaction with the baby and birthing process and to encourage bonding between mother and child.

Training Classes

In the training classes:

■ The father or some other person learns to act as a coach for the mother.
■ The mother learns ways of cooperating with her body during labor and delivery using special breathing and relaxation techniques.
■ The couple sees films of the birth process.
■ Vaginal and cesarean deliveries are discussed.
■ There are opportunities to ask questions of a trained professional.

Prenatal Testing

Techniques used to diagnose the possibility of complications can be done in the prenatal period. They include:

■ Weight measurement
■ Blood pressure measurement
■ Urine testing for the presence of albumin

Congenital abnormalities, those present at birth, can sometimes be identified through such prenatal testing as:

■ Ultrasound—a technique of using sound waves to identify gestational age (time of development) and defects in the structure of fetal organs.

■ Amniocentesis—a procedure in which a sterile needle is inserted into the fetal sac and cells are withdrawn for examination. Some genetic defects may be identified in this way.

■ Fetoscopy—a direct visualization of the fetus in the uterus through a small visualization instrument (endoscope). Blood abnormalities may also be identified from samples of the fetal blood that is withdrawn.

Labor and Delivery

When the mother reaches her due date and begins labor, she will experience contractions of her uterus. The uterine contractions:

■ Prepare the birth canal for passage of the baby.
■ Are irregular at first.
■ Become stronger and more regular and closer together as labor progresses.

Some families elect to have home deliveries. Most families prefer to be in a health facility when the:

■ Amniotic membrane ruptures.
■ Contractions are regular, sustained, and about 3 minutes apart.

The amniotic sac surrounds the developing fetus. It:

■ Maintains an even temperature.
■ Acts as a hydrostatic cushion.
■ Enables the fetus to grow and move freely.

The amniotic sac sometimes ruptures early in labor. When the sac ruptures, there is a rush of fluid from the vagina. If the membranes do not rupture, the physician may rupture them once the patient is in the hospital.

The length of labor varies. There are three stages of labor and delivery. They are dilation, expulsion, and placental.

Dilation

The dilation (opening) stage begins with the first regular uterine contractions. It ends when the cervix is fully dilated or opened. This may take 18–24 hours in a first pregnancy.

As the labor progresses, the cervix also thins (effaces) so that the fetus may move downward into the birth canal and out of the mother's body. The degree of dilation at any given time is measured by the nurse or physician. The nurse or physician places a gloved finger in the patient's vagina and measures approximately the size of the cervical opening. This procedure is called vaginal examination.

Relief of Discomfort

Drugs may be given to the mother in the labor and delivery phase to reduce pain. Three approaches are frequently employed for a vaginal delivery. They are:

1. Epidural—this is the most common technique. The anesthetic drug is introduced into the epidural space around the spinal cord. Since the drug is not introduced into the cerebrospinal fluid, its effect is more localized in the reproductive organs. The patient's legs can move, but they are weak. Women who are pregnant for the first time may be given this relief when they have reached 5–6 cm cervical dilation. Women who have had more than one pregnancy may have it started at 3–4 cm dilation without slowing the progress of labor. Controlled introduction of drugs through the epidural route can continue to offer relief throughout the delivery. Patients receiving epidural pain relief must be carefully monitored for changes in pulse and blood pressure. Report a drop in blood pressure to the nurse at once.

2. Regional caudal block—this technique introduces the drug into the cerebrospinal fluid. It affects a somewhat larger area, but the legs can still move. This form of relief is commonly known as a saddle block. This is usually given in the delivery room.

3. Pudendal block—this technique specifically blocks the function of the nerves that supply the perineum. This medication is usually administered in the delivery room.

When any of these procedures is used, the patient will not feel an episiotomy or its repair, but she will still be able to move her legs. The type of pain relief given to the mother during labor and delivery will determine the postpartum care she will receive.

Fetal Monitors

In many hospitals, a fetal monitor (instrument to check the well-being of the baby during labor), Figure 41–3, is attached either to the mother's abdomen or to the baby's head.

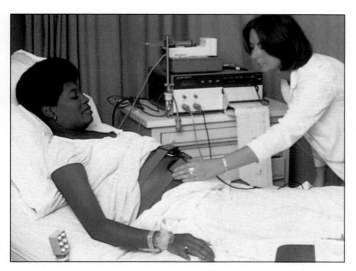

FIGURE 41–3. The fetal monitor allows the staff to evaluate the condition of the infant during labor. *(Photo courtesy of Memorial Medical Center of Long Beach, CA)*

The patient is moved to a special delivery room where sterile precautions can be carried out to protect both mother and child when the:

■ Cervix has fully dilated.
■ Baby has moved down through the birth canal.
■ Baby's head can be seen at the vaginal opening, Figure 41–4.

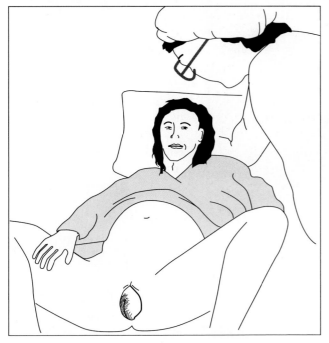

FIGURE 41–4. The baby's head is seen at the vaginal opening just before delivery.

Expulsion

Expulsion stage is the period extending from the point of full cervical dilation until the baby is delivered. This may be a period of 1–2 hours or more.

The baby moves down the birth canal. The mother is encouraged to help the process by "bearing down" with her abdominal muscles with each contraction. Figures 41–5 and 41–6 show the baby being assisted in delivery and rotated as the shoulders are presented.

During delivery it may be necessary to enlarge the vaginal opening. This is done by making a cut in the perineum. The cut is called an **episiotomy**. The episiotomy is sutured after delivery.

Forceps may be used at this stage to assist the delivery of the head. Once delivered, the baby is held head down to clear the respiratory tract, Figure 41–7.

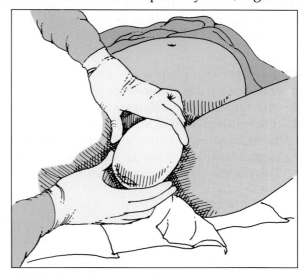

FIGURE 41–5. The baby's head emerges.

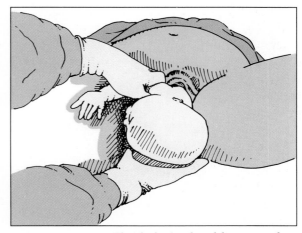

FIGURE 41–6. The baby's shoulders are then delivered.

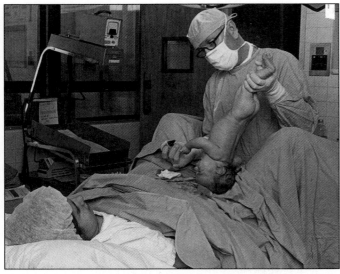

FIGURE 41–7. Immediately following delivery, the baby is held head down to clear the respiratory tract. The baby is also suctioned to clear mucus.

The baby is then usually placed on the mother's abdomen while the cord is clamped and cut. In addition:

- An Apgar score is determined.
- The mother is encouraged to hold her newborn, now called a neonate, to establish emotional bonding. This is done even when the baby is delivered by cesarean section.

Placental Stage

The placental stage lasts from the delivery of the baby through the delivery of the placenta. This is a short period. The placenta is usually delivered within an hour of the delivery of the baby.

In this stage, the placenta separates from the wall of the uterus. Uterine contractions push it downward and out through the birth canal. After the delivery of the placenta:

- If an episiotomy was needed, it is repaired.
- The mother's uterus is checked for firmness. Drugs may be given to help it contract to control bleeding.
- Both mother and child are identified with name tags before being separated.
- The baby may be footprinted along with the mother's thumbprint.
- The baby's eyes may be treated to prevent infection.
- The baby is transferred for neonatal care to the newborn nursery. The mother is moved to her room. In some hospitals, the mother and child are cared for in a single unit in the postpartum period. This encourages bonding between mother and child as the mother assists with the care. This form of care is called rooming in. Family members are encouraged to help in infant care, Figure 41–8.

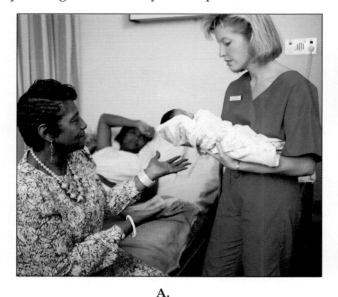

A.

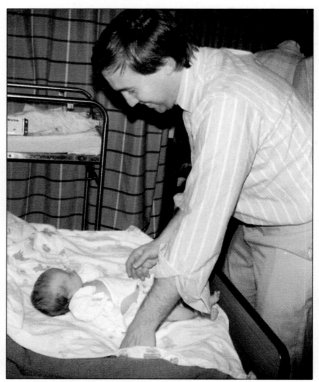

B.

FIGURE 41–8. When at-home delivery, a birthing center, or "rooming in" is chosen as a means of caring for the baby, family members are encouraged to participate in the infant's care.

In the last several years there has been a trend toward
- Making the delivery a family affair.
- Having the delivery take place at home, or in a homelike environment.
- Continuing to provide for the safety of both mother and infant.

These goals are being met in private homes or **birthing centers** (facilities that specialize in the birth process). Some birthing centers are part of a hospital; others are independent units close by clinical facilities.

Birthing rooms resemble a comfortable bedroom. The bed is constructed in such a way that, when needed, it can be easily converted into a delivery table. Immediate family members are encouraged to wait with the mother during labor. They may also remain during the actual delivery. One nurse is assigned, if possible, to assist the mother and family through the entire birthing process.

After the delivery, unless there are complications, the mother and baby remain in the same room and receive all of their care in this setting. Visiting hours are liberal and include the children of the family.

Unless there are complications, patients usually do not remain in the birthing center for more than 24 hours postpartum. Some patients do not stay more than 6 hours postpartum .

The costs are far less when compared to the cost of delivery in a conventional health care facility. Many people prefer the less formal environment of a birthing center for uncomplicated births.

Cesarean Birth

Cesarean delivery is another way of delivering a baby. The baby is delivered through an incision in the abdomen rather than through the birth canal. Between 20–30% of all deliveries in the U.S. are made in this way.

A spinal anesthetic is administered prior to the surgery. This type of procedure introduces the drugs into the cerebrospinal fluid and blocks sensation from the upper abdomen down to the toes. Until the anesthetic wears off, the patient will not be able either to feel or move her legs.

After the delivery, the mother sometimes is given a general anesthetic that allows her to sleep during the rest of the procedure.

Cesarean deliveries are performed when there is:
- Fetal distress
- A preterm infant
- Breech (nonhead first) presentation
- Prolonged rupture of the membranes
- Prolapsed cord
- Genital herpes
- Premature separation of the placenta
- Placenta previa
- Dysfunctional labor

The incision in the abdominal wall may be:
- Vertical along the midplane
- Transverse across the lowest and narrowest part of the abdomen (bikini cut)

The mother's coach or partner is encouraged to be in the operative area to offer emotional support while the cesarean is being carried out. The same basic activities are carried out in the operating room as are followed after a vaginal delivery.

After the surgery is complete, the baby is usually admitted to the nursery, Figure 41–9. The mother is moved to the recovery room for immediate post-anesthesia care. If the infant is in distress, it will be taken to the neonatal intensive care unit, Figure 41–10.

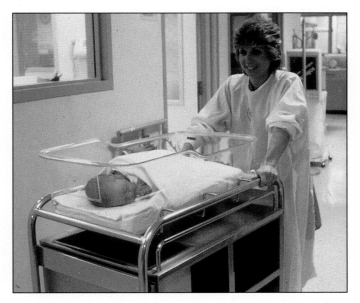

FIGURE 41–9. Babies are transported in their own bassinets from the delivery room to the newborn nursery. (*Photo courtesy of Memorial Medical Center of Long Beach, CA*)

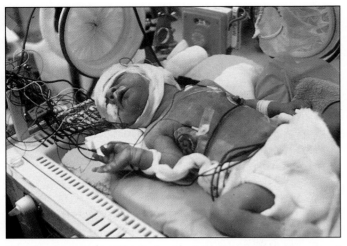

FIGURE 41–10. This baby has been moved to a neonatal intensive care unit following a cesarean delivery. The eyes are covered to protect them. *(Photo courtesy of Memorial Medical Center of Long Beach, CA)*

Postpartum Care

You may be assigned to assist with the care of the mother following delivery. This is known as the postpartum period.

With other team members, you will assist the mother from the stretcher into bed. A protective pad (Chux) may be placed under the patient's buttocks.

Anesthesia

If an anesthetic has been used, follow the procedures for postoperative care of surgical patients, which were covered in Unit 27.

- Keep the patient flat on her back.
- Make sure each patient has a fresh gown and the bed linen is kept clean.
- Check the blood pressure, pulse, and respirations as ordered until stable.
- Continue to monitor vital signs every four hours for 24 hours.
- If patients complain of being cold, an extra blanket may provide comfort.

If the patient does not become comfortable, inform the nurse.

Drainage

The Perineum.
- Carefully check the condition of the perineum and the perineal pad for the amount and color of drainage.
- When removing the pad, always lift it away from the body from front to back.
- Red vaginal discharge, called lochia, is expected. The amount of discharge and any clotting should be reported.

Initially, the lochia is bright red and moderate in amount. Over the next week, the lochia will lessen and become pink to pink-brown in color. A discharge that is yellowish-white or brown may continue 1–3 weeks after delivery and then stop. Note and report:

- Signs of tenderness
- Signs of inflammation
- Presence of an episiotomy

The Uterus

The size and firmness of the uterus should be checked and reported.

- A soft and enlarging uterus indicates excessive bleeding.

Massaging. The top of the uterus, the fundus, is massaged in a circular fashion while the opposite hand is held against the pubic bone. Massaging the fundus stimulates the uterine muscles to contract, firming the uterus. Be sure that your hospital policy allows nursing assistants to perform this procedure and that you are completely skilled before attempting to do it.

Measuring Height of Uterus. The level of the fundus is measured by placing the fingers lengthwise across the abdomen between the fundus and umbilicus. On the first post-partal day, the level of the fundus is at the umbilicus or may be one to two fingers below.

Cramping. As the uterus begins to return to its normal size, involution, the patient may experience strong uterine contractions or cramps. Cramping may also be associated with breast feeding. This is normal but be sure to report any complaints of pain to your team leader, who can administer medication for relief.

Voiding

The new mother should be encouraged to void within the first 6–8 hours after the delivery. Check carefully for signs of urine retention. These include:

- A uterus that is unusually high or pushed to one side
- Swelling noted just above the pubis

- Complaints of urgency, which is the need to void, but voidings of 200 ml or less

Be sure to report:
- Signs of possible urine retention immediately to the nurse so the patient's recovery will not be impeded
- Any inability to void within the first 8 hours postpartum
- Voidings of less than 100 ml

This is important since a full bladder can cause postpartum hemorrhage.

Ambulation

After the initial recovery period, many postpartum patients are up and about and care is self-directed. Unless otherwise indicated, the mother is allowed to dangle and then be up. In most cases, she will be able to care for most of her personal needs. Remember to check on the new mother, especially when she showers, as she may become faint. When the new mother is stronger, a visit to the nursery to see her new infant is a pleasurable experience.

Toileting and Perineal Care

The mother may be:
- Provided with a squeezable bottle, which is filled with warm tap water.

- Instructed to rinse the genitals and perineum after voiding or defecating.
- Instructed to gently pat, not wipe, the perineal area containing the stitches with tissue or special medicated pads, once only, from front to back. The tissue is discarded in the toilet.
- Taught to wash her hands before applying a fresh perineal pad.
- Taught not to touch the inside of the perineal pad.

If the perineum is very uncomfortable:
- Specially medicated pads may be used for cleansing. The procedure is always the same— front to back and discard.
- Anesthetic sprays may be ordered.
- Ice packs may be used to reduce edema and give comfort.

Patients should be cautioned to apply anesthetics and ointments after cleansing.

Sitting may be uncomfortable when an episiotomy has been performed. Instruct the mother to squeeze her buttocks together and hold them in this position until she is seated upright. This reduces tension on the suture line.

Before performing any patient care procedures, review the beginning procedure actions and procedure completion actions shown in Figure 41–11.

BEGINNING PROCEDURE ACTIONS	PROCEDURE COMPLETION ACTIONS
■ Wash your hands. ■ Assemble equipment needed. ■ Go to the patient's room, knock, and pause before entering. ■ Introduce yourself and identify the patient by checking the identification bracelet. ■ Ask visitors to leave and inform them where they can wait. ■ Care for equipment according to facility policy. ■ Provide privacy. ■ Explain what will happen and answer questions. ■ Allow patient to assist in procedure as much as possible. ■ Raise bed or table to comfortable working height.	■ Position patient comfortably. ■ Leave signal cord, telephone, and fresh water close at hand. ■ Return bed or table to lowest position. ■ Perform general safety check of patient and environment. ■ Wash your hands. ■ Report completion of task. ■ Let visitors know when they may reenter the patient's room. ■ Document action and your observations.

NOTE: Where there are open lesions, wet linen, or possible contact with patient body fluids or blood, disposable gloves are worn during the procedure. Put on gloves before contact with the patient or linen. Properly dispose of gloves after they are removed. ALWAYS APPLY UNIVERSAL PRECAUTIONS.

FIGURE 41–11. Beginning procedure actions and procedure completion actions

Breast Care

The mother's first milk is called colostrum. The colostrum:

■ Is watery.

■ Carries protective antibodies to the child.

■ Usually begins to flow about 12 hours after delivery. Lactation, the flow of milk, doesn't begin until the second or third postpartum day.

Keeping the breasts clean is especially important when the mother is planning to breast feed her baby.

■ The mother's hands and nipples should be washed just prior to feeding the baby.

■ During the shower, the mother should wash the breasts, using a circular motion from the nipples outward.

■ Creams are sometimes used between feedings to help the nipples remain supple.

■ Breast pads absorb milk leakage. They should be changed frequently.

■ The breasts should be supported by a well-fitted brassiere.

If the mother chooses not to breast feed:

■ The breasts should be washed daily with soap and water.

■ The breasts should be supported continuously by a well-fitted brassiere.

■ Medication to suppress milk production is sometimes ordered.

Mothers and healthy newborns, whose delivery is uncomplicated, do not remain in the hospital very long. They are able to go home within one day.

Neonatal Care

The newborn is admitted to the nursery where those procedures not carried out in the delivery room are completed. The physician or nurse will examine the baby and make an evaluation of the baby's condition, or status

Apgar Scoring

The Apgar score is an evaluation of the neonate. It is made at one minute and five minutes after birth. The areas evaluated are:

■ Heart rate

■ Respiratory effort

■ Muscle tone

■ Reflex, irritability

■ Color

A number value is applied to each assessment and recorded on a special form. For example, the neonate who has a heart rate less than 100 bpm, has slow respirations, offers slight resistance to limb extension, has a weak cry, and is pale and cyanotic would be rated as follows:

Heart rate	1
Respiratory effort	1
Muscle tone	1
Reflex, irritability	1
Color	0
Total	4

Totals indicate the infant's condition. A score of 7–10 indicates the infant is in good condition. A score of 4–6 indicates a fair condition. A score of 0–4 indicates a poor condition.

In the nursery:

■ The vital signs of the baby are determined.

■ Measurements of length and weight are taken.

If the newborn's status is stable:

■ If the eyes were not treated with silver nitrate drops or antibiotics in the delivery room and the footprints were not taken, Figure 41–12, these procedures will also be done at this time.

■ The baby is cleaned. Sometimes an admission bath using an antiseptic soap or oil is administered, but procedures for bathing newborns vary from hospital to hospital. In some hospitals, the bath is omitted and the cheesy material known as vernix caseosa is allowed to remain on the skin. The area around the cord is carefully cleaned with a solution prescribed by the facility, Figure 41–13.

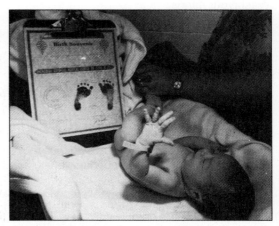

FIGURE 41–12. Footprinting is done in the delivery room or nursery. Note the name tag on the baby's arm. It matches the mother's identification band.

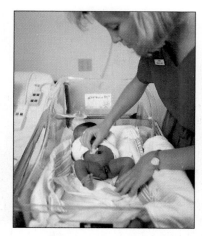

FIGURE 41–13. Carefully clean around the cord with solution prescribed by the facility.

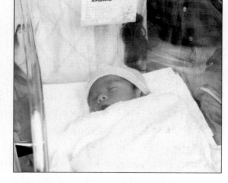

FIGURE 41–14. Babies tend to lose warmth through their heads so stockinette caps are used to cover them.

■ The baby is kept warm because a baby's temperature is not yet stabilized. The baby is dressed according to facility policy. A stockinette cap is placed on the head because much body heat can be lost through this surface, Figure 41–14.

■ The baby is placed on abdomen in crib or isolette, Figure 41–15.

■ Feeding is not usually started for 12 hours after birth. During these hours, the baby is monitored and observed carefully for successful, independent life. After 12 hours, the baby is either taken to breast or started on feedings of glucose and water. Babies whose mothers are unable to feed will be fed in the nursery.

■ Male babies may be circumcised before discharge. In **circumcision** the excess tissue (**foreskin**) is cut from the tip of the penis. This procedure is no longer performed routinely. However, the procedure is still routinely performed on male babies whose parents are members of Orthodox Jewish congregations.

■ Babies who are jaundiced may have their eyes protected and be placed under a special light (bili light) to help clear the levels of bilirubin in the skin.

Handling the Infant

Lifting, carrying, and positioning an infant must be done with care. Remember to:

■ Lift the baby by grasping the legs securely with one hand while slipping the other hand under the baby's back to support the head and neck, Figures 41–16 and 41–17.

■ Hold the baby securely.

■ Support the head, neck, and back at all times.

■ Back through doorways when carrying the baby.

■ Never turn your back on an infant when the infant is on an unprotected surface.

PKU Test

The baby's blood is tested to detect the presence of phenylketonuria (PKU), Figure 41–18. PKU is a congenital, hereditary abnormality. It may lead to mental retardation if undetected and not treated early. In PKU, normal protein digestion is not possible. The

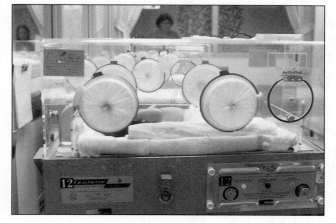

FIGURE 41–15. Babies may be cared for in isolettes that provide a controlled environment. (*Photo courtesy of Memorial Medical Center of Long Beach, CA*)

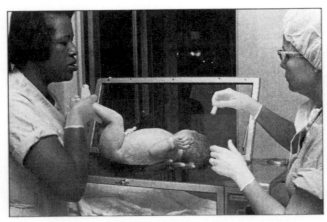

FIGURE 41–16. While grasping the legs securely, the other hand is slipped under the back to support the head and neck. Note the vernix caseosa on the infant's back.

disorder cannot be cured, but it can be controlled by a special diet.

Eye Care

This procedure is usually performed by the nurse. If you are assigned this responsibility, check your hospital policy. Silver nitrate ($AgNO_3$) in a 1% solution is commonly used, but other medications such as antibiotics may be ordered.

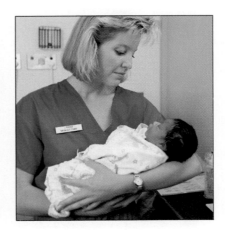

A. Cradle hold

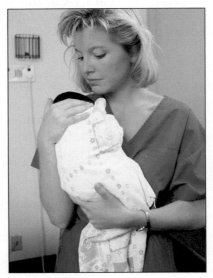

B. Shoulder hold

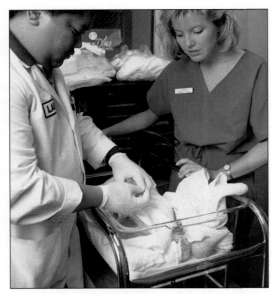

FIGURE 41–18. Blood is drawn from a heel stick to check for phenylketonuria (PKU). PKU is a congenital, hereditary abnormality that can lead to mental retardation if undetected and not treated early.

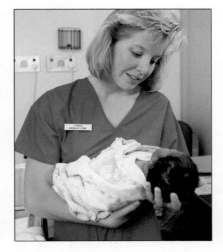

C. Football hold

FIGURE 41–17. Proper techniques for holding a baby

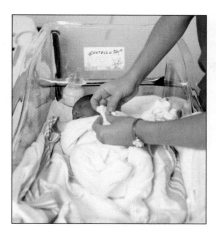

FIGURE 41–19. Dress the child in his/her own clothing.

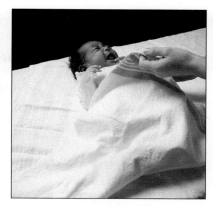

FIGURE 41–20A. Wrap the baby by placing infant on a receiving blanket that is placed so corners are at head and feet. Bring bottom corner up over infant.

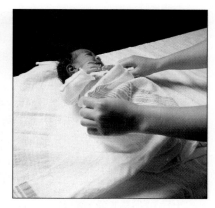

FIGURE 41–20B. Bring one side corner of blanket over infant.

Post Circumcision Care

The circumcision should be checked each time the diaper is changed and should be a routine part of that care. Observe the incision site for bleeding and report anything unusual. The crib identification should note the new circumcision. A note should be included on the nursery record as to the condition of the circumcision and first voiding after circumcision.

Discharge

To carry out the discharge procedure from a facility:

- Match the baby's identification with the mother's.
- Dress child in his/her own clothing, Figure 41–19. This may be done in the nursery or in the mother's room.
- Wrap the baby in a blanket, using the technique of "papoosing," as shown in Figures 41–20A through D.
- Check to be sure that the mother has received and understands any special discharge instructions. If not, inform the nurse.
- Check to be sure equipment or needed formula is ready. The parents and newborn are ready to go home, Figure 41–21.
- Transport the mother, carrying her baby, by wheelchair to the discharge area. Stay with them until they leave.

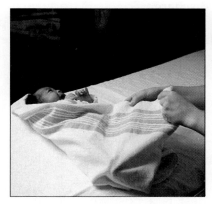

FIGURE 41–20C. Then bring the other side corner of blanket over the infant.

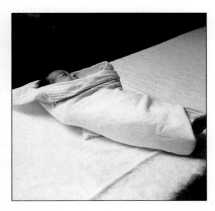

FIGURE 41–20D. Tuck final corner under infant. The infant is ready to be discharged.

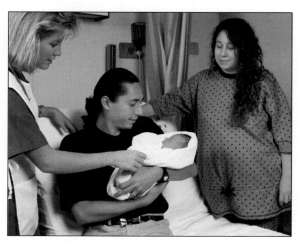

FIGURE 41–21. Parents prepare to leave the hospital with their newborn.

■ Record discharge information on the charts of both mother and child. Include the condition of each and the time of release.

Home Care

The discharged mother faces many new challenges. It will take approximately six weeks for her reproductive organs to recover. Home care of the mother includes:

■ Providing adequate nutrition
■ Allowing for sufficient rest
■ Attending to proper elimination
■ Providing emotional support during any transitory depression
■ Providing breast care, if nursing

SUMMARY

The care of the obstetrical patient is a specialized area of medicine. It includes:
■ Supervision of the health of the mother throughout the prenatal, labor and delivery, and postpartum periods to discharge
■ Care of the neonate
The nursing assistant may participate in this care under the close direction of the professional staff if facility policy permits.

A thorough understanding of your responsibilities and close attention to the details of care help ensure a successful and safe pregnancy and delivery.

All the procedures presented in this unit require advanced training and supervision before you attempt to perform them. In addition, you may do so only under proper authorization.

UNIT REVIEW

A. True/False. Answer the following statements true or false by circling T or F.

T   F   1. A positive pregnancy test is a positive sign of pregnancy.

T   F   2. You are responsible for noting and reporting the first postpartal voiding.

T   F   3. The care of the mother begins in the prenatal period.

T   F   4. The nurse or physician monitors the progress of labor by performing a vaginal examination.

T   F   5. Immediate postpartum lochia should be yellowish-white.

T   F   6. Massaging the cervix stimulates the uterine muscles to contract.

T   F   7. The Leboyer method is based on the principle of "birth without violence."

T   F   8. Ultrasound is a technique that is used to examine the baby before birth.

T   F   9. In the first pregnancy, the period of labor and delivery called expulsion lasts 18–24 hours.

T   F   10. As labor progresses, the uterine cervix becomes more and more tightened.

T   F   11. The shoulder hold is a safe way to hold and support an infant.

T   F   12. A newborn should be burped after each 2 ounces is taken during feeding.

T   F   13. The mother's hands and nipples should be washed prior to nursing the baby.

B. Matching. Match Column I with Column II.

Column I	Column II
_____ 14. surgery to remove the foreskin	a. lochia
	b. umbilical cord
_____ 15. maintains an even temperature for the baby	c. fundus
	d. lactation
_____ 16. mother's first postpartum breast secretions	e. colostrum
	f. circumcision
_____ 17. attachment between baby and placenta	g. vernix caseosa
	h. amniotic fluid
_____ 18. vaginal discharge following delivery	i. placenta

C. Completion. Complete the following statements in the space provided.

19. Five unusual findings made in the prenatal examination that should be reported to the nurse include:

    a. _____

    b. _____

    c. _____

    d. _____

    e. _____

20. The nursing assistant assigned to check the perineum of a postpartum patient should:

    a. _____

    b. _____

    c. _____

21. Reportable signs and symptoms that indicate the postpartum patient may be retaining urine include:

    a. _____

    b. _____

    c. _____

    d. _____

    e. _____

22. Two actions that must be taken to protect a newborn during weighing are:

    a. _____

    b. _____

23. Reportable observations regarding the newborn relate to:

    a. _____

    b. _____

    c. _____

    d. _____

Unit 42

The Pediatric Patient

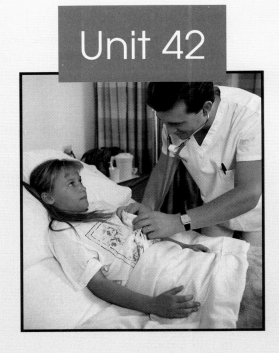

Judith A. DiNardo, MS, RN
Pediatric Staff Education Instructor
New England Medical Center Hospitals
Boston, MA

Linda M. Donovan, RN, BSN
Nurse Manager, Pediatrics Surgical Unit
Boston Floating Hospital for Infants and Children
New England Medical Center Hospitals
Boston, MA

OBJECTIVES

As a result of this unit, you will be able to:

- Spell and define terms.
- Describe the major developmental tasks for each pediatric age group.
- Describe how to foster growth and development for hospitalized pediatric patients.
- Describe how to maintain a safe environment for the pediatric patient.
- Discuss the role of parents and siblings of the hospitalized pediatric patient.
- Describe and demonstrate the proper procedure for admitting a pediatric patient.
- Describe and demonstrate the proper procedure for weighing the pediatric patient.
- Describe and demonstrate the proper procedure for measuring the vital signs of the pediatric patient: temperature, pulse, respirations, and blood pressure.
- Describe and demonstrate the proper procedure for bottle feeding an infant.
- Describe and demonstrate the proper procedure for burping an infant.
- Describe and demonstrate the proper procedure for changing the crib linens.

VOCABULARY

Learn the meaning and the correct spelling of the following words and phrases:

adolescence
adoptive parent
autonomy
biological parent
developmental
 milestones
developmental tasks
family
foster parent
initiative
legal custody
legal guardian
regress
stepparent

Children, like adults, get sick and require hospitalization for diagnosis and treatment of their illnesses. But children are different. They are not just small adults. Children can differ in age, in size, and in developmental level. When you work with children, you also will be working with the people who are most important to them—their parents or those responsible for their upbringing. When a child is sick and is hospitalized, the illness affects the entire family. The family is an important part of the child's life regardless of the child's age. When working with pediatric patients, you will need to include the parents in giving care to the child.

In today's society, the words *parents* and *family* can have different meanings. A child may live with one or both parents. The words *biological, adoptive, foster*, and *step* can refer to the various types of parents that may be part or all of a child's family. The terms are defined as follows:

- **Biological parent**—birth parent
- **Adoptive parent**—person who has assumed responsibility for parenting
- **Foster parent**—person who carries out parenting duties under the authority of a legal agency
- **Stepparent**—person who assumes the parenting role by marrying a birth or adoptive parent

Families may also include combinations of parents. For example, a child may live with a biological father and an adoptive or stepmother. Or a child may live with a single parent who could be either biological, adoptive, or foster. Other family arrangements may include the child living with a relative while the parent maintains legal custody of the child. **Legal custody** refers to the person who has the right to give consent for hospitalization and for the procedures that may be needed while the child is hospitalized. This person is known as the **legal guardian**. The child may live with someone other than the legal guardian.

The word **family** refers to the household unit in which the child lives. Members of the family may include the parents, siblings (biological, adoptive, or step), and/or other relatives or people in the household.

As a member of the health care team, it is important to identify the child's caretakers as well as that person who has legal custody.

This unit provides guidelines for the care of the hospitalized child. The nursing assistant must recognize that hospitalization may interrupt the child's normal growth and development. This is a traumatic time for the child. Suggestions are provided to show how the nursing assistant can assist and encourage the child's development during hospitalization.

Safety is an important part of providing care. This unit presents guidelines for creating a safe environment for each pediatric age group. Because families are important, suggestions are given for creating a family-centered approach to pediatric health care.

Pediatric Units

Pediatric units are typically set up in two ways:
1. According to specific age groups of children.

2. According to the types of patients, such as surgical, orthopedic, cardiac, and so on.

You may have the opportunity to work with children in a specific age group or you may work with children in a variety of age groups. Regardless of the ages of the children, working in pediatrics will offer you many rewards and challenges.

When a child is admitted to the hospital, you may be involved in the admitting procedure, Figure 42–1. A nurse will obtain a medical and social history from the parents. Information obtained will include the child's nickname, the ages and names of siblings, the child's likes and dislikes, and "normal times" and routines for meals, naps, and bedtimes. Any information that will make the child's hospital stay easier is marked in the history. Once the history is complete, you can continue with the admission procedure.

In this unit, guidelines are presented for caring for children by age groups. The groups are:
- Infancy (0–1 year)
- Toddler (1–3 years)
- Preschooler (3–6 years)
- School-age (6–12 years)
- Adolescent (13–18 years)

Refer to Figure 42–2 to review the beginning procedure actions and procedure completion actions.

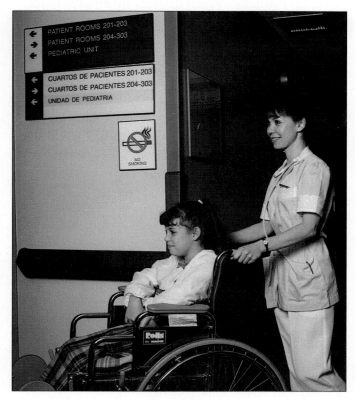

FIGURE 42–1. The nursing assistant is transporting an older child to the pediatric unit following admission.

BEGINNING PROCEDURE ACTIONS	PROCEDURE COMPLETION ACTIONS
■ Wash your hands. ■ Assemble equipment needed. ■ Go to the patient's room, knock, and pause before entering. ■ Introduce yourself and identify the patient by checking the identification bracelet. ■ Ask visitors to leave and inform them where they can wait. ■ Care for equipment according to facility policy. ■ Provide privacy. ■ Explain what will happen and answer questions. ■ Allow patient to assist in procedure as much as possible. ■ Raise bed or table to comfortable working height.	■ Position patient comfortably. ■ Leave signal cord, telephone, and fresh water close at hand. ■ Return bed or table to lowest position. ■ Perform general safety check of patient and environment. ■ Wash your hands. ■ Report completion of task. ■ Let visitors know when they may reenter the patient's room. ■ Document action and your observations.

NOTE: Where there are open lesions, wet linen, or possible contact with patient body fluids or blood, disposable gloves are worn during the procedure. Put on gloves before contact with the patient or linen. Properly dispose of gloves after they are removed. ALWAYS APPLY UNIVERSAL PRECAUTIONS.

FIGURE 42–2.   Beginning procedure actions and procedure completion actions

PROCEDURE 127

ADMITTING A PEDIATRIC PATIENT

1. Introduce yourself to the child and his parents.
2. Show them to the child's room and familiarize them with the unit.
3. Explain what you will do.
4. Wash your hands.
5. Place an identification band on the child.
6. Dress the child in his own pajamas or hospital clothing.
7. Obtain the child's height and weight. Record according to hospital policy. (Refer to Procedure 128.)
8. Measure the vital signs of the child. (Refer to Procedures 131–134 on pages 635–638.)
9. Obtain a urine specimen. (Refer to Unit 24.)
10. Wash your hands.
11. Assist the physician with examination of the child when necessary.
12. Explain rooming-in and visiting policies to parents.
13. If parents leave, stay with the child to provide comfort.

Developmental Tasks

For each age group, it is expected that the child will have reached a certain developmental level. Each level is characterized by physical and psychological tasks that the average child in the group can perform. If you understand the developmental tasks for each age group, it will be easier to find ways to help and encourage the child's development during hospitalization. The approaches suggested here may need to be personalized for each patient. Some children may appear younger than their stated age due to medical and/or emotional problems. It is also normal for children to regress (go backward) when hospitalized.

Caring for Infants (Birth–1 Year)

During the first year of life, the normal infant will:
■ Double birth length.
■ Triple birth weight.

■ Show progress in gaining mastery over his gross motor behavior beginning with head and moving down trunk toward feet.

The normal infant begins by gaining head control. The infant then progresses to rolling over, sitting up, crawling, and walking. These motor skills generally occur within specific weeks or months of the infant's life. Achieving these skills is referred to as the infant's **developmental milestones**. These milestones are outlined from birth through two years of age in Table 42–1.

Learning to trust is the primary psychosocial developmental task for the infant. All infants depend on others for all of their basic needs. They depend on others for their survival. How the infant's needs are met lays the foundation for the infant's developing personality.

Normally, the mother is the caretaker and prime source for developing the trust of the infant. However, when the infant is hospitalized, the hospital caretakers assume the role of substitute mother. A caretaker can continue to develop the infant's trust by

Table 42–1   Normal Age for Attainment of Major Developmental Milestones

Age	Motor Skill	Language	Adaptive Behavior
4–6 wk.	Head lifted from prone position and turned from side to side	Cries	Smiles
4 mo.	No head lag when pulled to sitting from supine position Tries to grasp large objects	Sounds of pleasure	Smiles, laughs aloud, and shows pleasure to familiar objects or persons
5 mo.	Voluntary grasp with both hands	Primitive sounds: "ah goo"	Smiles at self in mirror
6 mo.	Grasps with one hand Rolls prone to supine Sits with support	Range of sounds greater	Expresses displeasure and food preference
8 mo.	Sits without support Transfers objects from hand to hand Rolls supine to prone	Combines syllables: "baba, dada, mama"	Responds to "No"
10 mo.	Sits well Creeping Stands holding Finger-thumb opposition in picking up small objects		Waves "bye-bye," plays "patty-cake" and "peek-a-boo"
12 mo.	Stands holding Walks with support	Says two or three words with meaning	Understands names of objects Shows interest in pictures
15 mo.	Walks alone	Several intelligible words	Requests by pointing Imitates
18 mo.	Walks up and down stairs holding Removes clothes	Many intelligible words	Carries out simple commands
2 yr.	Walks up and down stairs by self Runs	Two- to three-word phrases	Organized play Points to some parts of body

Source: Mary Fran Hazinski, *Nursing Care of the Critically Ill Child*, (St. Louis: C.V. Mosby Company, 1984, p. 387).

responding to her cry and her needs. Trust is fostered by feeding, holding, touching, and talking to the infant, Figure 42–3, in addition to keeping her warm and dry.

It is important for the infant to have consistent mothering. Therefore, it is ideal to have the mother room-in with her infant. If this is not possible, an alternative approach is to have consistent caretakers for an infant. This means that every time a nurse or nursing assistant works, he will care for the same infants. Besides being consistent for the infant, it also allows the caretaker to become familiar with the infant as a unique person. Consistency is especially important when an infant is between six and seven months of age. At this age, the infant normally begins to display a fear of strangers.

Communicating With Infants

Working with infants can be challenging because the infant cannot tell the caretaker in words what she wants or needs. The infant communicates with her cry and body movements. The cry can vary depending on needs. Just as a mother learns to interpret the sound of her infant's cry, the caretaker will also learn to interpret the meanings of the cry by caring for the infant.

Infants respond to voices, faces, and touch. You should talk to the infant, Figure 42–4, whenever you are giving personal care such as bathing, feeding, and holding.

The Waking Hours

When the infant is awake, he/she needs to explore the environment. Age-appropriate toys are provided so that the infant can continue his/her development while in the hospital. Appropriate toys include colorful mobiles, rattles, and mirrors.

Importance of Families

Siblings of the infant should be allowed to visit while the infant is hospitalized. Toddlers and pre-schoolers engage in "magical thinking." In other words, they believe that if they wish the infant to be sick it happens, or if they wish the baby to be gone she won't be back. Therefore, it is important for both toddlers and preschoolers to see their infant sibling. If the mother is rooming-in with the infant, it is also important for toddlers and preschoolers to see and talk to their mother.

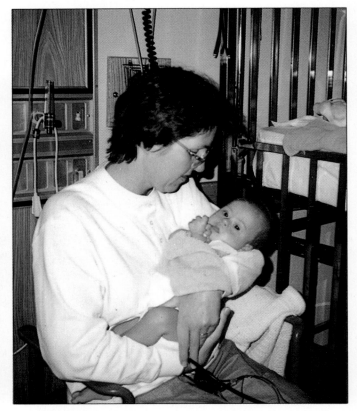

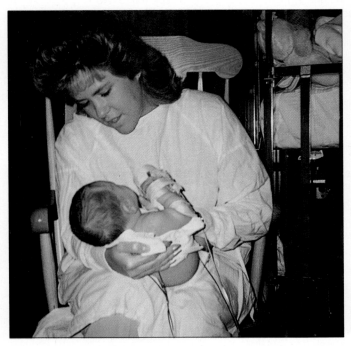

FIGURE 42–3. Holding and talking to the infant helps build trust between the infant and the care giver. Security and affection also are promoted by this contact.

FIGURE 42–4. Talk to the infant or child whenever care is being given or when you are holding the infant in a quiet moment.

Routine Procedures

When carrying out routine care of the infant, be sure that you hold the infant properly, Figure 42–5. (Refer to Unit 41.)

Before feeding the infant, organize his care so that after he has eaten he can be allowed to digest his food and sleep. You should not move him unnecessarily as it may cause him to vomit what he has just eaten. In organizing the care, you would weigh him, bathe him, diaper him, and dress him. Then change the crib linens, weigh him, and feed him.

The routine procedures covered at this time include:

- Procedure 128—Weighing the pediatric patient (infant and older children)
- Procedure 129—Changing crib linens
- Procedure 130—Changing crib linens (infant in crib)
- Procedure 131—Measuring temperature (rectal, oral, and axillary)
- Procedure 132—Determining heart rate (pulse)
- Procedure 133—Counting respiratory rate
- Procedure 134—Measuring blood pressure

Weighing the Infant

Routine care includes weighing the infant. This procedure should also be done before feeding.

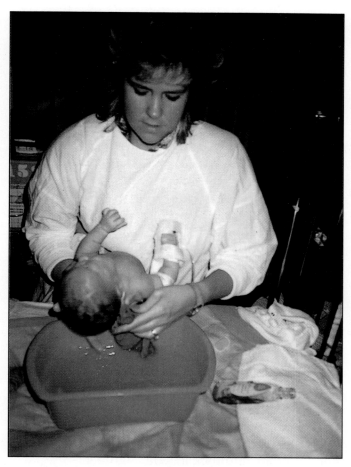

FIGURE 42–5. Always hold the infant properly during all care procedures. Note how the head is being supported while the nursing assistant washes the infant's head.

PROCEDURE 128

WEIGHING THE PEDIATRIC PATIENT

1. Wash your hands.
2. Place a small sheet or receiving blanket on the scale and balance the scale with the blanket on it.
3. Check the infant's previous weight.
4. Check the infant's identification band.
5. Remove the infant's diaper and shirt.
6. Place the infant on the scale, keeping a hand over the infant to prevent falling.
7. Move the bar to the correct weight until the scale balances.
8. Return the infant to his crib. Diaper and dress.
9. Record the infant's weight according to hospital policy.
10. Remove the linen from the scale and place in laundry receptacle.
11. Return the scale to its proper storage place.
12. Wash your hands.

Children and Adolescents: Use an upright scale if the child is able to stand.

1. Bring the scale to the bedside, if possible, and balance it.
2. Wash your hands.
3. Check the child's identification band.

continues

4. Check the child's previous weight.
5. Weigh the child in as few clothes as possible. Remove diaper and shoes or slippers.
6. Have the child stand on the scale. Move the bar to the correct weight until the scale balances.
7. Record the weight according to hospital policy.
8. Return the child to bed.

9. Return the scale to its proper storage place.
10. Wash your hands.

NOTE: If the toddler is unable to stand on his own, pick him up and step on the scale. Obtain the combined weight. Put the toddler back in bed and subtract your weight from the combined weight. The toddler's weight is the difference in weights.

PROCEDURE 129

CHANGING CRIB LINENS

1. Wash your hands.
2. Gather linens: i.e., sheet, blanket, shirt, diaper and pad. Do Steps 1 and 2 before bathing the infant.
3. After bathing infant, diaper and dress.
4. Place infant in stroller, playpen, or other safe place.
5. Strip linen from crib.
6. Place clean linen on bed and open sheet, hem side down.
7. Make one side of crib, miter corners top and bottom, and tuck in side, Figure 42–6A.
8. Pull down crib top, Figure 42–6B. Pull up crib side, Figure 42–6C.

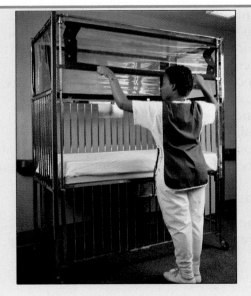

FIGURE 42–6B. Pull down crib top.

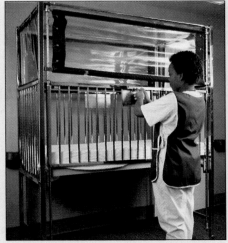

FIGURE 42–6C. Pull up crib side and check for security.

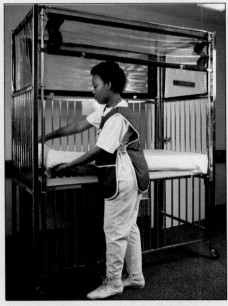

FIGURE 42–6A. Make one side of crib. Miter corners at the top and bottom and tuck under mattress.

9. Repeat Step 7 on opposite side of crib.
10. Place diaper pad on top of sheet, according to hospital policy.
11. Place clean blanket at bottom of bed.

12. Arrange bumper pads around sides of crib.
13. Wash your hands.
14. Return infant to crib, cover with blanket (if appropriate), and pull up crib side.

PROCEDURE 130

CHANGING CRIB LINENS (INFANT IN CRIB)

1. Wash your hands.
2. Gather linens: i.e., sheet, blanket, shirt, diaper and bathing equipment. Do Steps 1 and 2 before bathing infant.
3. After bathing infant, diaper and dress.
4. Pick up infant and hold in one arm.
5. With free hand, strip old linen off crib.
6. Place clean linen on mattress and open sheet, placing hem side down. Place infant on sheet.
7. Place one hand on infant and keep it on infant at all times.
8. Make one side of crib, miter corners top and bottom, and tuck in side.
9. Remove hand from infant and pull up crib side.
10. Go around to other side of crib.
11. Take down crib side, place one hand on infant, and repeat Step 8.
12. Place diaper pad under infant and cover with blanket, if appropriate.
13. Arrange bumper pads around crib, if appropriate.
14. Pull up crib side.
15. Wash your hands.

Determining Vital Signs

The infant's vital signs must be measured as outlined in the care plan. It is normal for an infant's heart to beat faster than an adult's. The normal ranges of heart rates and respiratory rates for each age group are listed in Figure 42–7. An increase in the infant's heart and respiratory rates can be caused by stress (crying, fever, and infection). Therefore, the pulse and respiratory rates should be taken when the infant is quiet, either awake or sleeping.

Age	Heart Rate	Respirations	Blood Pressure	
			Systolic	Diastolic
Infants	120–160	30–60	74–100	50–70
Toddlers	90–140	24–40	80–112	50–80
Preschoolers	80–110	22–34	82–110	50–78
School-age	75–100	18–30	84–120	54–80
Adolescents	60–90	12–16	94–140	62–88

NOTE: Pulse and respiration are taken for a full minute. The apical pulse is used with infants and young children.

FIGURE 42–7. Normal vital signs

PROCEDURE 131

MEASURING TEMPERATURE

Temperatures on children five years of age and under are usually taken rectally unless there is a medical reason against doing so. Axillary temperatures can be taken in place of rectal temperatures.

Rectal Temperature
All other vital signs should be measured before the temperature if a rectal temperature is to be measured.

1. Wash your hands and put on gloves.

continues

2. Check patient's identification band.
3. Explain to the parents and child what you will be doing.
4. Inspect thermometer for breaks.
5. Shake down thermometer.
6. Lubricate thermometer.
7. Lay child on back on bed or on stomach across your lap.
8. Insert thermometer 1/2 inch into rectum and hold. Hold child securely and gently so the child does not move about.
9. Leave in place for required amount of time (4–5 minutes). See your hospital policy.
10. Remove thermometer, wipe off lubricant, and read thermometer.
11. Report any deviations from normal according to hospital policy.
12. Remove gloves and wash your hands.
13. Record.

Oral Temperature
1. Explain to the parents and child what you will be doing.
2. Check patient's identification band.
3. Wash your hands.
4. Inspect thermometer for breaks.
5. Shake down thermometer.
6. Instruct the child to hold the thermometer under the tongue. If the child cannot hold the thermometer in the mouth, then obtain either a rectal or an axillary temperature.
7. Leave under the child's tongue for the required amount of time (usually 5–8 minutes).
8. Remove and read thermometer.
9. Report any deviations from normal according to hospital policy.
10. Wash your hands and record temperature value.

Axillary Temperature
1. Explain to the parents and child what you will be doing.
2. Check patient's identification band.
3. Wash your hands.
4. Inspect thermometer for breaks.
5. Shake down thermometer.
6. Place the thermometer in the child's arm pit.
7. Hold the child's arm close to the chest for the required amount of time (10 minutes).
8. Remove thermometer and read.
9. Report any deviations from normal according to hospital policy.
10. Wash your hands and record temperature value.

NOTE: If an electronic thermometer is used, follow the manufacturer's directions supplied with the equipment.

NOTE: In some facilities, aural thermometers are used to measure temperature.

PROCEDURE 132

DETERMINING HEART RATE (PULSE)

With infants and children, the easiest way to accomplish this is to place the stethoscope over the heart, Figure 42–8. This is called the apical pulse. It should be done when the child is quiet or at rest because stress and crying can result in a higher than normal reading.
1. Wash your hands.
2. Check patient's identification band.
3. Explain procedure to patient and/or his parents. Clean stethoscope earpieces and diaphragm with antiseptic wipe and dry. Allow the child to play with the stethoscope first.

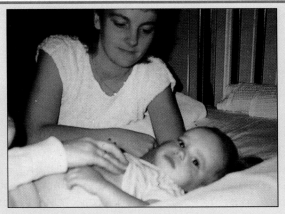

FIGURE 42–8. Measuring the apical pulse of a toddler

4. Rub the diaphragm of the stethoscope to warm it so that it will not be cold when placed on the child's chest.
5. Place the stethoscope over the patient's heart and count the number of beats you hear in a minute.
6. Report rates higher or lower than the normal for the appropriate age group according to hospital policy.

7. Clean stethoscope earpieces and diaphragm with antiseptic wipe and dry.
8. Wash your hands and record results.

The radial pulse can be used for children 6 years and over. The procedure used is the same as that for adults. Refer to Procedure 42 in Unit 15.

PROCEDURE 133

COUNTING RESPIRATORY RATE

Infants and toddlers use their abdominal muscles for breathing. To count the respiratory rate for this age group, look at the abdomen and chest and count the respirations for a minute.

To obtain the respiratory rate for preschoolers and older children follow Procedure 44 for adults, Unit 15, but count the respirations for a full minute.

PROCEDURE 134

MEASURING BLOOD PRESSURE

Measuring blood pressure may not always be required for all pediatric patients. If blood pressure is to be recorded, you must have the correct size cuff for the child, Figure 42–9. The cuff should cover two-thirds of the upper arm.
1. Select the correct cuff size for the patient.
2. Assemble all equipment. Clean stethoscope earpieces and diaphragm with antiseptic wipe and dry.
3. Wash your hands.
4. Check patient's identification band.
5. Explain the procedure to the child, e.g. "This will feel like a tight hug on your arm."
6. Wrap the cuff securely around the upper arm.
7. Feel for the brachial pulse.
8. Place stethoscope earpieces in ears and place diaphragm near pulse.
9. Pump up cuff until pulse is no longer heard. Release valve and listen for systolic and diastolic sounds.

10. Wash your hands and record results according to hospital policy.

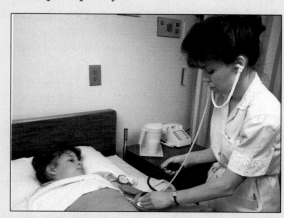

FIGURE 42–9. When measuring the blood pressure of an infant or child, make sure the proper sized cuff is used to ensure an accurate measurement.

Feeding

Feeding is important to the infant because it satisfies her hunger and sucking needs. Sucking provides the infant with a pleasant sensation whether she receives food with her sucking or not. The amount of time an infant needs to suckle will vary with each infant. Always provide the infant with the opportunity to suck. This is even more important if the infant cannot eat.

When feeding an infant:
- Hold the infant unless there is a medical reason for not doing so.
- If an infant cannot be held, the bottle should still be held for her while she eats.
- An infant should never be left in a crib with a bottle propped in the mouth. This is dangerous because the infant could get too much formula at one time, vomit, and choke.

- Holding the infant during a feeding also provides her with the close, physical contact of the person feeding her.
- During feeding and following feeding, the infant should be burped.

NOTE: If an infant cannot be fed, she should still be held and allowed to suck on a pacifier unless there is a medical reason to prevent removal of the infant from the crib.

PROCEDURE 135

BOTTLEFEEDING THE INFANT

1. Wash your hands.
2. Gather the infant's formula and diaper pad, washcloth, or bib.
3. Check the infant's identification band.
4. Pick up infant and hold to feed unless there is a medical reason for not doing so.
5. Sit in a chair or rocker.
6. Hold infant in the crook of your arm, with head of infant slightly raised, Figure 42–10.
7. Place a diaper, washcloth, or bib under infant's chin, covering chest.
8. Tip bottle so nipple is filled with formula.
9. Stroke side of infant's cheek closest to you, so the infant will automatically turn toward the side stroked and open mouth. Place nipple in infant's mouth.
10. If nipple is in mouth and infant is not sucking, gently lift up under the infant's chin to close mouth on nipple.
11. Hold bottle so nipple is filled with formula while infant feeds.
12. Feed infant the ordered amount of formula and burp according to infant's age and hospital policy. (See procedure following.)
    NOTE: Bottlefed infants swallow a lot of air while sucking. Burping, therefore, is important to remove the air from their stomachs.
13. If the infant starts to vomit while feeding, remove bottle and turn infant to side with head lowered to prevent aspiration. Seek appropriate help as needed.
14. After feeding, return child to crib and place on back or side.
15. Pull up crib side.
16. Wash your hands.
17. Record amount of formula infant took, according to hospital policy.

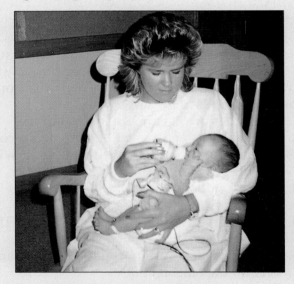

FIGURE 42–10. Hold the infant for bottlefeeding with head elevated. Make sure fluid always fills the nipple of the bottle while the infant sucks.

Burping

The frequency of burping the infant will depend on the age and the medical condition of the infant. Burping is important when bottlefeeding an infant because bottlefed infants swallow a lot of air when sucking. The infant can be burped as frequently as after every 1/2 ounce of formula. Older infants can be burped after 1–2 ounces during feeding, and at the conclusion of feeding. Refer to your hospital policy for the frequency of burping. There are two methods of burping the infant. (See Procedures 136 and 137.)

Breastfeeding

If the rooming-in or visiting mother is breastfeeding, she should be directed to an area where she can be assured of privacy as well as comfort. As a nursing assistant, you may be responsible for weighing the infant before and after feeding, according to your hospital policy. Refer to the weighing procedures given earlier in this unit.

When the infant is returned to his crib after feeding, he should not be placed on his back. Place the infant on his abdomen or on his side. A rolled blanket can be used to keep him on his side. This is done to prevent choking should he "spit up" or vomit.

PROCEDURE 136

BURPING (METHOD A)

1. Place diaper or cloth over your shoulder.
2. Lift infant up to shoulder, holding infant close to your chest, Figure 42–11.
3. Holding infant in place with one hand, use the other hand to gently rub or pat the infant's back until the infant burps.

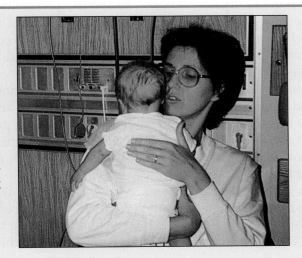

FIGURE 42–11. Burping the infant during and following feeding helps to eliminate air swallowed. Gently rub or pat the infant's back.

PROCEDURE 137

BURPING (METHOD B)

1. Place diaper, cloth, or bib under infant's chin.
2. Place child in sitting or upright position. Put one hand on the infant's chest supporting the infant's weight, Figure 42–12. With the other hand, gently rub or pat the infant's back until the infant burps.

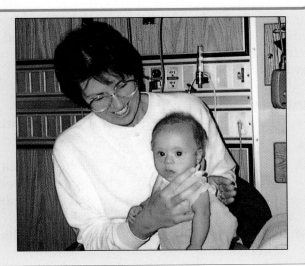

FIGURE 42–12. An alternative method of burping the infant. Remember to place a cloth or bib under the infant's chin.

Safety Guidelines

- Always keep crib side rails up.
- Always keep one hand on the infant when the crib side rail is down.
- Use crib bumpers or rolled blankets to prevent injury.
- Never tie balloons or toys to cribs.
- Never use toys with small removable parts or pointed objects.
- Never prop bottles.
- Never tape pacifiers in an infant's mouth.

Restraints

It is generally not necessary to obtain a physician's order to restrain an infant or a child. The infant or child is considered to be incompetent. Restraints can be used for the child's safety. Restraints are used to protect the child from injury to herself or to others, or to protect the child from injury due to equipment used in her care. Any child who is restrained in any way should be freed from restraints at least once per shift and allowed to exercise extremities under supervision. Restraints should never be tied to a cribside or bedrail, only to the bed or crib frame.

A jacket restraint is a sleeveless cloth garment. It is fitted to the child's chest and crosses in the back, out of the child's reach. It has long straps which can be tied under the mattress or through a chair. When they are tied this way, the child can move extremities, sit up, lay down in bed, or turn side-to-side without falling.

An extremity restraint is used on the child's arms/hands or legs/feet. Commercial restraints are available in sheepskin, Velcro, or disposable materials. This restraint is placed on the child's extremity according to the package directions. The ties are tied to the frame of the crib. For very small infants, the ties may be pinned to the mattress.

Summary of Nursing Assistant Tasks and Responsibilities When Caring for the Infant

- Maintain a safe environment.
- Provide information to the health team through monitoring of vital signs (temperature, pulse, respiration) weight, intake, and output.
- Provide routine care such as bathing, feeding, and changing.
- Collect and test specimens.
- Assist with treatments, examinations, and procedures.
- Provide warmth, security, and affection.

Caring for Toddlers (1–3 years)

The years between one and three can be a difficult time for a child to be hospitalized. This is the age when a child is trying to be independent and in control. Between 1-1/2 and 3 years of age the child:

- Increases motor coordination.
- Becomes more verbal.
- Becomes more inquisitive about his world.

At the same time, her parents are trying to toilet train her. They also are beginning to set limits on her behavior. The developmental task for the toddler is **autonomy** (independent action).

When caring for the toddler, allow him as much independence and choice as possible (within hospital policy guidelines). Avoid situations that could create a struggle between the care giver and the child. Expect delays when the toddler is feeding himself or bathing. Be sure to allow the toddler time to do these activities.

The Hospital Environment

When a toddler is hospitalized, it is important to provide an environment that allows as much independence and control as possible while ensuring safety. An example of this is the choice of bed (crib) that is provided for the toddler. If a crib is to be used, it should have a top and sides to prevent the child from climbing out and possibly falling, Figure 42–13. If the child has been sleeping in a bed at home, then it is more appropriate to provide a child-sized hospital bed with side rails, if available. Hospital policies vary, so check your hospital policy with reference to toddlers.

If the child is toilet trained, it is important to know the words the child uses for urination and bowel movements. It is also important to know if the child uses a potty chair or the toilet at home. You should try to provide the same arrangements for toileting in the hospital. It is not uncommon for a hospitalized child to regress. You should not be surprised if a toddler who is toilet trained starts to have "accidents" while in the hospital. Do not scold the child if this happens. The incident should be treated in a matter of fact manner. In addition, you will find that hospitalized toddlers may ask for a bottle or pacifier. Even though the

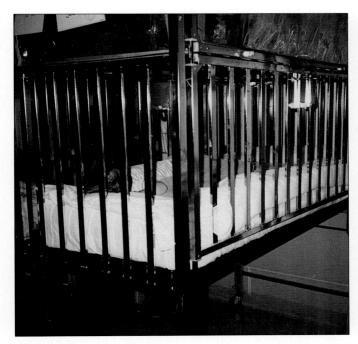

FIGURE 42–13. If the toddler is to use a crib while in the hospital, it should provide a safe environment to protect the toddler from falls. At the same time, it should provide room for freedom of movement (if medical condition permits).

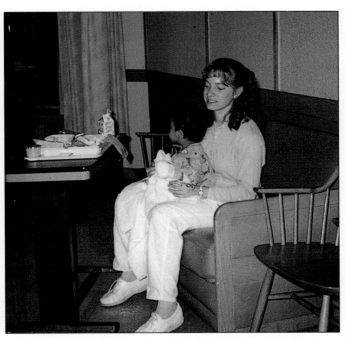

FIGURE 42–14. The nursing assistant can help the toddler with routine activities such as feeding, but it is important to allow the toddler as much independent action as possible. Do not hurry the toddler through mealtimes.

toddler may have been weaned from them, treat the request as normal. Do not try to reason with the child.

The Toddler's Need for Autonomy

The toddler is learning to be independent. He may want to feed, dress, and wash himself in the hospital. It will be your responsibility to help the toddler with these activities, Figure 42–14. You should allow him his independence. At the same time, you must keep him safe. For example, when bathing the toddler in the bath tub, you must never leave the toddler alone, even for a minute. Before you put the toddler in the bath tub, check the temperature of the bath water.

Emotional Reaction to Illness

Another important area in the care of toddlers concerns their feelings of responsibility for their own illnesses. You must stress that the illness is not the toddler's or anyone else's fault.

To overcome anxiety about routine procedures, allow the toddler to handle the equipment whenever possible. A few extra minutes spent to familiarize the toddler with the equipment may make the difference between a frightened child and an interested one, Figure 42–15.

The toddler will have a difficult time if separated from the mother. One way to prevent this is to permit the mother to "room-in." If this cannot happen, either because a parent cannot stay or hospital policy does not permit it, then parents should be encouraged to visit frequently. If a parent is not going to stay:

- Reassure the child that he will not be alone.
- Tell her the names of the people who will care for her.
- Encourage each person caring for the toddler to introduce himself when entering the room.
- Whenever possible, the toddler who does not have a parent staying with her should be placed in a room near the nurses' station.
- Encourage parents who can't visit to call or you can call the parents so the child can talk to them.

Routine Activities

Routines are important to toddlers. Ask the parents to describe the child's normal day. Try to follow the child's usual schedule as much as possible for eating, naps, toileting, and other activities. Ask the parents about the child's nickname, likes, dislikes, names of siblings and pets, and anything else the parents feel the nursing assistant should know about the child.

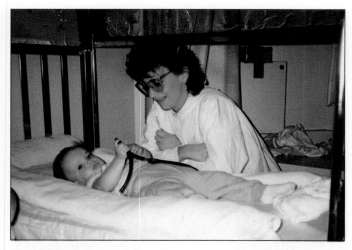

FIGURE 42–15. Allowing the toddler to become familiar with equipment used in routine care may help relieve anxiety about procedures to be performed. (Crib sides are down only to improve the visibility of the picture.)

Toddlers love to play but, because they have short attention spans, they cannot play with one toy for a long time. Plan for a variety of activities to keep the toddler amused. For example:

- Finger painting.
- Blocks.
- Trucks.
- Push-pull toys.
- Coloring.
- Reading of stories.
- Educational toys that teach how to dress, button, and zip can also be fun for the toddler. Stethoscopes, masks, and gloves make good hospital toys because they can allow the toddler to work out his fears.

Toddlers will not play together, but they will play near or next to each other.

Temper tantrums can be common with toddlers. If they occur, ignore the tantrum as long as the child cannot hurt herself or others. If a toddler is misbehaving, limits must be set in a firm, consistent manner.

When working with the toddler, remember that he is trying to be independent. Allow the toddler as much choice as possible. For example, at snack time ask if he wants an apple or a cracker. If no choice can be given, be firm and say what will occur. For example, "It's time to take your nap now." It is best to be truthful and to give simple explanations to toddlers. If the child is having a blood test, tell him just before it happens. It does not do any good to prepare toddlers in advance because they do not have any concept of time. Such advance warning only increases their anxiety.

Safety

The toddler has a natural curiosity and loves to explore. It is important to maintain a safe environment in the hospital.

Safety Guidelines

- All poisonous liquids should be kept in a locked container or cabinet.
- All open electrical sockets should have protective covers. Never leave toddlers unattended or unsupervised.
- Never leave toddlers alone in the bath tub or bathroom.
- Keep thermometers out of toddlers' reach.
- Keep crib sides and side rails up when the toddler is in bed.
- Never allow toddlers to play with balloons unless supervised.
- Avoid toys with sharp edges, long strings, or small removable parts.
- Keep doors to stair, kitchen, treatment, and storage areas closed and locked whenever possible.
- Keep doors to linen chutes locked.

Summary of Nursing Assistant Tasks and Responsibilities When Caring for the Toddler

- Maintain a safe environment.
- Provide information to the health team through monitoring of vital signs (temperature, pulse, and respiration), weight, intake, and output.
- Supervise/assist with routine care such as bathing, feeding, and dressing.
- Collect and test specimens.
- Assist with treatments, examinations, and procedures.
- Provide/assist with opportunities for play.
- Provide warmth, security, and affection.
- Promote independence by providing opportunities for choices.

Caring for Preschool Children (3–6 Years)

Developmental Tasks

Between the ages of 3 and 6 years the child's language, fine motor, and gross motor skills continue to increase with activity. The preschooler continues to develop independence, but the primary developmental task for the age group is **initiative** (to do things themselves). Children in this age group need to be able to initiate physical and intellectual activities to feel more competent. The preschooler learns her sex role in life by imitating the behavior of the same sex parent.

The preschooler needs his independence, but he still needs to feel safe and secure. The caretaker must provide the correct balance of independence and control for the preschooler. This is normally the job of the parents, but when the preschooler is hospitalized, you will be considered the caretaker.

Emotional Reactions to Illness

Preschoolers normally have many fears. One fear is that their body parts will be injured or changed. Because of this, the preschooler fears that if an adhesive bandage is taken off some of her will "leak out." Preschoolers cannot tell the difference between a "good hurt" and a "bad hurt"; that is, pain from a procedure versus pain from a spanking. Therefore, it is important to use simple, honest explanations when telling the preschooler what to expect.

Fear of the dark, night time, or of being alone are other normal fears for the preschooler. You can help reduce this fear by leaving a night light on. Another child in the room can also ease his fears. Be sure to leave the call bell within his reach. Sitting with him until he falls asleep will also help. Like the toddler, the preschooler can also benefit from having his mother room-in because he still fears separation.

"Magical thinking" and fantasy are still present in this age group. Therefore, it is important to stress to the preschooler that it is not her fault that she is sick and that she is not sick because she was bad. The preschooler needs to know that she will return home. She will not be forgotten and left in the hospital. Siblings should be allowed and encouraged to visit. In addition to easing separation from the family, this can also be a way of assuring the child that no one is taking her place at home.

Explaining Procedures

When telling a preschooler what to expect, simple, honest explanations work best. Choose your words carefully because the preschooler takes things literally (exactly as said).

- If surgery is being planned, it is important to show and tell the child what parts of his body will be involved in the procedure.

- Preschoolers have a limited concept of time, so when you explain when something will occur, use time references that are familiar to the child; i.e., meal time, nap time, or the time of a favorite TV show. For example, if the child is scheduled for an X-ray in the late morning, tell her that she will have it after breakfast or before lunch.
- Always explain to the preschooler what you are going to do. Do not assume that he will remember what you told him before. The preschooler needs to maintain some control. Therefore, allow him to make as many decisions as possible. Give him the opportunity to make a choice.
- Allow her to do as much of her own care as she can to make her feel independent.

Activities

Imagination and fantasy are part of the preschooler's world. Imaginary playmates are normal with the preschooler. These playmates may find their way to the hospital with the child. These playmates can vary in age and sex. They often have different or unusual sounding names. If the child talks about his imaginary friend, treat it matter of factly and listen. However, you need to be realistic. Do not agree to seeing or hearing this playmate. Just say that you know this playmate exists only in the child's imagination.

Play is important for the hospitalized preschooler. Play may give you clues about what the preschooler is thinking. The preschooler is more coordinated and can enjoy activities such as puzzles, coloring, and drawing. The preschooler enjoys imitating roles and playing with other children. Playing "house" and "doctor" are especially fun for this age group. Hand puppets are also a good way to talk to preschoolers because they relate directly to the character of the puppet.

You can help the preschooler deal with her hospital stay by maintaining consistency in her schedule and in the limits put on her behavior. Positive reinforcers such as hugs or stickers should be used as rewards for appropriate behavior.

Safety Guidelines

- Keep toys from cluttering walkways to prevent falls.
- Keep side rails on bed up at night.
- Keep beds in low position.
- Keep doors to kitchen and storage areas closed.

- Keep a night light on.
- Never leave the child unattended in the tub.
- Never allow children to run with popsicles or lollipops in their mouths.

Summary of Nursing Assistant Tasks and Responsibilities When Caring for the Preschooler

- Maintain a safe environment.
- Provide information to the health team through monitoring of vital signs (temperature, pulse, and respiration), weight, intake, and output.
- Supervise/assist with routine care such as bathing, feeding, and dressing.
- Collect and test specimens.
- Assist with treatments, examinations, and procedures.
- Provide/assist with opportunities for play.
- Provide warmth, security, and affection.

Caring for School-age Children (6–12 Years)

In general, the school-age years are a time of exceptionally good health, Figure 42–16. School-age children are more active, stronger, and more steady than younger children. They have had most childhood illnesses and have been immunized against the rest. The most common problems of these times involve the gastrointestinal system (for example, stomach aches) and the respiratory system (for example, colds and coughs).

Developmental Tasks

In this period, the child is striving to achieve a sense of accomplishment through an increasing number of tasks and completion of projects. He also continues to increase control over his environment and his independence. It is important to remember these tasks when caring for the school-age child.

The school-age child's reaction to hospitalization will be significantly different from that of the younger child. The school-age child is better able to handle the stress of illness and hospitalization.

The hospitalization of the school-age child presents her with an opportunity to:

- Explore a new environment.
- Meet new friends.
- Learn more about her body.

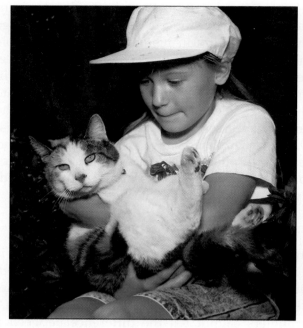

FIGURE 42–16. School-age children tend to be healthier than younger children but complain mostly of colds and stomachaches.

Psychosocial Adjustment

Separation from his parents will not be as difficult for the school-age child. However, those just entering this period may regress to a preschool level. These children will need their parents' presence.

The school-age child has left the security of home and entered the school system. In school, the child has begun to develop relationships with other children. In the hospital, she may respond more to the separation from her peers than from her parents. It is important to give these children opportunities to communicate with their schoolmates. For example, they can be helped to write letters and make phone calls. When possible, friends can visit. The older school-age child may welcome the opportunity to be away from his parents. In this situation, the child can test newly developed skills and increase independence. Children of this age group also need privacy. If their parents are present, they may not get privacy. Some parents may need to have their child's opposition to their staying explained in this context as they may see it as anger toward them.

Roommate selection is especially important for this age group. A roommate of approximately the same age will act as a diversion. With a roommate of the same age, the child will be able to continue work on the developmental task of learning to get along with others. Because the school-age child is seeking more independence, she may be reluctant to ask for help although she may need it. Her feelings may show themselves in different ways, such as:

- Irritability.
- Hostility toward her siblings.
- Other behavior problems. It is important as a care giver to observe and note these behaviors and bring them to the attention of your supervisor.

Resistance to bedtime may also become a problem during these years. In the hospital, it is important to be aware of the parents' rules and follow them. Learning rules is another developmental task of the school-age years.

Adjustment to Illness

Fears or stresses associated with an illness and subsequent hospitalization contribute to the school-age child's feelings of loss of control. By including this child in her care, you will help her to be a more cooperative patient, Figure 42–17. Procedures that we routinely do without explaining or without providing the child with options, such as using the bedpan, are particularly upsetting to the school-age child. This child is trying hard to act "grown up" but is not being given the chance. It is also important for this child's self-esteem that you do not scold him when he does lose control. It is best to just overlook the episode.

The school-age child is able to reason. She also understands the impact of her illness and the potential for disability and death. These children take an active interest in their health. Children of this age group are also interested in acquiring knowledge. You can help them gain information as well as deal with their fears by explaining all procedures in simple terms. This is also an appropriate age for playing with hospital equipment such as a stethoscope.

Pain is passively accepted by the school-age child. He is able to tell you where his pain is located and what it feels like. This child will hold rigidly still, bite his lip, or clench his fists when in pain in an effort to keep in control and to act brave. This child does well with distraction during painful procedures. During procedures, you should stay with him whenever possible to talk him through them. This child also tries to postpone all major procedures. For example, when it is time to go to a test, he will need to go to the bathroom. The care giver needs to put limits on the amount of postponements this child is allowed.

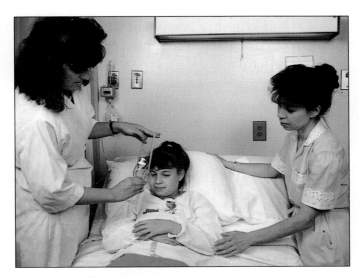

FIGURE 42–17. Explain procedures to the school-age child to give her a feeling of joining in her care.

Activities

Increased physical and social activities are characteristic of this period. Hospitalization does not usually provide school-age children with adequate diversions. School-age children may also miss the activities of school, although they usually deny this.

You should allow these children time during the day for their own work. This includes school work and visits with friends and other patients. Competitiveness is also characteristic of this period. It adds to the school-age child's need to stay up-to-date with school work. Having the play therapist at the hospital provide appropriate activities will help to reduce the stress the child feels.

Care givers should encourage the child to take part in her own care as part of her "work." Helping to make her bed or clean her room will make her feel useful. She should be held responsible only for tasks that are within her capabilities.

Physically, this child has entered a period of slow, steady growth. Although his growth has slowed, it is still important to maintain a balanced diet. School-age children tend to be less picky about what they eat. They are more willing to try new foods.

Safety Guidelines

- Never leave poisonous materials within reach.
- Keep side rails up when children are in bed.
- Monitor toys to ensure that they are not dangerous.

Summary of Nursing Assistant Tasks and Responsibilities When Caring for the School-age Child

- Maintain a safe environment.
- Provide information to the health care team through monitoring of vital signs (temperature, pulse, and respiration), weight, intake, and output.
- Supervise/assist with routine care.
- Collect and test specimens.
- Assist with treatments, examinations, and procedures.
- Provide explanations using proper names of body parts, drawings, and books.
- Encourage socialization with other children of similar age group.
- Provide time for school work and tutors.

Caring for the Adolescent (13–18 Years)

Adolescence is the transitional period from childhood into adulthood. Like school-age children, the adolescent is relatively healthy. The major health problems of this period are usually related to the drastic physical changes that occur during this time, to accidents, to sports injuries, or to chronic and/or permanent disabilities.

Psychosocial Development

Dealing with adolescents is especially difficult for heath care providers because:

- The adolescent is developing an identity and becoming increasingly independent.
- Being hospitalized forces the adolescent into a situation where she is now dependent on others to meet her needs. Because of this, it is important to allow the adolescent to make as many of her own decisions as possible. When this is not possible, keep the adolescent involved in the decision-making process.
- Adolescents have a difficult time with authority figures, Figure 42–18. As the care giver, you will represent authority to this child. You should not get into struggles with the adolescent. Limit the restrictions on them whenever appropriate.
- Adolescents are usually uncooperative. The best approach is to let the adolescent know, in

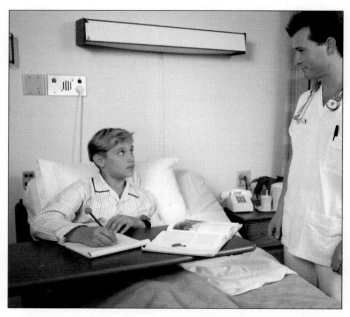

FIGURE 42–18. Adolescent patients sometimes have difficulty with authority figures and may be uncooperative. Be firm and persistent.

a nonthreatening way, what the rules of the unit are at the time of his admission. Speak to adolescents as you would to adults. Be as flexible as possible. For example, instead of struggling through the morning trying to get the adolescent up and washed, give him a list of things that need to be accomplished by a certain time. Then allow him the freedom to do things his way and in his order. At the time you had decided upon, check back with the adolescent to see that the tasks have been completed.

The most important people to adolescents are their friends. A hospital stay makes it more difficult for the adolescent to see friends. It is essential that you:

- Allow the adolescent time for visits.
- Permit phone calls, Figure 42–19.
- Introduce them to other patients their age.

Recognize that adolescents may not want to visit with others if illness has changed their appearance in any way. Body image is important at this age. You can promote a positive image by encouraging the adolescent to continue a normal grooming routine in the hospital. Also encourage the adolescent to wear clothes or her own pajamas. This will make her look and feel better about herself. Use the opportunity to teach good hygiene practices if the hospitalized adolescent does not already practice them. Ask a nurse to help you if you note that this is a problem for your patient.

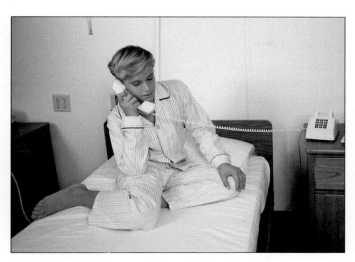

FIGURE 42–19. It is essential that you permit telephone calls so the adolescent can keep in touch with his friends.

Keep in mind that the adolescent is very aware of the changes taking place in his body whether they can be seen or not. It is important to provide the adolescent with privacy. Keep him covered as much as possible during procedures and examinations.

Nutrition and Activity

Adolescents go through a growth spurt. Girls are usually two years ahead of boys. Adequate nutrition and rest continue to be important. In the hospital, the importance of proper eating habits should be stressed to the adolescent. You should:

- Permit the adolescent to continue to make decisions about what and when she will eat unless it is medically unsafe.
- Recognize that adolescent girls are often on diets. Emotional problems related to weight are common.
- Be aware that adolescents frequently skip breakfast.

The adolescent often stays up late and likes to sleep late in the morning. Sleep requirements are decreased but a good night's sleep is essential. It is important to explain the routines of the unit and yet provide flexibility for the adolescent. For example, if the television must be turned off at a certain time, the adolescent should be encouraged to find another quiet activity such as listening to music with headphones if he does not want to go to sleep. Many hospitals have lounges exclusively for the use of this age group for that purpose and for socializing. Check with your supervisor to find out if there is a specific area for adolescents.

Safety Guidelines for the Adolescent

- Carefully check all electrical equipment that the adolescent may bring to the hospital—radios, hair dryers, and so on—to ensure that it is appropriate to use. Review hospital guidelines regarding use of electrical equipment with the patient.
- Review smoking policies with all adolescents.
- Reinforce to adolescents that alcohol or other drugs are illegal and are not permitted.
- Provide assistance with showers/bathing if the patient is incapacitated or weakened in any way. The adolescent may not ask for assistance.
- Reinforce the use of shoes or slippers to prevent injuries to the feet.
- Remind adolescents to keep staff informed of their whereabouts.
- Keep beds in low position to prevent falls.

Summary of Nursing Assistant Tasks and Responsibilities When Caring for Adolescents

- Maintain a safe environment.
- Orient the adolescent to unit and hospital rules.
- Provide information to the health team through monitoring of vital signs (temperature, pulse, and respiration), weight, intake, and output.
- Provide simple explanations to the adolescent.
- Assist with body hygiene to help maintain a positive self-image.
- Collect and test specimens.
- Assist with treatment, examinations, and procedures.
- Promote independence—allow adolescent as much control as possible over schedule of treatments, procedures, and so on.
- Encourage socialization with other adolescents.

SUMMARY

This unit provides the nursing assistant with information on giving safe care to the hospitalized pediatric patient. Because children differ in age, size, and developmental level, five developmental levels are described:

- Infancy
- Toddler
- Preschooler
- School-age
- Adolescent

For each age group, suggestions are offered to promote normal growth and development while maintaining a safe environment for the hospitalized pediatric patient.

Families are important to the pediatric patient. Because the family can also be affected by the child's hospitalization, suggestions are provided to promote and encourage a family-centered approach to care.

UNIT REVIEW

True/False. Answer the following statements true or false by circling T or F.

T F 1. Children normally may regress when hospitalized.

T F 2. The nursing assistant can foster an infant's sense of trust by keeping him warm and dry.

T F 3. The nursing assistant may assume the role of substitute mother.

T F 4. Between the ages of 6 and 7 months, the infant loses her fear of strangers.

T F 5. Following a feeding, the infant should be encouraged to play.

T F 6. Routine weighing of the infant should be carried out right after the 10 AM feeding.

T F 7. Pulse and respirations should be measured when the child is quiet or asleep.

T F 8. The school-age child has an average heart rate of 90–140 beats per minute.

T F 9. The respiratory rate of the toddler averages 30–60 respirations per minute.

T F 10. The systolic blood pressure of the child increases with age.

T F 11. Preschoolers normally have many fears.

T F 12. The preschooler learns his or her sex role in life by imitating the behavior of the opposite sex parent.

T F 13. The most common physical complaints of a school-age child are stomach aches and colds.

T F 14. The school-age child would be most comfortable sharing a room with a teenager.

T F 15. It is best to overlook the loss of self-control exhibited by the school-age child.

T F 16. The best way to measure a pulse rate in an infant or child is the apical method.

T F 17. The temperature of a child under five years of age should be measured using the rectal method.

T F 18. Sucking should only be encouraged when the infant is hungry.

T F 19. It is proper to prop a bottle so the infant can eat in his crib if you are very busy.

T F 20. After a feeding, the infant should be placed carefully on her back.

T F 21. To entertain an infant, tie a bright red balloon to the crib.

T F 22. The toddler should be placed in a crib with a top and sides as a safety measure.

T F 23. It is permissible to allow a toddler to play unsupervised in a bathtub for a short time before bathing him as long as the water is warm.

T F 24. Adolescents have a difficult time dealing with authority figures.

T F 25. Adolescents are particularly sensitive about changes in their body images.

B. Matching. Match the word in Column II with the phrases in Column I.

<table>
<tr><td colspan="2">Column I</td><td>Column II</td></tr>
<tr><td>_____</td><td>26. physical and psychological achievements</td><td>a. autonomy</td></tr>
<tr><td></td><td></td><td>b. regress</td></tr>
<tr><td>_____</td><td>27. achievement of skills characteristic of a specific age group</td><td>c. legal custody</td></tr>
<tr><td></td><td></td><td>d. developmental tasks</td></tr>
<tr><td>_____</td><td>28. a person married to a biological parent</td><td>e. biological parent</td></tr>
<tr><td>_____</td><td>29. moving backward</td><td>f. developmental milestone</td></tr>
<tr><td></td><td></td><td>g. stepparent</td></tr>
<tr><td>_____</td><td>30. person who has the right to consent to procedures for a hospitalization of a minor</td><td></td></tr>
<tr><td>_____</td><td>31. birth parent</td><td></td></tr>
<tr><td>_____</td><td>32. self-determination</td><td></td></tr>
</table>

Special Advanced Procedures

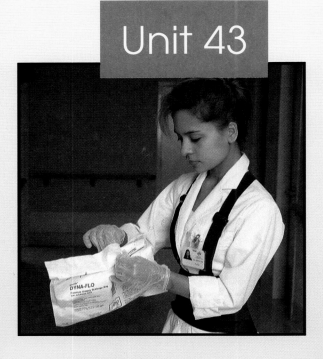

As a result of this unit—and with advanced training—you will be able to:

- Spell and define terms.
- Open and handle sterile equipment.
- Put on sterile gloves.
- Perform tracheal suctioning.
- Perform advanced urine and stool tests.
- Insert a rectal suppository.
- Give routine colostomy care.
- Give routine ileostomy care.
- Obtain a urine specimen from a closed urinary drainage system.

Learn the meaning and the correct spelling of the following words:

appliance	port
colostomy	sterile field
ileostomy	stoma

The responsibilities of nursing assistants vary throughout the nation. The scope and type of assignments that are given to nursing assistants are influenced by:

- Basic preparation
- Experience
- Specific advanced training in procedural skills
- Facility policy
- State laws that specify the range of practice of nursing assistants

Important principles to keep in mind are that:

- Some procedures considered routine for some workers would not be appropriate or permitted in other situations. Even basic procedures such as bed bathing might be restricted to nurses if the situation or patient conditions warrant such precautions.
- Under no circumstances must it be assumed that because the following procedures are included in this text that they should be assigned to all nursing assistants.
- Each facility has established policies and supervisory practices that are consistent with legal regulations and that ensure competency on the part of the care giver and safety for the patient/resident.

■ These procedures are to be carried out only after adequate practice with supervision and only in accord with specific facility policy. Additional information supporting these advanced procedures may be found in the units indicated.

Sterile Techniques

Sterile technique is an exacting procedure. *There can be no mistakes.* For this reason, usually only very specially trained people like you are given this responsibility. There will be times that you might be called upon to assist someone performing these duties or to perform them yourself. Therefore, you will need to develop an awareness of correct technique and be ready to assist without fear of contamination.

The term **sterile field** refers to an area of sterile equipment and materials. When working with a sterile field and sterile equipment, keep the following points in mind:

■ The sterile field may be a table covered with a sterilized sheet or a sterile towel placed on an over-bed table.

■ Only the center of the towel is actually used.

■ Equipment is kept two inches in from the edges all around as an added precaution.

■ Never reach for or pass anything that is unsterile over a sterile field. You might drop the unsterile article onto the field or touch the field. Instead, carry the unsterile object around the sterile field or hold it away from the sterile field.

■ If there is even a suspicion that anything unsterile has touched any part of the sterile field, the field must be considered contaminated. The entire setup must be discarded.

■ Coughing or sneezing while preparing a sterile field or after the field has been set up means contamination of the field.

■ Moisture means contamination. If a sterile towel is placed on an unsterile surface, any wetness on the towel means that the towel is contaminated. The towel and anything on the towel will be discarded.

Refer to Figure 43–1 to review the beginning procedure actions and procedure completion actions.

Opening a Sterile Package

Sterile equipment:

■ Is double wrapped in cloth or paper.

■ Is sealed.

■ Usually has a seal that changes color to indicate that the sterilizing process has been completed.

Before opening and using packaged sterile equipment:

■ Check the color code. If the color code has not changed or a seal does not look intact, do not consider the contents sterile.

BEGINNING PROCEDURE ACTIONS	PROCEDURE COMPLETION ACTIONS
■ Wash your hands. ■ Assemble equipment needed. ■ Go to the patient's room, knock, and pause before entering. ■ Introduce yourself and identify the patient by checking the identification bracelet. ■ Ask visitors to leave and inform them where they can wait. ■ Care for equipment according to facility policy. ■ Provide privacy. ■ Explain what will happen and answer questions. ■ Allow patient to assist in procedure as much as possible. ■ Raise bed or table to comfortable working height.	■ Position patient comfortably. ■ Leave signal cord, telephone, and fresh water close at hand. ■ Return bed or table to lowest position. ■ Perform general safety check of patient and environment. ■ Wash your hands. ■ Report completion of task. ■ Let visitors know when they may reenter the patient's room. ■ Document action and your observations.

NOTE: Where there are open lesions, wet linen, or possible contact with patient body fluids or blood, disposable gloves are worn during the procedure. Put on gloves before contact with the patient or linen. Properly dispose of gloves after they are removed. ALWAYS APPLY UNIVERSAL PRECAUTIONS.

FIGURE 43–1. Beginning procedure actions and procedure completion actions

■ Do not take a chance that items are sterile. If you have any questions, consider the package contaminated.

■ Touch only the outside of the package. Remember, only sterile surfaces may touch sterile surfaces.

PROCEDURE 138

OPENING A STERILE PACKAGE

NOTE: Background information is given in Unit 9.
1. Wash your hands.
2. Check tape seal to be sure color change indicating sterility has taken place.
3. Place package fold side up on a flat surface.
4. Remove tape.
5. Unfold flap farthest away from you by grasping outer surface only between thumb and forefinger, Figure 43–2A.
6. Open right flap with right hand using same technique, Figure 43–2B.
7. Open left flap with left hand using same technique, Figure 43–2C.

8. Open final flap (nearest you), Figure 43–2D. Touch only the outside of flap. Be careful not to stand too close. Do not allow uniform to touch flap as it is lifted free. Be sure the flaps are pulled open completely to prevent them from folding back up over the sterile field.

Once the sterile field is established, sterile materials may be added to the field. The following

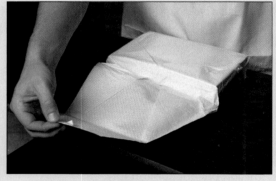

A. Open the top flap away from you; handle only the outside.

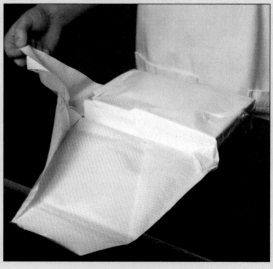

B. Open the right side. Do not touch the inside of folded-over portion.

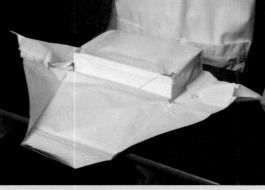

C. Open the left side drawing the left flap to the side.

FIGURE 43–2. Opening a sterile package

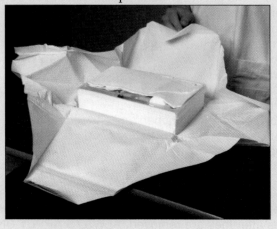

D. Without reaching over the sterile field, open the side toward you.

continues

procedure shows how this is done without contaminating the sterile field.

1. Wash your hands.
2. Check seal to be sure it is intact.
3. With two hands, grasp each side of separated end of package and gently pull apart, Figure 43–3A.

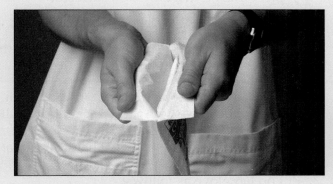

A. Open the package containing material or equipment without touching the inner contents.

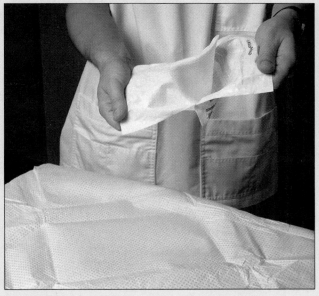

B. Expose contents over sterile field as you separate the package.

4. Open package until item is free of packaging material and hold over the sterile field, Figure 43–3B. Be sure you do not touch the sterile field
5. Drop contents of package into the sterile field, Figure 43–3C.
6. If article is to be taken from the package by the nurse or physician:
   a. Do not open the package until the nurse or physician is ready for it.
   b. Open package only enough to expose the end to be withdrawn without contamination.

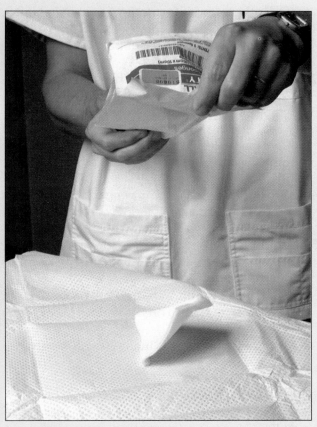

C. Turn package over and drop contents to sterile field without touching the field with the package and contaminating it.

FIGURE 43–3. Adding sterile material to the sterile field

Gloving

Gloves are sterilized in double-layered packages of cloth or paper. They are arranged so that:

- When opened, the gloves will be on the proper side for gloving.
- The palms will be up with thumbs pointing to outer edge.

- The wrist will be cuffed and folded over.

Keep in mind that:

- Once touched, the inside of the glove (the part that comes in contact with the skin) is considered contaminated.
- When putting on gloves, the most important principle to remember is that glove surfaces must touch only glove surfaces, and skin surfaces must touch only skin surfaces.

PROCEDURE 139

PUTTING ON STERILE GLOVES

NOTE: Background information is given in Unit 9.

1. Wash your hands and dry them thoroughly. Gloves will stick to moist hands. This will make them hard to put on.
2. Pick up wrapped gloves. Check seal for sterility. Open outer package, Figure 43–4A.
3. Open seal and open outer cover, touching outside of package only, by grasping either side of glove package. Holding each edge between the fingers, carefully pull the edges in opposite directions.
4. With one hand, remove inner package of gloves and place on inner surface of outer cover on flat surface.
5. Lift inner covering exposing gloves and allowing them to remain flat on the inside of inner covering, Figure 43–4B.
    - The gloves will now be flat with palm sides up.
    - The right glove is on the right and the left is on the opposite side.
    - If powder packet is included, lift free, without touching gloves.
    - Move away from gloves.
    - Gently sprinkle powder on hands.
    - Rub hands together to spread powder.
    - Drop packet in waste basket.
6. With left hand, pick up right glove. Proceed as follows:
    - Slip thumb of left hand inside edge of right glove at wrist. Grasp glove at edge. Fingers must not extend beyond the cuff or touch outside of glove, Figure 43–4C.
    - Lift glove free of covering and table and step back. Glove must not touch any unsterile surface.

- Curve right hand with thumb toward palm. Insert into glove with a rotating motion. Pull up with left hand, Figure 43–4D.
- Once in place, let go with left hand but *do not pull cuff over wrist*.

7. Put on left glove as follows:
    - Holding gloved fingers of right hand together, slide them under cuff of left glove, Figure 43–4E (your fingers will be pointed toward you). Thumb of right hand may touch only the rim of cuff for control.
    - Lift glove clear of table and wrapping.
    - Curve fingers of left hand, bending thumb slightly forward and insert in glove. As hand is inserted, spread fingers to slide into proper areas. Do not let the right gloved thumb touch the left, ungloved hand.
    - Cuff may be brought slightly down on wrist as long as the gloved hand never touches the inner cuff surface.
8. Adjust cuffs as follows:
    - Gloved fingers of right hand are slipped into cuff of left glove, adjusting the cuff by pushing downward toward arm, Figure 43–4F.
    - If gloves only are worn, a small rim of cuff may be left. It is, of course, not to be considered sterile.
9. Adjust fingers with a gentle, rotating motion, working from tips to base of fingers.

If gloves are included in a sterile, prepackaged procedure set, proceed as follows:

1. Wash your hands.
2. Remove lid, exposing sterile interior.
3. Follow Steps 6–9.
4. Sterile supplies within kit may then be handled with sterile, gloved hands.

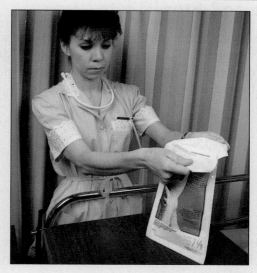

A. Open the outer cover by grasping the flaps between fingers of each hand and pulling in opposite directions.

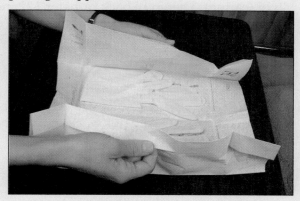

B. Open the inner package by holding the edges. Do not touch the inside of the wrapper.

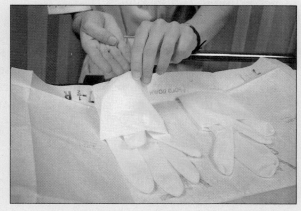

C. Grasp the cuff of the opposite glove. Lift free of wrapper. Tucking thumb of hand across the palm, slip fingers into the glove.

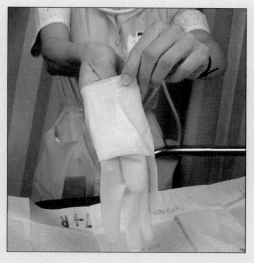

D. Holding edge of glove, pull over right hand.

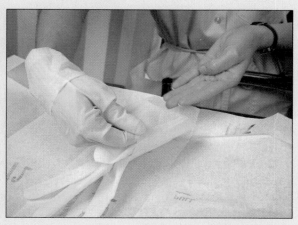

E. Slip gloved fingers under the cuff. Lift and slip fingers in, being careful that only glove surfaces touch glove surfaces and skin touches skin.

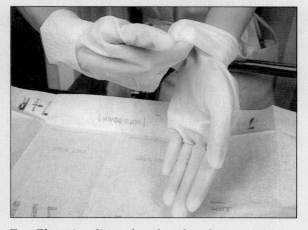

F. Glove is adjusted on hand and over wrist.

FIGURE 43–4. Procedure for putting on sterile gloves

Tracheal Suctioning

The nursing assistant who has been trained, has practiced with supervision, and has been determined to be competent in this skill may be assigned to apply suction to a patient who has collected secretions in the upper respiratory system.

Urine and Stool Tests

Special tests performed on urine and stool samples that may be part of your responsibility include the following three procedures. Additional information may be found in Unit 24 and Unit 38.

PROCEDURE 140

TRACHEAL SUCTIONING

1. Carry out each beginning procedure action.
2. Remember to wash your hands, identify the patient, and provide privacy.
3. Assemble equipment needed.
   - Sterile gloves
   - Sterile suction catheter
   - Y or vented connector
   - Box of tissues
   - Sterile cup
   - Sterile 5–ml syringe
   - Sterile normal saline/water
   - Suction source (separate machine or wall unit)
4. Establish a sterile field and open sterile equipment.
5. Position sterile equipment for easy access on bedside table.
6. Pour normal saline solution in cup.
7. Position the patient in high Fowler's position, if permitted. This will make the passage of the suction catheter easier.
8. Open the sterile catheter package so that the tip remains covered within the package.
9. Open vented Y tip. Leave open on sterile cover.
10. Turn on the suction machine. Pressure should not be greater than 120 mm Hg.
11. Put on sterile gloves.
12. Dip end of catheter into sterile saline/water. Then attach one end of Y connector to catheter. Attach the single end of Y tip to the suction.
13. Insert catheter gently into the larynx and then trachea, leaving vent open so no suction is applied.
14. Slowly advance catheter until it meets resistance at the level of the beginning of the bronchi (carina). Then pull back catheter 1/2 inch.
15. Once catheter is in place, put thumb over Y tip to begin suctioning. Continue for specified amount of time. Discontinue suctioning if patient shows any signs of distress. Notify nurse immediately.
16. Once suctioning is complete, remove catheter by gently rotating catheter. Suction oral pharynx.
17. Make patient comfortable.
18. Dispose of equipment or clean according to facility policy.
19. Note character and amount of secretions removed by suctioning. Dispose of secretions according to facility policy.
20. Remove and dispose of gloves according to facility policy.
21. Carry out procedure completion actions. Report completion of procedure (tracheal suctioning). Record date, time, procedure, character and amount of material suctioned, and patient reaction.

PROCEDURE 141

TESTING URINE WITH THE HEMACOMBISTIX®

NOTE: The HemaCombistix® is used to test for the presence of protein, blood, glucose, and for pH (acidity) of urine.

1. Wash your hands and assemble the following equipment:
   - Bottle containing HemaCombistix® reagent strips
   - Disposable gloves
   - Fresh sample of urine
2. Put on gloves.
3. Take reagent strips and sample to bathroom.
4. Remove cap and place top side down on table.
5. Shake bottle gently until reagent strips protrude from end.
6. Remove one reagent strip. Do not touch test areas of strip with fingers. Be sure your gloves are dry.
7. Dip reagent end of strip in fresh, well-mixed urine—remove immediately.
8. Tap edge of strip against container to remove excess urine.
9. Compare reagent side of test areas with corresponding color charts on the bottle at the time intervals specified. See Figures 43–5A and B.

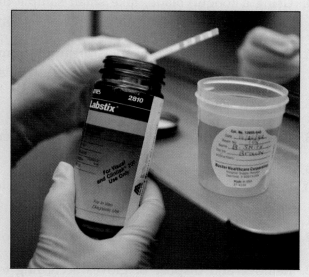

FIGURE 43–5A. HemaCombistix® results

10. Remove and dispose of gloves according to facility policy.
11. Remember to wash your hands, report completion of task, and document time, date, HemaCombistix® reactions (positive/negative), and patient reaction.

Test	Reaction Time	Results
Blood	30 sec.	Light blue green to deep blue
Glucose	10 sec. qualitative 30 sec. qualitative	Light blue to dark brown
Protein	Immediately	Yellow to green
pH	Immediately	Orange to blue

FIGURE 43–5B. HemaCombistix® results

PROCEDURE 142

TESTING FOR OCCULT BLOOD USING HEMOCCULT® AND DEVELOPER

1. Wash your hands and assemble the following equipment:
   - Bedpan with fresh specimen
   - Hemoccult® slide packet
   - Hemoccult® developer
   - Tongue blade
   - Paper towel
   - Disposable gloves

continues

2. Place paper towel on flat surface and open flap of Hemoccult® packet, exposing guaiac paper.
3. Put on gloves.
4. Using a tongue blade, take small sample of feces and smear on paper area marked *A*, Figure 43–6.
5. Repeat the procedure, taking fecal sample from a different part of the specimen and making smear in area *B*.
6. Close tab and turn packet over.
7. Open back tab.
8. Apply two drops of Hemoccult® developer directly over each smear. Time reaction.
9. Read results 30–60 seconds later.
10. Presence of blood is indicated by a blue discoloration around perimeter of smear.
11. Dispose of specimen.
12. Clean bedpan per facility policy and dispose of paper towel, packet, and tongue blade.
13. Remove and dispose of gloves according to facility policy.
14. Remember to wash your hands, report completion of task, and document time, date, Hemoccult® test (positive/negative), and patient reaction.

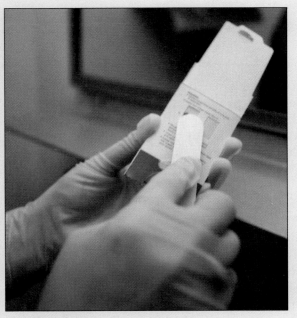

FIGURE 43–6. A small specimen of stool is placed on a special area of the card for an occult blood test.

PROCEDURE 143

TESTING FOR OCCULT BLOOD USING HEMATEST® REAGENT TABLETS

1. Wash your hands and assemble the following equipment:
   - Bedpan with fresh specimen
   - Hematest® filter paper
   - Glass or porcelain plate
   - Hematest® reagent tablet
   - Distilled water
   - Dropper
   - Disposable gloves
   - Tongue blade
2. Place Hematest® filter on a glass or porcelain plate.
3. Put on gloves.
4. Smear a thin streak of fecal material lightly on the filter paper. Do not use an emulsion or suspension.
5. Place the Hematest® reagent tablet on smear.
6. Place one drop of distilled water on the

Hematest® reagent tablet. Allow 5–10 seconds for the water to penetrate the tablet.
7. Then add a second drop so that the water runs down the side of the tablet onto the specimen and filter paper. Gently tap side of plate once or twice to knock off water droplets from top of tablet.
8. For up to 2 minutes, observe filter paper for color change.
9. Read reaction. A positive reaction is indicated by a blue halo forming on the paper towel around the smear.
10. Dispose of specimen and equipment per facility policy.
11. Remove and dispose of gloves according to facility policy.
12. Remember to wash your hands, report completion of task, and document time, date, Hematest® (positive/negative), and patient reaction.

Collecting a Specimen from a Closed Urinary Drainage System

At some time, it may be necessary to collect a fresh specimen of urine when the patient is on a closed urinary drainage system. Keep in mind that the:

■ Urine sample must be fresh.
■ Urine collected in the bag has accumulated over a period of time.
■ Specimen may not be taken from the bag.
■ Specimen must be taken from the catheter.

The procedure to be followed is determined by the type of Foley catheter that is in place.

■ If the catheter has a port (opening) for fluid withdrawal, Figure 43–7, follow Procedure 144.

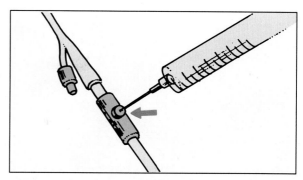

FIGURE 43–7. When the indwelling catheter has a sample port, the syringe is inserted in the port to gather the specimen.

The procedure must be carried out using proper techniques so as to avoid introducing infectious organisms into the system.

PROCEDURE 144

COLLECTING A URINE SPECIMEN THROUGH A DRAINAGE PORT

1. Carry out each beginning procedure action.
2. Remember to wash your hands, identify the patient, and provide privacy.
3. Assemble equipment needed:
   ■ Tube clamp
   ■ Completed label
   ■ Emesis basin
   ■ 10-ml syringe
   ■ Specimen cup and lid
   ■ 21–gauge or 22–gauge needle
   ■ Alcohol sponge
   ■ Gloves
4. Go to bedside half an hour before sample is to be collected.
5. Clamp the drainage tube.
6. Wash your hands. Return to bedside after 30 minutes.
7. Put on gloves.
8. Place emesis basin on the bed under the catheter drainage port.
9. Wipe the drainage port with an alcohol sponge, Figure 43–8.
10. Carefully remove the cap on the syringe. Do not contaminate the tip.
11. Attach needle carefully. Do not contaminate the needle tip.
12. Open the package containing the specimen container. Remove the lid and lay it top up on the bedside stand, Figure 43–9.
13. Insert the needle into the port and withdraw the specimen.
14. Carefully withdraw the needle.
15. Wipe the port with the alcohol sponge.
16. Transfer the urine sample to the specimen container, Figure 43–10.
17. Handling cover by top only, cover container.
18. Remove gloves and dispose of according to facility policy.
19. Remove the catheter clamp.
20. Complete information on label and put label on container. Compare label to the requisition to be sure that the information is complete and accurate, Figure 43–11.
21. Dispose of needle in proper container.
22. Carry out each procedure completion action. Remember to wash your hands, report completion of task, and document time, date, urine sample taken through drainage port, and patient reaction.
23. Follow instructions as to the care of the specimen.

continues

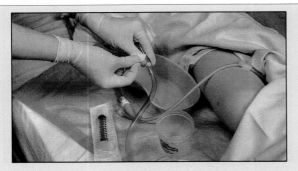

FIGURE 43–8. Wipe the port with an alcohol sponge.

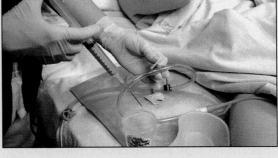

FIGURE 43–10. Transfer specimen to container.

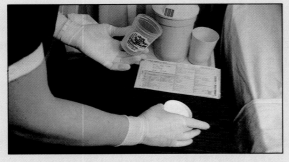

FIGURE 43–9. Remove lid of specimen jar and place it on stand.

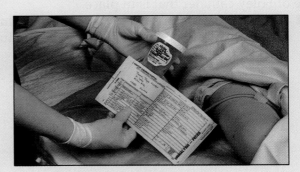

FIGURE 43–11. Complete label to conform to laboratory requisition.

Rectal Suppositories

Suppositories are given to stimulate bowel evacuation or to instill medications. Medicinal suppositories must be inserted by the nurse. You may be asked to insert suppositories that soften the stool and promote elimination.

PROCEDURE 145

SIDE **10**

INSERTING A RECTAL SUPPOSITORY

NOTE: Background information is given in Unit 38.

1. Carry out each beginning procedure action.
2. Remember to wash your hands, identify the patient, and provide privacy.
3. Assemble equipment needed:

- Suppository, as ordered
- Toilet tissue
- Bedpan and cover, if needed
- Lubricant
- Gloves

4. Help patient assume the Sims' position.

5. Expose buttocks only.
6. Put on gloves.
7. Unwrap suppository.
8. With left hand, separate the buttocks, exposing the anus.
9. Apply a small amount of lubricant to anus and insert the suppository. Suppository must be inserted deeply enough to enter the rectum beyond the sphincter (approximately 2 inches).
10. Encourage patient to take deep breaths and relax until the need to defecate is experienced, approximately 5–15 minutes.
11. Remove gloves and dispose of properly.
12. Adjust the bedding, helping patient to assume a comfortable position.
13. Place call bell near patient's hand, but check every 5 minutes.
14. Assist patient to bathroom or position on bedpan. Provide privacy.
15. Put on gloves. Once the patient is finished, assist with hygiene if necessary.
16. Observe results and note any unusual characteristics of stool. If stool is unusual, save and report to nurse.
17. Dispose of stool and clean equipment according to facility policy. Store equipment as required.
18. Remove and dispose of gloves according to facility policy.
19. Carry out each procedure completion action. Remember to wash your hands, report completion of task, and document time, date, suppository (type) inserted, results, and patient reaction.

Care of the Patient with a Colostomy

A colostomy is a semipermanent or permanent artificial opening into the colon through the abdominal wall. To make this possible, a section of the bowel is brought to the surface of the abdomen and an opening made. When there is the potential to reunite the bowel in the future, both segments are brought to the surface and two openings are made (this is called a double-barreled colostomy). This surgical procedure is performed frequently because of tumors that require the removal of a section of the colon, or because of disease such as ulcerative colitis. The opening in the abdominal wall is called a stoma. To collect the drainage from the stoma, a disposable or reuseable drainage pouch called an appliance is attached over the stoma and held in place with a belt or adhesive seal. Proper stoma care is required to maintain healthy tissue since the area around the opening comes into contact with the liquid or semiliquid stool.

The patient with a colostomy does not have normal sphincter control. At the stoma, there may be problems of:

■ Leakage
■ Odor control
■ Irritation of the surrounding area

There are several common colostomy sites, Figure 43–12. You can assist the colostomy patient by:

■ Keeping the area clean and dry.

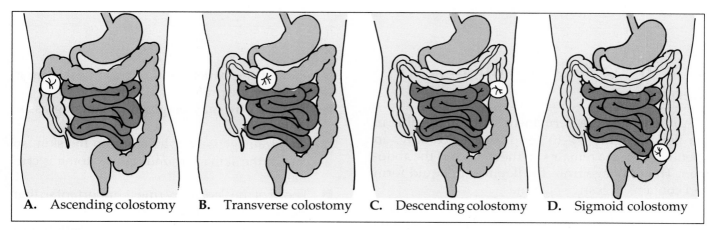

A. Ascending colostomy   **B.** Transverse colostomy   **C.** Descending colostomy   **D.** Sigmoid colostomy

FIGURE 43–12. Colostomy sites vary depending on the part of the bowel that needs to be removed. Area of colon removed is in blue.

■ Performing routine stoma care including removing drainage and/or replacing the appliance if your facility allows you to assist or give this care after you have had special training. Remember:

■ Initial irrigations will be performed by the nurse.
■ If the colostomy is to be permanent, patients are taught to carry out the irrigation procedure for themselves.

PROCEDURE 146

GIVING ROUTINE STOMA CARE (COLOSTOMY)

1. Carry out each beginning procedure action.
2. Remember to wash your hands, identify the patient, and provide privacy.
3. Assemble equipment needed:
    ■ Washcloth and towel
    ■ Basin of warm water
    ■ Bed protector
    ■ Bath blanket
    ■ Disposable colostomy bag and belt
    ■ Bedpan
    ■ Disposable gloves
    ■ Skin lotion as directed
4. Replace top bedding with the bath blanket.
5. Place bed protector under the patient's hips.
6. Put on disposable gloves.
7. Remove the soiled disposable stoma bag (appliance) and place in bedpan—note amount and type of drainage.
8. Remove belt that holds stoma bag and save if clean.
9. Gently clean area around stoma with toilet tissue to remove feces and drainage. Dispose of tissue in bedpan.
10. Wash area around stoma with soap and water. Rinse thoroughly and dry.
11. If ordered, apply skin lotion lightly around the stoma—too much lotion may interfere with proper seal of fresh ostomy bag.
12. Position clean belt around patient—inspect skin under belt for irritation or breakdown.
13. If necessary, remove and replace adhesive wafer. Place clean ostomy bag over stoma and secure belt.
14. Remove bed protector. Check to be sure bottom bedding is not wet. Change if necessary.
15. Replace bath blanket with top bedding, making patient comfortable.
16. Gather soiled materials and bedpan. Take to utility room. Dispose of materials according to facility policy.
17. Empty, wash, and dry bedpan. Return to patient's unit.
18. Remove and dispose of gloves properly.
19. Carry out each procedure completion action. Remember to wash your hands, report completion of task, and document time, date, ostomy care, lotion applied (if any), type and amount of drainage, condition of stoma and surrounding tissue, and patient reaction.

Care of the Patient with an Ileostomy

An ileostomy is a permanent artificial opening in the ileum, Figure 43–13. As in the colostomy, an opening or stoma remains on the surface of the abdomen. The drainage from the ileum is in liquid form and contains digestive enzymes.

Care of the patient with an ileostomy has some similarities and some differences with the care given to the colostomy patient.

■ Care of the patient with a fresh ileostomy is given by the professional nurse.
■ Routine care may be given by nursing assistants.
■ The drainage is very irritating to the skin, so care of the skin surrounding the stoma is crucial.
■ The fit of the ileostomy ring is important so that leakage doesn't occur, Figure 43–14. This is true for both the disposable and reusable types of appliances.

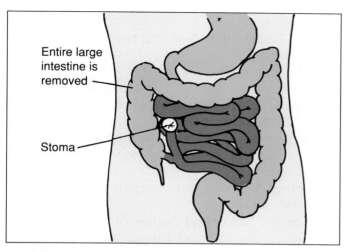

FIGURE 43–13. An ileostomy brings a section of the ileum through the abdominal wall.

FIGURE 43–14. Stoma protector and drainage bag *(Photo courtesy of Hollister Corporation)*

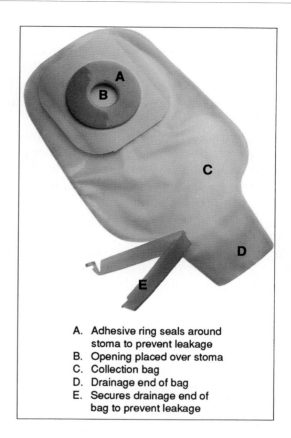

A. Adhesive ring seals around stoma to prevent leakage
B. Opening placed over stoma
C. Collection bag
D. Drainage end of bag
E. Secures drainage end of bag to prevent leakage

PROCEDURE 147

ROUTINE CARE OF AN ILEOSTOMY (WITH PATIENT IN BED)

1. Carry out each beginning procedure action.
2. Remember to wash your hands, identify the patient, and provide privacy.
3. Assemble equipment needed:
   - Basin of warm water
   - Bed protector
   - Bath blanket
   - Bedpan/cover
   - Disposable gloves
   - Fresh appliance and belt
   - Clamp for appliance
   - Prescribed solvent/dropper
   - Cotton balls
   - Deodorant (if permitted)
   - Cleansing agent
   - Karaya ring
   - 4 × 4 gauze squares
   - Toilet tissue
   - Paper towels
4. Raise opposite side rail for safety. Elevate head of bed and assist patient to turn on side toward you.
5. Replace bedding with bath blanket.
6. Place bed protector under patient.
7. Put on disposable gloves.
8. Place bedpan on bed protector against patient.
9. Place end of ileostomy bag in bedpan. Open clamp and allow to drain. Note amount and character of drainage.
10. Wipe end of drainage sheath with toilet paper and move out of drainage. Place tissue in bedpan. Cover bedpan.
11. Disconnect belt from appliance and remove from patient. Place on paper towels.
12. With dropper, apply a small amount of solvent around the ring of the appliance. This will loosen it so it can be removed. Wait a few seconds. Do not force the appliance free.
13. Cover stoma with gauze.
    - Carefully inspect skin area around stoma.
    - If the area is irritated or skin is broken, cover patient with bath blanket, raise side rail, and lower bed.
    - Remove gloves and dispose of properly.
    - Wash your hands.
    - Report to the nurse for instructions.
    - Put on fresh gloves before continuing procedure.

continues

14. Gently cleanse the area around the stoma with cotton balls. Use recommended cleansing agent. Gently pat dry.
15. Remove gauze from stoma and place in paper towels.
16. If appliance is used with a Karaya ring, moisten ring, allow it to become sticky, and apply to stoma. If appliance uses paper-covered adhesive strip around the stoma opening, remove paper and apply around stoma.
17. Clamp appliance bag, add deodorant, and apply to ring.
18. Adjust a clean belt in position around the patient and connect it to the appliance.
19. Remove covered bedpan and place on chair on paper towels.
20. Remove bed protector and place on bedpan.

■ Check bottom bedding to make sure it is dry.
■ Change, if necessary.
21. Replace bath blanket with top bedding.
22. Gather soiled materials and bedpan.
■ Take to utility room.
■ Dispose of according to hospital policy.
■ If belt and bag are reusable, wash and allow to dry.
23. Empty, wash, and dry bedpan. Return to patient's unit.
24. Remove gloves and dispose of properly.
25. Carry out each procedure completion action. Remember to wash your hands, report completion of task, and document time, date, ileostomy care, character and amount of drainage, and patient reaction.

PROCEDURE 148

ROUTINE CARE OF AN ILEOSTOMY (IN BATHROOM)

1. Carry out each beginning procedure action.
2. Remember to wash your hands, identify the patient, and provide privacy.
3. Assemble equipment needed.
   ■ Disposable gloves
   ■ Fresh appliance and belt
   ■ Bath blanket
   ■ Clamp for appliance
   ■ Cotton balls
   ■ Solvent/dropper
   ■ Deodorant
   ■ Cleansing agent
   ■ Karaya ring
   ■ 4 × 4 gauze squares
   ■ Paper towels
4. Take equipment to patient's bathroom.
5. Assist patient into robe and slippers.
6. Assist patient into bathroom. Position on toilet.
7. Place bath blanket over patient's legs. Raise gown and roll at waist, exposing appliance. Instruct patient to separate legs.
8. Put on gloves. Open ileostomy appliance, directing drainage into toilet, Figure 43–15. Note character and amount of drainage.

9. With dropper, apply a small amount of solvent around the Karaya gum ring to loosen from skin. Do not force from skin.
10. Cover stoma with gauze sponge to collect drainage.
11. With cotton balls, cleanse area around stoma with warm water and soap or cleansing agent (if skin area is broken, report to nurse for instructions). Pat area dry.

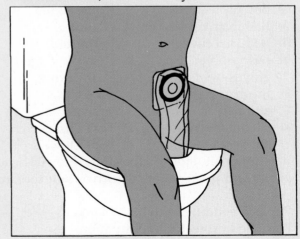

FIGURE 43–15.   Direct the end of the drainage bag into the toilet.

12. Remove gauze from stoma and place in paper towels.
13. If appliance is used with a Karaya ring, moisten ring, allow to become sticky, and apply to stoma. If appliance uses paper-covered adhesive strip around the stoma opening, remove paper and apply around stoma.
14. Clamp appliance bag and apply to ring.
15. Remove gloves and dispose of properly.
16. Adjust clean belt in position around the patient, and connect it to the appliance.
17. Remove bath blanket, and assist patient to wash hands and return to bed.
18. Clean patient's bathroom. Wash belt and appliance, if reusable, and allow to dry.
19. Carry out each procedure completion action. Remember to wash your hands, report completion of task, and document time, date, ileostomy care, character and amount of drainage, and patient reaction.

Remember, all the procedures presented in this unit require advanced training and close supervision before you attempt to perform them. In addition, you can do so only when properly authorized.

SUMMARY

As a nursing assistant you should be willing to learn and grow in your chosen field, always bearing in mind your ethical and legal limitations.

■ Material in this unit introduces techniques that may be assigned to the experienced nursing assistant who has received advanced training and who has demonstrated skill and proficiency.

■ These procedures must be carried out under proper supervision and authorization, since any errors might result in a greater likelihood of injury to the patient or inaccuracy of test results.

UNIT REVIEW

A. True/False. Answer the following statements true or false by circling T or F.

T F 1. All nursing assistants are assigned the task of carrying out sterile procedures.

T F 2. Nursing assistants should follow established policies of their own facilities in carrying out assigned tasks.

T F 3. Nursing assistants should not carry out any procedure they have not been taught and in which they have not received supervision.

T F 4. If you have a sterile field open, you may reach over the field as long as you don't touch anything.

T F 5. Sterile technique is an exacting technique.

T F 6. The outer six inches of any sterile field are considered unsterile.

T F 7. When performing tracheal suction, it is best to position the patient in a high Fowler's position, if possible.

T F 8. It is impossible to safely collect a sample of urine from a closed urinary drainage system.

T F 9. Once touched, the inside of sterile gloves are contaminated.

T F 10. Sterile equipment is double wrapped in paper or cloth.

B. Matching. Match Column I with Column II.

Column I	Column II
_____ 11. a process that destroys all organisms	a. occult
	b. ileostomy
_____ 12. artificial opening in large intestine	c. stoma
_____ 13. artificial opening in small intestine	d. suppository
	e. colostomy
_____ 14. hidden	f. contamination
_____ 15. stool softener	g. sterilization

C. **Multiple Choice.** Choose the answer that best completes each of the following sentences by circling the proper letter.

16. You select presterilized sponges for a dressing and find the seal broken. You should
    a. use the sponges.
    b. reseal the package.
    c. not use the sponges.
    d. None of the above.
17. An ileostomy as compared to a colostomy
    a. has more liquid drainage.
    b. tends to be more irritating.
    c. has drainage containing digestive enzymes.
    d. All of the above.
18. When assigned to insert a lubricating suppository, position the patient in the
    a. Sims' position.
    b. lithotomy position.
    c. high Fowler's position.
    d. None of the above.
19. Lubricating suppositories should be inserted in an adult
    a. 1/2 inch.   c. 2 inches.
    b. 1 inch.   d. 4 inches.

20. You are giving routine stoma care to the colostomy patient and find the stoma red and irritated. You should
    a. complete the procedure.
    b. clean the area with alcohol.
    c. apply powder and attach the ostomy bag.
    d. cover the area and notify the nurse.
21. You prepared a sterile field using a sterile towel on the overbed table. You recognize the sponges can no longer be considered sterile because they are
    a. 1 inch from the towel edge.
    b. 3 inches from the towel edge.
    c. 4 inches from the towel edge.
    d. in the center of the towel.
22. When opening a wrapped sterile package, first unwrap the
    a. left side.
    b. side nearest to you.
    c. right side.
    d. side farthest away from you.

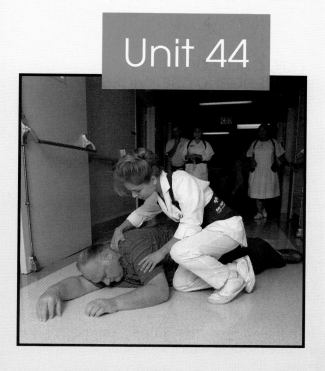

Response to Basic Emergencies

VOCABULARY

Learn the meaning and the correct spelling of the following words and phrases:

cardiac arrest	seizure
cardiopulmonary	shock
resuscitation (CPR)	urgent care
first aid	victim

All emergency situations develop rapidly and unpredictably. Emergency situations can occur at any time to anyone. Examples include:

- Automobile accidents
- Strokes
- Suddenly feeling weak
- Fainting and falling

Being Prepared

While working in the hospital or long-term care facility, you are always close to professional medical help. When you witness an accident away from the medical facility, however, professional help is not always readily available. Whatever course of action you choose, the victim (person needing help) should not be placed in additional jeopardy.

First-aid techniques are taught by the American Red Cross as a specific course. You should take the course to be thoroughly and properly trained in these skills. In addition, both the American Red Cross and the American Heart Association provide instruction and certification in cardiopulmonary resuscitation

OBJECTIVES

As a result of this unit, you will be able to:

- Spell and define terms.
- Recognize emergency situations that require urgent care.
- Be able to assess situations and determine the sequence of appropriate actions to be taken.
- Recognize the need for CPR.
- List the steps to be taken when performing the Heimlich maneuver.
- Identify the signs and symptoms of common emergency situations such as:
  — Fainting
  — Heart attack
  — Bleeding
  — Shock
  — Stroke
  — Seizure

(CPR). You are encouraged to sign up to learn this life-saving technique. Your course of instruction may require that you be certified in CPR. Your future employer may also require you to be certified.

At the Scene

As the first person to witness an accident or arrive on the scene, your action could save a life or prevent serious additional injury.

- Be prepared to offer assistance in any emergency situation.
- Always defer to someone who has the greater training and experience.

If you are able to react in an emergency situation, remember:

- Always keep calm so that your actions reflect clear thinking.
- Use a calm voice to talk to the victim and to instruct others in the area.
- Keep onlookers away.
- Proceed in a methodic, quiet way.

Seeking Assistance

In certain areas of the country, the emergency telephone number 911 can be dialed for help in case of an accident, Figure 44–1. In other areas, the closest sources of help are the:

- Police
- Local rescue squads
- Telephone operator, who can complete a call for you

When calling the emergency number, state:

- Your name
- Location
- Brief description of the scene
- Information about the type of injury
- Possible help you may need

First Aid

First aid includes:

- Immediate care for victims of injuries or sudden illness
- Care needed later if medical help is delayed or is not available

First aid will be needed for different conditions in a variety of situations. These conditions can range from the minor to the very severe. When you give first aid, you deal with the:

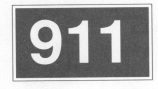

TO CALL FOR EMERGENCY SERVICES

911

FIGURE 44–1. 911 is a national emergency telephone number.

- Victim's emotional state
- Victim's physical injuries
- Management of the whole accident situation

Persons in life-threatening situations must be given immediate attention. Life-threatening situations include those in which a person:

- Has no airway
- Has stopped breathing
- Is in shock
- Has been poisoned
- Is choking
- Is bleeding profusely

Assessing the Situation

At the scene of an accident, proceed as follows:

- Assess the situation and determine the extent of injuries. Quickly take into account the number of victims, their potential injuries, and any dangerous factors at the scene.
  - For example, at the scene of an auto accident, there may be several victims. Some may be trapped in their vehicles, others may be lying on the highway. There may be cars burning and the danger of explosion. In this situation, you must first get yourself and the victims away from further danger.
  - In the medical facility, unless there is a fire, you usually will be dealing with a single victim. You will be able to focus on the needs of that individual. For example, you might enter a patient's room and, despite the fact that side rails are up at the bed, find a patient lying on the floor. Make a quick assessment as you signal for help, giving the patient's name and location, and describing the scene.

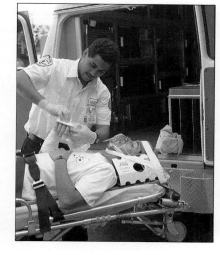

FIGURE 44–2. At the accident scene, emergency medical personnel assess the victim's needs and provide appropriate assistance.

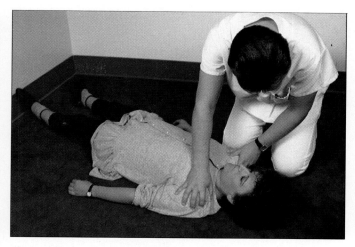

FIGURE 44–4. Determine if the patient is conscious.

■ Do not move the victim if professional help is available.
  — Keep the person quiet and calm until help arrives.
  — Try to maintain an even body temperature.
  — Provide urgent care if needed.
■ Activate the emergency medical service, Figure 44–2.
  — If you are in a home situation, make a quick evaluation and summon help if available.

  — A list of emergency numbers should be posted near the phone—911 is an emergency telephone number. If it is in use in your area, it can be used to call for help in a real emergency. When using 911, make sure to give the:
■ Location of the emergency.
■ Closest cross street.
■ Telephone number where call is made.
■ Type of emergency.
■ Number of persons needing help.
■ Extent of first aid given.
■ Other information requested by person answering; let the emergency medical service answerer hang up first.

Emergency Care

Emergency care is care that must be given right away to prevent loss of life.
■ If you are out in the community or in the health care facility, ask someone nearby to summon help.
■ Do not leave people who need urgent care to get help yourself, Figure 44–3.
■ As help is on the way, check, in the following order, the:
  — Degree of consciousness, Figure 44–4.
  — Airway/breathing capability
  — Rate of heart beat
  — Signs of bleeding
  — Signs of shock
■ Do not move the person if you do not have to.
■ Do not allow the person to get up and walk around.
■ Check for other injuries.

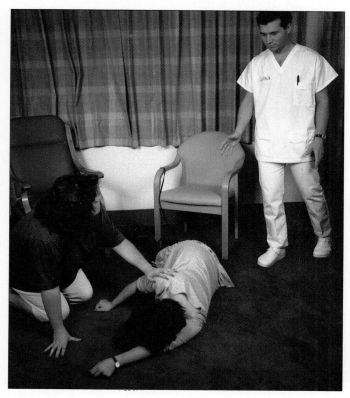

FIGURE 44–3. In an emergency, keep calm. Do not panic. Do not leave the victim alone but summon help.

Choking

A person chokes when the throat is occluded (closed up or blocked) and air cannot get into the airway. In this situation, you must take quick, decisive action.

■ The airway can be blocked by the accumulation in the back of the throat of:
   — Any foreign body   — Food
   — Blood   — Vomitus

■ Tilting the head back can sometimes clear the airway since positioning in this way pulls the tongue forward.

■ If the person can speak and is coughing vigorously, do not intervene. Coughing is the most effective way to dislodge materials from the airway. Stay close by and encourage coughing.

■ A complete blockage is signaled by the person being unable to speak, high-pitched sounds on inhalation, and grasping the throat in the universal distress signal, Figure 44–5.

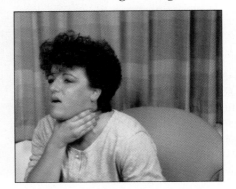

FIGURE 44–5. The distress signal of choking

PROCEDURE 149   **OBRA**   **SIDE 10**   

HEIMLICH MANEUVER—ABDOMINAL THRUSTS

1. Ask the person if he is choking.
2. If the person starts to cough, wait.
3. If the person cannot speak, cough, or breathe, but is conscious, apply subdiaphragmatic abdominal thrusts, until the foreign body is expelled:
   a. Stand behind victim and wrap arms around victim's waist.
   b. Clench fist, keeping thumb straight, Figure 44–6A.
   c. Place fist, thumb side in, against abdomen slightly above navel.
   d. Grasp clenched fist with opposite hand, Figure 44–6B.
   e. Thrust forcefully with thumbside of fist against midline of abdomen, slightly above navel, inward and upward, Figure 44–6C. Keep your elbows bent and extended away from your body. You do not want to "hug" the victim since the thrust will not be as effective. Be sure you are below the tip of the sternum (xiphoid process).

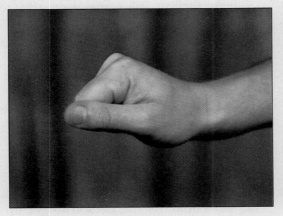

A.

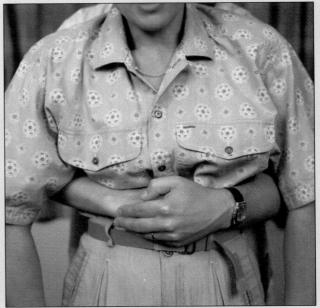

B.

FIGURE 44–6. Abdominal thrust

4. Keep thrusting if object has not been dislodged. If the person begins to cough forcefully, wait.
5. Continue Heimlich maneuver until obstruction is expelled or victim becomes unconscious. If victim becomes unconscious, continue alternating the following steps in rapid sequence:
   — Abdominal thrusts
   — Finger sweep to remove foreign body from mouth
   — Rescue breathing (Head tilt/chin lift and try to give two breaths.)

NOTE: Chest thrusts are used when pressure to the abdomen would be harmful or impossible. Chest thrusts are used if the choking person is in late pregnancy or if the victim is so large you are unable to get your arms around him. Follow Steps 1 and 2, then:

6. Stand behind victim.
7. Place arms around victim directly under the victim's armpits.
8. Form fist as previously described and place thumbside of fist against breastbone (sternum), level with the armpits.
9. Grasp fist in opposite hand and administer firm thrusts, pulling straight back toward you.

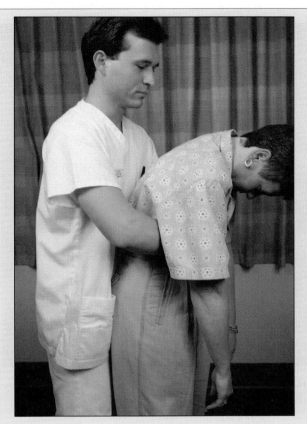

C.

SIDE
10

PROCEDURE 150 | OBRA

ASSISTING THE ADULT WHO HAS AN OBSTRUCTED AIRWAY AND BECOMES UNCONSCIOUS

1. Activate EMS system.
2. Turn victim on back, tip the head back and check for signs of breathing.
3. If the victim is not breathing, try to give two slow breaths. If the air does not go in, retilt head and try again. If the air still does not go in, begin with five abdominal thrusts.
4. Straddle the victim's thighs, Figure 44–7, and administer 5 subdiaphragmatic abdominal thrusts, as follows:
   a. Place the heel of one hand on the victim's abdomen slightly above the navel. Hand should be flat with fingers pointing toward victim's head.
   b. Place your other hand in a similar position over the first.
   c. Keep your elbows straight with your shoulders directly over the victim's abdomen. Press inward and upward with 5 quick thrusts. Keep hands centered on person's abdomen.
5. To remove the object, follow these steps:
   a. With face up, grasp tongue and jaw between thumb and index finger, opening mouth and drawing jaw forward.
   b. Insert index finger of other hand down along side of cheek toward the base of the tongue. Bend finger and sweep with a hooking motion.

continues

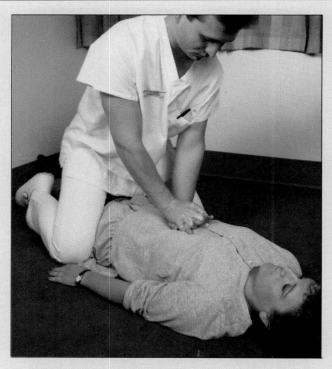

FIGURE 44–7. Abdominal thrusts with victim lying down

c. Attempt to bring the foreign object up into the mouth if you can see it.
d. Be careful not to force the object deeper into the throat.
e. If the object can be brought into the mouth, remove it.

6. Attempt giving breaths. If airway is still obstructed, give five abdominal thrusts, sweep the mouth, and try to ventilate. Keep repeating these steps until the object moves and the victim can be ventilated or help arrives (EMS).
7. To give chest thrusts, proceed as in applying external chest compression as you learned in your CPR training.
8. Check again for foreign body using finger sweep of mouth. Grasp the tongue and lower jaw between thumb and fingers.
   a. Pull upward.
   b. With the index finger of your other hand, follow down along the inside of one cheek, toward the base of the tongue.
   c. Sweep in from the side (hooking motion).
   d. Do not poke straight in because that may push the object down.
   e. Use a hooking action, across toward the other cheek, to loosen and remove the object.
9. After sweeping in the mouth, tip the head back, lift the chin, and try to give breaths. If air will not go into the lungs, repeat abdominal thrusts, finger sweeping, and breaths.

NOTE: A victim who is given mouth-to-mouth breathing or abdominal thrusts may vomit. Roll a victim who vomits away from you on one side and clean out the mouth with your fingers. Then roll the victim back and continue repeating the sequence of breaths, thrusts, and finger sweeps.

Airway Obstruction

Relief of obstruction should only be attempted if:
■ The cough becomes ineffective.
■ There is increased respiratory difficulty, accompanied by a high-pitched noise while inhaling.

In children under one year of age, a combination of 5 back blows and 5 chest thrusts is best. If you can see foreign body, remove it but *do not* perform finger sweeps.

In older children, use the adult procedure for relief of airway obstruction. But, do *not* use a blind finger sweep. Use finger to remove obstruction only if you can see it.

Bleeding

Remember that if the person is conscious, the extent of injuries is likely to be far less severe than if the person is unconscious. With the unconscious person, the next imminent threat to life is the loss of blood. Bleeding is usually easy to see. Sometimes, however, the bleeding is internal. Internal bleeding will only be evidenced by the signs of shock as they are described in the next section. Examine the person for evidence of bleeding. Take the following steps to prevent additional loss:

- Identify the location of bleeding area.
- Have victim apply continuous pressure over bleeding area, if able.
- If not, apply continuous, direct pressure over bleeding area with a pad or even your hand, if necessary, Figure 44–8.
- Call for help.
- If seepage occurs, increase the padding and pressure.
- If there are no broken bones and there is no pain, raise the wounded area above the level of the heart, but do not release pressure. This will help to reduce bleeding.
- Support the elevated area.
- Use binding of some kind to hold the padded pressure if there is bleeding from more than one area.

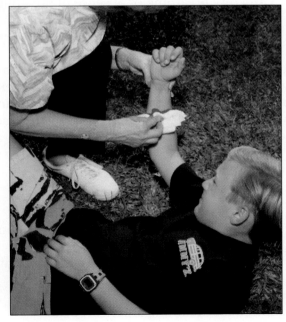

FIGURE 44–8. Apply direct pressure over bleeding area.

- If you have learned the location of the major blood vessels which control blood flow to an area and direct pressure seems ineffective, apply pressure over the appropriate vessel to stem hemorrhage.
- Keep the person comfortably warm and quiet until help arrives.

NOTE: People who are bleeding are often very frightened. Their anxiety contributes to the development of shock. Continuous reassurance is essential.

Shock

Shock is defined as a disturbance of the oxygen supply to the tissues and return of blood to the heart. It can follow:

- Any severe injury
- Cardiac arrest
- Acute hemorrhage
- Severe pain
- Excessive loss of body fluids as seen in severe burns

Signs and Symptoms of Shock

Early signs and symptoms include:
- Pale, cold skin that is moist to the touch
- Complaints of feeling weak
- Weak, rapid pulse
- Rapid and irregular breathing
- Restlessness and anxiety
- Perspiration

Later signs of shock include:
- Mottled skin
- Lack of response
- Sunken eyes with pupils that are dilated and vacant expression
- Loss of consciousness
- Drop in body temperature

Preventive Measures

Anxiety contributes to the situation, but shock can be prevented if steps are taken early. Prevention of shock includes controlling situations that could trigger it.

- Call for help—activate emergency medical system.
- Keep the person lying down and quiet.
- Maintain normal body temperature. Provide light warmth if needed.
- Position person with the feet and legs slightly higher than body and head (Trendelenburg position), unless contraindicated by specific

injury. This assures improved circulation to vital organs.

— If burn areas are involved, however, the area should be elevated unless it causes the person pain.

— If fractures are involved, make sure the part is splinted (braced) before positioning the person to prevent shock.

■ Intravenous fluids to improve circulatory volume and low volumes of oxygen will be given.

— This equipment will be readily at hand in a care facility.

— In the community, the emergency personnel answering the call will bring the supplies necessary to manage fluid and oxygenation.

■ Give small amounts of fluids by mouth if help is delayed over an hour and the person's condition seems to be deteriorating. A solution of tepid water, salt, and baking soda can be given.

■ Fluids should not be given if:
— Surgery is possible.
— There is abdominal injury.
— The person is likely to vomit.
— The person is apt to convulse.
— The person is unconscious.

■ Continue to monitor pulse and respirations.

Unless shock is controlled, death can occur. Until help arrives, your care can often make the difference between life and death.

Fainting

When the blood supply to the brain is reduced for a short time, the person loses consciousness. This is called fainting. Fainting is usually a temporary condition. It is corrected as soon as blood flow to the brain is restored.

Unfortunately, when consciousness is lost, the person is likely to fall and injuries can occur. Patients who are ambulating for the first time should be assisted. If fainting occurs, and the patient falls, do not try to hold the patient upright. Ease the patient to the floor to prevent injury. Assist patients who are *feeling* faint to a safe position.

The patient who is sitting and feels faint, light-headed, dizzy, and nauseated should be encouraged to lower her head between her knees. Pallor, cold skin, perspiration, or visual changes also signal fainting. To provide assistance to a fainting person, the nursing assistant should:

■ Help the patient to assume a protected position sitting or lying down.
■ Loosen tight clothing.
■ Position head lower than heart to encourage cerebral blood flow.
■ Allow person to rest for at least 10 minutes.
■ Maintain normal body temperature.
■ Call for additional help.
■ Monitor pulse and respirations.

Heart Attack

Heart attacks can occur in any age group, but the high-risk group includes those who:

■ Are overweight
■ Smoke
■ Have atherosclerosis
■ Remain immobile for long periods
■ Are older
■ Have diabetes
■ Have a history of heart disease

Signs and Symptoms

Signs and symptoms include:

■ Crushing pain that can radiate up the jaw and down the arm or heaviness in chest.
■ Perspiring, skin cold and clammy.
■ Nausea and vomiting.
■ Pale to grayish color of the face.
■ Difficulty breathing or absence of breathing.
■ Loss of consciousness.
■ Irregular pulse or loss of pulse. The loss of heart function is called cardiac arrest.

At other times, the pain of the attack may resemble indigestion and the person remains conscious. Do not be fooled into thinking that the degree of pain indicates the severity of the attack. Both victims need immediate attention.

Action

In the health care facility:

■ Immediately signal for help.
■ Stay with the patient if the patient is conscious.
■ Help keep him calm.
■ Elevate the head of the bed to assist breathing.
■ Provide oxygen, if available.

If the patient is unconscious:

■ Check for breathing and heart beat.
■ If necessary, institute CPR, if you have been trained, until a professional takes charge.

In the community and if the person is conscious, proceed as follows.

1. Assess the situation.
2. If possible, activate the emergency medical system.
3. Allow the person to sit up or assume a position of comfort. Loosen clothing about the neck.
4. Keep onlookers away.
5. Provide fresh air but keep the person comfortably warm.
6. Monitor pulse and respirations.
7. Be prepared to initiate CPR.

In the community, if the person is unconscious, follow Steps 1 and 2. Then:

3. Check for breathing and heart beat.
4. If heart beat is present but breathing has ceased, establish an open airway, and institute mouth-to-mouth resuscitation.
5. If breathing and heart beat have ceased (cardiac and respiratory arrest), institute CPR until a professional takes charge.

Stroke

A stroke (cerebral vascular accident or CVA) occurs when there is an interference with normal blood circulation to the brain. It usually is caused by a clot that has lodged in a cerebral vessel or by a blood vessel that has ruptured.

Signs and Symptoms

The severe stroke victim usually:
■ Experiences seizure activity
■ Loses consciousness
■ Experiences difficulty breathing
■ Develops paralysis on one side of the body and of the muscles of either side of the face
■ Has unequal pupil reaction

The stroke patient with a less severe stroke may experience:
■ Disorientation
■ Dizziness
■ Headache
■ Slurred speech
■ Memory loss
■ Loss of consciousness

Action

First aid includes:
■ Maintaining an airway

■ Providing mouth-to-mouth breathing as needed
■ Administering CPR, if needed (qualified individual)
■ Positioning person on one side so fluids will drain from the mouth
■ Maintaining normal body temperature
■ Keeping the person quiet until help arrives or transportation to a medical facility can be arranged

Seizures (Convulsions)

Seizures or convulsions are sometimes seen when there is:
■ Omitted antiseizure medications.
■ Drug overdose.
■ Head injury.
■ Degenerative brain disease.
■ Stroke.
■ Infectious disease and fevers.
■ Tumors.
■ Hypoglycemic reactions.
■ Seizure disorder. Seizure disorder is largely controlled today with medication, but unusual stress, medication omission, and other factors can cause a convulsion.

Signs and Symptoms

Seizures do not always follow the same pattern. Their range may be:
■ A momentary loss of contact with the environment, (*petit mal*), in which there are no random or uncontrolled movements but the person seems to stare blankly.
■ A grand mal form in which:
— Consciousness is lost.
— The person falls.
— The person becomes rigid.
— Uncontrolled voluntary movements occur.
— Frothing at the mouth occurs.
— The person becomes cyanotic.
— The person loses control of bladder and/or bowel function

Gradually the seizure lessens and the person recovers. The person is usually:
■ Confused
■ Disoriented for a period of time
■ Very tired

Action

If you witness a seizure, take the following steps:
- Do not restrain the movements.
- Protect from injury. For example, move any objects that might cause injury.
- Loosen clothing around the neck.
- Maintain an airway by positioning. Do not try to put anything in the mouth.
- Cradle head.
- Observe seizure.

After Seizure Activity Stops

- Turn person to the side so fluid or vomitus can drain freely after the movements subside.
- Give mouth-to-mouth resuscitation if breathing is not resumed following the seizure.
- Allow the person to rest undisturbed.
- Stay with patient but summon medical assistance.
- Report and record seizure activity: time, length of seizure, body parts or activity involved.

Electric Shock

Electric shock can occur in the:
- Community when high-tension wires are knocked down in accidents or storms
- Health facility because of frayed wires and faulty outlets or fixtures

Severe burns and cardiac and respiratory arrest can result from electric shock. You must protect yourself as you try to rescue the victim.

Action

- Turn off the source of electricity from the terminal source, such as at a fuse box, before touching the person, if possible.
- If the source of electricity cannot be controlled, try to move the victim away with some non-conductive material. Dry wood is a good non-conductor, a broom handle, for example.
- Once free of electrical source, check victim for breathing and pulse.
- Summon medical help.
- Administer CPR, if necessary.
- Once breathing and heart function are restored, check for burns and other injury. Keep person lying down and comfortable.
- Give first aid for burns or other injuries.

SUMMARY

Emergency situations can occur without warning at any time. A person who has been specially trained in the techniques of first aid can be of great service.
- Never overestimate your abilities.
- Use the special skills you have been taught wisely.

Special training will enable you to assess injuries and know the proper steps to follow in:
- Calling for help
- Carrying out life-saving skills such as mouth-to-mouth resuscitation
- Controlling bleeding
- Administering CPR
- Helping stroke, heart attack, and electrically shocked victims

UNIT REVIEW

A. True/False. Answer the following statements true or false by circling T or F.

T F 1. You need no special instruction to give CPR.

T F 2. CPR is needed if heart and circulation fail.

T F 3. The Heimlich maneuver is used to stop bleeding.

T F 4. The person in shock should be kept quiet and lying down.

T F 5. When controlling bleeding, the part should be elevated.

B. Matching. Match Column I with Column II.

Column I

_____ 6. person needing first aid

_____ 7. bleeding to excess

_____ 8. care given when victim has no breathing or heart beat

_____ 9. signaled by a drop in blood pressure

_____ 10. emergency care

Column II

a. arrest

b. first aid

c. victim

d. CPR

e. contraindicated

f. hemorrhage

g. splintered

h. shock

C. Multiple Choice. Choose the answer that best completes each of the following sentences by circling the proper letter.

11. An organization that offers instruction in CPR is the
    a. American Diabetes Association.
    b. American Association of Nurses.
    c. Association for the Blind.
    d. American Heart Association.

12. First aid is care given
    a. immediately to victims of injury.
    b. immediately to victims of sudden illness.
    c. if medical help is delayed.
    d. All of the above.

13. Which of the following is a life-threatening situation requiring intervention? A person who
    a. broke a finger.
    b. fell and bruised a knee.
    c. is in shock.
    d. is coughing.

14. The first step you should take when arriving on the scene of an accident is to
    a. stop a passerby.
    b. assess the situation.
    c. move the victims to one side.
    d. help the victims get up and walk.

15. To assist a person who has fainted
    a. help the person to stand up and walk to circulate the blood.
    b. cover the person with several blankets.
    c. loosen tight clothing.
    d. position the person's head higher than the heart.

16. To assist the person experiencing a seizure, you should
    a. keep the person as active as possible.
    b. restrain the person's movements.
    c. keep the head straight.
    d. maintain an airway and protect person from injury.

17. You suspect the patient is in shock because the
    a. blood pressure is elevated.
    b. face is flushed.
    c. skin is cold and clammy.
    d. pulse is full and bounding.

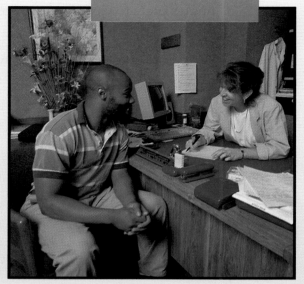

Employment Opportunities

OBJECTIVES

As a result of this unit, you will be able to:

- ■ Spell and define terms.
- ■ List nine objectives to be met in obtaining and maintaining employment.
- ■ Follow a process for self-appraisal.
- ■ Name sources of employment for nursing assistants.
- ■ Prepare a résumé and a letter of resignation.
- ■ List the steps for a successful interview.
- ■ List steps for continuing development in your career.

VOCABULARY

Learn the meaning and the correct spelling of the following words:

job interview	reference
networking	résumé

Having completed a program as a nursing assistant, you are now ready to look for employment. You will want to be as successful as an employee as you were as a student.

Meet the objectives presented in this unit of study and the task will be made much easier.

As an employed nursing assistant, you will receive hepatitis B vaccine at your employer's expense. In addition you will be tested yearly for tuberculosis. Both of these procedures are protective for you and for your patients.

Objective 1: Self-appraisal

The first objective is to determine your personal assets and limitations that could influence your choice of employment. To do this:

- ■ Divide a piece of paper into three columns.
- ■ Title one column *assets*, one *limitations*, and one *solutions*.
- ■ Honestly review all of the positive contributions you can make to an employment situation and list them. For example:

— Your preference in the care of certain patients
— Your caring attitude
— Special skill you have with particular patients
— Your personal appearance
■ Frankly review all the limitations that might make certain employment less obtainable. For example, consider:
— Home responsibilities
— Specific hours you can work
— Transportation problems
— Physical limitations
■ Review possible solutions so that you reduce the number of limitations. The fewer limitations you have at the beginning of your job search, the more you expand the possibilities for employment.

Make your lists, review them, and add to them over several days.

Objective 2: Search for All Employment Opportunities

Having thought through your assets and limitations and found as many solutions to the limitations as possible, you are ready to search for employment possibilities. Possible sources for the search process are all the agencies or facilities that employ nursing assistants:

■ Physicians' offices
■ Blood banks
■ Clinics
■ Hospices
■ Homes for aged/disabled
■ Nursing homes
■ Hospitals
■ Home health care agencies
■ Rehabilitation centers
■ Telephone directory—select facilities that meet your specific needs for available transportation or specific type of care.
■ Classified ads—found in the newspaper
— Look for facilities in your area.
— Consider the type of work you are willing to do.
— Consider the shifts that have openings.
— Note the person to contact for an interview or additional information.
■ Facility in which you received your clinical experience

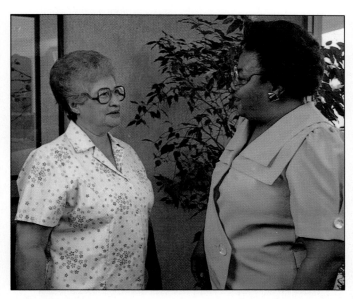

FIGURE 45–1. Friends, classmates, and colleagues are valuable sources of information about potential jobs.

— Administrators sometimes offer jobs to new nursing assistants who trained in their facility.
— Job openings may be posted on the employee bulletin board.
■ Friends and colleagues
— Friends may know of possible openings.
— Colleagues may put you in touch with others who may have potential job connections, Figure 45–1.
— A current term for these activities is networking

Objective 3: Assemble a Proper Résumé

A résumé is a written summary of work and educational history, Figure 45–2. You should:
■ Prepare several copies.
■ Always keep a copy for yourself.
■ Type the résumé for a neat appearance.
■ Carry a copy whenever you seek employment.
■ Use the résumé as a ready reference when you fill out forms.
■ Update the résumé regularly.
The résumé should be carefully prepared to include:
■ Your name, address, and telephone number.
■ Your educational background.
— List your most recent education first.
— Give dates.
— Include a brief summary of the content.

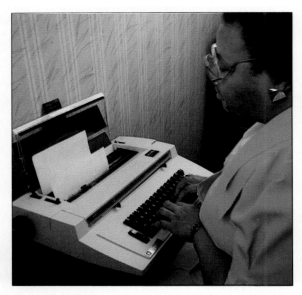

FIGURE 45–2. Carefully prepare a résumé and keep it current.

■ Your work history over the last five years, especially if it gives evidence of successful experiences in the same or related areas as the job for which you are applying.
■ Proof of being on the State Nurse Aide Registry.
■ List of any continuing education classes you have attended.
■ Other experiences you have had. Include jobs that show initiative, reliability, trustworthiness, and worthwhile ways you have spent your time.
■ References—a list of three people who know you and can verify your abilities.
■ Some personal information that indicates your interests and activities.

It is not necessary to include the following in your résumé, although some of this information may be shared during the interview:
■ Age
■ Marital status
■ Religion
■ Sex
■ Height
■ Weight

Objective 4: Validate References

References are people who know you and who would be willing to comment either in writing or verbally over the telephone about you and your abilities. Be sure to include accurate titles, names, addresses, and telephone numbers when listing these references.

References:
■ Should give you permission to use their names, Figure 45–3.
■ Should know you well enough to make an honest evaluation.
■ Should not be related to you.
■ May need to have their memories refreshed about dates of employment or experiences you have stated in your résumé.

Objective 5: Make Specific Applications for Work

Handle this part of the job search process in a business-like way by:
■ Selecting three facilities that interest you most.
■ Calling and asking for the director of nursing or personnel department.
■ Telling the person who answers that you are interested in learning if there are any openings for a nursing assistant, and if so, what application procedure is to be followed.
■ Being prepared to answer questions about your preparation and experience. Have your résumé in your hand.
■ Making an appointment for an interview if possible. A job interview is an opportunity for the person applying for a job and the employer's representative to learn about each other. Each person has the opportunity to ask questions to determine if the job seeker has the qualifications that match the needs of the job available.
■ Completing an application form, Figure 45–4A and B. Use your résumé to be sure you com-

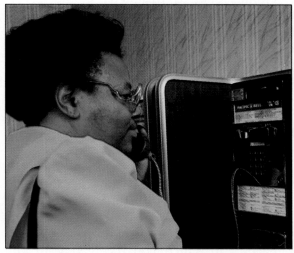

FIGURE 45–3. Get permission before using names for references.

CUSHMAN MANAGEMENT ASSOCIATES   **EMPLOYER:**

APPLICATION FOR EMPLOYMENT

We are an equal opportunity employer. Federal and state laws prohibit discrimination in employment practices based on race, color, religion, sex, age, handicap, disability, or national origin. No question on this application is asked for the purpose of limiting or excluding any applicant's consideration for employment
because of his or her race, color, religion, sex, age, handicap, disability, or national origin.

Name: Last	First	Middle	Social Security No.	Telephone No.
Address: Street	City	State Zip Code	Licensed Nurses Only	
			Mass. Reg. No.	Date Granted:
If your records may be under a name other than indicated above, please specify:			Last Renewal:	Expiration Date:

Are you a citizen of the United States? ☐ yes ☐ no	If you are not a U.S. Citizen, do you have the legal right to remain permanently in the United States? ☐ yes ☐ no	Explain
Are you between the ages of 18 and 70? ☐ yes ☐ no	Do you know of any fact that would limit or impair your ability to perform the functions of the job you are applying for? ☐ yes ☐ no	Describe
Date of last Physical Examination:	Family Physician:	I authorize my doctor to release to you the results of my pre-employment and subsequent medical examinations, and to discuss those results with you. ☐ yes ☐ no

Position desired: Hours desired: Salary expected:

Specialized training or experience
not shown on other side of form:

Where now employed?	Reason for desiring change:

Have you ever pleaded guilty   ☐ yes   If yes to either, please explain:
or been convicted of a felony?   ☐ no

or a misdemeanor other than a first conviction
for drunkenness, simple assault, speeding, minor   ☐ yes
traffic violations, affray, or disturbance of the peace ☐ no
within the past 5 years?

In case of emergency notify	name	relationship
	address	telephone

*I authorize the schools, employers, and individuals listed in this application to release any information regarding my previous employment,
character, general reputation and personal characteristics.   ☐ yes ☐ no

I certify that the statements I have made in this application are true and hereby grant the employer permission to verify the accuracy and completeness of this
information and to investigate all references and educational records. I understand that any false or misleading statements made by me on this application or in
conjunction with my physical examination will be sufficient cause for the rejection of this application or for immediate dismissal if such false or misleading
information is discovered after my employment. If I am accepted for employment, I agree to abide by the rules and regulations of the employer.

Signed _____

Date _____

"It is unlawful in Massachusetts to require or administer a lie detector test as a condition of employment or continued employment. An employer who violates this
law shall be subject to criminal penalties and civil liability".

E-2

FIGURE 45–4A. On application forms, answer all questions to the best of your ability. Be sure the information is
accurate. *(Form courtesy of Danvers Twin Oaks Nursing Home.)*

EDUCATION

Name and Location of Schools or Colleges	Major Subject	Did You Graduate?	College Degree	Period of Attendance From	To

FORMER EMPLOYERS AND EXPERIENCE (References)

	Name and Address	Nature of Experience	Period From	To	Salary	Reason for Leaving
1.						
2.						
3.						
4.						

PERSONAL REFERENCES   (Not Relatives)

	Name	Address	Phone	Business
1.				
2.				

(APPLICANT PLEASE DO NOT WRITE IN SPACE BELOW)

Interview by _____ Date _____ 19____

Date to Start Work _____ 19 ____ Department _____

Position _____ Temporary _____ Permanent ____

Starting Salary/Wage _____ _____

Remarks _____

_____

_____

_____

REFERENCE CHECK

EMPLOYER #1 _____

_____

#2 _____

_____

#3 _____

_____

PERSONAL #1 _____

_____

#2 _____

_____

COMPLETED BY_____

EXIT INTERVIEW

RESIGNED   RELEASED   ON LEAVE   CIRCLE RATING

Ability as _____	Excellent	Poor	Good	Fair	Average
Ability to work in a group _____	Average	Good	Poor	Excellent	Fair
Cooperation with others_____	Good	Fair	Average	Poor	Excellent
Intelligence; ability to grasp ideas _____	Poor	Good	Fair	Average	Excellent
Personality_____	Good	Average	Poor	Excellent	Fair
Initiative; Leadership _____	Fair	Good	Excellent	Average	Poor
Stability; Dependability; Punctuality _____	Average	Poor	Fair	Good	Excellent
Character; Integrity; Honesty _____	Excellent	Good	Average	Fair	Poor
Personal Appearance_____	Fair	Average	Excellent	Poor	Good

Interview by_____ Date _____

Reason for Leaving _____

Additional Comments_____

FIGURE 45–4A.   Continued. *(Form courtesy of Danvers Twin Oaks Nursing Home)*

EMPLOYMENT APPLICATION
(PLEASE TYPE OR PRINT IN INK)

CHARTER SUBURBAN HOSPITAL
16453 South Colorado Avenue
Paramount, California 90723

PERSONAL DATA

LAST NAME	FIRST		TELEPHONE ( )	DATE
ADDRESS	STREET	CITY	STATE	ZIP	HOW LONG?
PREVIOUS ADDRESS	STREET	CITY	STATE	ZIP	HOW LONG?

OTHER NAMES UNDER WHICH YOU HAVE WORKED | HOW WERE YOU REFERRED TO US FOR EMPLOYMENT?

POSITION DESIRED:

1ST CHOICE: 2ND CHOICE: | DATE YOU CAN START:

SHIFT YOU CAN WORK:

☐ DAYS , ☐ P.M.s ☐ NIGHTS ☐ WEEKENDS

ARE YOU APPLYING FOR: ☐ FULL-TIME ☐ PART-TIME
☐ ON CALL/FLOAT ☐ TEMPORARY

SOCIAL SECURITY NUMBER
__ __ __

DO YOU HAVE THE LEGAL RIGHT TO WORK IN THIS COUNTRY? ☐ YES ☐ NO

ARE YOU UNDER 18 YEARS OLD? ☐ YES ☐ NO

LIST FRIENDS & RELATIVES (STATE RELATIONSHIP) EMPLOYED BY THIS HOSPITAL | TRANSPORTATION AVAILABLE? ☐ YES ☐ NO

HAVE YOU EVER BEEN CONVICTED OF A FELONY? IF YES, DESCRIBE THE CIRCUMSTANCES:
(A FELONY CONVICTION WILL NOT AUTOMATICALLY DISQUALIFY YOU FOR EMPLOYMENT)_____

EDUCATION

	NAME AND LOCATION	CIRCLE LAST YEAR COMPLETED	DATE LAST ATTENDED	MAJOR FIELD OF STUDY	DIPLOMA OR DEGREE RECEIVED
HIGH SCHOOL		1 2 3 4	✕		
COLLEGE OR UNIVERSITY		1 2 3 4			
PROFESSIONAL TRAINING		YEARS ATTENDED			
GRADUATE SCHOOL					
OTHER					

OFFICE SKILLS (CLERICAL APPLICANTS ONLY)

☐ TYPING_____WPM   ☐ DICTAPHONE   ☐ MEDICAL TERMINOLOGY
☐ SHORTHAND/SPEEDWRITING_____WPM   ☐ KEYPUNCH   ☐ OTHER_____
☐ 10 KEY ADDING MACHINE   ☐ PBX

PROFESSIONAL LICENSURE

TYPE	LICENSE NUMBER	STATE	EXPIRATION DATE

AP1018

FIGURE 45–4B. On application forms, answer all questions to the best of your ability. Be sure the information is accurate. *(Form courtesy of Charter Suburban Hospital)*

EMPLOYMENT (LIST MOST RECENT FIRST)

MAY WE CONTACT PRESENT EMPLOYER? ☐ YES ☐ NO

FROM MO YR / TO MO YR	EMPLOYER'S NAME	POSITION & DUTIES	PRESENT OR LAST SALARY	REASON FOR LEAVING
STREET ADDRESS	CITY STATE			
PHONE NO. ( )	SUPERVISOR'S NAME & TITLE			
FROM MO YR / TO MO YR	EMPLOYER'S NAME			
STREET ADDRESS	CITY STATE			
PHONE NO. ( )	SUPERVISOR'S NAME & TITLE			
FROM MO YR / TO MO YR	EMPLOYER'S NAME			
STREET ADDRESS	CITY STATE			
PHONE NO. ( )	SUPERVISOR'S NAME & TITLE			
FROM MO YR / TO MO YR	EMPLOYER'S NAME			
STREET ADDRESS	CITY STATE			
PHONE NO. ( )	SUPERVISOR'S NAME & TITLE			
FROM MO YR / TO MO YR	EMPLOYER'S NAME			
STREET ADDRESS	CITY STATE			
PHONE NO. ( )	SUPERVISOR'S NAME & TITLE			

DO YOU HAVE A MEDICAL/PHYSICAL CONDITION WHICH COULD LIMIT YOUR JOB PERFORMANCE?

☐ YES ☐ NO. IF "YES", PLEASE EXPLAIN:_____

_____

_____

I CERTIFY THAT ALL STATEMENTS MADE ON THIS APPLICATION ARE TRUE AND THAT ANY MISSTATEMENTS MAY BE CAUSE FOR TERMINATION OR DENIAL OF EMPLOYMENT WITH CHARTER SUBURBAN HOSPITAL. PERMISSION IS GRANTED TO INVESTIGATE AND VERIFY EMPLOYMENT AND EDUCATION. I UNDERSTAND THAT EMPLOYMENT WITH CHARTER SUBURBAN HOSPITAL IS CONTINGENT UPON PASSING AN ANNUAL HEALTH ASSESSMENT THEREAFTER.
CHARTER SUBURBAN HOSPITAL IS AN EQUAL OPPORTUNITY EMPLOYER.

_____ _____ _____
SIGNATURE   DATE

FIGURE 45–4B. Continued. *(Form courtesy of Charter Suburban Hospital)*

plete the form. Make sure the information is accurate, spelled correctly, complete and neat.

■ Learning the name of the person to whom you are speaking.

■ Thanking the person speaking with you by name.

Repeat the steps until you land the job.

Objective 6: Participate in a Successful Interview

Approach the interview in three steps.

1. Preparation:
    ■ Plan what you will wear.
    ■ Do not overdress, but be neat and clean.
    ■ Check your clothes for loose or lost buttons or stains.
    ■ Be sure to take a bath and use deodorant.
    ■ Brush teeth.
    ■ Make sure fingernails are short and clean.
    ■ Polish your shoes.
    ■ Make sure your hair is neat.
    ■ Be sure if you have a beard or a mustache that it is trimmed.
    ■ Do not chew gum.
    ■ Prepare a list of questions you want to ask.
    ■ Have your résumé in hand.

2. Actual interview:
    ■ Be on time.
    ■ Offer a firm handshake.
    ■ Stand until you are invited to sit.
    ■ Remember you are selling yourself.
    ■ Be careful of body language.
    ■ Share information willingly with the interviewer, Figure 45–5.

■ Use your list to learn information important to you such as:
    — Responsibilities (ask for a job description)
    — Hours of work
    — Uniform regulations
    — Opportunities for future assistance/ financial aid to further your education
    — Starting salary
    — Fringe benefits such as health insurance
    — Schedule of raises
■ At the end of the interview:
    — Thank the interviewer whether you are hired or not.
    — Leave a copy of the résumé for future reference.

3. After the interview, when you get home:
    ■ Write a short thank-you note to the person who interviewed you, Figure 45–6, thanking her for her time and the opportunity to be considered for the job.
    ■ Review in your mind the interview. Plan changes you would make to improve future interviews.

Objective 7: Keep the Job

You can make your new position secure if you:
■ Arrive on time prepared to work.
■ Follow policies and procedures outlined in your orientation.
■ Follow the rules of ethical and legal conduct.
■ Recognize your limitations and seek help.
■ Have an open and positive attitude.

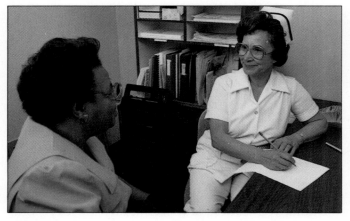

FIGURE 45–5. You have to sell yourself and your services during the interview.

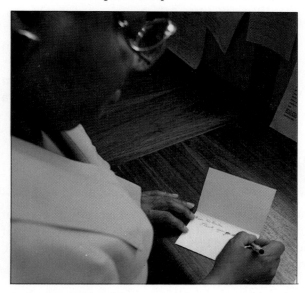

FIGURE 45–6. Write a thank-you note after the interview. It helps the interviewer remember you.

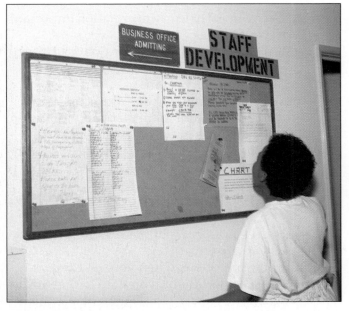

FIGURE 45–7. Once employed, take advantage of staff development programs to advance your education.

Objective 8: Continue to Grow Throughout Your Career

You will continue to grow if you take advantage of each new experience and opportunity you find.

- Keep your certificate current.
- Seek out knowledgeable staff members and watch and learn by their example.
- Don't be afraid to ask questions at the appropriate times.
- Use the nursing medical literature to learn more about the conditions of the patients.
- Participate in care conferences with an open mind so that each conference can become a learning experience for you.

SUMMARY

Finding the right employment after completion of your nursing assistant program can be made easier if you set objectives and meet each one in a systematic fashion.

The steps to take include:

- Appraising your assets and limitations
- Searching the job market

- Complete 24 hours of continuing education each year, Figure 45–7.
- Investigate the possibilities of advancing your formal education by:
  — Enlisting in general education courses offered at the high school or college in your area.
  — Taking courses in communication, listening, English, and psychology.
  — Participating in in-service education programs at your facility or at nearby hospitals.
  — Enrolling in minicourses offered by hospitals on subjects of general public interest, such as hypertension, weight control, and diabetes.
  — Selecting books at the library that pertain to health issues.
  — Researching programs that can prepare you for professional advancement into the ranks of LVN or RN.

Objective 9: Resign Properly from Employment

When you are ready to leave your present situation, you should do so pleasantly and properly.

- Give as much notice as possible—usually equal to the time of the pay period.
- Submit a letter of resignation and include:
  — Date
  — Salutation to the director of nursing
  — Brief explanation of your reasons for leaving
    NOTE: Even if you feel upset by something that happened, make your reasons positive in nature.
  — Date your resignation is to be effective
  — Thank-you for the opportunity to have worked and grown with the experience of working in that facility
  — Your signature

- Securing and holding the position
- Properly resigning when it is time to make a career change

Learning is a life-long process. It may involve additional education and the ability to leave one position to move to another.

UNIT REVIEW

A. True/False. Answer the following statements true or false by circling T or F.

T F 1. The employer may ask your religion during an interview.

T F 2. In making a self-appraisal, you need only list the things you could provide an employer.

T F 3. What you wear to an interview isn't important.

T F 4. The availability of transportation needs to be considered when choosing a job.

T F 5. The interview should provide you with information about the exact responsibilities you will have.

T F 6. Checking with the administrator of the facility in which you had your clinical experience for job possibilities is proper.

T F 7. If you fail to get the job after the interview, there is nothing left for you to do about the situation.

T F 8. At the end of every interview, you should thank the interviewer even if you didn't get the job.

T F 9. Participation in care conferences can be a way to continue to grow.

T F 10. When resigning, give ample notice.

B. Multiple Choice. Choose the answer that best completes each of the following sentences by circling the proper letter.

11. The first step in finding a job is
    a. making phone calls.
    b. doing a self-assessment.
    c. looking in the paper.
    d. writing letters to friends.

12. Jobs can be found through
    a. classified ads.
    b. networking with friends.
    c. telephone directories.
    d. All of the above.

13. A compilation of your work history is called a/an
    a. résumé.
    b. interview.
    c. summary.
    d. None of the above.

14. Which of the following would you include in your résumé?
    a. Marital status
    b. Religion
    c. Weight
    d. Address

15. Before putting a reference name down
    a. ask permission.
    b. call the prospective employer.
    c. tell the person you are going to use his name.
    d. All of the above.

C. Completion. Complete the following statements in the space provided.

16. You need to assess your strengths and limitations as a nursing assistant. Explain how you could proceed: _____

_____

17. Ten sources of employment opportunities for a nursing assistant in search of work are:
    a. _____
    b. _____
    c. _____
    d. _____
    e. _____
    f. _____
    g. _____
    h. _____
    i. _____
    j. _____

18. You are going on an interview. The information you will want to learn includes:
    a. _____
    b. _____
    c. _____
    d. _____
    e. _____
    f. _____
    g. _____

SELF-EVALUATION Section 11

A. Match the terms in Column I with the statement in Column II.

Column I	Column II
_____ 1. occult	a. arrest
_____ 2. Leboyer method	b. hemorrhage
_____ 3. ostomy	c. incision in perineum
_____ 4. episiotomy	
_____ 5. lochia	d. first breast milk
_____ 6. excessive blood loss	e. birth without violence
_____ 7. colostrum	f. vaginal discharge
_____ 8. suppository	g. hidden
_____ 9. postpartum	h. a cone-shaped solid mass inserted into the rectum for lubrication
_____ 10. stoppage	i. after birth
	j. artificial opening

B. Choose the phrase that best completes each of the following sentences by circling the proper letter.

11. You observe someone having a convulsion. You should
    a. restrain the movements.
    b. force something between the teeth to prevent injury to the tongue.
    c. move articles away that the patient might strike.
    d. encourage the patient to be active following the attack.
    e. keep the person flat on his back following the attack.

12. Your patient has just returned from delivery, looks pale, complains of feeling cold, and begins to shiver. You suspect
    a. she is excited about the delivery.
    b. she is just tired.
    c. she needs something to eat.
    d. she is in danger of shock.
    e. she is really all right and can safely be left alone.

13. When removing and replacing a perineal pad
    a. both sides may be handled.
    b. draw it forward before lifting.
    c. ignore the type of drainage.
    d. lift from the body from front to back.
    e. gloves need not be used.

14. In assisting the nursing mother
    a. use a very tight brassiere.
    b. do not use breast pads since leaking is normal.
    c. assist the mother to wash her hands prior to feeding.
    d. remind her to take her milk suppression medication.
    e. do not wash the breasts frequently.

15. When giving routine ileostomy care you should
    a. not wear gloves.
    b. leave unit unscreened.
    c. dry area around stoma briskly.
    d. not examine drainage.
    e. No answer applies.

16. Employment opportunities may be found
    a. in the classified ads.
    b. through friends.
    c. in the facilities in which you trained.
    d. by networking.
    e. All of the above.

17. When using a Hematest® reagent tablet to check feces for occult blood, add to the tablet and fecal smear
    a. 1 drop of water.   d. 4 drops of water.
    b. 2 drops of water.   e. 5 drops of water.
    c. 3 drops of water.

18. When putting on sterile gloves
    a. leave hands a little moist.
    b. set up a sterile field to open the gloves.
    c. pick both gloves up at the same time.
    d. touch only the inside cuff of the glove with your bare hands.
    e. spread fingers and slip into first glove.

19. A sterile field has been set up and you are to add some 4 × 4 sponges. You
    a. may reach over the sterile field as long as you don't touch it.
    b. place sponges at least 1/2 inch from the edge.
    c. may place the unopened package on the field.
    d. place sponges at least 2 inches away from the edge of the field.
    e. No answer applies.

20. Shock is a life-threatening situation. You would do which of the following?
    a. Elevate the head.
    b. Apply external heat in the form of hot water bags.
    c. Raise the feet and legs.
    d. Restrict all fluids.
    e. Give ice water.

21. Your first task in an emergency is to
    a. move the victims.
    b. assess the situation.
    c. call for help.
    d. ask the victim what happened.
    e. No answer applies.

22. To provide an open airway
    a. place one hand on the throat and one on the forehead.
    b. lift the neck gently and push down on the chin.
    c. lift the neck gently and push down on the forehead.
    d. put both hands under the shoulders.
    e. raise the arms over the head.

23. The easiest way to determine an accurate pulse rate on an infant or child is to
    a. have someone hold the child down.
    b. measure an apical pulse.
    c. measure a radial pulse.
    d. measure a temporal pulse.
    e. measure the blood pressure first.

24. Which of the following are nursing assistant responsibilities when caring for an infant?
    a. maintaining a safe environment.
    b. weighing the infant.
    c. bathing the infant.
    d. collecting specimens.
    e. all of the above.

25. A patient who is choking begins to cough. You had best
    a. administer chest thrusts.
    b. sweep her mouth.
    c. strike her sharply on the back between the shoulder blades.
    d. encourage her to continue coughing.
    e. encourage her to drink water.

26. You sneezed when setting up a sterile field. This means
    a. only the center is sterile.
    b. the outer two inches must now be considered contaminated.
    c. the field can still be used.
    d. the whole set up is considered contaminated.
    e. other materials can still be added to the field.

27. When putting on a sterile glove, the ungloved hand may touch the
    a. inner surface of the glove cuff.
    b. outer surface of the glove cuff.
    c. only the fingertips of the glove.
    d. glove only with a hand covered by another sterile glove.
    e. No answer applies.

28. When inserting a catheter to perform tracheal suctioning, make sure the
    a. Y vent is closed.
    b. Y vent is open.
    c. catheter stays in the nasal area.
    d. catheter is kept dry.
    e. No answer applies.

29. When collecting a urine specimen from a closed drainage system with a sampling port, the nursing assistant must
    a. clamp the drainage tube.
    b. clean the drainage port with an antiseptic wipe.
    c. use a needle to draw the sample.
    d. None of the above.
    e. All of the above.

30. The person you are eating with suddenly begins to choke and grasps his throat. You should
    a. run for help.
    b. start CPR.
    c. use the Heimlich maneuver.
    d. ignore him.
    e. None of the above.

COMPREHENSIVE

FINAL EVALUATION

A. IN EACH QUESTION, SELECT THE BEST ANSWER.

1. **Special health services offered in the community include**
   a. safe drinking water.
   b. statistical services.
   c. immunization procedures.
   d. X-rays.
   e. All of these.

2. **The national health agency is called**
   a. WHO.
   b. the Federal Bureau of Health.
   c. the U.S. Statistical Bureau.
   d. The U.S. Public Health Service.
   e. The National Public Health Service.

3. **Nursing assistants are most often employed in**
   a. homes for the aged.
   b. local health departments.
   c. The World Health Organization.
   d. state sanitation departments.
   e. statistical gathering agencies.

4. **The immediate supervisor of the nursing assistant is**
   a. another nursing assistant.
   b. an RN.
   c. an orderly.
   d. an MD.
   e. None of these.

5. **A nursing assistant failed to check the temperature of an enema solution and the patient was burned. This is a case of**
   a. malpractice.
   b. negligence.
   c. carelessness.
   d. aiding and abetting.
   e. dishonesty.

6. **The nursing assistant starts an intravenous infusion and the patient develops an infection. This is a case of**
   a. malpractice.
   b. negligence.
   c. carelessness.
   d. aiding and abetting.
   e. dishonesty.

7. **The nursing assistant feels unsure of how to manipulate the Circ-O-lectric® bed. She should**
   a. ask another assistant for instructions.
   b. try anyway.
   c. omit turning the patient.
   d. ask the nurse for help.
   e. tell the patient she doesn't know how to manipulate the bed.

8. **The patient offers the nursing assistant a little extra money for the care received. The nursing assistant should**
   a. accept and say nothing.
   b. accept and share with other team members.
   c. refuse courteously.
   d. refuse and abruptly walk out of the room.
   e. pretend the offer wasn't heard.

9. **The nursing assistant learns that the patient has several bank accounts. The assistant should**
   a. inform the charge nurse.
   b. share the information with coworkers.
   c. tell the family this information.
   d. keep this information secret.
   e. let only his family know this information.

10. **The nursing assistant learns that the patient is concerned about the cost of hospitalization. The assistant should**
    a. inform the charge nurse.
    b. share the information with coworkers.
    c. tell the family this information.
    d. keep this information secret.
    e. let only her family know this information.

11. **The patient is terminal and begs the nursing assistant to "pull the plug." The assistant should**
    a. do as asked so the patient will not suffer longer.
    b. explain that God makes those decisions and tell the patient to pray.
    c. report the incident to the team leader.
    d. tell the family.
    e. call a clergy person of the nursing assistant's faith to talk to the patient.

12. **Good grooming is seen when the nursing assistant has**
    a. long, flowing hair.
    b. short, well-kept, clean nails.
    c. bright red nail polish.
    d. dirty shoes and laces.
    e. failed to use a deodorant.

13. **Another nursing assistant asks you to help move a patient up in bed. You should**
    a. refuse. It's not your assignment.
    b. agree to help but be annoyed.
    c. say you are doing more than your share already.
    d. agree in a courteous manner.
    e. say you can only help if the other nursing assistant will do part of your assignment.

14. **Your team leader needs a specimen taken to the laboratory "stat" and asks you to do so.**
    a. You tell her you can't; you are too busy.
    b. You ask another nursing assistant to take the specimen.
    c. You follow directions but give a patient status report to your team leader before leaving.

d. You take the specimen and deliver it upon completion of your assignment.

e. You take the specimen and leave the floor immediately without reporting.

15. **Your patient is very irritable this morning and complains about how slow you are. You know that**
   a. illness brings out the best in people.
   b. people sometimes direct their frustrations about their illness toward other people.
   c. you had better rush the care.
   d. you had better get help to finish the care.
   e. the patient is being unfair and you tell him so.

16. **Which of the following could act as a fomite?**
   a. Drinking cup   d. Dressings
   b. Bedpan   e. All of these.
   c. Instruments

17. **In carrying out the handwashing procedure,**
   a. it is alright to leave suds on the soap.
   b. rinse hands with fingertips down.
   c. rinse hands with fingertips straight up.
   d. use very hot water.
   e. turn faucets on and off with your bare hands.

18. **The best temperature for the patient's room is about**
   a. 65°F.   c. 70°F.   e. 80°F.
   b. 68°F.   d. 75°F.

19. **A patient is being visited by her clergy. You should provide privacy by**
   a. drawing the curtains.
   b. asking the other patients to leave.
   c. asking the other patients not to listen.
   d. telling the cleric to speak softly.
   e. doing nothing.

20. **Your attitude is reflected in your**
   a. courtesy.
   b. cooperation.
   c. emotional control.
   d. tact.
   e. all of these.

21. **Nursing assistants communicate their feelings by**
   a. facial expressions.   d. body language.
   b. choice of words.   e. All of these.
   c. touch.

22. **Your patient has difficulty sleeping. You should consider**
   a. noise in the unit.   d. All of these.
   b. pain.   e. None of these.
   c. worry and anxiety.

23. **The nursing assistant can increase the patient's sense of security by**
   a. hanging his clothes in the closet.
   b. responding angrily to a refusal to cooperate.
   c. providing opportunities for the patient to talk.
   d. taking every remark by the patient personally.
   e. doing every aspect of care that the patient could do.

24. **The nursing assistant demonstrates proper body mechanics by**
   a. having sloping shoulders.
   b. using the right muscles to do the job.
   c. using the smaller back muscles to lift heavy objects.
   d. bending from the waist when picking up objects.
   e. keeping feet close together when picking up an object.

25. **The nursing assistant will turn patients frequently when they are unable to change their own position**
   a. to prevent contractures.
   b. to improve circulation.
   c. to prevent decubitis ulcers.
   d. All of these.
   e. None of these.

26. **The patient is severely burned and unable to turn herself. Which type of bed would most likely be used for such a patient?**
   a. Closed bed   d. Open bed
   b. Circ-O-lectric® bed   e. Gatch bed
   c. Orthopedic bed

27. **Toepleats are put in the occupied bed to prevent**
   a. decubitus.   d. pressure on the chest.
   b. footdrop.   e. None of these.
   c. wristdrop.

28. **The proper temperature for bath water is**
   a. 85°F.   c. 105°F.   e. 125°F.
   b. 95°F.   d. 115°F.

29. **During the bath procedure, other care is given, which includes**
   a. care of teeth.   d. range of motion
   b. care of nails.   exercises.
   c. care of hair.   e. All of these.

30. **Your patient will be most apt to require special mouth care if**
   a. he is unconscious.
   b. he drinks lots of fluids.
   c. he is receiving an IV.
   d. he can't get out of bed.
   e. None of these.

31. **To protect the patient's dentures**
   a. leave them uncovered in the bedside table.
   b. use hot water to clean dentures.
   c. use a heavy stream of water and toothpaste.
   d. store in a denture cup.
   e. wash only the front surfaces.

32. **Which of the following foods would be permitted on a light diet?**
   a. Fried fish
   b. Bran flakes
   c. Applesauce
   d. Broiled pork chops
   e. Green salad with blue cheese dressing

33. **The patient orders read "NPO after 4 PM." This means that the nursing assistant will**
    a. withhold dinner.
    b. force fluids.
    c. encourage patient to ambulate.
    d. do range of motion exercises.
    e. change the patient's diet.

34. **The patient has an order for a clear liquid diet. Which of the following would you omit from the tray?**
    a. Coffee with cream   d. Tea with sugar
    b. Ginger ale   e. None of these.
    c. Strained carrot juice

35. **The patient has dentures and a soft diet has been ordered. What should be omitted from the tray?**
    a. Coffee with cream and sugar
    b. Cooked, sieved peaches
    c. Fried eggs
    d. Toast
    e. Cream of Wheat

36. **You are assigned to give postmortem care. You assemble equipment to**
    a. give a bed bath.
    b. give afternoon (PM) care.
    c. determine vital signs.
    d. care for the body after death.
    e. None of these.

37. **The most accurate temperature reading is taken**
    a. orally.   d. axillary.
    b. rectally.   e. aurally.
    c. vaginally.

38. **A temperature of 98.6°F is equal to**
    a. 32°C.   c. 37°C.   e. 41°C.
    b. 35°C.   d. 39°C.

39. **An oral thermometer should be left in place before reading for**
    a. 1 minute.   d. 4 minutes.
    b. 2 minutes.   e. 5 minutes.
    c. 3 minutes.

40. **When measuring a blood pressure**
    a. apply the cuff 4 inches above the elbow.
    b. first determine the palpated systolic pressure.
    c. pump the gauge up quickly to 180-mm Hg and then release.
    d. place the stethoscope bell over the radial artery.
    e. make sure the cuff is very tight.

41. **A blood pressure of 80/30 should be reported since the patient is probably suffering from**
    a. bradycardia.
    b. tachycardia.
    c. hypertension.
    d. hypotension.
    e. None of these.

42. **The nursing assistant would record vital signs on the**
    a. physician's progress report.
    b. graphic chart.
    c. physical and history.
    d. operative record.
    e. X-ray record.

43. **Your patient is to be transferred to ICU. You would assist in transporting her to the**
    a. isolation care unit.
    b. intermediate care unit.
    c. intensive care unit.
    d. isotope unit.
    e. None of the above.

44. **Your patient is to have f.f. and receive solids *ad. lib.* You will**
    a. encourage the patient to eat but withhold liquids.
    b. place an NPO sign on the bed.
    c. caution the patient to limit his drinking to two glasses of water every eight hours.
    d. encourage fluids and let the patient eat what he wishes.
    e. let the patient drink anything he wants but restrict solid food.

45. **When giving an oral report, include the patient's**
    a. name, age, weight.
    b. name, marital status, diagnosis.
    c. name, location, dependents.
    d. location, diagnosis, age.
    e. name, location, diagnosis.

46. **SOAPE charting is**
    a. procedure oriented.
    b. problem oriented.
    c. order oriented.
    d. using only the graphic chart.
    e. only valid if block printed.

47. **Important rules to remember about charting include**
    a. erasures are permitted.
    b. each entry must be signed.
    c. spaces may be left safely.
    d. entries need not be dated or timed.
    e. All of these.

48. **The time 1 PM is expressed in international time as**
    a. 0100.   c. 1000.   e. 1300.
    b. 0101.   d. 1100.

49. **In which quadrant is the appendix located?**
    a. Upper right   d. Lower left
    b. Upper left   e. Retroperitoneal space
    c. Lower right

50. **Which of the following represents normal body defenses?**
    a. Unbroken skin   d. White blood cells
    b. Gastric juice   e. All of these.
    c. Saliva

51. The patient is on her abdomen with arms flexed and hands under her face, which is turned to one side. This position is
    a. semi-Fowler's.
    b. Sims'.
    c. prone.
    d. Trendelenburg.
    e. dorsal lithotomy.

52. The patient is going to surgery. Which of the following would you check?
    a. The chart for proper records
    b. Presence of prosthesis
    c. Removal of makeup including nail polish
    d. Bed rails up and in high position
    e. All of these.

53. TED hose or elastic bandages are used postoperatively to
    a. support the neck.
    b. support the leg veins.
    c. reduce the flow of blood to the legs.
    d. reduce the flow of blood to the arms.
    e. support the joints during initial ambulation.

54. The patient has small, solid, raised red spots all over the chest. These are best described as
    a. decubiti.
    b. pustules.
    c. papules.
    d. macules.
    e. vesicles.

55. The patient with emphysema is receiving oxygen by nasal cannula. Which of the following precautions should be followed?
    a. No smoking allowed.
    b. Use only woolen blankets.
    c. Keep O_2 running while operating electric equipment.
    d. All of these.
    e. None of these.

56. The patient is recovering from an attack of congestive heart failure. Which of the following applies?
    a. Weigh the patient at the same time daily.
    b. Carefully monitor I & O.
    c. Low-salt diet.
    d. Assist patient by oxygen and positioning.
    e. All of these.

57. Your patient has a fractured femur and is currently in traction. Which of the following applies?
    a. Check for areas of pressure or irritation.
    b. Allow feet to press gently against end of bed.
    c. Keep weights balanced on the floor.
    d. Periodically remove traction to relieve pressure.
    e. All of these.

58. Your patient has diabetes mellitus. Which of the following nursing care will you give?
    a. Strain all urine.
    b. Test urine for acetone.
    c. Serve a high-carbohydrate diet.
    d. Restrict fluids.
    e. All of these.

59. Your patient has had surgery to remove a cataract. You remember that
    a. the patient must avoid abrupt movements.
    b. you should encourage the patient to cough.
    c. glasses will no longer be needed.
    d. hearing will be improved.
    e. paralysis is a frequent complication.

60. Your patient has an order for a Harris flush. You know that
    a. the temperature of the solution should be 115°F.
    b. approximately 1500 ml will be needed.
    c. the tube should be inserted 4 inches.
    d. The container should be raised 5 inches above the hips and then lowered the same distance.
    e. None of these.

61. Your patient has a douche ordered. You know that
    a. the temperature of the solution is 105°F.
    b. the procedure is simple and will not require draping.
    c. the perineum should be cleansed.
    d. this is a sterile procedure.
    e. the patient should assume the prone position.

62. To be successfully employed, you should
    a. only be late for work occasionally.
    b. perform your work as you were taught.
    c. remember you have learned all you will ever have to know.
    d. set your own rules of ethical conduct.
    e. display a negative attitude.

63. When writing a letter of resignation, you should include
    a. the date of the letter.
    b. a salutation to the director of nursing.
    c. a brief explanation of your reasons for leaving.
    d. the date the resignation is effective.
    e. All of these.

64. Which of the following is not a stereotype of the patient in a long-term care facility? They
    a. are not competent to make decisions.
    b. have health needs requiring assistance.
    c. are all old.
    d. have no one who cares about them.
    e. have no interest in sex.

65. You can give your best care to a long-term care patient by recognizing that
    a. admission represents financial stress.
    b. a reversion to childlike behavior signals frustration or fear.
    c. the patient needs to be permitted to make choices.
    d. the patient can participate to some extent in his own care.
    e. All of these.

66. When providing care for older persons, you should remember that they may
    a. sleep less at night but need naps during the day.

b. have a more rapid sensory response to stimuli.
c. have more acute hearing as they age.
d. suddenly increase in height by 1–1½ inches.
e. experience a gradually increasing appetite.

67. **The older person has psychological needs, which include the need to be**
a. loved.
b. able to express love.
c. recognized as worthy.
d. physically and financially secure.
e. All of these.

68. **You best encourage proper nutrition in the elderly when you**
a. serve large meals twice a day.
b. do all the feeding yourself.
c. offer fluids frequently between meals.
d. deep fry foods so they have a pleasing color.
e. None of these.

69. **You may receive a home care assignment**
a. from a private agency that employs you.
b. because the family independently hires you.
c. because the family is a member of an HMO that employs you.
d. because you are employed by an agency that receives Medicare reimbursement.
e. All of these.

70. **Which characteristics will be most helpful when working in a private home? Being**
a. a self-starter.
b. one who needs constant supervision.
c. rigid in your approach to how things should be done.
d. poorly organized.
e. critical.

71. **Which duties would be part of your responsibilities as a nursing assistant?**
a. Washing windows
b. Preparing meals for the client
c. Waxing floors
d. Moving heavy furniture
e. Settling family disputes

72. **Which duties would *not* be part of your functions as a nursing assistant?**
a. Making decisions for a client capable of doing so
b. Light housekeeping
c. Shopping for meals
d. Assisting the client in carrying out ADL
e. Maintaining a safe environment

73. **Sources of danger in the home to be avoided include**
a. allowing clutter to develop.
b. leaving dirty dishes in the sink.
c. overloading electrical outlets.
d. leaving food out.
e. All of these.

74. **One source of updating or learning first-aid skills might be the**
a. American Health Association.
b. American Red Cross.
c. Tuberculosis Association.
d. American Diabetes Association.
e. National Multiple Sclerosis Society.

75. **If you come upon an accident, remember to**
a. speak quickly and excitedly.
b. allow onlookers to form a protective circle.
c. keep calm.
d. take care of the person closest to you first.
e. None of these.

76. **The national emergency number to call is**
a. 911.   c. 211.   e. 742.
b 468.   d. 555.

77. **At the scene of an accident, you should**
a. keep the person quiet.
b. maintain an even body temperature.
c. provide urgent care if necessary.
d. activate the emergency medical service if necessary.
e. All of these.

78. **Nursing assistant duties when caring for a pregnant woman in the first trimester would include**
a. checking the level of the fundus.
b. weighing the patient.
c. advising the patient about proper diet.
d. listening for the fetal heart sounds.
e. checking the patient's temperature.

79. **Signs and symptoms in a pregnant woman that must be reported include**
a. elevated blood pressure.
b. vaginal bleeding.
c. swelling of the hands and feet.
d. complaints of dizziness.
e. All of these.

80. **A patient who has received medication to relieve the discomfort of labor and delivery by epidural route will, when returned to the postpartum floor,**
a. be sound asleep.
b. be able to move her legs.
c. not be able to feel her arms.
d. not be able to feel her legs.
e. not be able to move her toes.

81. **The pregnant woman may undergo a cesarean section if the**
a. mother is overdue.
b. parents want to select the birth date.
c. membranes are intact.
d. fetus is in distress.
e. mother is in active labor.

82. **When examining the postpartum patient's perineum, you should make a report to the nurse if there is**
a. a red lochia.

b. signs of inflammation.
c. a swollen episiotomy.
d. a foul odor.
e. All of these.

83. **Which of the following represents a major stress factor?**
   a. A visit from a grandchild
   b. Loss of a spouse
   c. Getting a new job
   d. Getting a promotion

84. **The person who involuntarily excludes a painful experience from memory is using the defense mechanism of**
   a. denial.   c. projection.
   b. suppression.   d. repression.

85. **A nursing assistant is reprimanded for displaying an uncaring attitude and explains to his coworkers that it is really the patient's fault for being so grouchy. He is using the defense mechanism of**
   a. projection.   c. denial.
   b. reaction formation. d. repression.

86. **You best relate to a demanding patient by**
   a. telling her she will get care when it is her turn.
   b. trying to establish a person-to-person rapport.
   c. ignoring her since all patients get that way sometimes.
   d. being just as demanding as she is.

87. **Your patient is constantly by the sink washing his hands. You know he has been found guilty of child abuse. You might think he is using the defense mechanism of**
   a. conversion.   c. compensation.
   b. fantasy.   d. undoing.

88. **A test performed to diagnose the presence of HIV infection is**
   a. biopsy   d. all of the above
   b. culture   e. none of the above
   c. ELISA

89. **Perineal care means to wash the area**
   a. under the arms
   b. from shoulder to waist
   c. including the genitals and anus
   d. of the buttocks
   e. under the breasts

90. **When giving male perineal care**
   a. gloves are not needed
   b. reposition foreskin after cleansing if uncircumcised
   c. do not wash scrotum
   d. use a large amount of liquid soap
   e. none of the above

91. **When giving female perineal care the nursing assistant should**
   a. use gloves
   b. not use heavy soap application

c. cleanse vulva from pubis toward anus
d. all of the above
e. none of the above

92. **A trochanter roll is**
   a. best made with a sheet
   b. rolled against the patient's feet
   c. rolled against the patient's back
   d. best made from a bath blanket
   e. best made with a towel

93. **Blood loss may be measured by**
   a. marking dressings
   b. measuring with a graduate pitcher.
   c. measuring amounts in hemovac container
   d. all of the above
   e. wringing out the dressing

94. **A special bed filled with sandlike material through which dry warm air circulates is known as the**
   a. Clinitron Air Fluidized therapy unit
   b. Circ-O-lectric bed
   c. Stryker frame
   d. Electric bed
   e. Gatch bed

95. **When using a gait belt the nursing assistant should**
   a. be sure the belt is very tight
   b. adjust the belt just under the axilla
   c. make the belt loose enough to slip fingers between patient and belt
   d. hold belt with an overhand grasp
   e. hold belt with both hands.

96. **The aural thermometer measures temperature of the**
   a. tympanic membrane   d. axilla
   b. oral cavity   e. vagina
   c. rectal cavity

97. **To help prevent falls in a long-term facility**
   a. increase noise and activity.
   b. help residents to get up quickly.
   c. encourage blue/green color schemes.
   d. use tub or shower chairs.
   e. none of these.

98. **To prevent thermal injuries**
   a. follow procedures accurately.
   b. check food temperature before feeding.
   c. follow smoking policy of the facility.
   d. do not use microwave ovens to heat food.
   e. all of these.

99. **When handling soiled linen in an isolation unit, the nursing assistant should**
   a. shake the linen
   b. bag outside the room
   c. fold the dirtiest side outward
   d. single bag soiled Linen
   e. none of the above

100. **Isolation cover gowns should be**
  a. made of moisture resistant material
  b. used when soiling with secretions is likely
  c. used when soiling with excretions is likely
  d. all of the above
  e. none of the above

101. **In which situation should the nursing assistant use gloves**
  a. serving food
  b. giving an enema
  c. giving a routine backrub
  d. carrying out range of motion exercises
  e. ambulating a patient

102. **Which of the following applies to immunization**
  a. vaccines exist for all infectious diseases
  b. vaccine is available for Hepatitis B
  c. vaccine is unavailable for Rubella
  d. vaccines make people more susceptible to an infection
  e. none of the above

103. **Which of the following are "at risk" for infections.**
  a. aged people
  b. young babies
  c. patients with chronic respiratory problems
  d. those infected with HIV
  e. all of the above

104. **An important way to protect yourself from pathogens is to**
  a. keep active and get little sleep
  b. stay on a calorie limited diet
  c. manage stress
  d. all of the above
  e. none of the above

105. **The patient reports feeling anxious, is dyspneic, cyanotic and has a feeling of heaviness in his chest. The nursing assistant should**
  a. let the patient up to ambulate
  b. report immediately to the nurse
  c. lower the head of bed
  d. encourage the patient to take deep breaths
  e. none of the above

106. **The depressed patient may be treated with**
  a. antidepressants
  b. electroshock therapy
  c. talk therapy
  d. all of the above
  e. range of motion exercises

107. **Tuberculosis is often seen today among those who are**
  a. malnourished
  b. debililated
  c. aged
  d. HIV positive
  e. all of the above

108. **When delivering oxygen by nasal cannula the nursing assistant should**
  a. be sure straps are very tight
  b. check for sign of irritation where prongs touch patient
  c. clean only when removed
  d. all of the above
  e. none of the above

109. **The odometer of the nursing assistant's car read 45061 when leaving one client's home and 45068 on arrival at the second client's home. The total mileage traveled should be recorded as**
  a. 3 miles
  b. 5 miles
  c. 6 miles
  d. 7 miles
  e. 9 miles

110. **The basic guidelines for reality orientation include**
  a. speaking clearly and directly
  b. calling residents by pet names
  c. eliminating clocks and calendars
  d. speaking loudly so residents will better understand
  e. giving many directions at once

111. **Validation therapy is a technique which**
  a. helps disoriented people feel good about themselves
  b. denies feelings and memories
  c. denies people based in reality
  d. all of the above
  e. none of the above

112. **When caring for the patient with dementia the nursing assistant should**
  a. use logic to reason with resident
  b. keep the environment stimulating
  c. provide a structured but flexible routine
  d. avoid eye contact with the resident
  e. use physical force to make the resident cooperate

113. **A catastrophic reaction may be signaled by**
  a. increased physical activity
  b. increased talking or mumbling
  c. explosive behavior with physical violence
  d. all of the above
  e. none of the above

114. **To help decrease "sun downing" the nursing assistant might**
  a. feed the evening meal at least two hours before bedtime
  b. increase activity before bedtime
  c. increase the level of caffeine in the diet
  d. give a stimulating backrub
  e. play loud music at bed time

115. **When caring for the disoriented patient the nursing assistant should**
  a. speak slowly and clearly
  b. give two instructions at the same time
  c. use negative comments to change behavior
  d. frequently change the routine so it will not be boring
  e. use physical restraints

116. **Residents have the right to**
    a. full information about health care planning
    b. refuse treatment
    c. take part in the assessment and care planning
    d. make and receive communications
    e. all of the above

117. **Reality orientation helps the disoriented person**
    a. pronounce words correctly
    b. ignore people and place
    c. remain withdrawn
    d. use visual reminders and verbal clues
    e. remember his childhood

118. **Under OBRA Regulations, nursing assistants must**
    a. pass a competency test within four attempts.
    b. complete a 10 hour course
    d. complete a 50 hour course
    d. complete a written and skill test
    e. have a pleasing personality

119. **The Omnibus Budget Reconciliation Act of 1987 is Federal legislation which is also called the**
    a. Hemodialysis Safety Act
    b. Nursing Home Reform Act
    c. The Acute Care Facility Act
    d. the Home Nursing Act
    e. the Nursing Assistant Registration Act

120. **The best way to keep track of wandering residents is to**
    a. use a restraint jacket
    b. apply a sensor around the patient's ankle
    c. keep the patient in bed
    d. paint the exit doors bright red
    e. use a gait belt

121. **Immobility can cause**
    a. pressure sores
    b. restricted circulation.
    c. loss of muscle tone
    d. decreased sensory awareness
    e. all of the above

122. **When restraints *must* be used**
    a. check residents at least every 2 hours
    b. release the restraints every 4 hours
    c. keep the resident in a sitting position
    d. apply restraints according to manufacturer's directions
    e. isolate the resident so other residents won't be disturbed

123. **The nursing assistant can be an effective member of the interdisciplinary team by**
    a. learning about the resident
    b. attending care conferences
    c. recognizing the importance of all team members
    d. getting to know the family
    e. all of the above

124. **It is important to follow techniques which prevent infection transmission in a long term care facility because the elderly**
    a. are more susceptible to infection
    b. bladder empties more efficiently
    c. have a stronger cough reflex
    d. pay close attention to their diets
    e. are more active

125. **The nursing assistant can help prevent infections by helping residents**
    a. maintain adequate fluid intake
    b. maintain proper nutrition
    c. perform exercise programs
    d. all of the above
    e. none of the above

126. **The risk of a resident falling is increased when**
    a. environments are poorly controlled
    b. staff delay attending to resident needs
    c. assistive mobility devices are securely applied
    d. fever medications are taken by the elderly
    e. staff members carefully monitor residents

127. **People with Alzheimer's disease may, after onset, live**
    a. only briefly
    b. only one year
    c. up to two years
    d. up to ten years
    e. up to twenty years

128. **Alzheimer's disease is**
    a. the least common form of dementia
    b. a condition which only affects people one to 5 years
    c. progressive and cannot be cured
    d. known to be caused by a virus
    e. known to be inherited

129. **Which of the following is sexually transmitted**
    a. Chlamydia
    b. HIV
    c. Trichomonas
    d. Gonorrhea
    e. all of the above

130. **When the patient is receiving a feeding the nursing assistant should keep the**
    a. head of the bed elevated 50° during the feeding
    b. patient flat during the feeding
    c. tubing free of kinks
    d. tubing open between feedings
    e. feeding flowing readily by using force

131. **If the patient is receiving fluids through an infusion pump and the alarm sounds. The nursing assistant should**
    a. notify the nurse
    b. call the doctor
    c. do nothing since the alarms often go off and mean nothing
    d. stop the infusion
    e. flush the infusion line with water

132. The daily calcium requirement for post-menopausal women is
a. 1000 mg   c. 1500 mg
b. 1200 mg   d. 2500 mg

133. When feeding a patient who has had a stroke
a. elevate the foot of the bed
b. direct food toward the unaffected side
c. give only thick liquids
d. direct food to the affected side
e. none of the above

134. Which of the following foods would be included in a low fat diet
a. vegetables and fruits
b. jam, jellies
c. cereal, pasta
d. fish
e. all of the above

B. ANSWER THE FOLLOWING STATEMENTS TRUE (T) OR FALSE (F).

You have been assigned to a patient who is terminally ill. Statements 135 to 139 apply to this assignment.

T   F   135. When in the denial stage of grieving, the patient accepts that her death is inevitable.

T   F   136. The patient who says "You really aren't trying to help me" is probably in the stage of anger.

T   F   137. The patient who is writing her will may have reached the stage of bargaining.

T   F   138. Patients with a terminal diagnosis move through the process of grieving in an orderly manner, one step at a time.

T   F   139. The family and staff also move through the same stages of grieving as the patient but not necessarily at the same rate.

T   F   140. It is permissible to reach over a sterile field when adding sterile sponges.

T   F   141. If a sterile towel is placed on an unsterile surface and becomes wet, it must be considered contaminated.

T   F   142. Always check to see that the color-coded autoclave tape has changed colors before considering a package sterile.

T   F   143. Sterile technique is not needed when collecting a sample of urine from a urinary drainage system that has a port.

T   F   144. The patient with a colostomy may experience problems of leakage, odor control, and irritation around the stoma.

You have been asked to prepare an isolation unit. Statements 145 to 148 apply to this assignment.

T   F   145. Place the proper color barrier sign on the door.

T   F   146. Stock a table or cart just inside the door with isolation gowns.

T   F   147. Line the wastepaper basket inside the room with a plastic bag.

T   F   148. Prepare a basin of disinfectant and leave it near the sink in the room.

T   F   149. The infant is able to smile, laugh aloud, and show pleasure to familiar objects by the age of four months.

T   F   150. The twelve-month-old infant can usually walk without help.

T   F   151. Hospitalization is particularly traumatic for a child.

T   F   152. A toddler is safest in a crib with sides and top.

T   F   153. The teenager is most often hospitalized for accidents, such as sports injuries.

T   F   154. The disoriented person has impaired judgment, memory and orientation.

T   F   155. Disposable gloves should be worn when handling wet soiled linen.

T   F   156. All patients are shaved prior to surgery.

T   F   157. A urinary drainage tube should be coiled on the bed with a straight drop to the drainage bag.

T   F   158. The glucometer measures the level of blood acetone.

T   F   159. An arm with an atrial-venous shunt for dialysis may be used to measure a blood pressure.

T   F   160. Always use a gait belt if a resident has problems with balance, coordination or strength.

T   F   161. Spasticity is common in paralyzed limbs.

T   F   162. All patients or residents should be encouraged to let the nursing assistant carry out most of the activities.

T   F   163. The homemaker assistant gives direct nursing assistant care to home clients.

T   F   164. When ambulating a resident, always stand on the resident's strongest side.

T   F   165. Medications sometimes act as chemical restraints.

T   F   166. Protection of the disoriented person is the nursing assistant's primary responsibility.

T F 167. Sexuality is a characteristic that defines the maleness or femaleness of each person.

T F 168. People over 65 have no interest in sexual activity.

T F 169. A special sensor may be attached to the leg or wrist to keep track of a wandering resident.

T F 170. Reminiscing is a waste of time.

T F 171. Medicare is a government program that partially pays for the health care for persons over 65 and for those who are permanently disabled.

T F 172. Passive range of motion exercises are usually carried out by the physical therapist or the registered nurse.

C. I. MATCH THE FOLLOWING PHRASES AND TERMS.

_____ 173. Bisexuality
_____ 174. Homosexuality
_____ 175. Fomite
_____ 176. Ombudsman
_____ 177. DRG
_____ 178. Advance Directive
_____ 179. Living Will
_____ 180. DNR
_____ 181. POMR
_____ 182. Power of Attorney

a. diagnosis related grouping
b. patient advocate
c. sexual attraction to members of both sexes
d. problem oriented medical records
e. a document which specifies exactly what a person wants at time of death
f. sexual attraction between same sexes
g. a contaminated article
h. a document giving one person the legal right to make decisions for another
i. a document signed before diagnosis of a terminal illness permitting a physician to respect a person's wishes regarding dying care
j. means no extraordinary means should be used to resuscitate a person to prevent death

II. MATCH THE FOLLOWING PHRASES AND TERMS.

_____ 183. Atelectasis
_____ 184. Rales
_____ 185. Dyspnea
_____ 186. Prosthesis
_____ 187. Hypochondriasis
_____ 188. Singultus
_____ 189. Receptive aphasia
_____ 190. Gait belt
_____ 191. Hemovac drain
_____ 192. Expressive aphasia

a. difficult breathing
b. an artificial body part
c. transfer belt
d. means a person cannot comprehend communication
e. closed drainage system
f. magnification of physical ailments
g. collapsed lung tissue
h. gurgles heard in the chest
i. hiccups
j. means the person cannot properly form thoughts or express them in a coherent way

III. MATCH THE FOLLOWING PHRASES AND TERMS.

_____ 193. Solid wastes
_____ 194. Abnormal shortening of muscle fibers
_____ 195. Intravenous infusions
_____ 196. Armpit area
_____ 197. External reproductive organs
_____ 198. Intake and output
_____ 199. Area around nail beds
_____ 200. An item that can be thrown away
_____ 201. Artificial teeth
_____ 202. Nutrient that provides energy

a. expendable
b. genitalia
c. carbohydrate
d. contracture
e. dentures
f. minerals
g. feces
h. I & O
i. IV
j. axilla
k. cuticle

IV. MATCH THE FOLLOWING SETS.

____ 203. Poisons produced by microbes
____ 204. Bacteria that grow in clusters
____ 205. Procedures used to prevent germs from spreading
____ 206. One-celled microbes that cause malaria and diarrhea
____ 207. Disease-producing microbes
____ 208. Contaminated articles
____ 209. Machine used to sterilize equipment
____ 210. Organisms that grow best in absence of oxygen
____ 211. Rod-shaped microbe
____ 212. Resistant forms of bacteria

a. anaerobe
b. fomites
c. spores
d. autoclave
e. aerobes
f. staphylococci
g. medical asepsis
h. pathogens
i. bacteria
j. toxins
k. protozoa

V. MATCH THE FOLLOWING VALUES.

____ 213. 1 minim
____ 214. 16 minims
____ 215. 1 ounce
____ 216. 1 pint
____ 217. 1 quart
____ 218. 2.2 pounds
____ 219. 1 inch
____ 220. 1 foot
____ 221. 3 feet
____ 222. 3 kilograms

a. 500 ml
b. 2.5 centimeters
c. 90 centimeters
d. 1 ml
e. 30 centimeters
f. 6.6 pounds
g. 0.0616 milliliters
h. 1000 milliliters
i. 2 quarts
j. 1 kilogram
k. 30 ml

VI. MATCH THE FOLLOWING TERMS AND DEFINITIONS.

____ 223. Language impairment
____ 224. Used to listen to body sounds
____ 225. Used to provide continuous, constant temperature
____ 226. Cancer of the blood
____ 227. Used to determine blood pressure

a. aphasia
b. sphygmomanometer
c. leukemia
d. stethoscope
e. Aquamatic K-pad®

D. COMPLETION

228. List eight steps to be included at the beginning of every procedure.

a. _____
b. _____
c. _____
d. _____
e. _____
f. _____
g. _____
h. _____

229. List eight steps to be carried out to complete each procedure.

a. _____
b. _____
c. _____
d. _____
e. _____
f. _____
g. _____
h. _____

230. Name ten areas of special nursing practice

a. _____
b. _____
c. _____
d. _____
e. _____
f. _____
g. _____
h. _____
i. _____
j. _____

231. Complete the chart by listing observations related to each system:

System	Significant observations
a. Integumentary	_____
b. Musculoskeletal	_____
c. Circulatory	_____
d. Respiratory	_____
e. Nervous	_____
f. Urinary	_____
g. Digestive	_____

232. List ten negative effects of immobility.

    a. _____
    b. _____
    c. _____
    d. _____
    e. _____
    f. _____
    g. _____
    h. _____
    i. _____
    j. _____

233. List four ways the nursing assistant can help relieve patient frustration.

    a. _____
    b. _____
    c. _____
    d. _____

234. List three basic steps to learning.

    a. _____
    b. _____
    c. _____

235. Write three techniques the nursing assistant can use to improve note taking.

    a. _____
    b. _____
    c. _____

236. Name 4 distractions to comprehensive hearing.

    a. _____
    b. _____
    c. _____
    d. _____

237. List the steps in the nursing process and explain two actions a nursing assistant does to support the process.

    Steps   **Nursing assistant actions**

    a. _____
    b. _____
    c. _____
    d. _____
    e. _____

238. Describe the attitude a nursing assistant should display.

    _____
    _____
    _____
    _____

239. List three articles usually carried in a home health aid kit.

    a. _____
    b. _____
    c. _____

240. List three characteristics of each stage of Alzheimer's Disease.

Stage	Characteristics
I	a. _____
	b. _____
	c. _____
II	d. _____
	e. _____
	f. _____
III	g. _____
	h. _____
	i. _____

241. Explain the relationship of the acronym RACE and fire control by indicating what each letter represents.

    a. R _____
    b. A _____
    c. C _____
    d. E _____

E. IN EACH OF THE FOLLOWING SITUATIONS, INDICATE IF YOU BELIEVE THE ACTION TAKEN BY THE NURSING ASSISTANT WAS PROPER.

a. Yes   b. No

a b 242. Since she felt tired in the morning, the nursing assistant didn't take time to remove the bright red nail polish she had worn to a party last night before reporting to duty.

a b 243. A nursing assistant overheard the social worker talking about a patient's dwindling financial reserves. He shared this information with coworkers at coffee break time.

a b 244. The patient being cared for is very irritable to the nursing assistant. The nursing assistant's response is "We've all got problems."

a b 245. The patient is receiving an intravenous feeding and the needle site looks red and swollen. The nursing assistant reports this fact immediately to the nurse.

a b 246. The postsurgical patient's blood pressure has dropped from 118/80 to 98/50. The nursing assistant believes this is alright since the patient is just back from surgery. The information is recorded but not reported.

a b 247. The nursing assistant notices that a postural support seems too tight on a patient who is not part of her assignment. She feels that since it is someone else's patient she can safely ignore the situation.

a b 248. A nursing assistant makes it a routine part of the care he gives to offer water each time he contacts a patient unless otherwise prohibited by the patient's condition or orders.

a b 249. The nursing assistant observes another nursing assistant treating and handling a patient in a rough manner. Since the other nursing assistant is her friend, she says nothing.

a b 250. The nursing assistant learns that her patient had an abortion two years ago and disapproves. She visits this patient less often than her other patients.

a b 251. The nursing assistant notices that a wheel of a patient's walker is loose but since it is not his patient he does not report the observation to the nurse.

a b 252. The patient is 12 years old and small in stature. The nursing assistant measured the patient's blood pressure with an adult blood pressure cuff.

a b 253. The nursing assistant knows her patient has tested HIV positive and has not told his wife. Although she sees his wife daily, she makes no mention of this information to the wife.

a b 254. The patient complains about a "heaviness" in her chest but the nursing assistant overheard someone say that this patient was a hypochondriac so she doesn't feel it is necessary to report the complaint to the nurse.

a b 255. The disoriented resident believes she is in school and that the nurse is her teacher. The patient becomes very agitated when the nursing assistant, trying to orient her to reality, argues with her.

PROCEDURE
EVALUATION

Student _____

NOTE: Procedures required for OBRA certification are printed in color. The number in parentheses following the procedure title is the number of the procedure in the text.

PROCEDURE*	Satisfactory	Marginal	Unsatisfactory
Admitting a Pediatric Patient (127)			
Admitting the Patient (49)			
Applying a Disposable Cold Pack (90)			
Applying a Behind-the-Ear Hearing Aid (112)			
Applying a Moist Compress (95)			
Applying a Warm Water Bag (91)			
Applying an Aquamatic K-Pad® (92)			
Applying an Ice Bag (89)			
Applying Elasticized Stockings (99)			
Assisting Patient to Brush Teeth (68)			
Assisting Patient to Deep Breathe and Cough (97)			
Assisting Patient to Get Out of Bed and Ambulate (28)			
Assisting Patient Who is Out of Bed to Ambulate (29)			
Assisting the Patient in Initial Ambulation (101)			
Assisting the Patient Into a Chair or Wheelchair (15)			
Assisting the Independent Patient From Wheelchair to Bed (21)			
Assisting the Patient into Bed From a Chair or Wheelchair (19)			
Assisting the Patient to Dangle (100)			

*Procedures required for OBRA certification are printed in color. Number in parentheses following procedure title is the number of the procedure in the text.

703

PROCEDURE	Satisfactory	Marginal	Unsatisfactory
Assisting the Patient to Move to the Head of the Bed (12)			
Assisting the Patient to Sit Up in Bed (11)			
Assisting the Patient Who Can Feed Self (78)			
Assisting the Resident Who Ambulates With a Cane or Walker (103)			
Assisting the Adult Who Has an Obstructed Airway and Becomes Unconscious (150)			
Assisting With Routine Oral Hygiene (66)			
Assisting With Special Oral Hygiene (67)			
Assisting With the Tub Bath or Shower (56)			
Assisting With the Use of the Bedside Commode (75)			
Bathing a Patient in a Century Tub (59)			
Bottlefeeding the Infant (135)			
Breast Self-Examination (125)			
Burping (Method A) (136)			
Burping (Method B) (137)			
Care of Eyeglasses (104)			
Care of Resident With an Artificial Eye (105)			
Care of the Falling Patient (30)			
Caring for Dentures (69)			
Caring for Linen in the Isolation Unit (7)			
Changing Crib Linens (129)			
Changing Crib Linens (Infant in Crib) (130)			

PROCEDURE	Satisfactory	Marginal	Unsatisfactory
Cleaning Glass Thermometers (41)			
Collecting a 24-hour Urine Specimen (86)			
Collecting a Clean-Catch Urine Specimen (84)			
Collecting a Fresh Fractional Urine Specimen (85)			
Collecting a Routine Urine Specimen (82)			
Collecting a Routine Urine Specimen From an Infant (83)			
Collecting a Specimen in the Isolation Unit (6)			
Collecting a Sputum Specimen (88)			
Collecting a Stool Specimen (87)			
Collecting a Urine Specimen Through a Drainage Port (144)			
Collecting Urinary Drainage in a Leg Bag (123)			
Counting Respirations (44)			
Counting Respiratory Rate (Pediatric) (133)			
Counting the Apical Pulse (43)			
Counting the Radial Pulse Rate (42)			
Determining Heart Rate (Pulse) (132)			
Discharging the Patient (51)			
Disconnecting the Catheter (121)			
Dressing and Undressing the Patient (65)			
Emptying a Urinary Drainage Unit (124)			
Feeding the Helpless Patient (79)			
Giving a Back Rub (70)			

PROCEDURE	Satisfactory	Marginal	Unsatisfactory
Giving a Bed Bath (57)			
Giving a Bed Shampoo (64)			
Giving a Commercially Prepared Enema (116)			
Giving a Harris Flush (Return-Flow Enema) (118)			
Giving a Nonsterile Vaginal Douche (126)			
Giving a Partial Bath (58)			
Giving a Rotating Enema (117)			
Giving a Soapsuds Enema (115)			
Giving an Emollient Bath (107)			
Giving an Oil-Retention Enema (114)			
Giving and Receiving the Bedpan (73)			
Giving and Receiving the Urinal (74)			
Giving Daily Care of the Hair (72)			
Giving Female Perineal Care (60)			
Giving Foor and Toenail Care (63)			
Giving Hand and Fingernail Care (62)			
Giving Indwelling Catheter Care (120)			
Giving Male Perineal Care (61)			
Giving Postmortem Care (106)			
Giving Routine Stoma Care (Colostomy) (146)			
Handwashing (1)			
Heimlich Maneuver—Abdominal Thrusts (149)			

PROCEDURE	Satisfactory	Marginal	Unsatisfactory
Independent Transfer, Standby Assist (18)			
Inserting a Rectal Suppository (145)			
Inserting a Rectal Tube and Flatus Bag (119)			
Lifting a Patient Using a Mechanical Lift (22)			
Log Rolling the Patient (27)			
Making a Closed Bed (52)			
Making an Occupied Bed (54)			
Making the Surgical Bed (55)			
Measuring a Rectal Temperature (Electronic Thermometer) (38)			
Measuring a Rectal Temperature (Glass Thermometer) (37)			
Measuring an Axillary or Groin Temperature (Glass Thermometer) (39)			
Measuring an Axillary Temperature (Electronic Thermometer) (40)			
Measuring an Oral Temperature (Electronic Thermometer) (36)			
Measuring an Oral Temperature (Glass Thermometer) (33)			
Measuring an Oral Temperature (Plastic Thermometer) (35)			
Measuring and Recording Fluid Intake (80)			
Measuring and Recording Fluid Output (81)			
Measuring and Weighing the Patient in Bed (47)			
Measuring Blood Pressure (134)			

Measuring Temperature (131)
    Axillary
    Oral
    Rectal			

PROCEDURE	Satisfactory	Marginal	Unsatisfactory
Measuring Temperature Using a Sheath-Covered Thermometer (34)			
Moving a Helpless Patient to the Head of the Bed (13)			
One Person Transfer From Wheelchair to Bed (20)			
One Person Transfer With Transfer Belt (17)			
Opening a Sterile Package (138)			
Opening the Closed Bed (53)			
Performing Postoperative Leg Exercises (98)			
Performing the Warm Arm Soak (94)			
Performing the Warm Foot Soak (93)			
Performing Range of Motion Exercises (Passive) (108)			
Providing Bedtime (PM) Care (77)			
Providing Early Morning (AM) Care (76)			
Putting on Sterile Gloves (139)			
Putting on a Cover Gown (3)			
Putting On and Taking Off a Disposable Paper Face Mask (5)			
Removing a Behind-the-Ear Hearing Aid (113)			
Removing Contaminated Cover Gown, Gloves, and Mask (4)			
Removing Contaminated Disposable Gloves (2)			
Replacing a Urinary Condom (122)			
Routine Care of an Ileostomy (in Bathroom) (148)			

PROCEDURE	Satisfactory	Marginal	Unsatisfactory
Routine Care of an Ileostomy (With Patient in Bed) (147)			
Shaving a Patient (71)			
Shaving the Operative Area (96)			
Taking Blood Pressure (45)			
Testing for Occult Blood Using Hematest® Reagent Tablets (143)			
Testing for Occult Blood Using Hemoccult® and Developer (142)			
Testing Urine for Acetone: Ketostix® Strip Test (111)			
Testing Urine with the HemaCombistix® (141)			
Tracheal Suctioning (140)			
Transferring a Conscious Patient From a Bed to Stretcher (23)			
Transferring a Conscious Patient From a Stretcher To Bed (24)			
Transferring an Unconscious Patient From a Bed to Stretcher (26)			
Transferring an Unconscious Patient or a Patient Unable to Assist From Stretcher to Bed (25)			
Transferring a Resident From Bed to Chair or Chair to Bed (for the Frail Elderly) (102)			
Transferring the Patient (50)			
Transporting a Patient by Stretcher (32)			
Transporting a Patient by Wheelchair (31)			
Transporting the Patient in Isolation (8)			
Turning the Patient Away From You (10)			
Turning the Patient Toward You (9)			

PROCEDURE	Satisfactory	Marginal	Unsatisfactory
Two Person Transfer With Transfer Belt (16)			
Using Accu-Chec III® (110)			
Using a Transfer (Gait) Belt (14)			
Using a Glucometer 3® (109)			
Weighing and Measuring the Patient Using an Upright Scale (46)			
Weighing a Patient on the Wheelchair Scale (48)			
Weighing the Pediatric Patient (128)			

Student _____

Area/Agency _____

Teacher will initial and date observations of clinical performance. Summary and comments can then be made and the performance record signed by both teacher and student.

EVALUATIONS OF CLINICAL PERFORMANCE

AREAS OF EVALUATION	Satisfactory	Marginal	Unsatisfactory
PERSONAL CHARACTERISTICS			
Attendance			
Flexibility			
Grooming			
Interpersonal relationships			
Promptness			
Response to criticism			
EXECUTION OF NURSING CARE			
Acceptance of responsibility			
Accuracy; safety			
Energy level; productivity			
Knows limitations; seeks appropriate guidance			
Observational skills			
Organization; use of time			
Theoretical knowledge			
COMMUNICATION			
Oral			
Written			

COMMENTS (Strengths and Weaknesses): _____

_____

_____

Clinical Rating:
Satisfactory _____
Marginal _____
Unsatisfactory _____

Teacher's Signature _____ **Student's Signature** _____ **Date** _____

GLOSSARY

Abbreviation (ah-**BREE**-vee-ay-shun)—shortened form of a word or phrase

Abdomen (**AB**-doh-men)—area of trunk between thorax and pelvis

Abduction (ab-**DUCK**-shun)—movement away from midline or center

Abuse (ah-**BYOUSE**)—improper treatment or misuse

Accelerated (ack-**SELL**-er-ay-ted)—increased motion, as in pulse or respiration

Accommodation (ah-**KOM**-moh-**day**-shun)—adjustment

Acidosis (ah-sih-**DOH**-sis)—pathological condition resulting from accumulation of acid or depletion of alkaline reserves in the blood and body tissues

Acquired immune deficiency syndrome (AIDS) (ah-**KWIRED** ih-**MYOUN** dih-**FISH**-en-see **SIN**-drohm) (ayds)—an infectious disease caused by human immunodeficiency virus (HIV)

Active listening (**ACK**-tiv **LISS**-en-ing)—listening with personal involvement

Activities of daily living (ADL) (ack-**TIV**-ih-tees of **DAY**-lee **LIV**-ing) (ay-dee-ell)—the activities necessary for the resident to fulfill basic human needs

Acute (ah-**KYOUT**)—having severe symptoms

Adaptations (ad-dap-**TAY**-shuns)—adjustments

Adaptive equipment (ah-**DAP**-tiv ee-**KWIP**-ment)—items altered to make them easier to use by those with functional deficits

Addison's disease (**AD**-ih-sons dih-**ZEEZ**)—disease caused by the underfunctioning of the adrenal glands

Adduction (ad-**DUCK**-shun)—movement toward midline or center

ADL (ay-dee-ell)—activities of daily living

Admission (ad-**MIH**-shun)—procedure carried out when patient first arrives at the facility

Adoptive parent (ah-**DOP**-tiv **PAIR**-ent)—a person who is a parent through a legal adoption procedure

Advance directive (ad-**VANS** dih-**RECK**-tiv)—a document signed before the diagnosis of a terminal illness when the individual is still in good health, indicating the person's wishes regarding care during dying

Advocate (**AD**-voh-kit)—one who promotes the welfare of another

Aerobic (air-**OH**-bick)—microorganisms that live best where plenty of oxygen is available

AFB (ay-eff-bee)—acid-fast bacillus

Afterbirth (**AF**-ter-burth)—the placenta through which the unborn child is nourished

Agency (**AY**-jen-see)—a business or company

Agent (**AY**-jent)—a person or substance by which something is accomplished

Agitation (aj-ih-**TAY**-shun)—a state in which behavior is irregular and erratic

Aiding and abetting (**AYD**-ing and ah-**BET**-ing)—not reporting dishonest acts that are observed

Akinesia (ah-kih-**NEE**-zee-ah)—abnormal absence or poverty of movement

Alcoholism (**AL**-koh-hall-izm)—a dependency on alcohol

Alignment (ah-**LINE**-ment)—keeping a resident in proper position

Allergen (**AL**-er-jen)—substance that causes sensitivity or allergic reactions

Allergies (**AL**-er-jeez)—abnormal and individual hypersensitivities

Alveoli (al-**VEE**-oh-lee)—tiny air sacs that make up the bulk of the lungs

Alzheimer's disease (**ALZ**-high-mers dih-**ZEEZ**)—a neurological condition in which there is gradual loss of cerebral functioning

Ambulation (am-byou-**LAY**-shun)—ability to walk

Ambulatory (**AM**-byou-lah-tor-ee)—walking about

AM care (ay-em kair)—care given in the early morning when the patient first awakens

Amenorrhea (ah-**MEN**-or-ree-ah)—without menstruation

Amino acid (ah-**MEAN**-oh **AH**-sid)—basic component of proteins

Amniocentesis (am-nee-oh-sen-**TEE**-sis)—transabdominal perforation of the amniotic sac to obtain a sample of the amniotic fluid

Amniotic fluid (am-nee-**OT**-ick **FLEW**-id)—fluid in which the fetus floats in the mother's womb

Amniotic sac (am-nee-**OT**-ick sack)—sac enclosing the fetus suspended in amniotic fluid

Amputation (am-pyou-**TAY**-shun)—removal of a limb or other body appendage

Anaerobic (an-er-**OH**-bick)—organisms that grow best where there is little oxygen

Anaphylaxis (an-ah-fih-**LACK**-sis)—severe, sometimes fatal, sensitivity reaction

Anatomy (ah-**NAT**-oh-mee)—study of the structure of the human body

Ancillary (**AN**-sill-**lar**-ee)—offering or providing help

Anemia (ah-**NEE**-mee-ah)—deficiency of quality or quantity of red blood cells in the blood

Anesthesia (an-es-**THEE**-zee-ah)—loss of feeling or sensation

Aneurysm (**AN**-you-rizm)—sac formed by dilation of the wall of a blood vessel (usually an artery) and filled with blood

Angina pectoris (an-**JYE**-nah or **AN**-jih-nah **PECK**-tor-is)—acute pain in the chest caused by interference with the supply of oxygen to the heart

Anorexia (an-or-**RECK**-see-ah)—lack or loss of appetite for food

Anterior (an-**TEER**-ee-er)—in anatomy, in front of the coronal or ventral plane

Antibody (**AN**-tih-bod-ee)—a protein that is produced in the body in response to invasion by a foreign agent. It reacts specifically with the foreign agent

Anti-embolism hose (an-tih-**EM**-bohl-izm hohz)—elasticized stockings used to support the leg blood vessels

Antipyretic (an-tih-pie-**RET**-ick)—drug given to reduce an elevated body temperature

Antiseptic (an-tih-**SEP**-tick)—anti-infectious agent used on living tissue

Anuria (ah-**NEW**-ree-ah)—no urine

Anus (**AY**-nus)—outlet of the rectum lying in the fold between the buttocks

Apathy (**AP**-ah-thee)—indifference; lack of emotion

Apgar score (**AP**-gar skor)—method for determining an infant's condition at birth by scoring heart rate, respiratory effect, muscle tone, reflex irritability, and color

Aphasia (ah-**FAY**-zee-ah)—language impairment; loss of ability to comprehend normally

Apical pulse (**AP**-ih-kal puls)—pulse rate taken by placing stethoscope over tip of heart

Apnea (ap-**NEE**-ah)—period of no respiration

Apprehensive (ap-ree-**HEN**-siv)—fearful

Aquamatic K-Pad® (**ack**-kwah-**MAT**-ick **KAY**-pad)—commercial unit for applying heat or cold

ARC (AIDS related complex) (ay-are-see) (ayds ree-**LAY**-ted **KOM**-plex)—conditions suffered by persons who are HIV positive before true onset of AIDS

Arrest (ah-**REST**)—to stop suddenly

Arteriosclerosis (are-tee-ree-oh-skleh-**ROH**-sis)—general term meaning a narrowing of the blood vessels, which can result in subsequent tissue hypoxia and degeneration and hardening of the arterial walls and sometimes of the heart valves

Artery (**ARE**-ter-ee)—vessel through which the blood passes away from the heart to various parts of the body

Arthritis (are-**THRIGH**-tis)—joint inflammation

Ascites (ah-**SIGH**-teez)—fluid accumulation in the abdomen

Asepsis (ah-**SEP**-sis)—without infection

Aseptic technique (ah-**SEP**-tick tek-**NEEK**)—technique used to destroy microorganisms and prevent their transmission

Aspirate (**ASS**-pih-rayt)—to withdraw

Aspiration (ass-pih-**RAY**-shun)—drawing foreign materials into the respiratory tract

Assault (ass-**SALT**)—attempt or threat to do violence to another

Assessment (ah-**SESS**-ment)—act of evaluating

Assimilate (ah-**SIM**-ih-layt)—absorb

Assistive devices (ah-**SIS**-tiv dih-**VICE**-es)—equipment used to help people be more effective in their physical activity

Asthma (**AZ**-mah)—chronic respiratory disease characterized by bronchospasms and excessive mucous production

Atelectasis (at-ee-**LECK**-tah-sis)—collapse of lung tissue

Atherosclerosis (ath-er-oh-skleh-**ROH**-sis)—degenerative process involving the lining of arteries, in which the lumen eventually narrows and closes; a form of arteriosclerosis

Atrium (**AY**-tree-um)—one of the two upper chambers of the heart

Atrophy (**AT**-roh-fee)—shrinking or wasting away of tissues

Attitude (**AT**-ih-tood)—an external expression of inner feelings about self or others

Auditory (**AWE**-dih-**toh**-ree)—hearing

Aura (**AWE**-rah)—peculiar sensation preceding the appearance of more definite symptoms in a convulsion or seizure

Aural temperature (**AWE**-ral **TEM**-per-ah-ty-our)—temperature of tympanic membrane blood vessels within ear

Ausculatory gap (aws-**KUL**-ah-**toh**-ree gap)—sound fadeout for 1–15 mm Hg mercury pressure, which then begins again. Sometimes mistaken as the diastolic pressure

Autoclave (**AWE**-toh-klayv)—machine that sterilizes articles

Autoimmune (**awe**-toh-im-**MYOUN**)—presence of antibodies against component(s) of body

Automatic speech (**awe**-toh-**MAT**-ick speech)—involuntary speech associated with brain injury

Autonomic nervous system (**awe**-toh-**NOM**-ick **NER**-vus **SIS**-tum)—that portion of the nervous system that controls the activities of the organs

Autonomy (awe-**TON**-oh-mee)—self-determination

Axillae (ack-**SILL**-ee)—plural of axilla; armpits

Axillary (**ACK**-sih-**lair**-ee)—pertaining to the axilla

Axon (**ACK**-son)—extension of neuron that conducts nerve impulses away from the cell body

Bacilli (bah-**SILL**-eye)—rod-shaped bacteria

Bacteria (back-**TEE**-ree-ah)—a form of simple microbes

Bacteriocide (back-**TEE**-ree-oh-side)—agent that destroys bacteria

Balanced suspension skeletal traction (**BAL**-anst sus-**PEN**-shun **SKEL**-eh-tal **TRACK**-shun)—type of traction used to reduce serious fractures in which there is one primary line of traction and extra weight and ropes provide suspension and countertraction

Bargaining (**BAR**-gan-ing)—stage of the grieving process in which the individual seeks to form a pact that will delay death

Barrier (**BAIR**-ee-er)—gown, mask, or gloves or combination of these articles worn by health care providers to prevent contact with pathogens spread by blood and other body fluids

Baseline assessment (**BAYS**-line ah-**SESS**-ment)—initial observations of the patient and condition

Bath itch—condition that affects the less oily elderly skin; characterized by tiny red eruptions and itching

Battery (**BAT**-er-ee)—an unlawful attack upon another person

Benign (bee-**NINE**)—nonmalignant tumor

Bile (byl)—secretion of the liver, needed to prepare fats for digestion

Biohazard (**bye**-oh-**HAZ**-ard)—laboratory specimens or materials contaminated with body fluids and their containers that have the potential to transmit disease

Biological parent (bye-oh-**LOJ**-ih-kul **PAIR**-ent)—natural parent who contributed sperm or an ovum to the development of the fetus

Biopsy (**BYE**-op-see)—removal and examination of a piece of tissue from the living body

Bisexuality (bye-sex-you-**AL**-ih-tee)—having sexual interest in both sexes

Blood-borne pathogen (blud born **PATH**-oh-jen)—disease causing microbe transmitted by contact with human blood

Blood pressure (blud **PRESH**-ur)—pressure of blood exerted against vascular walls

Body language (**BAH**-dee **LAN**-gwihj)—use of facial expression, body positions, and vocal inflections to convey a message

Body mechanics (**BAH**-dee mih-**KAN**-icks)—using muscles correctly to move or lift heavy objects properly

Bolus (**BOH**-lus)—soft mass of food that is ready to be swallowed

Bowel (**BOW**-el)—intestine

Bowman's capsule (**BOH**-manz **KAP**-sy-oul)—tubule surrounding the glomerulus of the nephron

Box (square) corner (bahx [skwair] **KOR**-ner)—one type of corner used in the making of a hospital bed

Brachial artery (**BRAY**-kee-al **ARE**-ter-ee)—main artery of the arm

Bradycardia (brad-ee-**KAR**-dee-ah)—unusually slow heartbeat

Bridging (**BRIHJ**-ing)—supporting the body on either side of the affected area to relieve pressure on the area

Bronchitis (brong-**KEYE**-tis)—inflammation of the bronchi

Burnout (**BURN**-out)—loss of enthusiasm and interest in an activity

Bursae (**BUR**-see)—small sacs of fluid found around joints

Bursitis (bur-**SIGH**-tis)—condition in which the bursae become inflamed and the joint becomes very painful

Cachexia (kah-**KEK**-see-ah)—state of malnutrition, emaciation and debility, usually in the course of a prolonged illness

Calibrated (**KAL**-ih-bray-ted)—marked in increments (measured amounts)

Cancer (**KAN**-sir)—malignant tumor; malignancy

Capillary (**KAP**-ih-**lair**-ee)—hairlike blood vessel; link between arterioles and venules

Carbohydrates (kar-boh-**HIGH**-drayts)—energy foods; used by the body to produce heat and energy for work

Carbon dioxide (**KAR**-bon dye-**OX**-side)—gas that is a waste product in cellular metabolism

Carcinogen (kar-**SIN**-oh-jin)—agent capable of causing malignant changes in tissue

Carcinoma (kar-sih-**NOH**-mah)—malignant tumor made up of connective tissue enclosing epithelial cells

Cardiac arrest (**KAR**-dee-ack ah-**REST**)—sudden and often unexpected stoppage of effective heart action

Cardiac cycle (**KAR**-dee-ack **SIGH**-kul)—all (mechanical and electrical) events that occur between one heart contraction and the next

Cardiac decompensation (**KAR**-dee-ack **dee**-kom-pen-**SAY**-shun)—another name for congestive heart failure

Cardiogram (**KAR**-dee-oh-gram)—record of cardiac pulsation produced by cardiograph

Cardiopulmonary resuscitation (CPR) (**kar**-dee-oh-**PULL**-moh-nair-ee ree-sus-ih-**TAY**-shun) (see-pee-are)—emergency medical procedure undertaken to restart and sustain heart and respiratory functions

Care plan (kair plan)—nursing plan for care of resident in long-term care facility

Caries (**KAIR**-eez)—tooth decay or cavities

Cartilage (**KAR**-tih-lij)—type of body tissue

Cast (kast)—rigid covering to keep a joint or other body part immobile

Cataract (**KAT**-ah-ract)—opacity of the lens of the eye, resulting in loss of vision

Catastrophic reaction (kat-ah-**STROH**-fick ree-**ACK**-shun)—severe and unpredictable violent behavior of a person with dementia

Category-specific isolation precautions (KAT-ih-**gor**-ee spih-**SIF**-ick eye-soh-**LAY**-shun pree-**KAW**-shuns)—isolation precaution system that groups diseases that require similar isolation procedures

Catheter (KATH-ih-ter)—tube for evacuating or injecting fluids

Causitive agent (KAWZ-ah-tiv AY-jent)—etiology of a specific disease process

Cell (sell)—basic unit in the organization of living substances

Cellulose (SELL-you-lohs)—basic substance of all plant foods, which can supply the body with roughage

Celsius scale (SELL-see-us skale)—scale for measuring temperature

Centimeter (SEN-tih-mee-ter)—one-hundredth of a meter

Cerebellum (ser-eh-BELL-um)—portion of the brain lying beneath the occipital lobe; coordinates muscular activities and balance

Cerebrospinal fluid (ser-eh-broh-SPY-nal FLEW-id)—water cushion protecting the brain and spinal cord from shock

Cerebrovascular accident (ser-eh-broh-VASS-kyou-lar ACK-sih-dent)—stroke; disorder of the blood vessels of the brain resulting in impaired cerebral circulation

Cerebrum (SER-eh-brum)—largest part of the brain, consisting of two hemispheres separated by a deep longitudinal fissure; controls all mental activities

Cervical (SER-vih-kal)—pertaining to the neck

Cervix (SIR-vicks)—neck of the uterus

Chain of infection (chayn of in-FECK-shun)—process or events involved in the transmission and development of an infectious disease

Chancre (SHANG-ker)—shallow, craterlike lesion; primary lesion of syphilis

Character (of pulse) (KAIR-ack-ter of puls)—rhythm and volume of pulse

Chart—record of information concerning patient

Cheeking (CHEEK-ing)—storing food in one side of the mouth

Cheyne-Stokes respiration (chain-stohkes res-pih-RAY-shun)—periods of apnea alternating with periods of dyspnea

CHF (see-aytch-eff)—congestive heart failure

Cholecystectomy (koh-lee-sis-TECK-toh-mee)—surgical removal of a diseased gallbladder and stones

Cholecystitis (koh-lee-sis-TIE-tis)—inflammation of the gallbladder

Cholelithiasis (koh-lee-lih-THIGH-ah-sis)—formation of stones in the gallbladder

Chromosome (KROH-moh-sohm)—rod-shaped body appearing at time of cellular division in the nucleus; contains the genes or hereditary factors

Chronic (KRON-ick)—persisting over a long period of time

Chronologic (kron-oh-LOJ-ick)—in sequential order by date or age

Chyme (kighm)—semiliquid form of food as it leaves the stomach

Chymopapaine (kigh-moh-pah-PAY-in)—an enzyme used to dissolve the protein in a ruptured disc

Circ O lectric® bed (sirk-oh-LET-rick bed)—special kind of bed that is used when a patient cannot be turned within the bed

Circumcision (sir-kum-SIJ-un)—removal of the end of the prepuce by a circular incision

Clean-catch urine specimen (kleen katch YOU-rin SPES-ah-men)—sample of urine taken midstream after the patient has been specifically cleansed

Clean technique (kleen tek-NEEK)—technique that limits potential pathogens but does not ensure the destruction of all organisms

Client (KLIGH-ent)—resident

Client care record (KLIGH-ent kair RECK-ord)—documentation of care provided in the home situation

Climacteric (kligh-MAK-ter-ick)—menopause; the combined phenomena accompanying cessation of the reproductive function in the female or diminution of testicular activity in the male

Climax (KLIGH-max)—period of greatest intensity during sexual stimulation or intercourse

Clinical thermometer (KLIN-eh-kul ther-MOM-eh-ter)—instrument used to measure body temperature

Clitoris (KLIT-oh-ris)—small, cylindrical mass of erotic tissue; part of the external female reproductive organs analogous to the penis in the male

Closed bed (klohzd bed)—bed with sheets and spread positioned to the head of the bed; unoccupied

Closed (oblique) fracture (klohzd [ah-BLEEK] FRACK-sure)—fracture in which bones remain in proper alignment

CNS (see-en-ess)—central nervous system

Cocci (KOCK-sigh)—round bacteria

Cognitive (KOG-nih-tiv)—mental

Coitus (KOH-ih-tus)—sexual intercourse; copulation

Colloidal (kuh-LOY-dal)—pertaining to a colloid (gelatinous substance)

Colon (KOH-lon)—large intestine

Colony (KAWL-oh-nee)—group of organisms derived from a single organism

Colostomy (koh-LAHS-toh-me)—artificial opening in the abdomen for the purpose of evacuation of feces

Colostrum (kuh-LAWS-trum)—secretion from the lactiferous glands of the mother before the onset of true lactation two or three days after delivery of a baby

Colporrhaphy (kohl-POOR-ah-fee)—suturing of the vagina; surgical procedure used to tighten vaginal walls

Comatose (KOH-mah-tohs)—unconscious; in a coma

Combining form (kom-BYN-ing form)—word part that can be used with other word parts to form a variety of new words

Comminuted fracture (KOM-ih-new-ted FRACK-shur)—fracture in which the bone is broken or crushed into small pieces

Commode (kum-MOHD)—portable toilet

Communicable (kuh-MYOU-nih-kah-bul)—capable of being transferred from one person to another directly or indirectly; for example, infectious disease

Communication (kuh-myou-nih-KAY-shun)—exchanging messages

Compensation (kom-pen-SAY-shun)—in psychology, the act of seeking a substitute for something unacceptable or unattainable

Competency (KOM-peh-ten-see)—capability

Complete fracture (kom-PLEET FRACK-shur)—separation of the ends of bone at the fracture site

Compound fracture (kom-pownd FRACK-shur)—fracture in which the broken bone protrudes through the skin

Comprehension (kom-prih-HEN-shun)—capacity of the mind for understanding

Compression fracture (kom-PRESH-un FRACK-shur)—fracture in which bone is crushed

Confidential (kon-fih-DEN-shall)—keeping what is said or written to oneself; private; nonsharing

Congenital (kon-JEN-ih-tal)—condition present at birth

Congestive heart failure (kon-JES-tiv hart FAIL-your)—condition resulting from cardiac output inadequate for physiological needs, with shortness of breath, edema, and abnormal retention of sodium and water in body tissues

Conjunctiva (kon-junk-TIGH-vah)—mucous membrane that lines the eyelids and covers the eye

Connective tissue (kuh-NECK-tiv TISH-you)—tissue that holds other tissues together and provides support for organs and other body structures

Constipation (kon-stih-PAY-shun)—difficulty in defecating

Constriction (kon-STRICK-shun)—narrowing; compression

Contaminated (kon-TAM-ih-nay-ted)—unclean; impure; soiled with germs

Continent (KON-tih-nent)—able to control elimination of feces and urine

Continuum (kon-**TIN**-you-um)—continuous related series of events or actions

Contract (**KON**-tract)—agreement between two or more people, especially one that is written

Contracture (kon-**TRACK**-shur)—permanent shortening or contraction of a muscle due to spasm or paralysis

Contraindicated (kon-trah-**IN**-dih-kay-ted)—harmful remedy or treatment

Convalescent home (kon-vah-**LESS**-ent hohm)—long-term care facility

Convulsion (kon-**VUL**-shun)—involuntary muscle spasm

COPD (see-oh-pee-dee)—chronic obstructive pulmonary disease; for example, pulmonary emphysema

Coping (**KOHP**-ing)—handling or dealing with stress

Copulation (kop-you-**LAY**-shun)—sexual intercourse; coitus

Cornea (**KOR**-nee-ah)—transparent portion of the eye through which light passes

Coronary embolism (**KOR**-uh-nair-ee **EM**-boh-lizm)—blood clot lodged in a coronary artery

Coronary occlusion (**KOR**-uh-nair-ee uh-**KLEW**-zhun)—closing off of a coronary artery

Coronary thrombosis (**KOR**-uh-nair-ee throm-**BOH**-sis)—blood clot within the vessel

Cortex (**KOR**-tex)—outer portion of a kidney

Countertraction (kown-ter-**TRACK**-shun)—providing opposing balance to traction; used in reduction of fractures

Cranial (**KRAY**-nee-al)—pertaining to the cranium or skull

Critical list (**KRIT**-ih-kul list)—list that patients are placed on when they are dangerously or terminally ill

Croupette (krew-**PET**)—type of crib that is enclosed to provide moisture and/or oxygen to an infant or child

Cryosurgery (kry-oh-**SIR**-jer-ee)—destruction of tissue by application of extreme cold

Culturing (**KUL**-tyour-ing)—taking a sample from the affected area to discover the cause of infection by growing the organisms

Cushing's syndrome (**KUSH**-ingz **SIN**-drohm)—condition that results from an excess level of adrenal cortex hormones

Cuticle (**KYOU**-tih-kul)—base of the fingernail

CVA (see-vee-ay)—cerebrovascular accident

Cyanosis (sigh-ah-**NOH**-sis)—bluish skin discoloration caused by lack of oxygen

Cystitis (sis-**TIE**-tis)—inflammation of the urinary bladder

Cystocele (**SIS**-toh-seel)—bladder hernia

Cystoscopy (sis-**TOS**-koh-pee)—procedure using cystoscope for visualization of the urinary bladder, ureter, and kidney

Cytoplasm (**SIGH**-toh-plazm)—protoplasm of a cell outside the nucleus

Dangling (**DANG**-gling)—sitting up with legs hanging over the edge of the bed

Day care center (day kair **SEN**-ter)—place where senior citizens may go for various services

Debilitating (dee-**BILL**-ih-tayt-ing)—weakening

Debride (day-**BREED**)—to remove foreign material and devitalized tissue

Debridement (day-**BREED**-ment)—removal of foreign matter or devitalized tissue

Deconditioning (dee-kon-**DISH**-un-ing)—reversing a learned response

Decubitus (pl. decubiti) ulcer (dee-**KYOU**-bih-tus [dee-**KYOU**-bih-tie] **UL**-sir)—dermal ulcer, bedsore or pressure sore

Defamation (def-eh-**MAY**-shun)—something harmful to the good name or reputation of another; slander

Defecation (def-eh-**KAY**-shun)—bowel movement that expels feces

Defense mechanism (dee-**FENS MECK**-ah-niz-em)—psychological reaction or technique for protection against a stressful environmental situation or anxiety

Degeneration (dee-jen-er-**AY**-shun)—deterioration of tissues from a more to less functional status

Degenerative joint disease (dee-**JEN**-er-ah-tiv joynt dih-**ZEEZ**)—deterioration of the tissues of the joints

Dehydration (dee-high-**DRAY**-shun)—excessive water loss

Delirium (dih-**LEER**-ee-um)—disordered mental condition in which speech is incoherent, fever may occur, and illusions, delusions, and hallucinations may be experienced

Delusion (dee-**LEW**-zhun)—false belief

Dementia (dee-**MEN**-she-ah)—progressive mental deterioration due to organic brain disease

Dendrite (**DEN**-dryt)—branch of a neuron that conducts impulses toward the cell body

Denial (dih-**NIGH**-al)—unconscious defense mechanism in which an occurrence or observation is refused recognition as reality in order to avoid anxiety or pain

Dentures (**DEN**-churz)—artificial teeth

Depilatory (dee-**PILL**-ah-tor-ee)—substance used to remove body hair

Depreciate (dih-**PREE**-she-ayt)—treat as being of less value

Depressant (dee-**PRESS**-ant)—drug that slows down body functions

Depression (dee-**PRESH**-un)—morbid sadness or melancholy

Dermal ulcer (**DER**-mul **UL**-sir)—bedsore or decubitus ulcer

Development (dee-**VEL**-op-ment)—gradual growth

Developmental milestones (dee-vel-op-**MEN**-tal **MYL**-stohns)—achieving specific skills at a particular age level

Developmental tasks (dee-vel-op-**MEN**-tal tasks)—in psychology, tasks that are normally carried out as steps in personality development

Diabetes mellitus (die-ah-**BEE**-teez **MEL**-ih-tus)—disorder of carbohydrate metabolism

Diabetic coma (die-ah-**BET**-ick **KOH**-mah)—comatose state of acidosis due to diabetes mellitus

Diagnosis (die-ahg-**NOH**-sis)—art or method of identifying or recognizing a disease

Dialysis (die-**AL**-ih-sis)—diffusion of solutes through a semipermeable membrane, passing from an area of higher concentration to an area of lower concentration

Diaphoresis (die-ah-foh-**REE**-sis)—profuse sweating

Diarrhea (die-ah-**REE**-ah)—watery stool

Diastole (die-**AS**-toh-lee)—period during which the heart muscle relaxes and the chamber fills with blood

Diastolic pressure (die-ah-**STOL**-ick **PRESH**-ur)—refers to period of cardiac ventricular relaxation

Diathermy (**DIE**-ah-ther-mee)—treatment with heat

Digestion (die-**JEST**-shun)—process of converting food into an assimilable form

Dilate (**DIE**-layt)—to enlarge, as capillaries

Dilation stage (die-**LAY**-shun stayj)—stage of labor in which the opening to the cervix enlarges

Diplo- (**DIP**-loh)—arranged in pairs, such as diplococci; bacteria that are arranged in groups of two

Direct cause (of disease) (die-**RECT** kaws [of dih-**ZEEZ**])—immediate or exact cause of a disease process

Directive (die-**RECK**-tiv)—serving or qualified to direct; statement of direction

Disability (dis-ah-**BILL**-ih-tee)—persistent physical or mental defect or handicap

Discharge (dis-**CHARJ**)—procedure carried out as the patient leaves the hospital

Disease (dih-**ZEEZ**)—definite marked process having a characteristic train of symptoms

Disease-specific isolation precautions (dih-**ZEEZ** spih-**SIF**-ick **eye**-soh-**LAY**-shun pree-**KAW**-shuns)—system of isolation precautions that considers precautions for each disease individually

Disinfectant (**dis**-in-**FECK**-tant)—agent that kills germs

Disinfection (**dis**-in-**FECK**-shun)—process of destroying pathogenic organisms or agents

Disk—flat plate on which computer information is stored

Disorientation (dis-**oh**-ree-en-**TAY**-shun)—loss or recognition of time, place, or people

Displacement (dis-**PLAYZ**-ment)—unconscious defense mechanism in which an emotion, such as anger, is directed at the wrong person

Disposable (dis-**POSE**-ah-bul)—not reusable after one use

Disruption (dis-**RUP**-shun)—interference with the normal progress of events

Distal (**DIS**-tal)—farthest away from a central point, such as point of attachment of muscles

Distention (dis-**TEN**-shun)—the state of being stretched out (distended)

Diuresis (**die**-you-**REE**-sis)—increase of output of fluids by the kidneys

Diurnal (die-**UR**-nal)—daily

Diverticula (**die**-ver-**TICK**-you-lah)—small blind pouches that form in the lining and wall of the colon

Diverticulitis (**die**-ver-tick-you-**LIE**-tis)—inflammation of diverticula

Diverticulosis (**die**-ver-tick-you-**LOH**-sis)—presence of many diverticula

DNR (dee-en-are)—do not resuscitate when cardiac and respiratory arrest occur

Dorsal (**DOR**-sal)—posterior or back

Dorsal lithotomy position (**DOR**-sal lih-**THOT**-oh-mee pih-**ZISH**-en)—person is positioned on back with knees flexed and well separated; feet are usually in stirrups

Dorsal recumbent position (**DOR**-sal ree-**KUM**-bent pih-**ZISH**-en)—person is flat on back, knees flexed and slightly separated with feet flat on bed

Dorsiflexion (dor-sih-**FLECK**-shun)—toes pointed up

Double bagging (**DUB**-ul **BAG**-ging)—technique in which a contaminated article is placed in a plastic bag that is then placed in a second protective covering to prevent transmission of infectious organisms

Drainage (**DRAYN**-aj)—systematic withdrawal of fluids and discharges from wounds, sores, or body cavities

Drawsheet (**DRAW**-sheet)—sheet folded under the patient and extending from above the shoulder to below the hips

DRG (dee-are-jee)—diagnosis-related grouping

Drip chamber (drip **CHAYM**-ber)—part of the IV equipment found between the bag of solution and the tube leading to the patient

DSD (dee-ess-dee)—dry, sterile dressing

Due date (dew dayt)—expected date of delivery

Duodenal ulcer (**dew**-oh-**DEE**-nal **UL**-sir)—ulcer on the mucosa of the duodenum due to the action of gastric juice

Dura mater (**DEW**-rah **MAY**-ter)—outer layer of the brain and spinal cord

Dyscrasia (dis-**KRAY**-zee-ah)—abnormality or disorder of the body

Dysmenorrhea (**dis**-men-oh-**REE**-ah)—painful menstruation

Dyspepsia (dis-**PEP**-see-ah)—indigestion

Dysphagia (dis-**FAY**-jee-ah)—difficulty in swallowing

Dyspnea (**DISP**-nee-ah)—difficult or labored breathing

Dysuria (dis-**YOU**-ree-ah)—painful voiding

Edema (eh-**DEE**-mah)—excessive accumulation of fluid in the tissues

Efface (eh-**FAYS**)—thinning of the cervix during labor

Ejaculation (ee-**jack**-you-**LAY**-shun)—forcible, sudden expulsion of semen from the male penis

EKG (ee-kay-jee)—electrocardiogram. *See* Cardiogram

Elasticity (ee-las-**TIS**-ih-tee)—ability to stretch

Electrolytes (ee-**LECK**-troh-lights)—compounds that play an essential role in regulating body chemistry

Electronic thermometer (**ee**-leck-**TRON**-ick ther-**MOM**-eh-ter)—battery-operated clinical thermometer that uses a probe and records the temperature on a viewing screen in a few seconds

Elimination (ee-**lim**-ih-**NAY**-shun)—excretion; discharge from the body of indigestible materials and of waste products of body metabolism

Embolus (**EM**-boh-lus)—mass of undissolved material carried in the bloodstream and frequently causing obstruction of a vessel

Emesis (**EM**-eh-sis)—act of vomiting

Emesis basin (**EM**-eh-sis **BAY**-sin)—utensil for catching vomitus

Emollient (ee-**MOL**-ee-ent)—agent that softens and soothes the part when applied locally

Empathy (**EM**-pah-thee)—intellectual understanding of something in another person that is foreign to one's self

Emphysema (em-fih-**SEE**-mah)—chronic obstructive pulmonary disease in which the alveolar walls are destroyed

Endocrine gland (**EN**-doh-krin gland)—gland that secretes hormonal substances directly into the bloodstream; ductless gland

Endometrium (en-doh-**MEE**-tree-um)—mucous membrane lining the inner surface of the uterus

Endoscope (**EN**-doh-skohp)—instrument for examining the interior of the body

Enema (**EN**-eh-mah)—injection of water into the rectum and colon; used to help the bowels eliminate feces

Epidermis (ep-ih-**DER**-mis)—top layer of skin

Epididymis (**ep**-ih-**DID**-ih-mis)—elongated, cordlike structure along the posterior border of the testes in the ducts of which the sperm is stored

Epilepsy (**EP**-ih-**lep**-see)—noninfectious disorder of the brain manifested by episodes of motor and sensory dysfunction, which may or may not be accompanied by convulsions and unconsciousness

Episiotomy (eh-**piz**-ee-**OT**-oh-mee)—incision of the perineum at the end of the second stage of labor to avoid tearing of the perineum

Epithelium (ep-ih-**THEE**-lee-um)—tissues characterized by tightly packed cells with a minimum of intracellular material; forms epidermis and lines all hollow organs and passages of respiratory, digestive, and genitourinary systems

Equilibrium (**ee**-kwih-**LIB**-ree-um)—sense of balance

Erythrocyte (eh-**RITH**-roh-sight)—red blood cell

Eschar (**ES**-kar)—slough of tissue produced by burning or by a corrosive application

Estrogen (**ES**-troh-jen)—hormone produced by ovaries

Ethical code (**ETH**-ih-kal kohd)—rules of moral, responsible conduct

Etiology (**ee**-tee-**OL**-oh-jee)—cause of a disease

Eustachian tube (you-**STAY**-kee-an tewb)—auditory tube; leads from the middle ear to the pharynx

Evaluation (ee-val-you-**AY**-shun)—judgment

Eversion (ee-**VER**-zhun)—turning outward

Exchange list (ecks-**CHAYNJ** list)—list of measured foods that allows equivalent exchanges between foods within a designated food group

Excise (eck-**SIZE**)—remove by cutting

Excoriated (ecks-**KOR**-ee-ay-ted)—superficial loss of substance such as that produced by scratching the skin

Excreta (ecks-**KREE**-tah)—excretions such as feces

Expectorate (eck-**SPECK**-toh-rayt)—to spit (to bring up sputum)

Expiration (ecks-pih-**RAY**-shun)—exhalation

Exposure incident (ecks-**POH**-zhur **IN**-sih-dent)—an occurrence where there has been possible personal contact with infectious material

Expulsion stage (eck-**SPUL**-shun stayj)—stage of labor and delivery during which the fetus is expelled

Extended care facility (ecks-**TEN**-ded kair fah-**SILL**-ih-tee)—long-term care facility

Extension (ecks-**TEN**-shun)—movement by which the two ends of any jointed part are drawn away from each other

External urinary meatus (ecks-**TER**-nal **YOU**-rin-**air**-ee mee-**AY**-tus)—opening to the outside of the urethra

Facility (health care) (fah-**SILL**-ih-tee [hellth kair])—an agency that provides health care

Fahrenheit scale (**FAR**-en-hight skale)—scale used in the United States and England to express temperature

Fallopian tube (fal-**LOH**-pee-an tewb)—*See* Oviduct

False imprisonment (fawls im-**PRIH**-son-ment)—unlawfully restraining another

Fanfold (**FAN**-fold)—procedure for folding a sheet

Fasting (**FAST**-ing)—act of not eating

Fats—nutrient used to store energy

Fecal impaction (**FEE**-kul im-**PACK**-shun)—condition in which feces are wedged tightly in the bowel

Feces (**FEE**-sees)—semisolid waste eliminated from the body

Femur (**FEE**-mur)—thigh bone

Fetoscopy (fee-**TOS**-koh-pee)—examination of the fetus while in utero

Fetus (**FEE**-tus)—child in utero from the third month to birth

Fever (**FEE**-ver)—abnormally high body temperature

First aid—emergency care and treatment of an injured person before complete medical and surgical care can be secured

Flagged (flagd)—marked in a special way to call attention to it

Flatulence (**FLAT**-you-lens)—excessive gas in the stomach and intestines

Flatus (**FLAY**-tus)—gas or air in the stomach or intestines; air or gas expelled by way of any body opening

Flexible (**FLECK**-sih-bul)—ability to bend in different directions

Flexion (**FLECK**-shun)—decreasing the angle between two bones

Flora (**FLOH**-rah)—normal population of organisms found in a given area

Flowmeter (**FLOH**-mee-ter)—instrument for controlling gas flow in oxygen equipment

Flow rate (floh rayt)—rate at which oxygen or liquids are administered to the patient

Flow sheet (floh sheet)—a clinical record of ongoing patient care and progress

Foley catheter (**FOH**-lee **KATH**-eh-ter)—indwelling catheter placed in the urinary bladder to remove urine continuously

Fomite (**FOH**-might)—any object contaminated with germs, and thus able to transmit disease

Footboard (**FOOT**-bord)—appliance placed at the foot of the bed so the feet rest firmly against it and are at right angles to the legs

Forcing fluids (**FORS**-ing **FLEW**-ids)—notation meaning the patient must be encouraged to take as much fluid as possible

Foreskin (**FOR**-skin)—prepuce; loose tissue covering the penis and clitoris

Foster parent (**FOS**-ter **PAIR**-ent)—parent figure assigned by an agency

Fracture (**FRACK**-shur)—break in the continuity of bone

Frequency (**FREE**-kwen-see)—occurrence repeated often

Fundus (**FUN**-dus)—portion of uterus superior to point of entrance of oviducts

Fungus (**FUN**-gus)—class of organisms to which mold and yeast belong

Fusion (**FYOU**-zhun)—combining into a single unit

Gait (gayt)—manner of walking

Gait belt (gayt bellt)—belt placed around the patient's waist to assist in ambulation

Gallbladder (**GAWL**-blad-der)—small, sac-like organ in which bile is stored; found on the underside of the liver

Gangrene (**GANG**-green)—death and putrefaction of body tissue caused by stoppage of circulation of blood to an area

Gastrectomy (gas-**TRECK**-toh-mee)—surgical removal of part or all of the stomach

Gastric (**GAS**-trick)—pertaining to the stomach

Gatch bed—bed fitted with a jointed back rest and knee rest; patient can be raised to a sitting position and kept in that position

Gavage (gah-**VAHZH**)—feeding through a tube

General anesthetic (**JEN**-er-al **an**-es-**THET**-ick)—gas that induces a state of unconsciousness and insusceptibility to pain

Genes (jeenz)—units of heredity arranged into a linear fashion along a chromosome

Genetic (jeh-**NET**-ick)—pertaining to or carried by a gene or genes

Genital (**JEN**-ih-tul)—pertaining to reproduction

Genitalia (jen-ih-**TAIL**-ee-ah)—reproductive organs

Geriatrics (jer-ee-**AT**-ricks)—care of the elderly

Gerichair (**JER**-ee-chair)—chair or wheelchair with table or tray attached to it

Germs (jerms)—pathogenic microorganisms

Gestational age (jes-**TAY**-shun-al ayj)—age of development of a new individual within the uterus from conception to birth

Glaucoma (glaw-**KOH**-mah)—increased intraocular pressure that ultimately results in loss of vision

Global aphasia (**GLOH**-ball ah-**FAY**-zee-ah)—loss of all language ability

Glomeruli (gloh-**MER**-you-lie)—blood vessels that branch to form balls of capillaries in the cortex

Glossary (**GLOSS**-ah-ree)—alphabetical list of terms and explanations

Glucometer (glew-**KOM**-eh-ter)—instrument used to measure the level of blood sugar

Glucose (**GLEW**-kohs)—simple sugar; also called dextrose

Glycogen (**GLIGH**-koh-jen)—polysaccharide that is the chief carbohydrate storage material

Glycosuria (gligh-koh-**SOO**-ree-ah)—sugar in the urine

Gonads (**GOH**-nads)—reproductive organs; ovaries and testes

Gonorrhea (gon-oh-**REE**-ah)—sexually transmitted disease that causes an acute inflammation

Grand mal seizure (grand mawl **SEE**-zhur)—major epileptic seizure attended by loss of consciousness and convulsive movements

Graphic chart (**GRAF**-ick chart)—patient care record on which vital signs and sometimes other information are recorded

Greenstick fracture (green-stick **FRACK**-shur)—breaking of a bone on one side only, most often seen in children

Groin (groyn)—depression between the thigh and trunk

Gurney (**GUR**-nee)—equipment used to transport a patient; a stretcher

Halitosis (hal-ih-**TOH**-sis)—offensive odor to breath

Hallucination (hah-**loo**-sih-**NAY**-shun)—idea or perception that is not based on reality

Hand-over-hand technique (hand oh-ver hand tek-**NEEK**)—technique in which an instructor or care giver places his or her hand over the hand of a learner or patient to guide an activity

Harvest (**HAR**-vest)—to remove donor organs

Health (hellth)—state of physical, mental, and social well-being

Heart (hart)—hollow, muscular organ lying slightly to the left of the midline of the chest

Hematuria (hem-ah-**TOO**-ree-ah)—blood in the urine

Hemiplegia (hem-ee-**PLEE**-jee-ah)—paralysis on one side of the body

Hemoptysis (he-**MOP**-tih-sis)—expectoration of blood

Hemorrhage (**HEM**-or-ij)—escape of blood from blood vessels

Hemorrhoids (**HEM**-oh-royds)—varicose veins in the rectum

Hepatitis B virus (HBV) (hep-ah-**TIE**-tis bee **VY**-rus) (aytch-bee-vee)—organism that causes a serious form of infectious liver inflammation

Herniation (her-nee-**AY**-shun)—abnormal protrusion of an organ or other body structure

Hernia (**HER**-nee-ah)—protrusion or projection of a stomach organ through the wall or cavity that normally contains it

Herniorrhaphy (**her**-nee-**OR**-ah-fee)—surgical operation for hernia

Herpes simplex (**HER**-peez **SIM**-plex)—acute infectious viral disease

Hiatal hernia (high-**AY**-tal **HER**-nee-ah)—protrusion of a stomach portion through the esophageal hiatus of the diaphragm

Home health assistant (hohm hellth ah-**SIS**-tant)—nursing assistant who practices under supervision in a client's home

Home health services (hohm hellth **SIR**-vih-sez)—help provided after an acute hospitalization

Homemaker assistant (**HOHM**-may-ker ah-**SIS**-tant)—person who provides home management help to a client in the client's home

Horizontal recumbent position (supine) (hor-ih-**ZON**-tal ree-**KUM**-bent poh-**ZISH**-un)—patient is positioned flat on the back, arms extended by the sides, and legs extended

Hormone (**HOR**-mohn)—secretion of endocrine gland; substance produced by endocrine gland

Hospice (**HOS**-piss)—special facility or arrangement to provide care of terminally ill people

Hospital (**HOS**-pit-ul)—facility for the care of the sick or injured

Host (hohst)—animal or plant that harbors another organism

Human immunodeficiency virus (HIV) (**HUE**-man im-**myou**-noh-dee-**FISH**-en-see **VY**-rus) (aytch-eye-vee)—virus that causes acquired immunodeficiency disease (AIDS)

Hydrochloric acid (high-droh-**KLOR**-ick **AH**-sid)—acid produced by the stomach

Hydronephrosis (high-droh-neh-**FROH**-sis)—increasing pressure of urine that causes pressure on the kidney cells and results in their destruction

Hyperalimentation (**high**-per-**al**-ih-men-**TAY**-shun)—technique in which high density nutrients are introduced into a large vein

Hyperbaric chamber (**high**-per-**BAIR**-ick **CHAYM**-ber)—sealed enclosure for the raising of the level of oxygen in a patient's tissues

Hypercalcemia (**high**-per-kal-**SEE**-mee-ah)—excess calcium in the bloodstream

Hyperextension (**high**-per-ecks-**TEN**-shun)—excessive extension (straightening) of a limb or part

Hyperglycemia (**high**-per-gligh-**SEE**-mee-ah)—excessive levels of blood sugar

Hyperopia (**high**-per-**OH**-pee-ah)—farsightedness

Hypersecretion (**high**-per-see-**KREE**-shun)—excessive secretion

Hypersensitivity (**high**-per-sen-sih-**TIV**-ih-tee)—state of altered reactivity in which the

body reacts to a foreign agent more strongly than normal or in an abnormal way

Hypertension (**high**-per-**TEN**-shun)—high blood pressure

Hyperthermia (**high**-per-**THER**-mee-ah)—greatly increased temperature

Hyperthyroidism (**high**-per-**THIGH**-royd-izm)—excessive functioning of the thyroid gland

Hypertrophy (high-**PER**-troh-fee)—increase in the size of an organ or structure that does not involve tumor formation

Hypochondriasis (**high**-poh-kon-**DRY**-ah-sis)—abnormal concern about one's health

Hypoglycemia (**high**-poh-gligh-**SEE**-mee-ah)—abnormally low level of sugar in the blood

Hyposecretions (**high**-poh-sih-**KREE**-shuns)—less than normal production of secretions

Hypotension (**high**-poh-**TEN**-shun)—low blood pressure

Hypothermia (**high**-poh-**THER**-mee-ah)—greatly reduced temperature

Hypothermia/hyperthermia blanket (**high**-poh-**THER**-mee-ah/**high**-per-**THER**-mee-ah **BLAN**-ket)—a fluid filled blanket, the temperature of which can be raised or lowered

Hypothyroidism (**high**-poh-**THIGH**-royd-izm)—condition due to deficiency of the thyroid secretion, resulting in a lower basal metabolism

Hypoxia (high-**POX**-ee-ah)—lack of adequate oxygen supply

Hysterectomy (his-teh-**RECK**-toh-mee)—surgical removal of the uterus

Icon (**EYE**-kon)—image or figure. As used in this text, refers to images used on computers that represent various functions

ICU (intensive care unit) (eye-see-you) (in-**TEN**-siv kair **YOU**-nit)—hospital unit that provides care for critically ill patients

Ileostomy (ill-ee-**OS**-toh-mee)—incision of the ileum

Illusion (il-**LOO**-zhun)—mental impression derived from misinterpretation of an actual sensory stimulus

Immobilization (im-**moh**-bill-ih-**ZAY**-shun)—making of a part or limb immovable, usually in a cast

Immune response (im-**MYOUN** rih-**SPONS**)—response of the body to elements recognized as nonself with the production of antibodies and the rejection of the foreign material

Immunization (**IM**-myou-nigh-**zay**-shun)—process of making a person more resistant to an infectious agent

Impaction (im-**PACK**-shun)—condition of being tightly wedged into a part (as feces in the bowel)

Implementation (im-plih-men-**TAY**-shun)—to put into effect

Impotence (**IM**-poh-tens)—inability to perform sexually

Incarcerated (strangulated) hernia (in-**KAR**-sir-**ayt**-ed [**STRANG**-you-lay-ted] **HER**-nee-ah)—abnormal constriction of part of the intestinal tract that has herniated

Incentive spirometer (in-**SEN**-tiv spih-**ROM**-eh-ter)—apparatus that is used to encourage better ventilation

Incontinence (in-**KON**-tih-nens)—inability to control defecation or urination

Incontinent (in-**KON**-tih-nent)—act of defecating or urinating uncontrollably

Increment (**IN**-kreh-ment)—amount of increase in measurements

Indwelling catheter (**IN**-dwell-ing **KATH**-ih-ter)—Foley catheter that remains in the patient's bladder to drain the urine

Infarction (in-**FARK**-shun)—death of tissue

Infection (in-**FECK**-shun)—invasion and multiplication of any organism and the damage caused by this in the body

Inferior (in-**FEER**-ee-or)—below another part

Infirm (in-**FERM**)—one who is ill or unable to care for himself or herself

Inflammation (**in**-flah-**MAY**-shun)—tissue reaction to injury either direct or referred

Informed consent (in-**FORMD** kon-**SENT**)—permission given after full disclosure of the facts

Infusion (in-**FYOU**-zhun)—introduction of a solution into a vein by gravity; for example, an intravenous infusion (IV)

Initiative (in-**ISH**-ee-ah-tiv)—action of taking the first step or initial action

Insertion (in-**SIR**-shun)—distal point of attachment of skeletal muscle

Inspiration (in-spih-**RAY**-shun)—drawing of air into the lungs (inhalation)

Insulin (**IN**-soo-lin)—active antidiabetic hormone secreted by the islets of Langerhans in the pancreas

Insulin dependent diabetes mellitus (IDDM) (**IN**-soo-lin dee-**PEN**-dent die-ah-**BEE**-teez **MEL**-ih-tus) (eye-dee-dee-em)—form of diabetes mellitus that requires insulin administration as part of the therapy

Intake and output (I & O) (**IN**-tayk and **OUT**-put) (eye & oh)—recording of the amount of fluid ingested and the amount of fluid expelled by a patient

Integument (in-**TEG**-you-ment)—the skin

Interdisciplinary team (in-ter-**DISS**-ih-plin-air-ee teem)—group of different professionals who each contribute their expertise to the care of a single person

Intermittent positive pressure breathing (IPPB) (in-ter-**MIT**-ent **POS**-ih-tiv **PRESH**-ur **BREE**-thing) (eye-pee-pee-bee)—technique for assisting breathing

Interpersonal relationships (in-ter-**PER**-son-al rih-**LAY**-shun-ships)—how people interact with each other

Intervention (in-ter-**VEN**-shun)—actions that influence the eventual outcome of a situation

Intimacy (**IN**-tih-mah-see)—feelings of closeness and familiarity

Intracranial pressure (in-trah-**KRAY**-nee-al **PRESH-**ur)—pressure exerted within the cranium

Intravenous infusion (IV) (in-trah-**VEE**-nus in-**FYOU**-zhun) (eye-vee)—nourishment given through a sterile tube into a vein

Invasion of privacy (in-**VAY**-zhun of **PRIGH**-vah-see)—taking liberties with the person or personal rights of another

Invasive (in-**VAY**-siv)—characterized by invading or spreading

Involution (in-voh-**LOO**-shun)—reduction in the size of the uterus following delivery

Iodine (**EYE**-oh-dine)—element needed for proper function of the thyroid gland

Iris (**EYE**-ris)—colored portion of the eye

Irrigate (**EAR**-ih-gayt)—to wash out

Ischemia (is-**KEE**-mee-ah)—deficient blood supply to body tissues

Ischemic (is-**KEE**-mick)—having inadequate blood flow to an area

Islets of Langerhans (**EYE**-lets of **LANG**-ger-hans)—cells in the pancreas that produce insulin

Isolation (eye-soh-**LAY**-shun)—place where the patient with easily transmitted disease is separated from others

Isolation technique (eye-soh-**LAY**-shun tek-**NEEK**)—special procedures carried out to prevent the spread of infectious organisms from an infected person

Isolette (eye-soh-**LET**)—type of environmentally controlled unit that is used to house a newborn infant

IV standard (eye-vee **STAN**-dard)—pole usually made of stainless steel, that can be attached to the bed or stand on the floor

Jacksonian seizure (jack-**SOH**-nee-an **SEE**-zhur)—type of convulsive seizure that is a progression of involuntary clonic movements with retention of consciousness

Jaundice (**JAWN**-dis)—yellowing of the skin

Job description (job dih-**SKRIP**-shun)—duties and responsibilities involved in a position

Joint (joynt)—point of articulation between bones

Kardex (**KAR**-dex)—type of file in which nursing care plans are kept

Ketosis (kee-**TOH**-sis)—abnormal levels of ketones in the blood; complication of diabetes mellitus

Keyboard (**KEE**-bord)—row of keys on a computer used to input information

Kidneys (**KID**-nees)—two glandular, bean-shaped bodies, purplish-brown in color, situated in back of the abdominal cavity, one on each side of the spinal column, that excrete waste matter in the form of urine

Knee-chest position (nee-chest poh-**ZISH**-un)—patient is positioned on abdomen with knees drawn up toward abdomen and with legs separated; arms are brought up and flexed on either side of the head that is turned to one side

Koran (kuh-**RAN**)—Muslim sacred book

Kyphosis (kigh-**FOH**-sis)—hunchback

Labia majora (**LAY**-bee-ah mah-**JOR**-ah)—two large, hair-covered, liplike structures that are part of the vulva

Labia minora (**LAY**-bee-ah mih-**NOR**-ah)—two hairless, liplike structures found beneath the labia majora

Labor (**LAY**-bor)—physiological process by which the fetus is expelled from the uterus at term

Lactation (lack-**TAY**-shun)—function of secreting milk

Laminectomy (lam-ih-**NECK**-toh-mee)—transection of a vertebral lamina

Lateral (**LAT**-er-al)—body parts away from the midline

Legal custody (**LEE**-gul **KUS**-toe-dee)—condition of having the right to consent to hospitalization and of giving permission for procedures

Legal guardian (**LEE**-gul **GAR**-dee-an)—person who has the legal right to make decisions for another person

Lesions (**LEE**-zhuns)—abnormal changes in tissue formation

Leukemia (loo-**KEE**-mee-ah)—malignant disease of the blood-forming organs, characterized by abnormal proliferation and distortion of the leukocytes in the blood and bone marrow

Leukocyte (**LOO**-koh-sight)—white blood cell

Leukorrhea (loo-koh-**REE**-ah)—white vaginal discharge

Lever (**LEV**-er)—bar or rodlike structure that operates on a fixed axis or fulcrum and is used to lift weight

Liable (**LIE**-ah-bul)—legally responsible

Libel (**LIE**-bul)—any oral or written defamatory statement

Licensed practical nurse (LPN); licensed vocational nurse (LVN) (**LICE**-enst **PRACK**-tih-kul nurs) (el-pee-en); (**LICE**-enst voh-**KAY**-shun-al nurs) (el-vee-en)—graduate of a one-year certificate program who must pass a state exam before being permitted to practice nursing

Libido (lih-**BEE**-doh)—sex drive

Life care facility (life kair fah-**SILL**-ih-tee)—apartment homes that offer health care and recreational facilities for the elderly

Life support system (life suh-**PORT SIS**-tum)—equipment needed to sustain life when vital signs are inadequate

Ligament (**LIG**-ah-ment)—band of fibrous tissue that holds joints together

Lithotripsy (**LITH**-oh-trip-see)—the crushing of calculi such as kidney stones

Litter (**LIT**-er)—equipment used to transport a patient; also called a gurney or stretcher

Living will (**LIV**-ing will)—written statement, usually by those who are terminally ill, requesting not to be kept alive on life support systems when their faculties have failed

Local anesthetic (**LOH**-kul an-es-**THET**-ick)—type of anesthetic for which the action is confined to a limited area. The anesthetic is usually given by injection and the patient remains awake

Lochia (**LOH**-kee-ah)—discharge from the uterus of blood, mucus, and tissue during the puerperal period

Logo (**LOW**-goh)—symbol that identifies a business, company, or organization

Long-term care facility (lawng turm kair fah-**SILL**-ih-tee)—facility that provides care for patients with long-standing disabilities; can be terminal care

Lubricant (**LOO**-brih-kant)—substance applied to a part to improve the ease of movement between touching parts; also substances secreted by the body for the same purpose

Lumpectomy (lum-**PECK**-toh-mee)—excision of abnormal tissue such as a "lump" in the breast

Lymph (limpf)—fluid found in lymphatic vessels

Macule (**MACK**-youl)—flat, discolored spot on the skin

Maladaptive behavior (mal-ah-**DAP**-tiv bee-**HAY**-vyour)—inappropriate reaction due to mental breakdown

Malignancy (mah-**LIG**-nan-see)—cancerous condition which, if left untreated, leads to death

Malignant (mah-**LIG**-nant)—cancerous

Malnutrition (mal-new-**TRISH**-un)—lack of necessary food substances in the body, or improper absorption and distribution of them

Malpractice (mal-**PRACK**-tis)—poor or improper medical treatment; for example, when a nursing assistant gives improper care or care for which the nursing assistant has not been instructed

Mammogram (**MAM**-oh-gram)—X-ray examination of the breasts

Mastectomy (mass-**TECK**-toh-mee)—excision of the breast

Masturbation (mass-tur-**BAY**-shun)—sexually stimulating self

Maternity (mah-**TER**-nih-tee)—related to pregnancy

Meatus (mee-**AY**-tus)—tubelike opening

Mechanical lift (mih-**KAN**-ih-kul lift)—apparatus used to assist in lifting and transferring a patient

Meconium (mih-**KOH**-nee-um)—first feces of the newborn infant which consists of salts, mucus, bile, and epithelial cells. Color is greenish-black to light brown

Medial (**MEE**-dee-al)—close to the midline of the body or structure

Medicaid (**MED**-ih-kayd)—federal- and state-funded program that pays for medical costs for those whose income falls below a certain level

Medical asepsis (**MED**-ih-kul ah-**SEP**-sis)—procedures followed to keep germs from being spread from one person to another

Medicare (**MED**-ih-kair)—federal program that assists persons over 65 years of age with hospital and medical costs

Medulla (meh-**DOOL**-ah)—forms part of the brain stem

Medulla (of kidney) (meh-**DOOL**-ah) (of **KID**-nee)—renal pyramids

Melanin (**MEL**-ah-nin)—dark pigment normally formed in the skin and hair

Membranes (**MEM**-brains)—tissue sheets that line the cavities

Menarche (meh-**NAR**-kee)—beginning of the menstrual function

Meninges (meh-**NIN**-jeez)—three-layered serous membrane covering the brain and spinal cord

Meningitis (men-in-**JIGH**-tis)—inflammation of the meninges

Menopause (**MEN**-oh-pawz)—period when ovaries stop functioning and menstruation ceases; climacteric

Menorrhagia (men-oh-**RAY**-jee-ah)—excessive bleeding during menstruation

Menstruation (men-stroo-**AY**-shun)—loss of an unneeded part of the endometrium following the release of an ovum and lack of conception

Mental illness (**MEN**-tal **ILL**-ness)—behavioral maladaptations

Menu (**MEN**-you)—as used in the text, a list of possible computer functions

Metabolism (meh-**TAH**-bohl-izm)—sum total of the physical and chemical processes and reactions taking place in the body

Metastasis (meh-**TAS**-tah-sis)—spreading of cancer to other body parts from a primary location

Metastasize (meh-**TAS**-tah-size)—to spread (cancer) to other body parts

Metric system (**MET**-rick **SIS**-tum)—system of weights and measurements based on the meter; all units based on some power of ten

Microbes (**MY**-krohbs)—tiny organisms that can be seen only with a microscope

Microorganisms (**my**-kroh-**OR**-gan-izms)—tiny organisms that can be seen only with a microscope, particularly bacteria

Micturition (**mick**-too-**RISH**-un)—urination

Midriff (**MID**-rif)—middle part of the body between the chest and waist

Mineral (**MIN**-er-al)—inorganic chemical compound found in nature; many are important in building body tissues and regulating body fluids

Mitered corner (**MY**-terd **KOR**-ner)—one type of corner used in making a facility bed

Mitosis (my-**TOH**-sis)—division of the cytoplasm and nucleus in the cell

Mobility (moh-**BILL**-ih-tee)—ability to move or to be moved easily from place to place

Monitor (**MON**-ih-tor)—apparatus that can observe and record information constantly

Morbidity (mor-**BID**-ih-tee)—state of being diseased; conditions inducing disease

Moribund (**MOR**-ih-bund)—dying

Mortality rate (mor-**TAL**-ih-tee rayt)—proportion of deaths in the population

Mottling (**MOT**-ling)—discoloration of skin or irregular areas

Mucolytic (myou-koh-**LIH**-tick)—destroying or dissolving mucus

Mucous (**MYOU**-kus)—pertaining to or resembling mucus; also, secreting mucus

Mucus (**MYOU**-kus)—secretion of mucous membranes; thick, sticky fluid

Multiple sclerosis (**MUL**-tih-pul skleh-**ROH**-sis)—disease characterized by hardened patches scattered throughout the brain and spinal cord that interfere with the nerves in those areas

Muscular tissue (**MUSS**-kyou-lar **TISH**-you)—tissues that have ability to shorten and lengthen

Myocardial infarction (**my**-oh-**KAR**-dee-al in-**FARK**-shun)—formation of an infarct in the heart muscle due to interruption of the blood supply to the area

Myocardium (**my**-oh-**KAR**-dee-um)—heart muscle

Myopia (my-**OH**-pee-ah)—nearsightedness

Nasogastric (NG) tube (nay-zoh-**GAS**-trick [en-jee] toob)—soft rubber or plastic tube that is inserted through the nostril and into the stomach

Necrosis (neh-**KROH**-sis)—tissue death

Negligence (**NEG**-lih-jents)—failure to give care that is reasonably expected of a nursing assistant

Neonate (**NEE**-oh-nayt)—newborn baby

Neoplasia (nee-oh-**PLAY**-zee-ah)—new, uncontrolled tissue growth; tumor

Neoplasm (**NEE**-oh-plazm)—new growth; tumor

Nephritis (nih-**FRIGH**-tis)—inflammation of the kidney

Nephron (**NEF**-ron)—microscopic kidney units that produce urine

Nerve (nurv)—bundle of nerve processes (axons and dendrites) that are held together by connective tissue

Nerve impulse (nurv **IM**-puls)—electrical wave that transmits a message

Nervous tissue (**NUR**-vus **TISH**-you)—highly specialized tissue capable of conducting a nerve impulse

Networking (**NET**-werk-ing)—line of communication between individuals with a common interest or goal

Neuron (**NEW**-ron)—cell of the nervous system

Neurotransmitter (new-roh-**TRANS**-mit-er)—chemical compound that transmits a nervous impulse across cells at a synapse

No-code order (no cohd **OR**-der)—an order not to resuscitate a patient

Nocturia (nock-**TUR**-ee-ah)—excessive urination at night

Noninvasive (non-in-**VAY**-siv)—remaining localized and not spreading

Nonpathogen (non-**PATH**-oh-jen)—microorganism that is not capable of producing disease

Nonverbal communication (non-**VER**-bal kom-**myou**-nih-**KAY**-shun)—communication transmitted through nonverbal ways, such as facial expression and body language

Nosocomial (noh-soh-**KOH**-mee-al)—pertaining to or originating in a facility, hospital, or infirmary

NPO (en-pee-oh)—nothing by mouth

Nucleus (**NEW**-klee-us)—part of the cell that directs the activities of the cell

Nurse Aide Competency Evaluation Program (NACEP) (nurs ayd **KOM**-peh-ten-see ee-**val**-you-**AY**-shun **PROH**-gram) (en-ay-see-ee-pee)—test taken by the nursing assistant which, when passed successfully, entitles the nursing assistant to certification

Nursing assistant (**NUR**-sing ah-**SIS**-tant)—person who assists, under supervision, with the care of the sick and infirmed

Nursing care plan (**NUR**-sing kair plan)—plan developed to direct the patient's care

Nursing home (**NUR**-sing hohm)—facility that provides room and board and some nursing care; also called convalescent home

Nursing process (**NUR**-sing **PRAH**-sess)—framework for nursing action

Nursing team (**NUR**-sing teem)—members of the nursing staff who provide patient care

Nutrient (**NEW**-tree-ent)—nourishing substance or food

Nutrition (new-**TRISH**-un)—process by which the body uses food for growth and repair and to maintain health

OB (oh-bee)—obstetrics

Obese (oh-**BEES**)—overweight

Objective observations (ob-**JECK**-tiv ob-sir-**VAY**-shuns)—observations made through the senses of the observer

Observation (ob-sir-**VAY**-shun)—noticing something

Obstetrical (ob-**STET**-ree-kal)—pertaining to pregnancy, labor, and delivery

Obstruction (ob-**STRUCK**-shun)—blockage in a passageway

Occult blood (ah-**KULT**-blud)—blood in such minute quantity that it can only be recognized by microscope or chemical means

Occupational exposure (ock-kyou-**PAY**-shun-al ecks-**POH**-zhur)—coming into contact with infectious materials during the performance of a person's job

Occupational Safety and Health Act (ock-kyou-**PAY**-shun-al **SAYF**-tee and hellth act)—known as OSHA—the regulations on occupational health and safety that must be followed by every facility

OD (oh-dee)—as used in the text, pertains to the right eye

Olfactory (ol-**FACK**-toh-ree)—pertaining to the sense of smell

Oliguria (ol-ih-**GYOU**-ree-ah)—scant urine

Ombudsman (**AHM**-buds-man)—patient advocate

Omnibus Budget Reconciliation Act (OBRA) (**OM**-nih-bus **BUD**-jet **reh**-kon-**sill**-ee-**AY**-shun akt) (oh-bee-are-ay)—law that regulates the education and certification of nursing assistants working in acute care and long-term care facilities

Oophorectomy (oh-of-oh-**RECK**-toh-mee)—surgical excision of an ovary

Open bed (**OH**-pen bed)—bed with top bedding fanfolded to bottom, ready for occupancy

Open fracture (**OH**-pen **FRACK**-shur)—broken bone in which part of the bone protrudes through the skin

Open reduction/internal fixation (**OH**-pen ree-**DUK**-shun/in-**TER**-nal fiks-**AY**-shun)—a surgical procedure to reduce a fractured bone. The skin is opened and the fracture realigned and held in place by screws, plates, and pins

Operative (**OP**-er-ah-tiv)—pertaining to an operation

Ophthalmoscope (oh-**THAL**-moh-skohp)—instrument for examining the eyes

OR (oh-are)—operating room

Oral hygiene (OR-al **HIGH**-jeen)—care of the mouth and teeth

Orally (**OR**-al-ee)—through the mouth

Oral report (**OR**-al ree-**PORT**)—verbal report

Orchiectomy (or-key-**ECK**-toh-mee)—excision of the testis

Organ (**OR**-gan)—any part of the body that carries out a specific function or functions, such as the heart

Organic mental syndrome (or-**GAN**-ick **MEN**-til **SIN**-drohm)—mental deterioration; general term that includes all dementia due to physical abnormalities of the brain

Orifice (**OR**-ih-fis)—body opening such as the nose or mouth

Origin (**OR**-ih-jin)—proximal point of attachment to skeletal muscle

Orthopedic (or-thoh-**PEE**-dick)—concerning orthopedics; prevention or correction of deformities

Orthopneic (or-thop-**NEE**-ick)—positioning of a patient by adjusting the over-bed table in such a way that the patient, supported by pillows, is able to lean on it

OS (oh-ess)—as used in the text, pertains to the left eye

Ossicles (**OS**-sih-kuls)—any small bones, such as one of the three bones in the ear

Osteoarthritis (**oss**-tee-oh-are-**THRIGH**-tis)—degenerative joint disease caused by disintegration of the cartilage that covers the ends of the bones

Osteoporosis (**oss**-tee-oh-poor-**OH**-sis)—most common metabolic disease of bone in the United States; characterized by a decrease in the mass of bony tissue; most commonly affects females past middle age

Ostomy (**OS**-toh-mee)—suffix meaning "to create a new opening"; for example, colostomy

Otitis media (oh-**TIGH**-tis **MEE**-dee-ah)—inflamed condition of the media part of the ear

Otosclerosis (oh-toh-sklee-**ROH**-sis)—formation of bone in the inner ear that causes the ossicles to be fixed

Otoscope (**OH**-toh-skohp)—instrument used to examine the ear

Outpatient surgery (**OUT**-pay-shent **SUR**-jer-ee)—short-term surgery

Output (**OUT**-put)—measured amount of fluid excreted in a given period of time

Ovaries (**OH**-vah-rees)—endocrine glands located in the female pelvis; female gonads

Ovulation (oh-vyou-**LAY**-shun)—lunar monthly ripening and rupture of the mature graafian follicle and the discharge of the ovum from the cortex of the ovary

Ovum (**OH**-vum)—female egg

Oxygen (**OK**-sih-jen)—gas that is essential to cellular metabolism and all life

Pacemaker (pacer) (**PAYS**-may-ker)—artificial device placed in the body to regulate the heartbeat

Pallor (**PAL**-or)—less color than normal for the skin

Palpated systolic pressure (**PAL**-pay-ted sis-**TOL**-ick **PRESH**-ur)—pressure indicated on the blood pressure gauge as the cuff is inflated and the radial pulse no longer can be felt

Panhysterectomy (pan-his-ter-**ECK**-toh-mee)—removal of the entire uterus

Pap smear (**PAP** smeer)—simple test used to detect cancer of the cervix

Papule (**PAP**-youl)—solid, elevated lesion of the skin

Paralysis (pah-**RAL**-ih-sis)—loss or impairment of the ability to move parts of the body

Paranoia (pair-ah-**NOY**-ah)—state in which one has delusions of persecution and/or grandeur

Paraplegia (pair-ah-**PLEE**-jee-ah)—paralysis of lower portion of the body and of both legs

Parasite (**PAIR**-ah-sight)—organism that lives within, upon, or at the expense of another organism known as the host

Parathormone (pair-ah-**THOR**-mohn)—hormone produced by parathyroid glands that regulates calcium and phosphorus blood levels

Parietal (pah-**RYE**-eh-tal)—pertaining to the walls of an organ or cavity

Pathogen (**PATH**-oh-jen)—microorganism or other agent capable of producing a disease

Pathology (pah-**THOL**-oh-jee)—disease

Patient (**PAY**-shent)—person who needs care; resident

Patient's Bill of Rights (**PAY**-shents bill of rights)—document developed by the American Hospital Association that describes the basic rights to which a patient is entitled

Pelvic belt traction (**PEL**-vick belt **TRACK**-shun)—special form of traction in which a belt, secured around a person's hips, is attached to ropes, pulleys, and weights

Pelvic inflammatory disease (PID) (**PEL**-vick in-**FLAM**-ah-toh-ree dih-**ZEEZ**) (pee-eye-dee)—inflammation of the pelvic organs

Pelvis (**PEL**-vis)—lower portion of the trunk of the body; basin-shaped area bounded by the hip bones, the sacrum, and the coccyx

Penis (**PEE**-nis)—male organ of copulation

Pepsin (**PEP**-sin)—enzyme produced in the stomach that begins protein digestion

Percussion (per-**KUSH**-un)—tapping a body part with the fingers to determine the size, position, or density of the organs underneath

Percussion hammer (per-**KUSH**-un **HAM**-mer)—instrument used to test reflexes

Pericardium (pair-ih-**KAR**-dee-um)—membranes that surround the heart

Perineum (pair-ih-**NEE**-um)—in the male, the area between the anus and scrotum; in the female, the area between the anus and vagina

Perioperative (pair-ee-**OP**-er-ah-tiv)—occurring in association with an operative procedure

Peripheral (peh-**RIF**-er-al)—pertaining to the outside or outer part

Peristalsis (per-ih-**STALL**-sis)—progressive, wavelike movement that occurs involuntarily in hollow tubes of the body, especially in the alimentary canal

Peritoneum (pair-ih-toh-**NEE**-um)—serous membrane lining the walls of the abdominal and pelvic cavities

Personality (per-son-**AL**-ih-tee)—sum of the behavior, attitudes, and character traits of an individual

Personal protective equipment (**PER**-son-al proh-**TEK**-tiv ee-**KWIP**-ment)—equipment such as waterproof gowns, masks, gloves, goggles, and other equipment needed to protect an employee from infectious material

Petit mal seizure (peh-**TEE** mawl **SEE**-zhur)—type of epileptic attack that is generally short in nature; absence attack

Phalanges (fah-**LAN**-jeez)—any bones of a finger or toe

Phantom pain (**FAN**-tom payn)—pain experienced in a body part that has been removed from the body as if the part were still attached

Phlegm (flem)—mucus

Physician (fih-**ZISH**-un)—licensed medical doctor

Physiology (fiz-ee-**OL**-oh-jee)—the science that deals with the functioning of living organisms

Physiotherapist (fiz-ee-oh-**THER**-ah-pist)—trained professional who provides therapy and exercise to maintain mobility

Pigmentation (pig-men-**TAY**-shun)—coloration of an area by pigment

Piles (pyls)—hemorrhoids

Pitting edema (**PIT**-ting eh-**DEE**-mah)—condition in which the tissue remains indented when presssure is applied to an edematous area

Pivot (**PIV**-ut)—to twist or turn in a swiveling motion

Placenta (plah-**SEN**-tah)—name given to the afterbirth

Placental stage (plah-**SEN**-tal stayj)—period of the delivery process during which the afterbirth is expelled from the uterus

Plane (playn)—imaginary line used to describe the relationship of one body part to another

Plantar flexion (**PLAN**-tar **FLECK**-shun)—extending the foot in a downward movement

Plasma (**PLAZ**-mah)—liquid portion of blood

Pleura (**PLOOR**-ah)—membranes that surround the lungs

PM care (pee-em kair)—care given to prepare the patient or resident for sleep

Pneumocystis carinii (new-moh-**SIS**-tis kah-**RIN**-ee)—protozoan frequently causing pneumonia in patients who are HIV positive

Pneumonia (new-**MOH**-nee-ah)—inflammation of the lungs

Podiatrist (poh-**DYE**-ah-trist)—physician specializing in foot problems

Polydipsia (pol-ee-**DIP**-see-ah)—excessive thirst

Polyphagia (pol-ee-**FAY**-jee-ah)—excessive ingestion of food

Polyuria (pol-ee-**YOU**-ree-ah)—excessive excretion of urine

POMR (pee-oh-em-are)—problem-oriented medical records

Port (port)—opening

Portal of entry (**POR**-tul of **EN**-tree)—area of body through which microbes enter and cause disease

Portal of exit (**POR**-tul of **EX**-it)—area of body through which disease-producing organisms leave the body

Positive signs of pregnancy (**POS**-ih-tiv sighns of **PREG**-nan-see)—hearing, seeing, or feeling a fetus

Postanesthesia care (post-an-es-**THEE**-see-ah kair)—care given to a patient following the administration of an anesthetic

Postanesthesia care unit (PACU) (post-an-es-**THEE**-see-ah kair **YOU**-nit) (pee-ay-see-you)—room where patients receive immediate care following surgery

Posterior (pos-**TEER**-ee-or)—back or dorsal

Postmortem (post-**MOR**-tem)—after death

Postmortem care (post-**MOR**-tem kair)—care given to the body after death

Postoperative (post-**OP**-er-ah-tiv)—after surgery

Postpartum (post-**PAR**-tum)—after parturition; after birth

Postural drainage (**POS**-chur-al **DRAYN**-aj)—technique of positioning the patient to encourage drainage of different areas of the pulmonary tree

Posture (**POS**-chur)—attitude or position of the body

Potentially infectious material (poh-**TEN**-shal-lee in-**FECK**-shus mah-**TER**-ee-al)—materials or equipment that could be a source of disease-producing organisms

Preadolescence (**pree**-ad-oh-**LESS**-ens)—years between the ages of 12 and 14

Predisposing cause (of disease) (**pree**-dis-**POS**-ing kawz [of dih-**ZEEZ**])—factors that contribute to the development of a condition

Prefix (**PREE**-fix)—term that is placed before a word that changes or modifies the meaning of the word

Prenatal (pree-**NAY**-tal)—before birth

Preoperative (pree-**OP**-er-ah-tiv)—period before surgery

Presbycusis (pres-beh-**KYOU**-sis)—impaired hearing, due to old age

Presbyopia (pres-bee-**OH**-pee-ah)—impaired vision resulting from the aging process

Pressure sore (**PRESH**-ur sor)—ulceration due to eschemia; decubitus

Presumptive signs of pregnancy (pree-**ZUMP**-tiv-sighns of **PREG**-nan-see)—indications seen early in pregnancy that may also be associated with other conditions; includes amenorrhea, morning sickness, fatigue, tender and full breasts

Probable signs of pregnancy (**PRAH**-bah-bul sighns of **PREG**-nan-see)—indications of pregnancy at a more advanced stage that may also accompany other conditions, including enlargement of the abdomen and positive pregnancy test

Probe (prohb)—as used in this text, long, slender part of an instrument; that portion of the electronic or aural thermometer placed into the patient

Problem-oriented medical record (POMR) (**PRAH**-blem **OR**-ee-en-ted **MED**-ih-kul **REH**-kord) (pee-oh-em-are)—form of documentation in which all recordings are organized around the strength or problem of the patient

Procedure (proh-**SEE**-jur)—series of steps outlining how and in what order and manner to do something

Process (**PRAH**-sess)—projection as from a bone; series of steps that may be taken as in the nursing process

Proctoscopy (prock-**TOS**-koh-pee)—instrumental inspection of the rectum

Progesterone (proh-**JES**-teh-rohn)—hormone produced by female ovaries

Prognosis (prog-**NOH**-sis)—probable outcome of a disease or injury

Progressive mobilization (proh-**GRESS**-iv moh-**bill**-ih-**ZAY**-shun)—gradual increase in activity

Projection (proh-**JECK**-shun)—unconscious defense mechanism in which an individual denies his/her own emotionally unacceptable traits and sees them as belonging to another

Pronation (proh-**NAY**-shun)—placing or lying in a face downward position; applied to the hand with the palms facing backward

Prone position (prohn poh-**ZISH**-un)—patient positioned on the abdomen, spine straight, legs extended, and arms flexed on either side of the head

Prostatectomy (pros-tah-**TECK**-toh-mee)—removal of all or part of the prostate gland

Prostate gland (**PROS**-tayt gland)—gland of male reproductive system that surrounds the neck of the urinary bladder and the beginning of the urethra

Prosthesis (pros-**THEE**-sis)—artificial substitute for a missing body part, such as dentures, hand, leg

Protein (**PROH**-tee-in)—basic material of every body cell; an essential nutrient

Protein bound iodine (PBI) (**PROH**-tee-in bownd **EYE**-oh-dine) (pee-bee-eye)—clinical test performed to determine thyroid function

Protozoa (proh-toh-**ZOH**-ah)—microscopic unicellular organism

Proximal (**PROX**-ih-mal)—closest to the point of attachment

Pruritus (prew-**RYE**-tus)—itching

Psychotic (sigh-**KOT**-ick)—completely out of touch with reality

Puberty (**PYOU**-ber-tee)—condition or period of becoming capable of sexual reproduction

Pubic (**PYOU**-bick)—concerning the pubes

Pulse (puls)—wave of pressure exerted against the walls of the arteries in response to ventricular contraction

Pulse deficit (puls **DEF**-ih-sit)—difference between contractions of the heart and pulse expansions of the radial artery

Pulse pressure (puls **PRESH**-ur)—difference between the systolic and diastolic pressures

Pustule (**PUS**-tyoul)—circumscribed pus-containing lesion of the skin

Pyloric sphincter (pie-**LOR**-ick **SFINK**-ter)—muscle at the exit point of the pylorus

Pyrexia (pie-**REX**-ee-ah)—fever

Quadrant (**KWAHD**-rant)—one of the four imaginary sections of the surface of the abdomen

Quadriplegia (kwahd-rih-**PLEE**-jee-ah)—condition of paralysis of all four limbs

Radial artery (**RAY**-dee-al **ARE**-ter-ee)—artery near the radius; commonly used to determine pulse

Radial deviation (**RAY**-dee-al dee-vee-**AY**-shun)—wrists are turned toward the thumb side

Radial pulse (**RAY**-dee-al puls)—pulse that can be measured by palpating the radial artery

Rales (rayls)—abnormal respiratory sound heard in auscultation of the chest

Range of motion (ROM) exercises (rainj of **MOH**-shun [are-oh-em] **ECK**-sir-size-es)—series of exercises specifically designed to move each joint through its range

Rapport (rah-**POOR**)—understanding between two persons

Rate (rayt)—valuation based on comparison with a standard

Rationalization (rash-un-al-ih-**ZAY**-shun)—unconscious defense mechanism in which one devises a logical, self-satisfying but incorrect explanation for one's behavior or feelings

Reaction formation (ree-**ACK**-shun for-**MAY**-shun)—repressing the reality of an anxiety-producing situation. The individual exhibits behaviors that are exactly opposite to the real feelings

Reality (ree-**AL**-ih-tee)—what is actually occurring; true in fact

Reality orientation (ree-**AL**-ih-tee or-ee-en-**TAY**-shun)—techniques used to help a person remain oriented to environment, time, and himself/herself

Recovery room (ree-**KOV**-er-ee room)—location where surgical patients are taken after surgery. They return to their rooms when their condition stabilizes

Rectocele (**RECK**-toh-seel)—protrusion of part of the rectum into the vagina

Rectum (**RECK**-tum)—lower part of the large intestine, about five inches long, between the sigmoid flexure and the anal canal

References (**REF**-er-en-sez)—in a résumé, statements about abilities and characteristics; persons who give such statements

Reflex (**REE**-flecks)—activity performed without conscious thought

Registered nurse (**REJ**-is-terd nurs)—specially educated person who is licensed to plan and direct the nursing care of patients

Regress (ree-**GRESS**)—to move in a backward fashion

Rehabilitative hospital (ree-hah-**BILL**-ih-**tay**-tiv **HOS**-pit-ul)—health care facility that offers specialized care to assist people regain optimum functioning

Reminiscing (reh-mih-**NISS**-ing)—thinking and talking about the past

Remission (ree-**MISH**-un)—period of decreased severity of symptoms in chronic disease

Renal calculi (**REE**-nal **KAL**-kyou-lee)—kidney stones

Renal colic (**REE**-nal **KOL**-ick)—spasm in area near kidney accompanied by pain

Replication (rep-lih-**KAY**-shun)—to reproduce exactly

Repression (ree-**PRESH**-un)—involuntary exclusion from awareness of a painful experience or conflict-creating memory, feeling, or impulse

Reservoir (**REZ**-er-vwar)—storage area; biologically, an animal or source that maintains infectious organisms that periodically can be spread to others

Resident unit (**REZ**-ih-dent **YOU**-nit)—room occupied by resident and his/her personal possessions; may be shared by other residents

Respiration (res-pih-**RAY**-shun)—process of taking oxygen into the body and expelling carbon dioxide

Respirator (res-pih-**RAY**-tor)—apparatus that assists the patient to breathe

Rest home (rest hohm)—long-term care facility

Restorative care (ree-**STOR**-ah-tiv kair)—care that emphasizes helping the person reach or maintain physical, mental, and psychological well-being

Restricted fluids (ree-**STRICK**-ted **FLEW**-ids)—limit to the amount of fluid intake

Résumé (**REH**-zoo-may)—short account of one's career and qualifications that is prepared by an applicant for a position

Retention (ree-**TEN**-shun)—inability to excrete urine that has been produced

Retinal degeneration (**RET**-ih-nal dee-jen-er-**AY**-shun)—breakdown and functional loss of the nervous layer of the eye

Retirement (ree-**TIRE**-ment)—period of time after leaving employment

Retrograde pyelogram (**RET**-roh-grayd **PIE**-eh-loh-gram)—moving backward of roentgen picture of the ureter and renal pelvis

Retroperitoneal space (ret-roh-**pair**-ih-toh-**NEE**-al spayce)—area of the anterior cavity behind the peritoneum; in it are the kidneys, aorta, and inferior vena cava

Reverse isolation technique (ree-**VERS** eye-soh-**LAY**-shun tek-**NEEK**)—requires that the environment, patient, and all objects coming in contact with the patient must be sterile or at least as free from microorganisms as possible

Rheumatoid arthritis (**REW**-mah-toyd are-**THRIGH**-tis)—autoimmune response that results in inflammation of the joints

Rhythm (**RITH**-um)—measured time or movement

Right lateral recumbent position (right **LAT**-er-al ree-**KUM**-bent poh-**ZISH**-un)—patient is turned on right side with the spine straight; left leg is slightly flexed and left arm is straight over hip; right arm is flexed

Rigor mortis (**RIH**-gor **MOR**-tis)—rigidity of skeletal muscles, developing six to ten hours after death

RN (are-en)—registered nurse

Rooming in (**ROOM**-ing in)—practice of having mother and neonate share a single room after delivery

Rotation (roh-**TAY**-shun)—act of turning about the axis of the center of a body, as in rotation of a joint

Rubra (**REW**-brah)—unusual redness or flushing of the skin

Sacrament of the sick (**SACK**-rah-ment of the sick)—last rites given by a clergyman to a person who is terminally ill (dying)

Saliva (sah-**LIE**-vah)—digestive secretion produced by the salivary glands and found in the mouth

Salpingectomy (sal-pin-**JECK**-toh-mee)—surgical removal of the fallopian tubes

Saprophyte (**SAP**-roh-fight)—organism that lives on dead matter or tissues

Sarcoma (sar-**KOH**-mah)—connective tissue tumor, often highly malignant

Scope of practice (skohp of **PRACK**-tis)—extent or range of permissible activities

Scrotum (**SKROH**-tum)—saclike pouch that holds the male gonads

Scultetus binder (skul-**TAY**-tus **BYN**-der)—band applied in overlapping strips in a shingle fashion

Sebaceous gland (seh-**BAY**-shus gland)—gland that produces a lubricating substance for the hairs

Secretion (see-**KREE**-shun)—product of glandular activity

Seizure (**SEE**-zhur)—sudden attack of a disease; a convulsion

Self-esteem (self-es-**TEEM**)—feeling of confidence about oneself

Semi-Fowler's position (**sem**-ee **FOWL**-ers poh-**ZISH**-un)—patient is positioned on the back, knees are slightly flexed, and head of bed is elevated 30–50 degrees

Senescent (seh-**NES**-ent)—aged

Senile dementia (**SEE**-nile dee-**MEN**-she-ah)—pronounced and abnormal loss of mental and emotional control in aged people

Serous fluid (**SEE**-rus **FLEW**-id)—thin, watery fluid produced by body cells

Setting exercises (**SET**-ting **ECK**-sir-size-es)—exercises that use isometric principles to contract muscles to maintain tone

Sexuality (**sex**-you-**AL**-ih-tee)—maleness or femaleness of an individual

Sexually transmitted disease (STD) (**SEX**-you-al-lee trans-**MIT**-ted dih-**ZEEZ**) (es-tee-dee)—disease that is passed from one individual to another through sexual contact

Shampoo (sham-**POO**)—to wash hair

Sharps—needles, knife blades, etc.

Shock (shok)—dangerous condition in which there is a disruption of the circulation that results in dangerously low blood pressure and an upset of all bodily functions

Short-term surgery (short turm **SUR**-jer-ee)—surgery performed on the day of admission. Patients are discharged the same or next day

Shroud (shrowd)—drape used in postmortem care

Side rails (side raylz)—sliding metal bar (bars) that may be pulled up on each side of the bed to prevent the patient from falling out of bed

Sigmoidoscopy (sig-moy-**DOS**-skoh-pee)—direct examination of the interior of the sigmoid colon

Sign (sighn)—any objective evidence of an abnormal nature in the body or its organs

Signing (**SIGHN**-ing)—using hands and facial expression to communicate without speaking words

Simple fracture (**SIM**-pul **FRACK**-shur)—fracture that does not produce an open wound in the skin

Simple goiter (**SIM**-pul **GOY**-ter)—thyroid gland hyperplasia unaccompanied by other signs or symptoms

Simple mastectomy (**SIM**-pul mas-**TECK**-toh-mee)—removal of the breast tissue without removing the underlying muscles

Sims' position (simz poh-**ZISH**-un)—patient is positioned on left side with left leg extended and right leg flexed; left arm is extended and brought behind back; right arm is flexed and brought forward

Singultus (sing-**GUL**-tus)—hiccup

Skilled care facility (skilld kair fah-**SILL**-ih-tee)—long-term care facility

Slander (**SLAN**-der)—false statement, oral or written, that injures the reputation of another person

SOAPE (es-oh-ay-pee-ee)—charting method; specific form of documenting observations and patient care; technique of documentation based on subjective and objective observations and assessment of the situation; a plan for treatment and evaluation of the effectiveness of treatment

Spasticity (spass-**TIS**-ih-tee)—continuous resistance to stretching by a muscle due to abnormally increased tension

Specimen (**SPESS**-ih-men)—small sample or part taken to show the nature of the whole

Speculum (**SPECK**-you-lum)—instrument used to dilate a body opening

Sperm (spurm)—male germ or reproductive cell

Sphincter muscle (**SFINK**-ter **MUS**-el)—circular muscle that constricts a passage or closes a natural orifice; when relaxed, it allows passage of materials

Sphygmomanometer (**sfig**-moh-mah-**NOM**-eh-ter)—instrument for determining arterial pressures; blood pressure gauge

Spica cast (**SPY**-kah kast)—body cast

Spinal anesthesia (**SPY**-nal an-es-**THEE**-zee-ah)—technique of providing anesthesia by introducing drugs into the spinal canal

Spirilla (spy-**RILL**-ah)—spiral-shaped bacteria

Spirometer (spy-**ROM**-eh-ter)—instrument for measuring air taken into and expelled from the lungs

Spore (spor)—dormant form of microbes that becomes active when conditions are favorable

Spouse (spows)—marriage partner; husband or wife

Sputum (**SPEW**-tum)—matter brought up from the lungs; phlegm

Staining (**STAYN**-ing)—laboratory technique used to make microbes more visible

Staphylo (**STAF**-ih-loh)—prefix meaning "in clusters"

Status (**STAY**-tus)—condition or state of health

Status epilepticus (**STAY**-tus ep-ih-**LEP**-tih-kus)—serious condition in which one epileptic-type seizure follows another

Stepparent (**STEP**-pair-ent)—person who is married to a child's natural parent

Sterile field (**STER**-ill feeld)—area considered free of all microbes

Sterile technique (**STER**-ill tek-**NEEK**)—technique that keeps an area free of microorganisms

Sterility (steh-**RILL**-ih-tee)—inability to produce offspring

Sterilization (**ster**-ih-lie-**ZAY**-shun)—process that renders an individual incapable of reproduction

Sterilize (**STER**-ih-lighz)—to make free of all microbes

Stertorous (**STER**-toh-rus)—snoring-type respirations

Stethoscope (**STETH**-oh-skohp)—instrument used in auscultation to make audible the sounds produced in the body

Stimulant (**STIM**-you-lant)—agent that produces stimulation or elicits a response

Stoma (**STOH**-mah)—artificial, mouthlike opening

Stool—another name for feces

Strepto (**STREP**-toh)—prefix meaning "in chains"

Stress incontinence (stress in-**KON**-tih-nens)—inability to hold urine when stressed, such as when coughing or laughing

Stressors (**STRESS**-ors)—situations, feelings, or conditions that cause a person to be anxious about his/her well-being

Stretcher (**STRECH**-er)—gurney or litter

Stroke (strohk)—cerebrovascular accident; damage to the blood vessels of the brain

Stryker frame (**STRY**-ker fraym)—special kind of bed that is used when a patient cannot be turned within the bed

Stump—distal end of a limb remaining after amputation

Subjective complaint (sub-**JECK**-tiv kom-**PLAINT**)—problem experienced personally by an individual

Subjective observations (sub-**JECK**-tiv ob-sir-**VAY**-shuns)—observations based on ideas perceived only by the individual involved

Sudoriferous glands (sue-doh-**RIFF**-er-us glandz)—glands that secrete perspiration

Suffix (**SUF**-fix)—term added to the end of a word that changes or modifies the meaning of the word

Suicide (**SOO**-ih-side)—self-destruction

Sundowning (**SUN**-down-ing)—behavior in which a person becomes more agitated and disoriented during the evening hours

Superimpose (**soo**-per-im-**POSE**)—put on top of something else

Superior (soo-**PEER**-ee-or)—toward the head; upward

Supination (sue-pih-**NAY**-shun)—act of turning the palm upward

Supine position (**SOO**-pine poh-**ZISH**-un)—lying with the face upward

Suppository (sup-**POZ**-ih-toh-ree)—medication used to help the bowels eliminate feces

Suppression (soo-**PRESH**-un)—consciously refusing to acknowledge unacceptable feelings and thoughts

Surgical asepsis (**SUR**-jih-kal ah-**SEP**-sis)—special techniques that maintain asepsis during surgical procedures

Surgical bed (**SUR**-jih-kal bed)—bed used for surgery

Susceptible host (sus-**SEP**-tih-bul hohst)—person who is more liable to contract a disease

Suspension (sus-**PEN**-shun)—temporary cessation

Symmetry (**SIM**-eh-tree)—correspondence in size, form, and arrangement

Sympathectomy (**sim**-pah-**THECK**-toh-mee)—excision or interruption of a sympathetic nerve

Symptom (**SIMP**-tum)—any perceptible change in the body or its functions that indicates disease or the phases of disease

Synapse (**SIN**-aps)—space between the axon of one cell and the dendrites of others

Syphilis (**SIF**-ih-lis)—infectious, chronic, venereal disease characterized by lesions that may involve any organ or tissue. It usually exhibits cutaneous manifestations, relapses are frequent, and it may exist asymptomatically for years

System (**SIS**-tem)—group of organs organized to perform a specific body function or functions; for example, the respiratory system

Systole (**SIS**-toh-lee)—contraction or period of contraction of cardiac muscle

Systolic pressure (sis-**TOL**-ick **PRESH**-ur)—pertaining to the pressure exerted during the contraction phase of the venticles

Tachycardia (**tack**-ee-**KAR**-dee-ah)—unusually rapid heartbeat

Tachypnea (**tack**-ip-**NEE**-ah)—respiratory pattern of rapid, shallow respirations

Tact—sensitive mental perception

Tasks of personality development (tasks of per-son-**AL**-ih-tee dee-**VEL**-op-ment)—growing stages through which personality is formed as described by Erickson

T-binder (tee-**BYN**-der)—T-shaped binder used to hold dressings in place on the male perineum

TED hose (TED hohs)—support hose

Tendon (**TEN**-don)—fibrous band of connective tissue that attaches skeletal muscle to bone

Terminal (**TER**-mih-nal)—final; life-ending stage

Testes (**TES**-teez)—male gonads; reproductive glands located in the scrotal sac

Testosterone (tes-**TOS**-teh-rohn)—hormone produced by the testes

Tetany (**TET**-ah-nee)—nervous condition, characterized by intermittent toxic spasms, that are usually paroxysmal and involve the extremities

Therapeutic (ther-ah-**PEW**-tick)—pertaining to results obtained from treatment; healing agent

Therapeutic diet (ther-ah-**PEW**-tick **DIE**-et)—treatment through specifically planned nutrition

Therapy (**THER**-ah-pee)—treatment designated to eliminate disease or other bodily disorder

Thermometer (ther-**MOM**-eh-ter)—instrument used to determine temperature

Thoracic (thor-**ASS**-ick)—pertaining to the chest

Thrombocyte (**THROM**-boh-sight)—blood platelet that is formed in the bone marrow and is important in blood clotting

Thrombophlebitis (throm-boh-flee-**BY**-tis)—development of venous thrombi in the presence of inflammatory changes in the vessel wall

Thrombus (**THROM**-bus)—blood clot

Thyroxine (thy-**ROCK**-sin)—hormone of the thyroid gland that contains iodine

TIA (transient ischemic attack) (tee-eye-ay) (**TRAN**-see-ent is-**KEE**-mick ah-**TACK**)—temporary decrease in blood flow to brain

Time and travel records (time and **TRAH**-vel **RECK**-ords)—records kept of the time spent with clients and the distance traveled between clients

Tipping (**TIP**-ping)—giving a sum of money for service rendered; not salary-connected

Tissue (**TISH**-you)—collection of specialized cells that perform a particular function; piece of paper used for cleansing; for example, toilet tissue, facial tissue

Toe pleats (toh pleets)—special folds made in top bedding to reduce pressure on toes

Total parenteral nutrition (**TOH**-tal pah-**REN**-ter-al new-**TRISH**-un)—meeting an individual's entire nutritional needs by providing high density nutrients directly into the bloodstream

Toxins (**TOCK**-sins)—microbes that produce poisons that travel to the central nervous system and cause damage

Transfer (**TRANS**-fer)—procedure followed when changing patient's location

Transfer belt (**TRANS**-fer belt)—gait belt that is used to assist and support patients during ambulation

Transient ischemic attack (TIA) (**TRAN**-see-ent is-**KEE**-mick ah-**TACK**) (tee-eye-ay)—temporary reduction of flow of blood to the brain

Transmission (trans-**MISH**-un)—transfer from one place or person to another

Transverse fracture (trans-**VERS FRACK**-shur)—fracture in which the break line is straight across the bone

Trapeze (trah-**PEEZ**)—horizontal bar suspended overhead down the length of the bed

Trauma (**TRAW**-mah)—wound or injury

Tremors (**TREM**-ors)—involuntary trembling

Trendelenburg position (tren-**DEL**-en-berg poh-**ZISH**-un)—patient is positioned with head lower than feet

Trimester (try-**MES**-ter)—period of three months

Trochanter roll (troh-**KAN**-ter rohl)—rolled sheet or bath blanket placed under the patient extending from waist to mid thigh; positioned against the hip to prevent lateral hip rotation.

Tubal ligation (**TOO**-bul lih-**GAY**-shun)—tying off a fallopian tube

Tubercle (**TO**-ber-kul)—small, rounded nodule formed by infection with *Mycobacterium tuberculosis*

Tuberculosis (too-ber-kyou-**LOH**-sis)—lung disease caused by a microorganism, easily transmitted to others by sneezing and coughing

Tumor (**TOO**-mor)—neoplasm

Turning sheet (**TURN**-ing sheet)—sheet used to turn a patient

Tympanic membrane (tim-**PAN**-ick **MEM**-brain)—membrane serving as the lateral wall of the tympanic cavity and separating it from the external acoustic meatus

Ulcer (**UL**-sir)—open sore caused by inadequate blood supply and broken skin

Ulceration (ul-sir-**AY**-shun)—development of an ulcer

Ulcerative colitis (**UL**-sir-ay-tiv koh-**LIGH**-tis)—inflammation of the colon resulting in the formation of ulcers

Ulnar deviation (**UL**-nar dee-vee-**AY**-shun)—with hand in supination, lateral movement of wrist

Ultrasound (**UL**-trah sownd)—mechanical radiant energy of a frequency greater than 20,000 cycles per second

Umbilical cord (um-**BILL**-ih-kul kord)—attachment connecting the fetus with the placenta. It is severed artificially at the birth of the child

Umbilicus (um-**BILL**-ih-kus)—depressed scar marking the site of entry of the umbilical cord in the fetus

Universal blood and body fluid precautions (you-nih-**VER**-sal blud and **BAH**-dee **FLEW**-id pree-**KAW**-shuns)—techniques used to prevent transmission of body fluids from one person to another

Upper respiratory tract infection (URI) (**UP**-per ree-**SPY**-rah-toh-ree tract in-**FECK**-shun) (you-are-eye)—infections involving the organs of the upper respiratory tract

Uremia (you-**REE**-mee-ah)—presence of excessive amounts of urea, a waste product, in the blood

Ureter (you-**REE**-ter)—narrow tube that conducts urine from the kidney to the urinary bladder

Urethra (you-**REE**-thrah)—mucus-lined tube conveying urine from the urinary bladder to the exterior of the body; in the male, the urethra also conveys the semen

Urgency (**UR**-jen-see)—need to urinate

Urgent care (**UR**-jent kair)—care that must be given right away to prevent loss of life

Urinalysis (you-rih-**NAL**-ih-sis)—laboratory analysis of the urine

Urinal (**YOU**-rih-nal)—vessel into which urine is voided (male)

Urinary bladder (**YOU**-rih-ner-ee **BLAD**-der)—receptacle for urine before it is voided

Urine (**YOU**-rin)—fluid secreted from the body by the kidneys

Uterus (**YOU**-ter-us)—organ of gestation

Vagina (vah-**JIGH**-nah)—tube that extends from the vulva to the uterine cervix; female organ of copulation that receives the penis during sexual intercourse

Vaginal examination (**VAJ**-ih-nal eg-**zam**-ih-**NAY**-shun)—examination of vaginal and pelvic organs

Vaginitis trichomonas (vaj-ih-**NIGH**-tis trick-oh-**MOH**-nas)—inflammation of the vaginal tract due to infection by a parasite, *Trichomonas vaginalis*

Validation therapy (val-ih-**DAY**-shun **THER**-ah-pee)—techniques used to help people feel good about themselves

Vas deferens (vas **DEF**-er-ens)—tube that carries sperm from the epididymis to the junction of the seminal vesicle; ductus deferens

Vasoconstriction (vas-oh-kon-**STRICK**-shun)—decrease in the caliber (inner diameter) of the blood vessels

Vasodilation (vas-oh-die-**LAY**-shun)—dilation of the blood vessels

Vector (**VECK**-tor)—carrier, such as an arthropod, that transmits disease

Vein (vain)—vessel through which blood passes on its way back to the heart

Venereal disease (VD) (vee-**NEE**-ree-al dih-**ZEEZ**) (vee-dee)—disease ordinarily acquired as a result of sexual intercourse with an individual who is infected

Venereal wart (vee-**NEE**-ree-al wart)—viral condition that can be sexually transmitted

Ventral (**VEN**-tral)—front; anterior

Ventricle (**VEN**-trih-kul)—small cavity or chamber, as in the brain or heart

Verbal communication (**VER**-bal kuh-**myou**-nih-**KAY**-shun)—transmitting messages using words

Verbal cues (**VER**-bal kyous)—words used to guide the thinking process of another

Vernix caseosa (**VER**-nicks kay-see-**OH**-sah)—sebaceous deposit covering the fetus due to secretions of skin glands

Vertebrae (**VER**-teh-bray)—backbones

Vertigo (**VER**-tih-goh)—sensation of rotation or movement of or about the person

Vesicle (**VES**-ih-kul)—blister-like skin lesion

Victim (**VICK**-tim)—someone who is injured unexpectedly, as in an accident

Virus (**VIGH**-rus)—specific, living, morbid principle by which an infectious disease is transmitted

Visceral (**VISS**-er-al)—pertaining to organs

Visceral muscles (**VISS**-er-al **MUSS**-sills)—muscles that operate without conscious control

Visual field (**VIZH**-you-al feeld)—refers to the area that can be seen

Vital capacity (**VIGH**-tal kah-**PASS**-ih-tee)—volume of air a person can forcibly expire from the lungs after a maximal inspiration

Vitality (**VIGH**-tal-ih-tee)—exuberant physical and mental strength; capacity for endurance

Vital signs (**VIGH**-tal sighns)—measurements of temperature, pulse, respiration, and blood pressure

Vitamin (**VIGH**-tah-min)—general term for various, unrelated organic substances found in many foods in minute amounts that are necessary for normal metabolic function of the body

Void (voyd)—to release urine from the bladder

Volume (**VOL**-youm)—capacity or size of an object or of an area; measure of the quantity of substance

Vomitus (**VOM**-ih-tus)—material vomited or brought up from the stomach

Vulva (**VUL**-vah)—external female genitalia

Vulvovaginitis (vul-voh-**vaj**-ih-**NIGH**-tis)—inflammation of the external female reproductive structures (vulva and vagina)

Wheal (wheel)—localized area of edema on the body surface, often associated with severe itching

Withdrawal (with-**DRAW**-al)—retreat from reality or from social contact associated with severe depression and other psychiatric disorders

Withhold (with-**HOLD**)—order to refrain from serving a patient or resident certain foods or all food

Word root—word form whose basic meaning can be used in forming new words by combining with prefixes or suffixes

INDEX

Note: Items in **bold type** are references to nursing assistant procedures. Items in *italics* are references to nontext material.

A

Abbreviations, 85, 91–93
  body parts, 91
  diagnosis, 91
  patient orders and charting, 91–92
  physical and history, 92
  places or departments, 92–93
  time, 93
Abdominal quadrants/regions, 44
Abdominal thrusts, choking, **670–671**
Abduction, in a diarthrotic joint, 61
Abuse, 34
  and the home care assistant, 478
  long term care facilities and, 425
Acceptance stage of grief, *463*, 464
ACCU-CHEK III®, **545–546**
Ace bandages, post-operative use of, 404
Acquired immunodeficiency syndrome (AIDS), *154*, 168, 604–605
Activities of daily living (ADLs), 438, 441
  Alzheimer's disease and, 455
Acute care hospitals
  nursing assistants and, 8
Acute disease, 98
Adaptive behaviors, *411*
Adaptive equipment. *See* Assistive devices
Addison's disease, 541
Adduction, in a diarthrotic joint, 61
Admission procedures, 266–269, **267, 269**
  admission kit, contents of, *267*
  baseline assessment, 265
  form, *268*
Adolescence
  growth and development in, 135
  nutrition and activity, 647
  psychosocial development, 646–647
  safety guidelines for, 647
Adoptive parent, 629
Adrenal cortex, 66, *67*
  common disorders of, 541
  glands, 66, *67*
  medulla, 66, *67*
Adrenalin, 67

Adrenocorticotropic hormone (ACTH), *66*
Adults, 135–136
  characteristics of mature, 427
Advanced directives, 458–459, 465
Advocate, defined, 426
Aerobic
  defined, *155*
  organisms, 154
Aerosol therapy, respiratory care and, 510
Afterbirth, 614
Agenesis of a kidney, 99
Aging
  circulatory system and, 56, 428
  effect on blood pressure, 56, 251, 428
  emotional adjustments to, 429–430
  endocrine system and, 68, 428
  gastrointestinal system and, 78, 428
  integumentary system and, 49, 428
  musculoskeletal system and, 64, 428
  nervous system and, 75, 428
  reproductive system and, 83, 428
  respiratory system and, 52
  urinary system and, 79–80, 428
    See also Elderly and chronically ill
Agitation
  Alzheimer's disease and, 456
  defined, 417
Aiding and abetting, 32
AIDS. *See* Acquired immunodeficiency syndrome (AIDS)
Air circulation, in the patient's room, 181
Airway, 672
  obstruction
    choking, 670
    Heimlich maneuver, abdominal thrust, **670–671**
    infant, *672*
    unconscious adult, assisting, **671–672**
Akinesia, 560
Alcoholism, 412–413
  alcohol-drug interactions, *412*
Allergen, 491
Allergies, 158, 491
Alveoli, 50, 51
Alzheimer's disease, 452–458
  activities of daily living, guidelines for, 455
  agitation, anxiety, and catastrophic reactions, 456

  hoarding, 456
  pacing, 455
  reality orientation (RO), 456–457
  reminiscing, 457–458
  stage I, 453–454
  stage II: moderate dementia, 454
  stage III: severe dementia, 454–455
  sundowning, 456
  validation therapy, 458
Ambulation, 404
  assisting in, **406–407**
  and the elderly, 440
  postpartum, 621
Amenorrhea, 83, 600
American Heart Association, 9
Amino acids, nutrition and, 338
Amniotic
  fluid, 614
  sac, 614
Amphiarthrotic joints, 60
Amputation, lower extremity, 535–536
Anaerobic
  defined, *155*
  organisms, 154–155
Anaphylactic shock, defined, 491
Anatomic position, 41
Anatomy, 41–44
  abdominal regions, 44
  cavities, 42–43
  membranes, 43
  planes of the body, 41–42
Anemia, 519–520
Aneroid gauge, 252, *253*
Anesthesia, 391–392
  for delivery, 616
Anger stage of grief, 462, *463*
Angina pectoris, 518
Ankle ROM exercises, *529*
Anorexia, from immobility, 198
Anterior planes, 41
Antibodies, 52, 104
Antidepressants, 414
Antidiabetic drugs, 543
Antidiuretic hormone (ADH), 66
Anus, *76*, 77
Anvil, 74
Anxiety
  Alzheimer's disease and, 456
  in the elderly, 430
Aortic semilunar valve, 54
Apgar scoring, neonates, 622
Aphasia, 449, 451, 558, 559

Apical pulse, 246
counting, **247**
Apnea, defined, 247
Apoplexy. *See* Stroke
Appendix, *76*, 77
Applications for employment, 680–681, *689–690*, *691–692*
Aquamatic K-pad®, 372
application, **377–378**
Aqueous humor, 73
Arachnoid mater, 72
Areola, 83
Arm soak, warm, **378–379**
Arterial circulation, *515*
Arteries
described, 52
elasticity and effect on blood pressure, 250
Arteriosclerosis, effect on blood pressure, 251
Arthritis, 530–531
Articles, containment of, 175, **176**
Artificial eye care, **453**
Asepsis, defined, 159
Aspiration, in the elderly, 435
Assault and battery, 33
Assistive devices
defined, 438
for self-feeding, *439*
walkers, *439*, *440*
Atheromas, described, 517
Atherosclerosis, 517
Auditory nerve, 75
Ausculatory gap, defined, 253
Autoclave, 163
Autoimmune reactions, 100
Autonomic nervous system (ANS), 72–73
Auxiliary structures, 50
Axons, *68*, 70
Azidothymidine (AZT), 605

B
Bacillus, 152
Back-lying position, 196, *197*
Back rubs, 314, **314–316**
Bacteria, 152
Balanced suspension cervical traction, 533–534
Bargaining stage of grief, 462, *463*
Barium enema, 103
Barium swallow, 103
Basal metabolism rate (BMR), 540
Bathing, 287–308
bed bath, giving, **290–296**
bed shampoo, **304–306**

Century tub, 297, **298**
dressing/undressing a patient, **306–308**
emollient bath, giving, **492–493**
foot and toenail care, **302–303**
hand and fingernail care, **301**
partial bath, giving, **296–297**
patient, 288
perineal care, 298
female, **299**
male, **300**
safety measures, 288
tub bath/shower, **289–290**
Bed cradle, 318–319
Bedpan, giving and receiving, **320–322**
Bedrest, dangers of, 198
Beds and bedmaking, 274–286
box (square) corner, 279
closed bed, 276
opening, **281**
making, **276–281**
mitered corner, 278, *278*
occupied bed, 282
making, **282–284**
for orthopedic patients, 534
surgical bed, 284–285
making, **284**
toepleats, *281*
types of beds, 274–276
unoccupied bed, 281
Bed shampoo, **304–306**
Bedside commode, assisting with use, **323**
Below the knee amputation (BKA), 536
Benign prostatic hypertrophy, 597, 599
Benign tumors, described, 100
Bicuspid valve, 54
Bile, 78
Binders, post-operative use of, 403–404
Biological parent, 629
Biopsy
breast, 600
defined, 506
Birthing center, *618*, 619
Bisexuality, defined, 142
Bladder spasm, 585
Bleeding, emergency procedures for, 673
Blindness, 564–565
Blood
abnormalities, 519–520
cells, 52–53
circulation, 52–53
described, 52
proteins, 78
vessels, 55, *57*, *58*

Blood and body fluid precautions, *171*
Blood glucose monitoring, 545
testing urine for acetone: Ketostix® strip test, **548**
using ACCU-CHEK III®, **545–546**
using a Glucometer 3®, **545**, *547*
Blood pressure, 56
cuff, *388*
described, 250–251
equipment, 251–252
factors influencing, *251*
gauge, how to read, 253
inaccurate readings, causes of, 253
measuring, 252–253, **253–255**
infant, **637**
Blood urea nitrogen (BUN), 585
BMR. *See* Basal metabolism rate (BMR)
Body
cavities of, 42–43
membranes, 43
organization
cells, 44–46
circulatory system, 52–56
endocrine system, 64–68
gastrointestinal system, 75–78
integumentary system, 47–49
musculoskeletal system, 56, 59–64
nervous system, 68–75
organs, 47, *48*
reproductive system, 80–83
respiratory system, 49–52
systems, 47, *49*
tissues, 46–47
urinary system, 78–80
pulse sites in, *245*
Body core, 230
Body defenses against disease, 104, 158
Body flora, 150
Body language, communications and, 112–113
Body mechanics, 193–199
for the nursing assistant
effective body movements, 194–195
posture, 194
for the patient, 196–198
body alignment and positioning, 196–198
dangers of bedrest and immobility, 198
Body parts, word roots for, 86–89
Bones, 56, 59–60
of the skeleton, *59*
of the skull, *60*
Bottlefeeding infants, **638**
Bowman's capsule, 79

Bradycardia, defined, 245
Brain, *552*
   CNS and, *69*
   described, 70
Breastfeeding, 639
Breasts, 83
   postpartum care of, 622
   self-examination, *602*
   tumors of the, 600–601
Breathing exercises, respiratory care and, 510
Bronchi, breathing and, 50
Bronchoscopy, 506
Burnout, 25
Burns
   classification of, 498–499
   rule of nines, 499
   treatment, 499
Burping infants, 638, **639**
Bursae, 60, 530
Bursitis, 530

C
Cachexia, 101
Calcium loss from bones, 198
Call bells, answering, 114
Calorie-restricted diet, 346
Cancer
   signs and symptoms of, 101
   types of
      breast, 600–601
      gastrointestinal system, 571–572
      sarcomas, 100
      skin, 444
      testes, 599
   tumors, 100–101
Candida albicans, 599
Capillaries, described, 52
Capsule, defined, *155*
Carbohydrates, nutrition and, 338
Carcinomas. *See* Cancers
Cardiac
   arrest, emergency procedures for, 674
   catheterization, 103
   muscle, 61
Cardiopulmonary resuscitation (CPR), 667–668
Cardiovascular system. *See* Circulatory system
Career ladder, 25
Care plan conference, 437
Caries, 310
Carriers of disease, 156
Casts, care of patients with, 532
Cataracts, 564

Catastrophic reaction, Alzheimer's disease and, 454
Category-specific isolation precautions, *170*, 171
Catheters, 399, 588
   care, 589, 591
      giving, **589–591**
   disconnecting, **591–592**
Caudal block, 616
Causative agent of disease, 155
Cavities, body, 42–43
Cecum, *76, 77*
Cells, 44–46
   cellular activity, 45–46
   division of, 44, *45*
Cellulose, 339
Celsius scale, 230
Centers for Disease Control and Prevention (CDC), 168, 170, 171
Centimeter/inch conversion chart, *260*
Central nervous system. *See* Nervous system
Century tub bathing, 297, **298**
Cerebellum, *69*, 70
Cerebral cortex, *69*, 70
Cerebral vascular accident (CVA)
   emergency procedures for, 675
Cerebrospinal fluid (CSF), 72
   examining, 563–564
Cerebrovascular accident (CVA), *556, 558–559*
Cerebrum, *69*, 70
Cervical traction, *533*
Cesarean birth, 619
Character, respiration, defined, 247
Charts
   components of, 124–125
   forms, 127–128
   graphic charts, 125–126, *129*
   guidelines for charting, 126–127
   intake/output chart, *126*
   nurses' notes, 126–127
   Problem-oriented Medical Record (POMR), 127–128
   SOAPIE approach, 127–128
   temperature, 242
Chemical studies, 103
Chemotherapy, described, 103
Chest tapping, respiratory care and, 510–511
Cheyne-Stokes respirations, 247
Children, growth and development of, 134
Chlamydia, 604

Choking, 670
   in the elderly, 435
   Heimlich maneuver-abdominal thrusts, **670–671**
Cholecystectomy, 573
Cholecystitis, 573
Cholecystogram, 573
Cholelithiasis, 573
Choroid, 73
Chromosomes, 44
Chyme, 77
Chymopapain, 535
Cigarette drain, 399
Circ-O-lectric® bed, 275
Circulation impairment, from immobility, 198
Circulatory system, 52–56
   aging and, 56
   arterial circulation, *515*
   blood, 52–53
      pressure, 56
      vessels, 55, *57, 58*
   cardiac cycle, 56
   common disorders, 513
      angina pectoris, 518
      atherosclerosis, 517
      blood abnormalities, 519–520
      congestive heart failure (CHF), 519
      hypertension, 517–518
      myocardial infarction (coronary heart attack), 518–519
      observations by nursing assistant, *517*
      peripheral vascular disease, 514–517
   diagnostic tests of, 514
   the heart, 54–55, *514*
   observation of, 117
   structure and function of, 52
   venous circulation, *516*
Circumcision, 623, 625
Cleanliness, of the patient's room, 181–182
Cleft lip, 99
Client care records, 482, *483*
Clinics
   nursing assistants and, 8
Clinitron bed, 275, *276*
Clitoris, 81
Closed beds, making, **276–281**
Closed fractures, defined, 531
Clostridium tetani, 154
Club foot, 99
Coccus, 152
Cochlea, 74
Coitus, 142

Cold therapy
   cooling baths, 380
   described, 371–372
   disposable cold pack application,
      374–375
   ice bag application, **373–374**
   types of, 372–373
Colectomy, 572
Colitis, 572
Colon, *76*, 77
Color blindness, 99
Color coding, for category-specific
      isolation, *170*
Colostomy, 572
   care of patient with, 582, 661–662
      routine stoma care, **662**
Colostrum, 622
Combining forms, 85, 86–89
Comfort devices
   bed cradle, 318–319
   footboard/footrest, 319
   pillows, 319
   routine positioning of patient, *319*
Commercially prepared enemas,
      giving, **579–580**
Comminuted fractures, defined, 531
Communicable diseases, isolation
      systems for, 171–172
Communication
   barriers to, 113
   body language and, 112–113
   call bells and, 114
   defined, 111
   improving, 113–114
   needs of the elderly, 449, 451–452
   nonverbal, 112–113
   oral report, 116
   with patients, 114
   the phone and, 115
   skills, 112–116
   with staff members, 115–116
   verbal, 112
   with visitors, 114–115
Community
   agencies, 8–10
   needs of, 8
Competency evaluation programs, 14,
      19
Complications, post-operative, *400*
Compound (open) fractures, defined,
      531
Compression fractures, defined, 531
Computerized axial tomography (CAT
      scan), described, 102
Computers, in health care, 123–124
Congenital abnormalities, defined, 99

Congestive heart failure (CHF), 519
Conjunctiva, 74
Connective tissue, *46*
Constipation
   in the elderly and chronically ill,
      431, 448–449
   from immobility, 198
Contact isolation, *170*
Continuous passive motion machine
      (CPM), 534
Contractures, from immobility, 198
Convulsions, 554
   emergency procedures for, 675–676
   seizure disorders, 561
Coping, assisting patients to, 410, 411
Coronal planes, 41, *42*
Coronary
   embolism, defined, 518
   heart attack, 518–519
   occlusion, defined, 518
   thrombosis, defined, 518
Coughing, assisting, post-operative
      care and, **401–402**
Cover gown, isolation techniques for,
      172–173, **173, 174**
Cranium, *69*, 70
Creatinine, 79
Croupettes, oxygen delivery and,
      508–509
Crusts, defined, 491
Cushing's syndrome, 541
CVA. *See* Cerebral vascular accident
      (CVA)
Cyanosis, 247
Cystitis, 585–586
Cystocele, 599
Cystoscopy, 103, 585
Cytoplasm, described, 44

D
Dangling, during post-operative
      recovery, 404, **406–407**
Deafness, described, 565
Death and dying
   discussion, 461–462
   hospice care, 467–468
   Kubler-Ross five stages of grief, 462,
      464, 464–465
   organ donations, 469
   physical changes of approaching
      death, 468
   postmortem
      care, 468–469, **470**
      examination, 469
   preparation for death, 464–465
   role of the nursing assistant, 466–467

Debriding, defined, 497
Deconditioning, and the elderly, 437
Decubitus ulcers
   assessing risk of, *494*
   avoiding, 493, 495, *496*
   described, 493
   development of, 496–498
   documentation of, *494*
   from immobility, 198
Deep breathing, assisting, post-
      operative care and, **401–402**
Defamation, 33
Defecation, 77
   diet and, 342
Defense mechanisms
   denial, 411
   other adaptive behaviors, *411*
   projection, 410
   reaction formation, 411
   repression, 410
   suppression, 410
Degenerative joint disease (DJD), 530
Dehydration, 354
Delivery, childbirth, 616–618
Delusions, defined, 418
Dementia, nursing care and
   dementia, defined, 452
   organic mental syndrome, defined,
      452
   See also Alzheimer's disease
Dendrites, *68*, 70, 74
Denial
   defined, 411
   stage of grief, 462, *463*
Denture care, 313, **313–314**, 446–447
Deoxyribonucleic acid (DNA), 44, *45*
Department of Health and Human
      Services, 14, 19
Depilatory, 393
Depressants, effect on blood pressure,
      251
Depression, 413–415
   drugs that may cause, 413–414
   signs and symptoms of, *414*
   stage of grief, 462, *463*, 464
Dermal ulcers. *See* Pressure sores
      (dermal ulcers)
Dermis, definition of, 47
Diabetes mellitus, 541–543
   antidiabetic drugs for, 543
   blood glucose monitoring, 545
      testing urine for acetone: Ketostix
         strip test, **548**
      using ACCU-CHEK III®, **545–546**
      using a Glucometer 3®, **545**, *547*

coma, 541
complications, 542
diet for, 345–346
disease mechanism, 541–542
the exchange systems, 542–543
and exercise, 543
types of, 542
Diagnosis of disease, 101–103
Diagnosis related grouping (DRGs), 124, 473
Diagnostic techniques/tests, 101–103
cardiovascular disease, 514
endocrine system, 540
gastrointestinal system, 573
invasive, 102–103
musculoskeletal system disorders, 530
noninvasive, 102
prenatal, 615–616
protocols for, 102
reproductive system, 597
urinary system, 585
Dialysis, renal, 586, 587
Diaphoresis, 354
measuring and recording
fluid intake, **355–356**
fluid output, **356–357**
Diaphragm, 51
Diarthrotic joints, 60–61
Diastolic pressure, 56, 252
Diathermy, 372
Diet
light, 344
liquid, 342–343
post-operative regime, *343*
regular, 342
soft, 343–344
special
calorie-restricted, 346
diabetic, 345–346, 542–543
low fat/cholesterol, 346
religious restrictions, 344, *345*
sodium-restricted, 346
therapeutic, 344–345
Digestion, defined, 336
Digestive system
observation of, 117
See also Gastrointestinal system
Dilatation and curettage (D&C), 597
Dilation, stage of delivery, 616
Discharge of patients, 270, **271–272**
neonate and mother, 625–626
release form, *271*
Disease
body defenses against, 104
causes of, 96–99

complications of, 98
course of, 98
defined, 95
diagnosis of, 101–103
infectious, process of, 155–158
prevention of, 159–165
process of, 99–101
risk factors for, 158
signs and symptoms of, 97
describing, 97–98
and therapy for, 103–104
Disease-specific isolation precautions, 171–172
Disinfection, 163
Disorientation, 415–417
Distension, defined, *400*
Diuresis, 354
Diurnal variation, 230
Diverticulitis, defined, 431
Diverticulosis, defined, 431
DNA, 44, *45*
Do not hospitalize, explained, 458
Do not resuscitate (DNR), defined, 458, 465
Dorsal lithotomy position, 387
Dorsal recumbent position, 196, *197, 319*, 385
Dorsiflexion, 529
Douche, vaginal, giving, **606–607**
Drainage
drainage/secretion precautions, *171*
postpartum care and, 620
post-operative, 399
from wound, output of, 357
Drawsheet, 203
Dressing/undressing a patient, **306–308**
Drugs, as cause of depression, 413–414
Duodenal
resection, 572
ulcer, 572
Duodenum, *76, 77*
Durable Power of Attorney, defined, 458, 465
Dura mater, 72
Dye studies, 103
Dying. *See* Death and dying
Dysmenorrhea, 83, 600
Dyspnea, 503
defined, 247
Dysuria, 585

E
Ear
care in the elderly, 447
common disorders

deafness, 565–566
hearing aids, *565*, **567**, **567–568**
otitis media, 565
otosclerosis, 565
structure of, 74–75, *554*
Edema, 354
EEG. *See* Electroencephalogram (EEG)
EKG. *See* Electrocardiogram (EKG)
Elasticized stockings, 404, **405–406**
Elbow extension, *526*
Elderly and chronically ill, 421–460
abuse of, 425
adulthood, characteristics of, 427
aging, effects of, 427–430
emotional adjustment to aging, 429–430
artificial eye care, **453**
assisting with cane or walker, **443**
communication needs, 449, 451–452
constipation and, 431
death and dying
advanced directives, 458–459
dementia, 452–458
Alzheimer's disease, 452–458
activities of daily living, guidelines for, 455
agitation, anxiety, and catastrophic reactions, 456
hoarding, 456
pacing, 455
reality orientation (RO), 456–457
reminiscing, 457–458
stage I, 453–454
stage II: moderate dementia, 454
stage III: severe dementia, 454–455
sundowning, 456
validation therapy, 458
elimination needs, 447–449
fecal incontinence and constipation, 448–449
urinary incontinence, 447–448
exercise and recreational needs, 436
eyeglass care, **452–453**
general hygiene, 441, 444–447
bathing, 444
eyes, ears, and nose care, 447
facial hair, 446
hair care, 446
hand and foot care, 445
mouth care, 446–448
skin care, 444
long term care facilities (LTCFs)
infection control in, 432–433
legislation affecting, 424
population in, 422–423

residents' rights, 424–426
    role of the nursing assistant in, 426
    safety in, 433–436
    types of, 422
nutritional needs of, 431–432
physical restraints and, 425
psychological needs, 452
restorative care, 437–441
    activities of daily living (ADLs),
        438, 441
    positioning and bed movement,
        440
    range of motion exercises, 440–441
    skills, 438, 440
    and sexuality, 430–431
    transfer from bed to chair or chair to
        bed, **442–443**
Electric bed, 275
Electric heating pad, using, 372
Electric shock, emergency procedures
    for, 676
Electrocardiogram (EKG or ECG), 102
Electroencephalogram (EEG), 102
Electromyogram (EMG), 102
Electroshock therapy, for depression,
    414
Elimination needs, 139
    bedside commode, assisting with
        use, **323**
    of the elderly, 447–449
        fecal incontinence and
            constipation, 448–449
        urinary incontinence, 447–448
    giving and receiving the bedpan,
        320–322
    giving and receiving the urinal, **322**
ELISA test, 605
Embolus, 402–403
Emergencies
    airway obstruction, **671–672**, 672
        infant, 672
    being prepared, 667
    bleeding, 673
    cardiopulmonary resuscitation
        (CPR), 667–668
    choking, 670
    described, 667
    electric shock, 676
    fainting, 674
    first aid, 668–669
    heart attack, 674–675
    Heimlich maneuver-abdominal
        thrusts, **670–671**
    at the scene, 668
    seeking assistance, 668
    seizures (convulsions), 675–676

shock, 673–674
stroke, 675
Emesis basin, *388*
EMG. *See* Electromyogram (EMG)
Emotional
    needs, 140–141
    stress, effect on blood pressure, 251
Employment opportunities, 679–686
    application forms, *689–690, 691–692*
    objectives
        applications for work, 680–681
        continue to grow in your career,
            686
        interviews, successful, 685
        keep the job, 685–686
        references, validating, 680
        resign properly, 686
        résumé, assembling a proper,
            679–680
    search for all opportunities, 679
    self-appraisal, 678–679
Endocardium, 54
Endocrine system, 64–68, *539*
    aging changes and, 68
    common disorders
        adrenal cortex, 541
        diabetes mellitus, 541–543
            antidiabetic drugs, 543
            blood glucose monitoring,
                545–548
            complications, 542
            disease mechanism, 541–542
            the exchange systems, 542–543
            and exercise, 543
            types of, 542
        hyperglycemia, 543–544
        hypoglycemia, 543
        parathyroid glands, 541
        thyroid gland, 540
    diagnostic techniques, 540
    functions of, 538, 540
    glands, 64–68, *539*
        adrenal, 66
        gonads, 66, 68
        and hormones secreted by, 66–67
        location of, *65*
        pancreas, *76, 78*
        parathyroids, 68
        pineal body, 66
        thyroid, 68
    islets of Langerhans, 68
Endogenous etiologies, 96
Enemas, 574–575, 579, 581
    giving
        oil-retention, **575–576**
        soapsuds, **577–578**

Enteral feeding, 337
Enteric precautions, 73, *171*
Environment
    observation of, 117–118
    patient, control of, 179–182
Enzymes, digestive, 75, 77, 572
Epidermis, definition of, 47
Epididymis, 80
Epidural anesthesia, 616
Epilepsy, 561–562
Episiotomy, 617
Epithelial tissue, *46*
Equilibrium, ear function and, 74
Equipment
    isolation precautions for, 175
    observation of, 117–118
    for patient care, cleaning,
        disinfecting, and
        sterilizing, 161–164
    for patient's room, cleaning and care
        of, 181–182
    for the physical exam, 387–388
    safety measures for care of, 182–183
Erikson's tasks of personality
    development, 136, *137*
Erythrocytes, 53
Eschar, defined, 499
Esophagectomy, 572
Esophagus, 75
Estrogen, 66, *67*
Ethical and legal issues, 27–38
    abuse-physical/verbal/psychological,
        34
    assault and battery, 33
    defamation, 33
    ethical/legal standards, 29
    ethical questions, 29
    ethics committees, 30
    false imprisonment, 33
    invasion of privacy, 33
    negligence, 32
    patient information, 30–31
    Patient's Bill of Rights, 27–29
    respect for life, 30
    respect for the individual, 30
    safety devices and restraints, 34–35
    theft, 32–33
    tipping, 31–32
Etiology, defined, 95
Eustachian tubes, 74
Exchange system, for diabetics,
    542–543
Excoriations, defined, 491
Excretory system. *See* Urinary system
Exercise
    in long term care facilities, 436

leg, postoperative, 402–403, **403**
    See also Range of motion exercises
        (ROM)
Exocrine glands, 48, 78
Exogenous etiologies, 96
Exposure incident, described, 169
Expressive aphasia, 559
Extension, in a diarthrotic joint, 60
Eye, *552*
    care
        elderly, 447
        neonate, 624
    common disorders of
        blindness, 564–565
        cataracts, 564
        retinal degeneration, 564
    described, 73–74
    effect of aging on, 428
Eyeglass care, 313, **452–453**

F
Facial hair, care of in the elderly, 446
Fahrenheit scale, 230
Fainting, emergency procedures for,
        674
Fallopian tubes, 81, *82*
Falls
    care of the falling patient, **222**
    preventing, 183
False imprisonment, 33
Families, 628–629
    meeting the needs of, 24
Fasting, effect on blood pressure, 251
Fats, nutrition and, 338, 339
Fecal
    impaction, from immobility, 198
    incontinence
        in the elderly, 448–449
            Hollister collector, usage
                guidelines, *450*
Federal/state regulations for
        certification, 19
Feeding restrictions, and the dying, 458
Fetal monitors, 616
Fetus. *See* Obstetrical patient
Fibrinogen, 78
Finger exercises, *527*
Fingernail
    care, giving, **301**
    effect of aging on, 428
Fire extinguishers, using, 187–188
Fire safety, 185–188
    fire extinguishers, using, 187–188
    hazards, 186
    oxygen precautions, 187, 506
    PASS, 188

prevention, 186
RACE, 187
smoking, 186
First aid, 668–669
First degree burns, described, 499
Flagella, defined, *155*
Flatulence, defined, 431
Flatus, 572
    bag, **581–582**
Flexion, in a diarthrotic joint, 60
Fluids
    intake/output
        guidelines for, 588
        measuring, **355–356, 356–357**
Fluoroscopy, described, 102
Foley catheters, 588, 659
Follicle-stimulating hormone (FSH),
        65, *66*
Fomites, defined, 156
Food, need for, 138
Food groups, nutrition and
    dairy, 341
    fruits, 340–341
    grains, 341
    meat, 342
    vegetables, 339–340
Food Guide Pyramid, 339, *340*
Foot and toenail care, **302–303**, 445
    foot soak, warm, **378**
    ROM exercises for feet, *529*
Footboard/footrest, 319
Footprinting, neonate, *622*
Foster parent, 629
Fractures
    care of patients
        in traction, 532–535
        with casts, 532
        treatment for, 531–532
        types of, 531
Frontal planes, 41
Functional nursing, 19
Fundus, 75, 620
Fungi, 153
Fusion, 535

G
Gait belt, 208
Gallbladder, *76*, 77–78
    conditions, 573
Gas-expelling methods, 581
Gastrectomy, 572
Gastric
    juice, 76
    resection, 572
    ulcer, 572
Gastrointestinal (GI) series, 573

Gastrointestinal system, 570
    aging changes and, 78
    common disorders
        gallbladder conditions, 573
        hernias, 573
        malignancies, 571–572
        ulcerations, 572–573
    diagnostic tests, 573
    digestive system, *571*
        and enemas, 574–575, 579, 581
            giving
                commercially prepared,
                    579–580
                Harris flush, **581**
                inserting rectal tube and
                    flatus bag, **581–582**
                rotating, **580**
    structure and function of, 75–78
    suppositories and, 582
Gastroscopy, 573
Gastrostomy tube, 337
Gatch bed, 274–275
Gavage, 138
    nutrition and, 337–338
General anesthetics, 391
Generalized seizures, 561
Genetic abnormalities, 99
    neoplasms, 100–101
Genital herpes, 603
Gerichair®, *436*
Glands
    described, 48–49
    endocrine, 64–68
        location of, *65*
    lacrimal, 74
    salivary, 75
Global aphasia, 559
Glomeruli, 79
Gloves, disposable, 654
    isolation techniques for, 173, **174**
    opening sterile gloves, 164
    putting on sterile gloves, **654, 655**
    removing contaminated, **161**
Glucagon, *67*, 68, 78
Glucometer 3®, using, **545**, *547*
Glycogen, 541
Glycosuria, 542
Goiter, 540
Gonads, 66, *67*, 68
Gonorrhea, 603
Governmental Agencies, nursing
        assistants and, 9
Grand mal seizures, 561
Greenstick fractures, defined, 531
Grooming, 21–22

Growth and development. *See* Human growth and development
Guidelines for Isolation Precautions in Hospitals, 170–171

H

Hair
  care, 317, **317**, 446
  described, 48
Halitosis, 310
Hammer, of the ear, 74
Hand care, giving, **301**, 445
Handwashing, 159–160
  procedure, **159**
Harris flush, giving, **581**
Harris splint, 534
Health and hygiene, 21–22
  in the long term care facility, 441, 444–447
    bathing, 444
    eyes, ears, and nose care, 447
    facial hair, 446
    hair care, 446
    hand and foot care, 445
    mouth care, 446–448
    skin care, 444
Health care
  delivery
    factors influencing
      computers, 123–124
      diagnosis related grouping (DRGs), 124
    facilities, nursing assistants and, 10–14
    Occupational Safety and Health Act (OSHA) regulations for, 168–169
  financing, 14–15
  trends in, 472–473
Health Care Financing Administration, 19
Health maintenance organization (HMO), 14
Hearing, 74
  common disorders of, 565–566
  deficits in the elderly, 428, 451
    guidelines for communicating with, *452*
Hearing aids
  applying, **567**, **567–568**
  care of, 566
  parts of, *565*
Heart, 54–55
  attack, emergency procedures for, 674–675
  cardiac cycle, 55, *56*

disorders
  congestive heart failure (CHF), 519
  myocardial infarction (coronary heart attack), 518–519
  valves, 54
Heart rate, measuring, infant, **636–637**
Heat cradles, 373
Heat therapy
  aquamatic K-pad®, application, **377–378**
  described, 371–372
  moist compress application, **379–380**
  types of, 372–373
  warm arm soak, **378–379**
  warm foot soak, **378**
  warm water bag application, **375–377**
Height/weight
  abbreviations for, 93
  measuring
    baseline, defined, 257
    mechanical lift scale, *258*
    patient in bed, **260–261**
    upright scale, *258*, **259–260**
    wheelchair scale, *258*, **261**
Heimlich maneuver-abdominal thrusts, **670–671**
HemaCombistix®, testing for urine, **657**
Hematest® reagent tablets, testing for occult blood, **658–659**
Hematuria, 585
Hemiplegia, 558
  neurological trauma, documentation for, *557*
Hemoccult® and developer, testing for occult blood, **657–658**
Hemophilia, 99
Hemoptysis, 505
Hemorrhage, 372
  effect on blood pressure, 251
Hepatitis, 168
  hepatitis B virus, *154*
Hereditary factors, effect on blood pressure, 251
Hernias, 573
  herniations, defined, 428
Herniorrhaphy, 573
Herpes, 603
  herpes simplex virus, *154*
Heterosexuality, defined, 141
High Fowler's position, 509
Hip
  fractures, 534–535
  ROM exercises for, *528*
Hoarding, Alzheimer's disease and, 456

Hollister drainable fecal incontinence collector, *450*
Home care
  avoiding liability, 478
  benefits of working in, 473
  the client, 473
  and elder abuse, 478
  health assistant
    characteristics of, 476
    duties of, 476–478
    and the nursing process, 474, 476
    types of, 473
  health team, 473–474
  housekeeping chores, 479–481
  infection control, 479
  record keeping, 482, *483*
  safety in the home, 478
  trends in health care, 472–473
Home health assistant aide, 473
Home health care aide, 473
Homemaker aide, 473
Homemaker assistant, 473
Homosexuality, defined, 142
Horizontal recumbent position, 196, *197*, 385
Hormones, 64–68
  female, 66, *67*
  pituitary, 64–66
Hose, anti-embolism, 404, **405–406**
Hospice care, 14, 467–468
Hospital beds, 180
  side rails, 180–181
Hospitals
  described, 10–11
  organization of, 11–13
Host, defined, 158
Housekeeping chores, in home care, 479–481
Human growth and development, 133–136
  adolescence, 135
  adulthood, 135
  defined, 131
  developmental milestones, *631*
  developmental tasks, 630
  infancy, 131–133
  maturity, 136
  middle age, 135–136
  old age, 136
  personality development, 136, *137*
  preadolescents, 134, *135*
  preschoolers, 133–134
  school-age children, 134
  tasks, 131
  toddlers, 133

Human needs, 130, 136–144
  emotional needs, 140–141
  fearful patients, dealing with,
      142–143
  human touch, 142
  intimacy needs, 141–142
  personality development, 136, *137*
  physical activity, 139–140
  physical needs, 137–140
  privacy needs, 142–143
  social needs, 144
  spiritual needs, 143
Hydrochloric acid, 572
  digestion and, 76
Hydronephrosis, 587
Hygiene. *See* Health and hygiene
Hyperalimentation, defined, 337
Hypercalcemia, 541
Hyperglycemia, 543–544
Hypersecretion, 540, 541
Hypersensitivity reactions, 100
Hypertension, 517–518
  defined, 252
Hyperthermia, 242
  blankets, 372, 381
Hyperthyroidism, 540
Hypertrophies, 540
Hypochondriasis, defined, 417
Hypoglycemia, 543
Hyposecretion, 540, 541
Hypotension, 252
Hypothermia, 241–242
  blankets, 372, 381
Hypothyroidism, 540
Hysterectomy, 600

I
Ice bag application, **373–374**
Ileostomy, 572
  care of patient with, 662–663
    patient in bathroom, **664–665**
    patient in bed, **663–664**
Ileum, *76, 77*
Immobility, dangers of, 198, *139–140*
Immunization, 164
Impaction, defined, 449
Incarcerated hernia, 573
Incentive spirometer, *510*
Inch/centimeter conversion chart, *260*
Increased intercranial pressure,
    554–557
Incus, 74
Infants, 131–133, 630–640
  airway obstruction in, *672*
  blood pressure, measuring, **637**
  breastfeeding, 639

burping, 638–639, **639**
  communicating with, 632
  crib linens, changing, **634–635**
  family importance to, 632
  feeding, 637–638, **638**
  heart rate (pulse), determining,
      636–637
  respiratory rate, counting, **637**
  restraints for, 640
  safety guidelines for, 640
  temperature, measuring, **635–636**
  urine specimen, collecting, **359–360**
  vital signs, determining, 635
  weighing, **633–634**
Infection control, in home care, 479
Infections, 100
Inferior planes, 41
Inflammation, 100
  described, 104
Influenza A virus, *154*
Infrared lamp treatments, 373
Insulin, *67, 68, 78,* 541, 543
  shock, 541
Insulin dependent diabetes mellitus
    (IDDM), 542
Integumentary system, 47–49, 489–490
  aging and, 49
  burns
    classification of, 498–499
    rule of nines, 499
    treatment, 499
  cross section of the skin, *490*
  emollient baths, giving, **492–493**
  glands of, 48–49
  lesions of
    care of, 491–492
    causes of, 491
    diagnosing, 491
    types, 490–491
  observation of, 117
  pressure sores (dermal ulcers)
    assessing risk of, *494*
    avoiding, 493, 495, *496*
    described, 493
    development of, 496–498
    documentation of, *494*
  structure and function, 47–48
Intercostal nerve, 51
Interdisciplinary team, 437
Intermittent positive pressure
    breathing (IPPB), 506, *507*
Interstitial cell-stimulating hormone
    (ICSH), 66
Interviewing, job opportunities and,
    685
Intestines, *76, 77*

Intimacy needs, 141–142
Intravenous infusion (IV), 138
  alternative nutrition and, 336–338
Intravenous pyelogram (IVP), 585
Intrinsic factor, digestion and, 76
Invasion of privacy, 33
Invasive tests and studies, 102–103
Involuntary muscles, 61
Involuntary seclusion, described, **425**
Iris, 74
Irritations, 100
Ischemia, defined, 99
Islets of Langerhans, 68
Isolation
  precautions, 168–170
    category-specific, 171
      color coding for, *170*
    disease-specific, 171–172
    procedure completion actions, 177
  systems, 170–172
  techniques, 172–177
    articles, containment of, 175, **176**
    cover gown, 172–173, **173, 174**
    equipment, 175
    gloves, 173, **174**
    handwashing, 172
    masks, 173, **174, 175,** *175*
    patient transporting, **176**
    specimen collection, **176**
  unit, 172
Isolettes, neonate, *623*

J
Jackson-Pratt (J-P) drain, 399
Jejunum, *76, 77*
Job attitude, 23
Joints, 60–61, *524*

K
Kaposi's sarcoma, 604
Ketosis, 541
Ketostix® strip test, **548**
Kidneys, 78–79
Kilogram/pound conversion chart, *259*
Knee-chest position, 385
Knee ROM exercises, *528, 529*
Kubler-Ross, Dr. Elisabeth, five stages
    of grief, 462, *464,* 464–465

L
Labia, 81
Labor, childbirth, 616–618
Lacrimal glands, 74
Lactation, 622
Lactogenic hormone (LTH), 66
Laminectomy, 535

Laryngoscopy, 103
Larynx, breathing and, 50
Learning process. *See* Study skills
Leboyer method of natural childbirth, 615
Left atrium (LA), 54
Left lateral recumbent position, 196–197, *319*
Left Sims' position, 574, *580*
Left ventricle (LV), 54
Legal guardian, defined, 437
Legal issues. *See* Ethical and legal issues
Legislation, affecting long-term care, 424
Lens of the eye, 74
Leukemia, 520
Leukocytes, 53
Leukorrhea, 603
Liability, avoiding, 478
Licensed practical/vocational nurse (LPN/LVN), 17, 25
Life stresses, *410*
Lifting patients. *See* Moving and lifting patients
Ligaments, 60, 64
Light diet, 344
Lighting, in the patient's room, 181
Linea nigra, 615
Linens, caring for in the isolation unit, **176**
Liquid diet, 342–343
Liquid stool, output of, 357
Lithotripsy, 587
Liver, *76*, 77–78
Living will, defined, 458, 465
Local anesthetics, 391–392
Lochia, 620
Logrolling patients, **219–220**
Long term care facilities (LTCFs)
    infection control in, 432–433
    legislation affecting, 424
    population in, 422–423
    resident's rights, 424–426
    role of the nursing assistant in, 8, 13–14, 426
    safety in, 433–436
    types of, 422
Lower extremity amputation, 535–536
Lower GI series, 103
Low fat/low cholesterol diet, 346
Lungs
    breathing and, 50
    described, 51
Luteinizing hormone (LH), 65, *66*
Lymphatic vessels, described, 52
Lymph nodes, described, 52

M

Magnetic resonance imaging (MRI), 102, 585
Malignancies
    of the gastrointestinal system, 571–572
    naming, 100–101
    tumors, described, 100
    See also Cancers
Malleus, 74
Malnutrition, and the elderly, 431–432
Mammography, 600
Masks, for oxygen delivery, 508
Maslow's hierarchy of needs, 136, *137*
Mastectomy, 600–601
Masturbation, 142
Maturity, 136
Measurements, abbreviations for, 93
Median planes, 41, *42*
Medicaid, 422
Medical asepsis, defined, 159–162
Medical specialties, 104, *105*
Medical terminology. *See* Terminology
Medicare/Medicaid, 14, 422
Medication restrictions, and the dying, 458
Medulla, *69*, 70
Melanin, 47
Membranes, 43, 47
Menarche, 83
Meninges, 43, 72
Meningitis, 563
Menopause, 83
Menorrhagia, 83, 600
Menstruation, 82–83
Mental abuse, described, 425
Mental health
    alcoholism, 412–413
    common life stresses, *410*
    coping, 410
        assisting patients to cope, 411
    defense mechanisms
        denial, 411
        other adaptive behaviors, *411*
        projection, 410
        reaction formation, 411
        repression, 410
        suppression, 410
    the demanding patient, 411–412
    described, 409–410
    maladaptive behaviors
        agitation, 417
        assessing patient, 413
        delusions, 418
        depression, 413–415
            drugs that may cause, 413–414

    signs and symptoms of, *414*
    described, 413
    disorientation, 415–417
    hypochondriasis, 417
    paranoia, 418
    reality orientation, 416
    suicide attempts, 415
    stresses, defined, 410
Mercury gravity gauge, 252, *253*
Messenger RNA, 45
Metabolic imbalances, 100
Methicillin resistant *Staphylococcus aureus* (MRSA), 154
Metric system conversion, 354
Metrorrhagia, 600
MI. *See* Myocardial infarction (MI)
Microorganisms, 150–155
    body flora, 151
    characteristics of, 151
    classification of, 151–155
    defined, 150
Microscopic studies, 103
Middle age, 135–136
Minerals, 339
Mistogen Units, oxygen delivery and, 508–509
Mitosis, 44, *45*
Moist compress application, **379–380**
Mold, 153
Moribund (dying) signs, 468
Morning sickness, 614
Mouth, 75, *77*
Mouth care, 446–448
Moving and lifting patients, 203–222
    assisting patient
        from bed to chair or chair to bed in LTCFs, **442–443**
        from bed to stretcher, **216, 218–219**
        from stretcher to bed, **217–218**, *218*
        into bed from chair or wheelchair, **212–213, 243**
        into chair or wheelchair from bed, **209–210**
        to get out of bed and ambulate, **220–221**
        to move to head of bed, **206, 207**
        to sit up in bed, **205**, *206*
        who is out of bed to ambulate, **221–222**
    care of the falling patient, **222**
    gait belt, *208*
    guidelines for safe transfers, *207*
    independent transfer, standby assist, **212**
    logrolling the patient, **219–220**

transfer belt, *208*
    one person, **211–212**
    two person, **210–211**
transporting patients, 220
    by stretcher, **224**
    by wheelchair, **223**
turning
    away from you, **204–205**
    toward you, **203–204**
using mechanical lift, **214–215**, *215, 216*
mRNA, 45
Mucous membranes, 43
Multiple sclerosis, 561
Muscles, 61, *62, 63,* 64
Muscular rigidity, 560
Muscular tissue, 46, *47*
Musculoskeletal system, 56, 59–64
    aging changes and, 64
    bones, 56, 59–60
        of the skeleton, *59, 523*
        of the skull, *60, 523*
    common disorders
        arthritis, 530–531
        bedmaking, for orthopedic
            patients, 532–535
        bursitis, 530
        diagnostic techniques for, 530
        fractures
            casts, care of patients in, 532
            of the hip, 534–535
            traction, care of patients in,
                532–535
            treatment, 531
            types of, 531
        lower extremity amputation,
            535–536
        ruptured or slipped disc, 535
    joints, 60–61, *524*
    muscles, 61, *62, 63,* 64, *524*
    observation of, 117
    range of motion exercises (ROM),
        524
        performing (passive), **525–530**
Myelogram, 103
Myocardial infarction (MI), 518–519
Myocardium, 54
Myopia, defined, 451
Myringotomy, 565

N
Nails
    care of, **301, 302–303**
    effect of aging on, 428
    fingernails, 47
    toenails, 47

Nasal
    cannula, for oxygen delivery, 508
    catheter, for oxygen delivery, 508
    cavities, breathing and, 50
    septum, 50
    speculum, *388*
Nasogastric tube, 572–573
National Council of State Boards of
    Nursing, Inc., 19
National Multiple Sclerosis Society, 9
Nebulizers, *510*
Necrosis, defined, 493
Negligence, 32
Neisseria gonorrheae, 152, *153*, 603
Neonatal intensive care unit, *620*
Neonates
    Apgar scoring, 622
    caring for, 622–625
    circumcision care, 623, 625
    discharging, 625–626
    eye care, 624
    home care, 626
    PKU test, 623–624
Neoplasms, 100–101
Nephritis, 586
Nephron, 79, *585*
Nerves, 69
    auditory, 75
    respiratory, 51
Nervous system, 68–75, 551
    aging changes and, 75
    autonomic nervous system (ANS),
        72–73
    brain, *552*
    central nervous system (CNS), 69–72
        brain, 70
        cerebrospinal fluid (CSF), 72
        meninges, 72
        spinal cord, 71–72
    common disorders
        aphasia, 558, 559
        of the ear, 565–567
        of the eye, 564–565
        increased cranial pressure,
            554–557
        meningitis, 563
        multiple sclerosis, 561
        Parkinson's syndrome, 560–561
        seizure disorder (epilepsy),
            561–562
        spinal cord injuries, 562–563
        spinal punctures, 563–564
        transient ischemic attack (TIA),
            559
    ear, structure of, 74–75
    eye, described, 73–74

nerves, 69
neurons, 69
observation of, 117
sensory receptors, 73
stroke (CVA), *556*, 558–559
Nervous tissue, 46, *47*
Neurons, 69, *552*
Noise reduction, in the patient's room,
    181–182
Noninsulin dependent diabetes
    mellitus (NIDDM), 542
Noninvasive tests and studies, 102
Nonprofit agencies
    nursing assistants and, 9
Nonverbal communications, 112–113
Normal values, observation of, 116–117
Nose
    care in the elderly, 447
    breathing and, 50
Nosocomial infection, defined, 154, 393
Notetaking skills, 2–3
NPO (nothing by mouth), 393
Nucleic acids, 45–46
Nucleus, described, 44
Nurse Aide Competency Evaluation
    Program (NACEP), 19
Nursing assistants
    the career ladder, 25
    career opportunities for, 14
    community agencies and, 8–10
    community needs and, 8
    described, 7–8
    facilities which employ, 8
    guidelines for, 21
    health care facilities and, 10–14
    long term care facility (LTCF) and,
        13–14
    personal health and hygiene, 21–22
    personal/vocational adjustments,
        22–25
        attitude, 23
        burnout, 25
        interpersonal relationships, 22–23
        meeting patient's needs, 23–24
        meeting the family's needs, 24
        patient relationship, 23
        reducing stress, 24–25
        staff relationships, 24
    role of, 16–26
        federal/state regulations and, 19
        in functional nursing, 19
        job description for a nursing
            assistant, 18
        lines of authority, 19–20
        nursing team, 16–17
        in primary nursing care, 18–19

and team nursing, 19
uniforms, 22
Nursing care
  bedtime (PM) care, 325–326, **328**
  early morning (AM) care, 325,
      326–327
  organization of, 18
Nursing care plan, 124–129
  charting forms
    Problem-oriented Medical Record
        (POMR), 127–128
    SOAPIE approach, 127–128
  Kardex, 124
  nurses' notes, 126–127
  patient's chart, 124–126
Nursing Home Reform Act, 424
Nursing Process, 118–123
  nursing action
    assessment, 118–122
    evaluation, 123
    implementation, 123
    planning, 122–123
Nursing specialties, 105
Nursing team, 17
Nutrients, in plasma, 52
Nutrition
  alternative, 336–338
  defined, 335
  diet
    light, 344
    liquid, 342–343
    post-operative regime, *343*
    regular, 342
    soft, 343–344
    special
      calorie-restricted, 346
      diabetic, 345–346, 542–543
      low fat/cholesterol, 346
      religious restrictions, 344, *345*
      sodium-restricted, 346
      therapeutic, 344–345
      supplemental nourishment,
          346–347
  digestion, defined, 336
  essential nutrients for, 338–339
  feeding, 348
    the helpless patient, **350–351**
    the patient who can self-feed,
        348–349
  food groups, 339
    dairy group, 341
    fruit group, 340–341
    grains, 341
    meat, 342
    vegetables, 339–340
  Food Guide Pyramid, 339, *340*

needs of the elderly, 431–432
normal, 336
water, providing, 347–348

O
Obesity, effect on blood pressure, 251
Objective observations, 97
Oblique fractures, defined, 531
Observations
  by body system, 117
  defined, 116
  of equipment/environment, 117–118
Obstetrical patient
  birthing center, *618*, 619
  breast care, 622
  Cesarean birth, 619
  labor and delivery, 616–618
    dilation, 616
    episiotomy, 617
    expulsion stage, 617–618
    fetal monitors, 616
    placental stage, 618
    relief of discomfort, 616
  postpartum care, 620–621
  prenatal care, 614
  prenatal testing, 615–616
  preparing for birth, 615
  signs of pregnancy, 614–615
  toileting and perineal care, 621
Obstruction, 100
Occult blood procedures, 365
  of normal values, 116–117
  testing
    using Hematest® reagent tablets,
        658–659
    using Hemoccult® and developer,
        657–658
Occupational exposure, defined, 168
Occupational Safety and Health Act
    (OSHA)
  regulations for health care facilities,
      168–169
Occupied beds, making, **282–284**
Oil-retention enemas, 449
  giving, **575–576**
Old age, 136. *See also* Aging; Elderly
    and chronically ill
Ombudsman, defined, 14, 426
Omnibus Budget Reconciliation Act of
    1987 (OBRA)
  and long term care facilities, 424
  and the training and certification of
      nursing assistants, 14, 19
Oophorectomy, 600
Open (compound) fractures, defined,
    531

Open reduction/internal fixation, 535
Ophthalmoscope, *388*
Oral hygiene
  assisting with
    brushing of teeth, **312–313**
    routine, **310–311**
    special, **312**
  denture care, 313, **313–314**
  described, 309–310
  eyeglass care, 313
Oral reports, 116
Organ donations, 469
Organic mental syndrome, defined, 452
Organisms, defined, 150. *See also*
    Microorganisms
Organs, 47
  of the abdominopelvic cavity, *48*
  placement in body cavities, *43*
Orthopneic position, 509
Ossicles, 74
Osteoarthritic joint disease (OJD), 530
Otitis media, described, 565
Otosclerosis, described, 451, 565
Otoscope, *388*
Outlines, how-to skills for, 3
Ovaries, 66, *67*, 81, *82*
Overhead trapeze, *533*
Ovulation, 82–83
Ovum, 68
Oxygen, need for, 137–138
Oxygen
  precautions, 187
  therapy
    delivery methods, 508–509
    fire safety and, 506
    giving, 506, 507
    intermittent positive pressure
        breathing (IPPB), 506, *507*
    maintaining an oxygen source,
        507–508
    maintaining moisture, 508
    oxygen tent, 509
Oxytocin, 66

P
Pacing, Alzheimer's disease and, 455
Pain
  blocking, with anesthetics, 391–392
    during childbirth, 616
  complaints of, 97–98
  effect on blood pressure, 251
  perception, in the surgical patient,
      391
  preventing and relieving in the
      dying, 459
Palliative care, therapy and, 104

Pancreas, *67, 68, 76, 78*
Panhysterectomy, 600
Pap smear, 597
    fixative, *387*
Papules, defined, 491
Paralysis, 554
Paranoia, defined, 418
Paraplegia, 562
Parasites, 151
    defined, *155*
Parasympathetic fibers, 72–73
Parathormone, *67, 68,* 541
Parathyroid glands, *67, 68*
    common disorders of, 541
Parents, 628–629
Parkinson's syndrome, 560–561
Partial seizures, 561
PASS, 188
Pathogens
    affect on body, 158
    blood-borne, 168, 169
    defined, 150
Pathology, defined, 95
Patient care
    bedtime (PM) care, 325–326, **328**
    early morning (AM) care, 325,
        326–327
    equipment, cleaning, disinfecting,
        and sterilizing, 161–164
Patient environment, control of,
    179–182
Patient information, legal issues and,
    30–31
Patients
    assessment, 118, *119–121*
    charts, 124–129
    communicating with, 114
    fearful, 142–143
    nursing care plan, 122–123, 124–129
    and relationships with the nursing
        assistant, 23–24
    transporting, in isolation, **176**
Patient's Bill of Rights, 27–29
Patient Self-Determination Act of 1990,
    465
Pearson attachment, 534
Pediatrics
    admitting a pediatric patient, **630**
    adolescents
        nutrition and activity, 647
        psychosocial development,
            646–647
        safety guidelines for, 647
    developmental milestones, *631*
    developmental tasks, 630

infant, 630–640
    blood pressure, measuring, **637**
    breastfeeding, 639
    burping, 638–639, **639**
    communicating with infants, 632
    crib linens, changing, **634–635**
    family importance to, 632
    feeding, 637–638, **638**
    heart rate (pulse), determining,
        636–637
    respiratory rate, counting, **637**
    restraints for, 640
    safety guidelines for, 640
    temperature, measuring, **635–636**
    urine specimen, collecting,
        359–360
    vital signs, determining, 635
    weighing, **633–634**
parents and families, 628–629
pediatric units, 629
preschool children
    activities for, 643
    developmental tasks, 642–643
    emotional reactions to illness, 643
    explaining procedures, 643
    safety guidelines for, 643–644
school-age children
    activities for, 645
    adjustment to illness, 645
    developmental tasks, 644
    psychosocial adjustment, 644–645
    safety guidelines for, 645
toddlers
    emotional reaction to illness, 641
    growth and development of, 133
    hospital environment and,
        640–641
    need for autonomy, 640, 641
    routine activities, 641–642
    safety guidelines for, 642
Pelvic belt traction, *533*
Pelvic examination, equipment for, *387*
Pelvic inflammatory disease (PID), 603
Penis, *80,* 81
Penrose drain, 399
Pepsin, 76
Percussion, respiratory care and, 510
Percussion hammer, 387
Pericardium, 43, 54
Perineal care, 298, 607
    female, **299**
    male, **300**
    postpartum, 621
Peripheral nervous system (PNS), 69
Peripheral vascular disease, 514–517
Peristalsis, 77, 572

Peritoneum, 43
Personality development, 136, *137*
Personal protective equipment (PPE),
    described, 169
Perspiration, output of, 357
Petit mal seizures, 561–562
Pharynx, 75
    breathing and, 50
Phonation, 50
Phrenic nerve, 51
Physical abuse, 34
    described, 425
Physical activity, need for, 139–140
Physical examination, 383–389
    dorsal lithotomy position, 387
    equipment for, 387–388
    knee-chest position, 385
    positioning the patient, 384–387
        dorsal recumbent position, 384
        horizontal recumbent position, 385
        modifications, 384
        prone position, 385
        Semi-Fowler's position, 386
        Sim's position, 386
        Trendelenburg position, 386
Physical needs, 137–140
Physical neglect, long term care
        facilities and, 425
Pia mater, 72
Pillows, used as comfort devices, 319
Pinna, 74
Pitocin, 66
PKU test, 623–624
Placenta, 614
Planes of the body, 41–42
Plantar flexion, 529
Plasma, 52
Platelets, 53
Pleura, 43, 51
Pneumocystis carinii, 604
Pneumonia, 503–504
    development of, from immobility,
        198
Poisonous substances, and safety
        concerns, 436
Polydipsia, 542
Polyphagia, 542
Polyuria, 542
Pons, *69,* 70
Populations, in long term care
        facilities, 422–423
Portals of entry/exit, disease, 156
Posterior planes, 41
Postmortem
    care, 468–469, **470**
    examination, 469

Post-operative regime (diet), *343*

Postural drainage, 511

Pound/kilogram conversion chart, *259*

Preadolescents, growth and development of, 134, *135*

Predisposing etiologies, 96

Prefixes, 85, 89–90

Pregnancy. *See* Obstetrical patient

Prenatal
    care, 614
    testing, 615–616

Presbycusis, defined, 451

Presbyopia, 451

Preschool children
    activities for, 643
    developmental tasks, 642–643
    emotional reactions to illness, 643
    explaining procedures, 643
    growth and development of, 133–134
    safety guidelines for, 643–644

Pressure sores (dermal ulcers)
    assessing risk for, *494*
    avoiding, 493, 495, *496*
    described, 493
    development of, 496–498
    documentation of, *494*

Privacy, respecting patients', 142–143

Private agencies, nursing assistants and, 9

Private room, defined, 180

Problem-oriented Medical Record (POMR), 127–128

Procedures, introduction to, 200–203
    beginning procedure actions, 201, *232*
    completion actions, 201–203, *232*

Proctoscopy, 573

Progesterone, 66, *67*

Prognosis, defined, 95

Projection, defined, 410

Prone position, 196, *197*, *319*, 385

Prostate
    conditions, 597, 599
    gland, 80–81

Prosthetic devices
    types of, 429
    artificial leg, 536

Protein bound iodine (PBI) test, 540

Proteins, nutrition and, 338

Proteolytic enzyme, 76

Prothrombin, 78

Protozoa, 151

Psychological
    abuse, 34
    needs, elderly and chronically ill, 452

neglect, long term care facilities and, 425

Puberty, 83

Pudendal block, 616

Pulmonary semilunar valve, 54

Pulse, 244–247
    apical, 246
        counting, **247**
    deficit, 246
    described, 245
    infant, measuring, **636–637**
    radial, counting, **245–246**
    sites in the body, *245*

Pupil of the eye, 74

Pustules, defined, 491

Pyelogram, 585

Pyloric sphincter, 76

Pylorus, 76

Pyrexia, 97

Q

Quadriplegia, 562

R

RACE, 187

Radial pulse, counting, **245–246**

Radiation therapy, 104

Radiographic techniques, 506

Rales, defined, 247

Range of motion exercises (ROM), 319, 524–530
    performing (passive), **525–530**

Rate, respiration, defined, 247

Reaction formation, 411

Reality Orientation (RO), 416
    Alzheimer's disease and, 456–457

Receptive aphasia, 559

Record keeping, for home care, 482, *483*

Recreational care, in long term care facilities, 436

Rectal tube, inserting, **581–582**

Rectocele, 599

Rectum, *76*, 77

Red blood cells, 53

References, validating, 680

Reflex arc, *553*

Registered nurse (RN), 17, 25

Regular diet, 342

Relationships
    interpersonal, 22–23
    meeting patient's needs, 23–24
    meeting the family's needs, 24
    with patient, 23
    with staff, 24

Religious-restricted diet, 344, *345*

Reminiscing, Alzheimer's disease and, 457–458

Renal calculi, 586–587

Renal dialysis, 586, 587

Reports, oral, 116

Repression, defined, 410

Reproductive system, 80–83, 597
    aging changes and, 83
    diagnostic techniques, 597
    female, *598*
        common disorders of
            breast surgery, 600–601
            cystocele, 599
            rectocele, 599
            tumors, 600
            vulvovaginitis, 599–600
        menstruation and ovulation, 82–83
        organs, 81–83
    male
        common disorders of
            cancer of the testes, 599
            prostate conditions, 597, 599
        lateral view, *597*
        organs, 80–81
        See also Sexually transmitted diseases (STD)

Reservoir of disease, 156

Resident's rights, 424–426

Resigning from employment, 686

Respiration, 244
    counting, **248**
    described, 247–248
    respiratory cycle, 51
    shallow, 247
    TPR readings, recording, *248*
    voice production and, 52

Respiratory isolation, *170*

Respiratory rate, measuring, infant, **637**

Respiratory system, 49–52
    aging changes and, 52
    asthma, 504
    bronchitis, 504
    chronic obstructive pulmonary disease (COPD), 504
    care of patients with, 504–505
    diagnostic techniques, 506
    emphysema, 504, *505*
    observation of, 117
    oxygen therapy for, 506–509
        delivery methods, 508–509
        fire safety and, 506
        giving, 507
        giving oxygen, 506
        intermittent positive pressure breathing (IPPB), 506, *507*

maintaining an oxygen source, 507–508
maintaining moisture, 508
oxygen tent, 509
pneumonia, 503–504
preventing transmission of infection, 502–503
reportables for, 503, *504*
respiratory positions, 509
structure and function of, 50–51
tuberculosis, 505–506
upper respiratory infections (URI), 503–504
voice production and, 52
Restorative care, in long term care facilities, 437–441
Restraints/safety devices, 34–35
examples of, 425
guidelines for use, 184, *185*
infant, 640
use of, in long term care facilities, 434–435
Résumés, 679–680
Retina, 73
Retinal degeneration, 564
Retrograde pyelogram, 585
Return-flow enema, giving, **581**
Rheumatoid arthritis, 530
Rhythm
pulse, defined, 245
respiration, defined, 247
Ribonucleic acid (RNA), *45*, 46
Ribosomal RNA, *45*
Right atrium (RA), 54
Right lateral recumbent position, 196, *197, 319*
Right ventricle (RV), 54
Rigor mortis, defined, 468
Risk factors for disease, 158
RNA, *45*, 46
ROM. *See* Range of motion exercises (ROM)
Roman numerals, 93
Rooming in, *618*, 619
Rotating enemas, giving, **580**
Rotation, in a diarthrotic joint, 61
Rubeola, *98*
Rule of nines, burns, 499
Ruptured disc, 535

S
Safety, 182–188
emergencies, 188
equipment and its care, 182–183
fire safety, 185–188
fire extinguishers, using, 187–188

hazards, 186
oxygen precautions, 187
PASS, 188
prevention, 186
RACE, 187
smoking, 186
guidelines
for the adolescent, 647
for infant care, 640
for moving or transporting patients, 183–184
for preschool care, 643–644
for school-age children, 645
for toddler care, 642
in the home, 478
in long term care facilities (LTCFs), 433–436
measures for bathing patients, 288
precautions when using thermometers, *234*
preventing falls, 183
restraints/safety devices, 184, *185*
Safety devices. *See* Restraints/safety devices
Sagittal planes, 41, *42*
Salivary glands, 75
Salpingectomy, 600
Saprophytes, defined, *155*
Sarcomas, 100
School-age children
activities for, 645
adjustment to illness, 645
developmental tasks, 644
psychosocial adjustment, 644–645
safety guidelines for, 645
Schwann cells, *68*
Sclera, 73
Scrotum, 68
Sebaceous (oil) glands, 48
Seclusion, described, 425
Second degree burns, described, 499
Secretions, 48
Seeing, 74
Seizure disorder (epilepsy), 561–562
Seizures, emergency procedures for, 675–676
Self-appraisal, 678–679
Self-esteem, 140–141
Semi-Fowler's position, 197, *319*, 386
Seminal vesicles, 80
Semiprivate room, defined, 180
Senile macular degeneration, 564
Sense organs, 48
Sensitivity responses, 158
Septum, 54
Serous membranes, 43

Sexual abuse, described, 425
Sexual intimacy, 141
Sexuality
effects of aging on, 429
and the older adult, 430–431
Sexually transmitted diseases (STD), 601–605
acquired immunodeficiency syndrome (AIDS), 604–605
chlamydia, 604
gonorrhea, 603
herpes, 603
syphilis, 603
trichomonas vaginitis, 602–603
venereal warts, 603
Shampoo, bed, **304–306**
Sharps, handling and disposing of, *169*, 170, *182*, 183
Shaving a patient, 316, **316–317**
surgical prep, 393–394, **394–395**
Shelter, need for, 137
Shock, emergency procedures for, 673–674
Shoulder abduction/adduction, *526*
Shoulder flexion, *526*
Sickle cell anemia, 99, 520
Side rails, 180–181, 434
Sigmoidoscopy, 103, 573
Signs, defined, 95
Sims' position, 197, 386
Singultus, defined, *400*
Sitting position, 197–198
Skeleton. *See* Musculoskeletal system
Skin, 47
aging and, 49
burns
classification of, 498–499
rule of nines, 499
treatment, 499
cross section of, *50, 490*
emollient baths, giving, **492–493**
glands of, 48–49
lesions of
care of, 491–492
causes of, 491
diagnosing, 491
types, 490–491
observation of, 117
pressure sores (dermal ulcers)
assessing risk of, *494*
avoiding, 493, 495, *496*
described, 493
development of, 496–498
documentation of, *494*
structure and function of, 47–49
Sleep, need for, 138–139

Slipped disc, 535
Smoking, patient safety and, 186
SOAPIE approach to charting, 127–128
Soapsuds enemas, giving, **577–578**
Social needs, 144
Sodium-restricted diet, 346
Soft diet, 343–344
Somatotropic hormone (STH), 65, *66*
Spasticity, 440
Specialties
  medical, 104, *105*
  nursing, 105
Specimens
  intake/output, 354
  routine, 354
  Sputum collecting, **365**
  stool, 364
    collecting, **364**
  urine collecting
    catheterized, 362
    clean-catch, **360–361**
    fresh fractional, **361–362**
    24-hour, **362–363**
    infant, **359–360**
    in the isolation unit, **176**
    routine, **357–358**
    through a drainage port, **659–660**
Speculum, *387, 388*
  defined, 388
Sperm, 68, 80, 83
Sphygmomanometer, 251–252
Spina bifida, 99
Spinal bed, 275
Spinal cord, *69*, 71–72
  injuries to, 562–563
Spinal punctures, 563–564
Spirillum, 152
Spiritual needs, 143–144
  providing for, 466
Spleen, described, 52
Spore, defined, *155*
Sputum specimens, collecting, **365**
Staff members, communicating with,
    115–116
Stapedectomy, 565
Stapes, 74
Staphylococcus aureus, 152, *153*
Status elipticus, described, 562
Stepparent, 629
Sterile field, 162
Sterile packages, opening technique,
    163
Sterile techniques, 162
  adding sterile materials to the field,
    652–653
  described, 651

gloving, 654
  putting on sterile gloves, **654, 655**
  opening a sterile package, **652**
  sterile field, defined, 651
  tracheal suctioning, **656**
Sterilization, 163
Sternal puncture, described, 102
Stertorous respirations, defined, 247
Stethoscope, 252, *388*
Stimulants, effect on blood pressure,
    251
Stirrup, 74
Stoma, 582
  care of patient with, 661–662, **662**
Stomach, 75–76
Stool specimens
  collecting, **364**
  occult blood procedures, 365
Strangulated hernia, 573
Streptococcus hemolyticus, 152, *153*
Stress, reducing, 24–25
Stretchers, moving and lifting patients
    with, **216–219**
Strict isolation, *170*
Stroke (CVA), *556*, 558–559
  emergency procedures for, 675
Stryker frame, 275
Study skills, 1–6
  active listening, 2
  careful practicing, 4
  hearing what is said, 2
  notetaking, 2–3
  outlines, 3
  processing information, 2
  references, 5
  studying effectively, 4
  textbook organization, *3*, 4–5
Subjective complaints, 97–98
Subtotal gastrectomy, 572
Sudoriferous (sweat) glands, 48
Suffixes, 85, 90
Suicide attempts, 415
Sundowning, Alzheimer's disease
    and, 454, 456
Superior planes, 41, *42*
Supination, 526
Supine position, 196, *197*
Supportive care,
  of the dying, 459
  therapy and, 104
Suppositories, rectal, 582, 660
  inserting, **660–661**
Suppression, defined, 410
Surgery, therapy and, 103
Surgical asepsis, 162
Surgical beds, making, **284**

Surgical patient
  and anesthesia, 391–392
  fears and concerns of, 390–391
  the operative period, 396
  pain perception, 391
  postoperative care, 396–408
    complications, *400*
    drainage, 399
    tubes, 398
  preoperative care, 392–396
    immediate, 395–396
    surgical prep area, 393–394
      shaving, **394–395**
  psychological needs, 392
  recovery
    binders, 403–404
    dangling, 404, **406–407**
    deep breathing and coughing,
      401–402
      assisting, **401–402**
    elasticized stockings, 404, **405–406**
    initial ambulation, 404
      assisting patient in, **407**
    leg exercises, 402–403
      performing, **403**
  teaching, 392
Symmetry, respiration, defined, 247
Sympathectomy, 517
Sympathetic fibers, 72–73
Symptoms, defined, 95
Synapse, 69
Synarthrotic joints, 60
Syphilis, 603
Systems of the body, *49*
  defined, 47
Systolic pressure, 56, 252

T
Tachycardia, defined, 245
Tachypnea, defined, 247
Talipes, 99
Talk therapy, for depression, 414
T-binders, 404
Team nursing, 19
TED hose, 404, **405–406**
Teeth, care of, 75, 446
Telephones
  answering, 115
  emergency numbers, list of, 478
Temperature
  abbreviations for, 93
  body, defined, 230
  control, 231
    cooling baths, 380
    hypothermia-hyperthermia
      blankets, 381

documentation, 242
hyperthermia, 242
hypothermia, 241–242
infants and children, 230
measuring, 231
  axillary or groin (electronic thermometer), **239**
  axillary or groin (glass thermometer), **239**
  infant, **635–636**
  oral
    glass thermometer, **234–235**
    plastic thermometer, **237**
    sheath-covered thermometer, **236**
  rectal (glass) thermometer, **237**
  of the patient's room, 181
  procedures review, 232
  thermometers
    cleaning glass, **240–241**
    reading, 232–233
    safety precautions when using, 234
    types of
      aural (ear), 232, 233
      disposable oral, 231
      electronic, 231, 232
      glass, 231
    values, 230
    when not to take, 233
Tendons, 64
Terminology, 85–108
  abbreviations, 85, 91–93
  combining forms, 85, 86–89
  prefixes, 85, 89–90
  suffixes, 85, 90
  word parts, 86–89
  word roots, 85, 86
Testes, 67, 68, 80
Testosterone, 67, 68
Tetany, 67, 68
Textbook organization, 3, 4–5
Theft, 32–33
Therapeutic diet, 344–345
Therapy, approaches to, 103–104
Thermal injuries, in the elderly, 435
Thermography, described, 102
Thermometers
  aural, 232, 233
  disposable, 231
  electronic, 231, 232
    using, **239**
  glass, 231
    using, **234–235, 237**
  plastic, using, **237**
  reading, 232–233

rectal, **237**
  sheath-covered, using, **236**
Third degree burns, described, 499
Thrombocytes, 53
Thrombophlebitis
  development of, from immobility, 198
  and use of elasticized stockings, 404
Thrombus, 402
Thrush, 197
Thyrocalcitonin, 68
Thyroidectomy, 540
Thyroid gland, 67, 68
  common disorders of, 540
Thyroid-stimulating hormone (TSH), 65, 66, 540
Thyroxine, 67, 68
TIA. See Transient ischemic attack (TIA)
Time, abbreviations for, 93
Time/travel records, home care, 482
Tipping, 31–32
Tissues, 46–47
Toddlers
  emotional reaction to illness, 641
  growth and development of, 133
  hospital environment and, 640–641
  need for autonomy, 640, 641
  routine activities, 641–642
  safety guidelines for, 642
Toenail
  care, giving, **302–303**, 445
  effect of aging on, 428
Toe ROM exercises, 530
Toileting, postpartum care and, 621–622
Tongue blade, 387
Total parenteral nutrition (TPN), 138, 337
Touch, need for, 142
Toxins, 158
Trachea, breathing and, 50
Tracheal suctioning, **656**
Traction, care of patients in, 532–535
Transfer belt, moving patients with, 208, **210–212**
Transfer of patients
  in isolation, **176**
  procedures for, 269–270, **270, 271**
  safety guidelines for, 183–184
  See also Moving and lifting patients; Transporting patients
Transient ischemic attack (TIA), 559
Transmission of disease, 156–157

Transporting patients, 220
  by stretcher, **224**
  by wheelchair, **223**
Transverse planes, 41, 42
Trauma, 100
Tremors, 560
Trendelenburg position, 386
Treponema pallidum, 603
Trichomonas vaginitis, 602–603
Tricuspid valve, 54
tRNA, 45
T-tube, 399
Tuberculosis, 505–506
Tumors, 100–101
Turning sheet, 203
Tympanic membrane, 74

U
Ulcerations, 572–573
Ulcerative colitis, 572
Ultrasound, described, 102
Ultraviolet lamp treatments, 373
Umbilical cord, 614
Uniforms, 22
United States Public Health Service, 9
Universal precautions, 161, 168–170. See also Isolation
Upper GI series, 103
Upper respiratory infections (URI), 503–504
Urea, 79
Ureters, 78
Urethra, 78
Uric acid, 79
Urinal, giving and receiving, **322**
Urinalysis, 357, 585
Urinary
  catheters, 588, 589, 591
    care, 589, 591
      giving, **589–591**
    disconnecting, **591–592**
  drainage systems (male), 591–594
    collecting urine in a leg bag, **593**
    condom, replacing, **592**
    emptying drainage unit, **594**
Urinary bladder, 78
Urinary incontinence, in the elderly, 447–448
Urinary meatus, 81
Urinary system, 78–80, 585
  aging changes in, 79–80
  common disorders
    cystitis, 585–586
    hydronephrosis, 587
    nephritis, 586
    renal calculi, 586–587

diagnostic techniques, 585
dialysis of, 586, 587
functions of, 584
kidneys, 78–79
nephron, *585*
nursing assistant responsibilities and, 588–594
  catheter care, 589–592
  urinary drainage and, 588, 591–594
observation of, 117
Urine
  described, 79
  production, 79
  testing
    for acetone, **548**
    with HemaCombistix®, **657**
Urine specimens. *See* Specimens
Uterine dressing forceps, *387*
Uterus, 81, *82*
  postpartum care of, 620

V

Vaccines, 164
Vagina, 81, *82*
Vaginal meatus, 81
Vaginal speculum, *387, 388*
  defined, 388
Vaginitis, 599–600, 602–603
Validation therapy, Alzheimer's disease and, 455
Valves, heart, 54
Vas deferens, 80
Vasoconstriction, 372

Vasodilation, 372
Veins, described, 52
Venereal warts, 603
Venous circulation, *516*
Ventricles, of the cerebrum, 72
Verbal abuse, 34, 425
Verbal communications, 112
Vernix caseosa, 622
Vertigo, during post-operative recovery, 404
Vesicles, defined, 491
Viruses, 153–154
  AIDS, 604–605
Vision
  effect of aging on, 428
  impaired, 451
Visitors, communicating with, 114–115
Vitamins, 339
Vitreous humor, 73
Voice production, 52
Voiding, postpartum care and, 620–621
Volume
  blood, and blood pressure, 250
  pulse, defined, 245
  respiration, defined, 247
Voluntary muscles, 61
Vomitus, output of, 357
Vulva, 81

W

Walkers, *439, 440*
Wards, defined, 180
Warm water bag application, **375–377**
Waste products, in plasma, 52

Water, providing, 347–348
Weight
  abbreviations for, 93
  measuring
    baseline, defined, 257
    mechanical lift scale, *258*
    patient in bed, **260–261**
    upright scale, *258*, **259–260**
    wheelchair scale, *258*, **261**
Weight loss, effect on blood pressure, 251
Western blot test, 605
Wheals, defined, 491
Wheelchairs
  assisting patient in
    into bed from wheelchair, **212–213, 243**
    into wheelchair from bed, **209–210**
  transporting by, **223**
White blood cells, 53
Wings incontinence briefs, *562*
Withdrawal, described, 430
Word parts, 86–89
Word roots, 85, 86
World Health Organization (WHO), 9
Wrist
  extension/flexion, *527*
  inversion/eversion, *528*

X

X ray, described, 102

Y

Yeast, 153